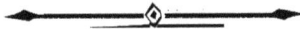

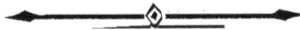

ISBN 978-1-330-27819-2
PIBN 10010972

1 MONTH OF
FREE
READING

at

www.ForgottenBooks.com

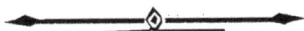

———◆———

By purchasing this book you are eligible for one month membership to ForgottenBooks.com, giving you unlimited access to our entire collection of over 1,000,000 titles via our web site and mobile apps.

To claim your free month visit:

www.forgottenbooks.com/free10972

A MANUAL

OF

OPERATIVE SURGERY.

BY

FREDERICK TREVES, F.R.C.S.,

SURGEON TO AND LECTURER ON ANATOMY AT THE LONDON HOSPITAL; MEMBER OF THE BOARD
OF EXAMINERS OF THE ROYAL COLLEGE OF SURGEONS.

WITH 422 ILLUSTRATIONS.

VOL. II.

PLASTIC SURGERY—OPERATIONS UPON THE NECK AND ABDOMEN—
OPERATIONS ON HERNIA—OPERATIONS UPON THE BLADDER,
SCROTUM, PENIS, AND RECTUM—OPERATIONS UPON
THE HEAD AND SPINE, THORAX, AND BREAST.

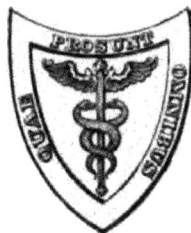

PHILADELPHIA:
LEA BROTHERS & CO.
1892.

CONTENTS.

Part VIII.
PLASTIC SURGERY.

Part IX.
OPERATIONS ON THE NECK.

Part X.

OPERATIONS UPON THE ABDOMEN.

Part XI.

OPERATIONS ON HERNIA.

Part XII.

OPERATIONS UPON THE BLADDER.

Part XIII.

OPERATIONS UPON THE SCROTUM AND PENIS.

Part XIV.

OPERATIONS UPON THE RECTUM.

Part XV.

OPERATIONS ON THE HEAD AND SPINE.

Part XVI.

OPERATIONS ON THE THORAX AND BREAST.

LIST OF ILLUSTRATIONS.

A MANUAL OF

OPERATIVE SURGERY.

Part VIII.

PLASTIC SURGERY.

CHAPTER I.

GENERAL PRINCIPLES.

PLASTIC surgery concerns itself with the remedy of certain congenital defects and malformations, such as hare-lip, cleft palate, and extroversion of the bladder, and with certain acquired defects and deformities, such as may follow the loss of parts by injury or ulceration, or the contraction incident to the formation of cicatrices.

The term "plastic surgery" appears to have been first used by Zeis about 1836, and although the majority of the operations included in that term are of modern origin, some few of them can claim great antiquity.

There is evidence to show that in the fifteenth century operations for the restoration of the nose were extensively performed. Gasparo Tagliacozzi's great work, "De Curt-orum Chirurgia per Institionem," was published in 1597, and with the name of this surgeon the Italian method of rhino-plasty has always been associated. Tagliacozzi's operations obtained, however, little hold in the surgical world, and appear to have been soon forgotten. The Indian method for the restoration of the nose is of great antiquity, and owed its origin to the frequent mutilation of the face as a punishment. The practice received little notice from Europeans until after

b

the publication of an article in the *Madras Gazette* in 1794.
The first rhinoplastic operation performed in England was
carried out in 1803, when the Indian method was employed.
Within modern times the progress of plastic surgery has been
very rapid, and since the introduction of antiseptic methods
in surgery, the results obtained have been infinitely improved.

Chelius, who gives an admirable account of the history of
this branch of operative work in the second volume of his
"Surgery" (South's edition), speaks of Graefe as "the actual
creator of plastic surgery in Germany."

With the name of Graefe must be associated the names of
Dieffenbach, Blandin, Roux, Langenbeck, Liston, and many
others.

General Principles.

1. The common feature which underlies plastic surgery, as
the term is usually understood, involves the ready and secure
union of refreshed or divided surfaces. The operations for the
most part concern the skin, and are dependent upon the
vascularity and elasticity of the skin, its mobility, the readiness with which wounds made in it unite, and the
comparative ease with which it may be displaced, and with
which it moulds and adapts itself to a new situation.

2. In the actual planning of incisions and the mapping
out of flaps, little can be done by following blindly any
especial method. Each case must be considered upon its
merits, and each operation arranged as the needs of the
particular case suggest. No branch of operative surgery
demands more ingenuity, more patience, more forethought, or
more attention to detail. In connection with certain operations it may almost be said that no two cases are alike.

3. As sound and rapid healing is essential in these
operations, it is of primary importance that the patient be in
the best possible health, and that the tissues in the operation
area be free from disease. Scar tissue can never be relied
upon, and it is needless to speak of the recklessness of plastic
operations in the vicinity of active syphilitic disease, or
lupus, or in aged or broken-down subjects. In many cases
the operation cannot be repeated: there is little before the
surgeon but success or a condition more lamentable than

mere failure. A plastic operation may leave the deformity in a worse condition than it was before the case was approached, and before the prospects of success are compromised the surgeon should be convinced that no possible element of failure has been overlooked.

4. In planning the flaps it is necessary that they be derived from sound tissues, that they be thick and include the subcutaneous tissue, that their vascularity be assured, and that they be so cut as to inflict the least possible damage upon the arteries which supply them.

The flap must be large enough, and as a rule should be one-sixth larger than the space it has to fill ; it must be gently handled, carefully adjusted, and most tenderly and precisely sutured. The pedicle of the flap must not be so twisted or extended as to occlude the nutrient vessel. It is of the utmost importance that there be no undue tension upon the parts, and that the edges of the wound are not merely dragged together.

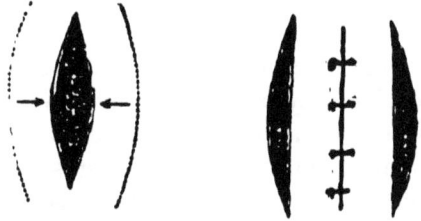

Fig. 221.

5. The margins of any surfaces of skin which are to be brought together must be evenly and liberally freshened. Throughout the whole progress of the case the strictest antiseptic precautions must be carried out, and the minutest care paid to the after-treatment.

In most cases union by first intention is aimed at, but, as is mentioned in a later section, this object may not be essential in all instances.

Methods.—The following are, very briefly, the chief methods made use of in plastic surgery. They must not be considered to represent either a complete system of operations or a series of rigid formulæ, but to rather form the groundwork of such varied procedures as the different classes of case to be dealt with demand.

1. THE DIRECT UNION OF FRESHENED EDGES WHICH ARE BROUGHT TOGETHER, ALL TENSION UPON THE PARTS HAVING BEEN RELIEVED.

B 2

This is applicable to small sinuses and fistulæ, to narrow linear and spindle-shaped gaps or fissures, and to such defects as the simpler forms of hare-lip.

The margins of the fissure or opening are freshened by removing the integument which covers them. The strip of skin to be removed is grasped and steadied with fine-toothed forceps, while the strip is severed with a narrow scalpel or sharp-pointed tenotome. The portion removed should include not only the skin but also the subcutaneous tissues, and must be so free that the raw edges which are to be united are made out of sound and vascular structures.

The edges of the fresh wound are carefully cleaned, bleeding is checked by the pressure of a sponge, and the margins are approximated by fine silkworm gut or silk sutures.

It is often well to leave the wound open for a while, to allow time for any bleeding to cease before the sutures are finally adjusted.

In the case of larger gaps, or of fissures in dense tissues, tension may be relieved by undermining the margins of the wound for a certain distance with the scalpel (subcutaneous detachment). If this be not sufficient, two parallel incisions may be made upon either side of the cleft, as shown in Fig. 221.

2. THE METHOD BY GLIDING OR LATERAL DISPLACEMENT.

Here the skin and subcutaneous tissues in the immediate vicinity of the defect or gap to be covered or closed are dissected up, and the tongue or strip of skin is so drawn upon and displaced as to occupy the freshened surface of the part to be covered.

In this case it must also be remembered that all edges and surfaces which are to be brought into contact must be liberally freshened. The strips of skin made use of to close the gap must be thick, and must include the subcutaneous tissues. The disposition of the strip must be influenced by convenience, by anatomical circumstances, and the arrangement of the blood-vessels. Bleeding should be checked before the sutures are drawn tight, and undue tension must not be allowed to fall upon the stitches.

A. **To close a Triangular Gap.**—1. If the gap be small,

and form an equilateral triangle, the area may be closed by uniting the sides or angles of the triangle.

2. If the defect be of larger size, one of the following methods may be made use of:—One side of the base of the triangle may be extended by an incision which cont nues the

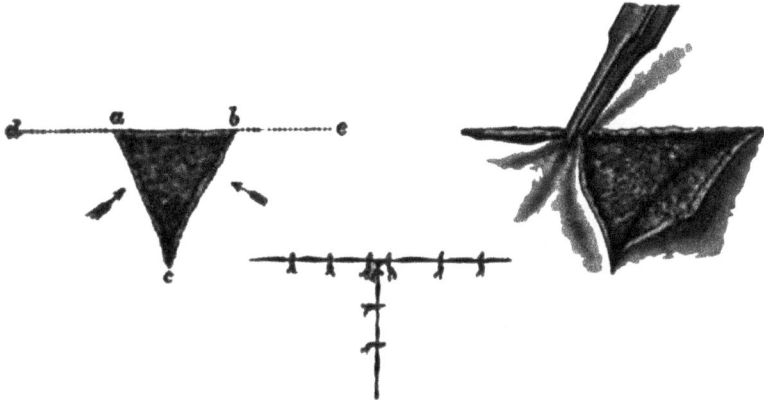

Fig. 222.—(*Löbker.*)

line of the base. The tongue of skin so marked out is freed by subcutaneous detachment, and the point of the freed flap is fixed to the angle on the undisturbed side of the base of the triangle. (*See* Fig. 222.)

3. The tissues upon both sides of the triangle may be freed in like manner (Fig. 222), so as to bring the two flaps together, *i.e.*, uniting the point *a* to the point *b*.

If necessary, the mobilisation of the tongues of integument may be aided by lateral parallel incisions made beyond the points *d* and *e*.

4. In order to conform with the natural line or disposition of the tissues or features, or to

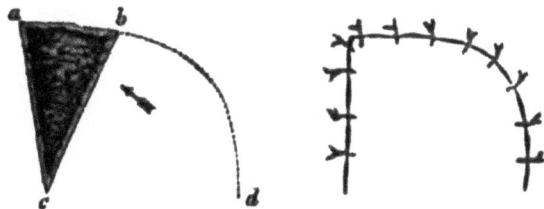

Fig. 223.—JAESCHE'S OPERATION. (*Löbker.*)

avoid nutrient vessels, a curved lateral incision (*b d*, Fig. 223) may be made, and the skin at *b* attached to the integument at *a*. This is known as Jaesche's operation.

b g, d h (Fig. 227). The two flaps, e a f c, b g d h, are detached, and are united along the margins, a c, b d. In many cases the formation of one lateral flap is sufficient, or the mobili-

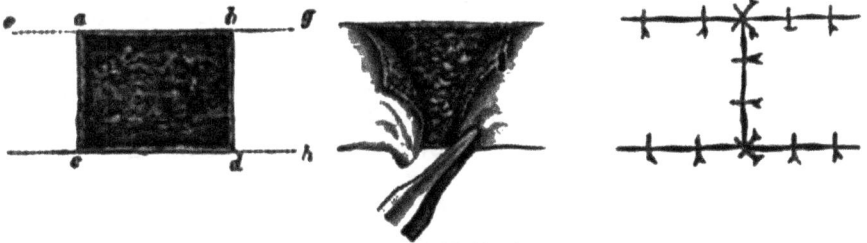

Fig. 227.—(*Löbker.*)

sation of the two strips of integument may be aided by parallel lateral incisions, made beyond the attached bases of the two flaps.

2. *Letenneur's Operation.*—The flap b e f g (Fig. 228) is

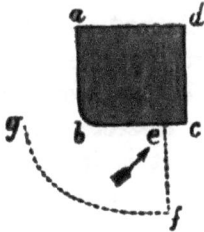

Fig. 228.

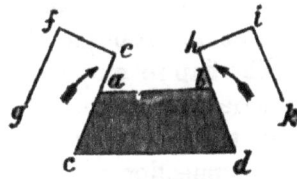

Fig. 229.

freed from below, and is displaced upwards until the margin e f can be sutured to the margin a d.

3. *Brüns' Operation.*—Two lateral flaps, a e f g, b h i k (Fig. 229), are marked out and detached, and are so brought

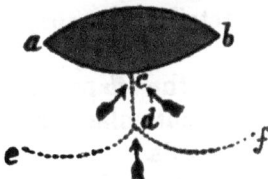

Fig. 230.

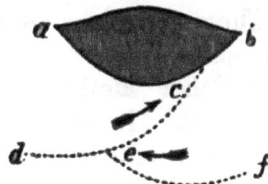

Fig. 231.

together that the borders e f and h i are united in the median line.

c. **To close Large Elliptical Defects.**—1. Simple curved flaps, such as $a\,c\,d\,e,\,b\,c\,d\,f$ (Fig. 230), may be cut and freed by subcutaneous detachment, and may then be displaced upwards, so as to close the raw area.

2. Two flaps, $a\,c\,d$ and $b\,e\,f$, may be fashioned as shown in Fig. 231, and after detachment may be so adjusted that the point c of the flap $a\,c\,d$ is raised, and attached to the angle b, while the gap left by its displacement is closed by the second flap, $b\,e\,f$. This is known as Weber's operation.

3. THE METHOD BY FLAP FORMATION.

Some of the methods just described may be properly considered as involving treatment by flap formation, and to be allied to what is known as the Indian operation; it is convenient, however, that the two sets of operations should be kept distinct.

The two chief methods of flap formation in plastic surgery are the Italian and the Indian.

1. **The Italian** or **Tagliacotian Method** involves the derivation of the flap from a distant part. In the restoration of the nose, for example, the flap may be obtained from the arm. The flap so employed is partially dissected up, and is left attached to the limb by its pedicle. It is in due course adjusted to its new situation, and after it has acquired a vascular connection with the tissues around the area it has to occupy, its connection with the arm is finally severed.

2. **The Indian Method** is understood to involve the derivation of the flap from the neighbouring integuments. Thus, in repairing defects of the nose the flap may be obtained from the forehead or cheek. A pedicle is formed, and the flap is drawn into its new position by torsion or gliding.

These operations are considered in detail in the chapter on Rhinoplasty.

3. **Other Methods** of disposing of the flaps may be mentioned. In the *reversed flap* the cuticular surface is directed inwards and its raw surface outwards.

In employing *superimposed*, or *double flaps*, the outer, raw or exposed surface of a reversed flap is covered by a second flap, the epidermic surface of which is turned outwards.

In Roux's method by *successive migration* the flap is

transferred from a distant part by stages. Thus a defect in the lip may be restored by a flap from the neck. This flap is first twisted transversely into a wound prepared for it, and as soon as union has occurred here is displaced upwards to the lower jaw, and thence to the lip.

The Treatment of the Flap.—In dealing with nearly all the cases in which a flap is fashioned, one of two methods may be followed:—(*a*) The flap may be at once fixed with sutures in its new situation, and to the newly-freshened surface prepared for it. (*b*) The implantation of the flap may be deferred until several days have elapsed, until its vitality is fully assured, and until its surface is granulating. The raw surface of the flap is prevented from acquiring attachments during the preparatory stage by the introduction of a piece of carbolised oil-silk beneath it. The detachment of the flap and its final severance may by this means be considerably postponed.

The advantages of this method are these:—The risks of sloughing of any part of the flap, and notably of its edges and free end, are greatly diminished. The flap is tested before it is employed. Instead of being transplanted just after it has been drained of blood and reduced in temperature, the flap is adjusted when it is vascular and the seat of an active repairing process. The treatment is certainly extended over a longer period of time, and involves greater inconvenience, and possibly more pain to the patient, but these drawbacks are considered to be more than met by the security given by the delay. This method has been carried out with great success by Thiersch in his operations for ectopia vesicæ (*Centralblatt für Chirurgie*, 1876, page 504). It has been strongly endorsed by Sir William MacCormac (*British Medical Journal*, Nov. 24th, 1888), and has been ably demonstrated by Mr. Croft, in the treatment of cicatricial deformities after burns. Mr. Croft's first operation by this method was carried out in 1880 (*Med.-Chir. Trans.*, vol. lxxii, 1889).

The details of this method are considered more fully in the following chapter on the treatment of cicatricial deformities.

CHAPTER II.

Plastic Operations for the Relief of Cicatricial Deformities after Burns.

The more gross variety of deformity which results from the contraction of the integuments after severe burns has been the subject of a great number of methods of treatment. It must be confessed that the results obtained have not been proportionate to the ingenuity and patience expended upon the treatment.

The contractions with which this chapter is mainly concerned are situated in the neck, face, or upper extremity. Various methods of extension, by means of screw apparatus, india-rubber bands, weights, etc., have been tried, but with little success. The same may be said of the treatment which consists in dividing the main contracting bands. Every variety of incision has been employed, a single large incision, multiple small incisions, subcutaneous sections, and cuts that have been placed in various relations with the line of the contracted band.

This method has been combined with extension and with forcible rupture, and has been aided by skin grafting, and every known means of securing rapid and complete healing.

The cicatrix has been entirely excised, and the gap left allowed to heal by granulation, or it has been partially excised, or has been so dissected up as to allow the contracted band to remain as a species of flap.

In these operations attempts have been made to lessen the area of the granulating surface by lateral incisions of various kinds made through the adjacent sound tissues, or by subcutaneous detachment of those tissues in one way or another.

In instances in which the deformity has attained to any magnitude it must be owned that these operations have met with but discouraging or very imperfect results.

Lastly come the various methods of dealing with these deformities by means of flap operations.

With these procedures the best results have been obtained. Very numerous methods of performing these operations have been devised. They need no especial mention, as they follow the ordinary principles of plastic repair by flap formation, and the points in which they differ from one another are of no great importance.

After an examination of the various operations described, and after a practical experience of some few of them, it has appeared to me that the most serviceable method at present available is that which has been so ably carried out by Mr. Croft.

The account which follows is derived from Mr. Croft's paper in vol. lxxii. of the *Med.-Chir. Trans.* (1889).

Mr. Croft has illustrated his procedure by an account of five cases, in all of which the treatment may be considered to have been successful.

The method consists of raising a strap or bridge of sound skin, which is left attached by its two extremities, but which is separated through the rest of its extent from the subjacent tissues by means of oiled silk.

After the process of granulation has been well established, the contracted structures are divided, and the bridge of skin, having been severed at one extremity, is made to occupy the gap formed by such division. The operation is indeed a flap operation, in which the attachment of the flap in its new situation is deferred until granulation has occurred.

The Operation as carried out by Mr. Croft.

The strap or bridge of skin to be . raised is cut where it can be taken free of scar tissue and well supplied with blood, yet sufficiently near to allow of its being twisted into its new bed. In the neck the bridge of skin may measure eight or nine inches in length. These bridges are cut as thick as possible, especially in their central parts (Fig. 232).

The bleeding from the flap and wound is carefully arrested before dressings are applied.

The sides of the wound are approximated by sutures, but tension from the stitches is avoided as much as possible.

With the object of promoting approximation or preventing retraction of the edges, these are also sutured to the muscle and fascia near the centre of the gaping wound.

This fixation of the edges is of assistance in limiting the extent of surface which has to heal by granulation.

The strap or bridge is left attached at either end.

The under-surface and edges of the bridge are to become covered by granulations. Care must be taken to prevent it from re-uniting, and especially that granulations do not spring up in the angles formed between the pedicles and the raw surface. In this situation there is not a little risk that the length of the span may become insidiously shortened.

A layer of oiled-silk protective dipped in carbolised oil is inserted between the raised skin

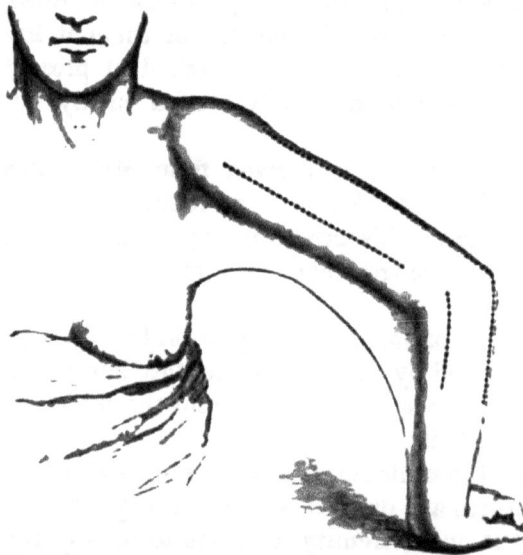

Fig. 232.—CROFT'S OPERATION FOR THE RELIEF OF CICATRICIAL DEFORMITY AFTER BURNS: POSITION OF BRIDGES OF SKIN IN A CASE OF BURN OF THE UPPER LIMB.

and the parts beneath it, and is carefully drawn under the pedicles.

The whole operation area is covered with a light antiseptic dressing, and the part is so secured as to keep the entire region at rest. A rigid fixation apparatus may be required, especially in young patients.

If all goes well, and no complication occurs, in a fortnight or three weeks' time it will be safe to proceed to the next stage of the operation—viz., that of cutting across the contracted scar and transplanting the strip of skin. In judging of the right moment for beginning the second stage, the surgeon must take into account the condition and extent of the granulating wound, the fresh loss of blood which must ensue in making a bed for the transplant, the extent of this fresh wound, and the influence that the operation will have upon the vitality of the transplant, which must now depend on one pedicle instead of on two.

At this second operation it is better first to cut through the contracted scar, and afterwards to cut across one end of the bridge. In dealing with the scar no tissue should be sacrificed. The scar tissue should be divided until healthy fat, fascia, or muscle is reached. All bleeding should have ceased before the final fixation of the transplant.

The bed and the flap must be made to agree in length, and for the most part in width, but the shape of the fresh wound cannot always be made to correspond exactly with the shape and extent of the transplant.

The form of the bridge will now have considerably changed from what it was when it was first cut. It will have become shorter and narrower and thicker.

The strap must be to a certain extent trimmed. The edges and granulating under surface at the free end, for a distance of about half the length of the strap, should be pared or freshened, so that a raw surface is presented for primary union.

In none of Mr. Croft's cases did the transplant correspond in its uniform width to the width of the bed for it. The latter always varied, except at the part which was to receive the free half or third of the flap.

It is enough to obtain primary union between the free end of the flap and the fresh wound. This union anchors the strap and fixes it in its place.

Union along the rest of the extent of the transplant is only a work of time. At first the transplant looks very ungainly and unpromising. As week after week goes by and healing takes place, the sausage-like thing flattens down and spreads out, until finally it may become twice as wide as it was originally cut.

The part of the transplant which causes anxiety is the

distal inch of it. This may slough to a slight extent, and union may therefore fail to take place. In consequence of this the strap may retract from its holding. It must then be kept in place by the troublesome process of strapping.

After healing has taken place, the surgeon must wait for about six months before he can judge of the final result of his operation.

CHAPTER III.

RHINOPLASTY.

A VERY large number of plastic operations, most of them ingenious and all more or less complex, have been designed to repair defects of the nose. The defect may be due to congenital deformity, or may depend upon injury, or upon the results of lupus, syphilis, or other destructive forms of ulceration. Any operation may be considered to be contraindicated in the case of partial or complete loss of the nose, the result of cancer.

The main flaps out of which the new organ is formed may be derived from the forehead, the cheek, the arm, or forearm. It is seldom that the whole of the nose is destroyed, and it will be evident that the least successful results follow in cases in which the bony parts of the nose have been lost.

In *complete rhinoplastic operations* it is assumed that the whole of the cartilaginous part of the organ, including the tip, the columna, the alæ, and more or less of the septum, are lost.

Partial rhinoplasty concerns itself with slighter defects, and is employed to replace the tip of the nose, or one ala or part of the septum, or to close a fistulous opening in the skin of the member.

Many of these minor operations are very successful, but many of the procedures which aim at the restoration of the entire nose do not give brilliant results.

Among the most excellent results obtained by rhinoplasty must be placed the very admirable series of cases published by Surgeon-Major Keegan in the *Lancet* for Feb. 21, 1891. (*See* Fig. 238.)

In cases in which the bony framework of the nose has been lost, or in which the patient is the subject of a "depressed nose"—as in congenital syphilis—the results are almost entirely unsatisfactory. An unsightly gap in the face may be closed in the one case, it is true, but it will be covered in by a flap of skin which is in time level with the cheek. In the case of the depressed nose it is a question whether the "improvement" merits that term, and to replace a flat area of integument by a rudimentary and imperfect ridge is to effect a doubtful change in the features.

Even in cases in which the nasal bones have survived, the results have often little to commend them. The new nose may be large and bulbous, or puny and abortive, and a feature which is unsightly may be replaced by one which is simply ridiculous. In the operations which involve the formation of a flap from the tissues of the face much additional disfigurement may result from an unsightly scar on the forehead or the cheek.

The results, however, obtained since improved methods of treating wounds have been introduced are certainly more encouraging.

It is true that the tissues of the face are admirably adapted for plastic procedures, and the actual surgical results, so far as healing is concerned, are often all that could be wished.

Before proposing a complete rhinoplastic operation, the use of an artificial nose carefully fashioned and coloured should be considered.

Within the last few years remarkable improvements have been effected in the manufacture of these artificial features. The best certainly look unnatural, but they are at least symmetrical and well-shaped, and do not look ridiculous.

By means of a spectacle-frame a very fair attachment of the upper part of the new member can be obtained, and in adult males a false moustache may be made to secure the lower attachment.

The special elements of failure in these operations are gangrene or sloughing of the flap, imperfect healing, secondary hæmorrhage, erysipelas, shrinking, or persistent œdema or distortion of the attached flap, and, lastly, a recurrence of the original disease.

COMPLETE RHINOPLASTY.

A selection from the extremely numerous operations

embraced by this title will be considered under the following headings:—

1. The Indian operation (flap taken from the forehead).
2. The Italian operation (flap taken from the upper limb).
3. The French operation (flap taken from the cheek).
4. Other operations.

1. The Indian Operation.

This procedure, as modified by modern and especially by German surgeons, may claim to be at present the best rhinoplastic operation. The flap is derived from the forehead, and is brought into place by torsion. One great objection to it is that a large and unsightly scar is left on the forehead. The operation is not applicable to cases in which the tissues of the forehead are un-sound, or are the seat of cicatrices.

First Stage.—The edges of the defect must be well and evenly freshened. The best results follow when the gap is triangular in outline, and in any case the outline of the area to be covered in should be made as nearly as possible triangular, the base of the triangle being towards the upper lip.

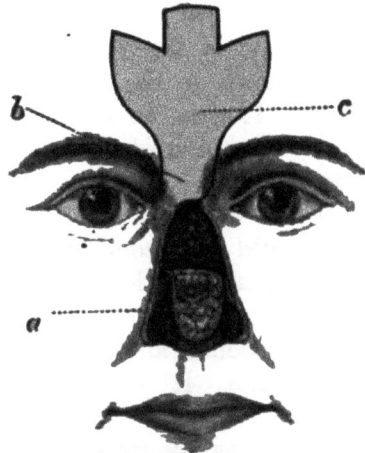

Fig. 233.—RHINOPLASTY.

a, Nasal flap ; *b,* Pedicle of frontal flap ; *c,* Frontal flap.

Second Stage.—When possible a small thin flap should be formed from the skin of the root of the nose. This flap should be quadrilateral, with the base or attached side downwards. It should be detached and turned downwards (*a,* Fig. 233), so that its raw surface is directed forwards.

This flap can only be used when the skin over the nasal bones is sound and healthy. It serves to increase the solidity of the new nose, and to form a further attach-ment for the frontal flap.

Third Stage.—The frontal flap is made. A model of
the new organ should have been already fashioned in
thin gutta-percha or plaster. This model when flattened
out is laid upon the forehead, and, guided by its outline,
the flap is marked out. The flap should be about a
third larger than the area of the defect, or in marking it
out in ink upon the forehead a quarter of an inch may
be allowed on each side of the prepared model. Enough
tissue must be provided to allow for the alæ and columna.
The upper extremity of the flap will reach about to the
border of the scalp. If the forehead be low the flap will
encroach upon the hair.

The apex or narrow part of the flap will be of course
at the root of the nose. The flap should include all the
tissues down to the pericranium, which must not be disturbed. It must be dissected up boldly and freely.

The formation of the pedicle or apex of the flap is important.

It is well that the incision marking one side of the
flap should be continued downwards into the recently
freshened area (*b*, Fig. 233).

By means of this incision the pedicle can be lifted
from the bones, and will contain the supra-trochlear artery
of one side. It is impossible that the pedicle can be so
made as to include the arteries of the two sides; and if
the plan just described be adopted, the compression of the
artery by the torsion of the pedicle is reduced to a minimum.

The side selected for the pedicle must of course depend
upon circumstances. Its width will be from 1 to 1½ c.m.
The incision marking the other side of the pedicle will
end at the inner side of the eyebrow, as shown in Fig. 233.

The flap is usually placed in or about the median line.
Some surgeons, and notably Dr. Keegan, direct the long axis
of the flap obliquely, so that its tissues are derived mainly
from one side of the forehead only. By this means it is
considered that the risk of compressing the artery of the
pedicle by torsion is minimised. The placing of the flap so
obliquely that its long axis is nearly parallel with the eyebrow
is, however, to be condemned.

The including of the pericranium in the flap, under

the impression that it would produce bone in the new situation, is a perfectly valueless proceeding, and may lead to some exfoliation of the frontal bone. The indisposition of the pericranium to form new bone is well known.

All bleeding must be arrested by sponge pressure or pressure forceps. No ligatures should be employed.

The shape of the flap may now be considered.

The outlines here described are those of (a) the triangular flap, (b) the pyriform flap of Dieffenbach, (c) Langenbeck's flap, and (d) Keegan's flap.

(a) The triangular flap conforms to the original plan of the operation, and is the basis of the many modifications.

Its outline is shown in Fig. 234, which represents the full size for an adult. The line d d indicates the median line of the dorsum of the new nose.

The upper border of the flap is divided into three parts by the two vertical incisions $a c$, $a c$.

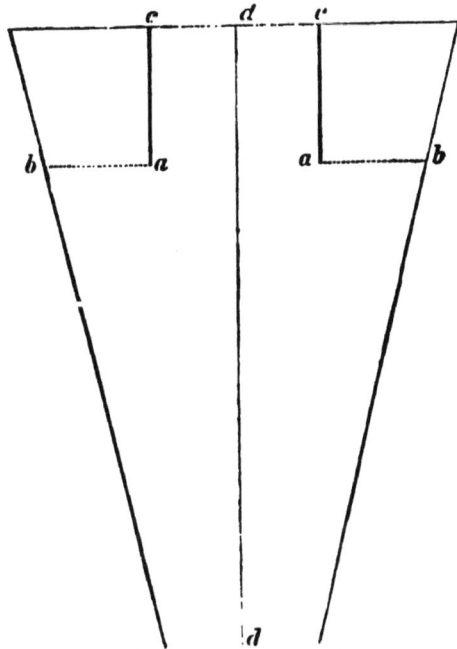

Fig. 234.—RHINOPLASTY: THE TRIANGULAR FLAP.
(Natural size.)

The median part is utilised to form the columna, and the two lateral parts to form the alæ.

The length of the central part must depend upon the profile of the features.

The lateral flaps are bent backwards along the lines $a b$, $a b$, so as to conform to the outline of the alar part of the nose. A narrow wedge-shaped piece of skin will probably have to be excised along the lines $a c$, $a c$.

(b) The pyriform flap of Dieffenbach is formed upon

c 2

the same plan as the above, its proportions are estimated in the same way, and the pedicle is arranged in the same manner. The outline of the flap is shown, of natural size, in Fig. 235. The incisions *a c, a c* are made as before in order to mark off a central segment for the columna. The lateral flaps are bent back in the direction of *c′ c′*, and are utilised to form the alæ.

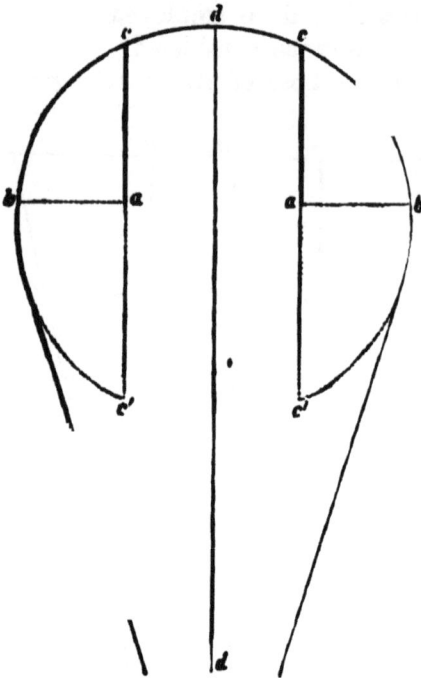

Fig. 235.—RHINOPLASTY: DIEFFENBACH'S FLAP.
(Natural size.)

(c) Langenbeck's flap has the outline shown in Fig. 236 (natural size). In its general proportions and in the disposition of its pedicle it follows the rules already laid down. The central segment *a c, c a* forms the columna, the lateral segments—which are bent backwards along the lines *a b, a b* —the alæ. This flap is in many respects the best of those described.

(d) Keegan's flap is described on page 25.

Fourth Stage.—The frontal wound is closed as far as is possible. If the triangular flap be used, the raw area can be closed in to a considerable extent. In Dieffenbach's flap the area can be but little diminished, while the most complete diminution of the raw gap can be effected when Langenbeck's or Keegan's method has been employed.

Fine harelip pins and silkworm-gut sutures may be used for this part of the 'operation.

By dealing with the frontal wound at this stage the bleeding is considerably diminished, and the surgeon has a clearer field for the manipulation of the flap.

Fifth Stage.—The flap is fixed into its new position. It is carefully twisted, and during this step the surgeon must hold in mind the possibility of occluding the nutrient artery by torsion.

The flap is secured in place by interrupted sutures of silkworm gut. These must not be too closely inserted, and no traction must be made upon them. The lateral parts of the flap are secured first, then the columna, and lastly the alæ.

If the columna has been provided for in the frontal flap as above described, then a suitable groove must be cut in the median part of the upper lip to receive it. If no columna can be obtained from

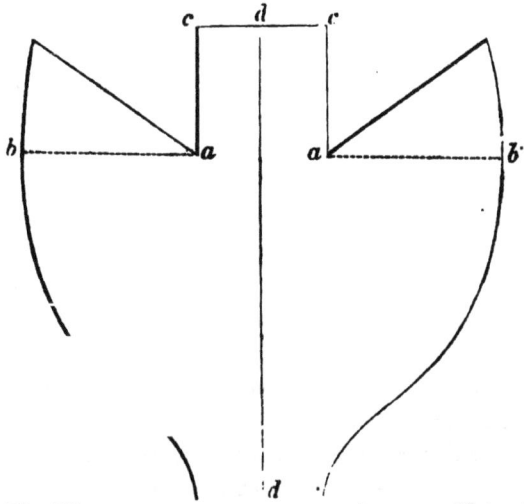

Fig. 236.—RHINOPLASTY: LANGENBECK'S FLAP. (Natural size.)

the tissues of the forehead, then it must be formed from the upper lip (page 22), either at once or at a later period.

If no columna be fashioned at this stage, then the flap must be carefully supported by a light plug of gauze, which should be changed frequently. If the septum of the nostrils be restored, then each of the new nostrils must be supported with pieces of drainage-tube of suitable size. These must be retained in position for some weeks.

A simple dry antiseptic dressing is applied, which is secured in place by a light gauze bandage.

The After-treatment is conducted upon general principles. Portions of redundant flap may have to be excised, or some slight secondary operations undertaken to improve the appearance of the new organ.

The pedicle may be severed at the end of three to four

weeks, and the wrinkled portion of protuberant skin which marks its position is excised in the form of a wedge-shaped piece to prevent the formation of a parrot-shaped nose.

Extensive skin grafting will be required for the granulating surface on the forehead.

Modifications of the Operation.

1. *The Frontal Flap may be Partially Detached at First,* and may have its upper attachment severed after its raw surface is granulating, and be then twisted into its new situation.

This modification has been already described (page 9).

Although this plan is admirably suited for some plastic operations, notably for such as are concerned in the relief of deformities produced by burns, it does not appear to be well adapted for this form of rhinoplasty, and it is to be noted that nearly every surgeon who has advocated the Indian method has carried out the immediate adjustment of the flap.

2. *The Formation of a New Columna from the Lip.*— In the description given above, provision for the new columna is made in fashioning the frontal flap. If, as is often the case, especially in patients with low foreheads, it is not possible to form the new septum from the frontal tissues the columna may be taken from the lip.

A narrow vertical strip (*b* c, *b* c, Fig. 247) of the median part of the upper lip is isolated by means of the scalpel.

This strip will be about one-fourth of an inch in width, will be quadrilateral, will be equal in length to the depth of the lip, and will include, at its free end, a part of the red margin of the lip. The little flap will be entirely free, except at its upper or nasal extremity, and to ensure its freedom the frænum of the lip, and the reflections of the mucous membrane from the lip to the maxilla, must be severed.

During the cutting of this thick but narrow strip of tissue the coronary arteries should be compressed by an assistant.

In males it is well to dissect off the skin, and with it the hair follicles.

The tip of the little flap is freshened, and is drawn forwards and fixed *in situ* to the tip of the nose.

It will be seen that the cutaneous surface of the flap

forming the new columna is turned upwards, *i.e.*, looks toward the nasal fossæ, while the mucous surface is directed downwards, *i.e.*, looks towards the chin. The flap is merely bent upwards, and is exposed to no torsion. The mucous membrane in time becomes thickened, and resembles skin.

After the columna has been fixed in position the gap in the upper lip is closed with sutures.

Volkmann, Bennett of Dublin, and others, are opposed to the formation of a special columna. They point out that the contraction of the deep surface of the frontal flap leaves an orifice none too large for the admission of air. The flap is allowed to hang freely downwards, and its extremity is not secured by sutures. The contraction of the flap leads to the formation of a definite tip to the new nose, the appearance of which, it is claimed, would not be improved by a columna.

3. *Operations to Prevent Depression of the New Nose* have led to numerous ingenious experiments and to many modifications of the original operation.

Supporting-plugs of amber or of gold have been employed, and various "nasal levers" have been devised, but the retention of these foreign bodies has caused intolerable irritation and ulceration.

Thiersch made two small longitudinal skin flaps from the edges of the gap to be closed, and, turning them both inwards, united them in the median line. The integumentary surfaces of the little flaps were thus turned inwards, the raw surfaces outwards. Upon this raw surface the frontal flap was allowed to rest, and from this small under-flap it obtained support.

Langenbeck cut, with a fine saw, lateral pieces of bone from the osseous margins of the nasal aperture. These, when sufficiently separated, were lifted up with an elevator, and were so placed with reference to one another that they acted like the beams of a roof to support the alæ and apex of the new nose.

4. *Keegan's Operation.*—This method of Rhinoplasty is thus described by Surgeon-Major Keegan in the *Lancet* for Feb. 21, 1891:—

The operation is begun by carrying two converging incisions (C A, H F, Fig. 237) from two points slightly external to the roots of the alæ nasi to two points about three-quarters of an inch apart on the bridge of the nose, where a pair of spectacles would rest. These two points on the bridge of the nose are now joined by a horizontal incision, A F. This horizontal incision is bisected, and a perpendicular incision (B D, E G) is drawn downwards from the point of bisection nearly as far as where the nasal bones join on to the cartilage of the nose. In other words, this perpendicular incision follows the course of the junction of the nasal bones, but is not carried down as far as their inferior borders. The skin and tissues are now

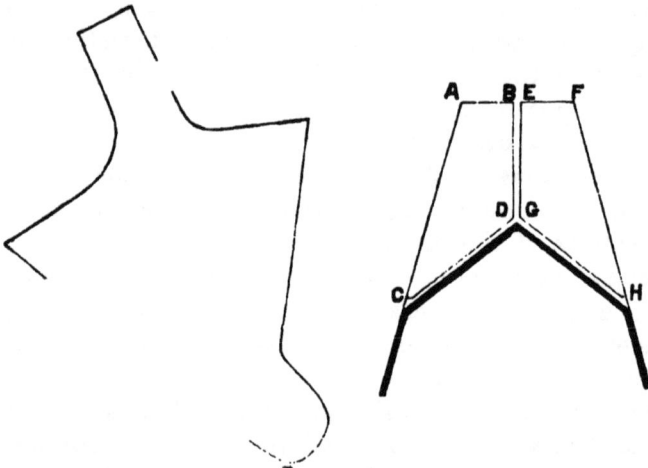

Fig. 237.—RHINOPLASTY. KEEGAN'S OPERATION: THE FLAP IS REDUCED IN SIZE. (From the *Lancet*, Feb. 21, 1891.)

dissected cautiously from off the nasal bones from above downwards in two flaps, A B C D and E F G H, as in Fig. 237. The two inferior borders of the flaps—viz., C D and G H—are not interfered with, and constitute the attachment of the flaps to the structures and tissues which clothe the inferior borders of the nasal bones, where they join on to the cartilage of the nose. If these two flaps are reflected downwards, so that their raw surfaces look forwards and their cuticular surfaces look backwards, it will be found that they overlap in the centre. The surgeon has therefore a redundancy of flap to deal with, a redundancy which he can utilise a little later when he has raised the flap from the forehead. He now proceeds to do so in the usual way. The root of the pedicle occupies the internal angle of the eye. The flap is inclined obliquely, and its outline is shown in Fig. 237. The pericranium is not disturbed. The sides of the gap now left in the forehead are approximated as quickly as possible by means of horsehair sutures, and it is surprising how small a raw surface is left behind on the forehead if the approximation of the sides of the gap be ·judiciously and expeditiously carried out. Attention is now directed to preparing a nidus or bed for the reception of the columna, and this does not require any description. The two flaps, A B C D and E F G H, which have been already raised from off the nasal bones, are now reflected downwards, and, as they overlap in the centre, two triangular-shaped pieces are cut away, and placed in the middle of the gap left in the forehead, in order to expedite the process of cicatrisation in the frontal scar. The forehead flap is now brought down over the nasal bones, and rests inferiorly on the two reflected flaps, A B C D and E F G H, taken from off the nasal bones. The raw surface of the frontal flap, inferiorly, lies on the raw surfaces of the two reflected nasal flaps, and the nostrils of the newly-formed nose are therefore lined inside with the skin or cuticular sides of the reflected nasal flaps. The free inferior margins of the forehead flap and the nasal flaps are now brought together by horsehair sutures. The columnar portion of the forehead flap is now fixed in the bed prepared for it by sutures, and the two original incisions drawn from the root of the alæ nasi on either side to the bridge of the nose are now deepened and bevelled off for the reception of the sides or lateral margins of the forehead flap. The sides or lateral margins of the forehead flap are most accurately attached by means of horsehair sutures to the bed prepared for them. Two pieces of drainage-tubing are inserted in the newly-formed nostrils. Strips of lint on which some boracic ointment has been smeared are placed over the junction of the lateral margins of the new nose to the cheeks, and also on the gap left behind on the forehead, and cotton-wool is applied over all.

Dr. Keegan divides the pedicle of the new nose at the end of a fortnight. The drainage-tubes which occupy the new nostrils are removed after ten days.

Dr. Keegan's paper is illustrated by a number of portraits of patients before and after operation, and the results obtained are in every respect most admirable.

Two of the portraits in question are reproduced in Fig. 238.

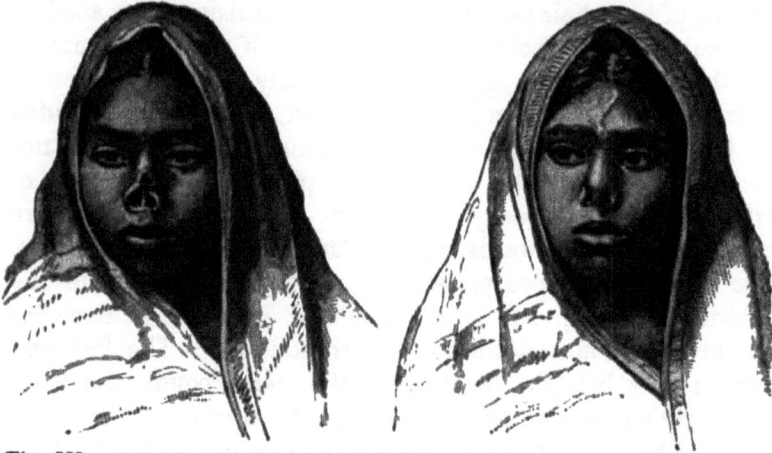

Fig. 238.—KEEGAN'S METHOD OF PERFORMING RHINOPLASTY: PORTRAITS OF THE SAME PATIENT BEFORE AND AFTER OPERATION. (From the *Lancet*, Feb. 21, 1891.)

Verneuil's Operation, for the treatment of "depressed nose," by means of a modified frontal flap, is described on page 33.

2. The Italian Operation.

This elaborate operation is very rarely performed at the present day, and is only considered to be indicated when the tissues of the forehead or of the cheek are not available for the formation of a flap.

The procedure is throughout extremely irksome. The flap obtained is not so well adapted for rhinoplasty as is a flap obtained from the forehead, and undergoes very considerable shrinking and atrophy. It would be of little purpose to give any description of the original operations as they were carried out in the 16th century.

The only notable example of the Italian method in recent times is, so far as I am aware, that carried out by Sir William MacCormac in 1877.

The procedure cannot be better illustrated than by a transcript of Sir William MacCormac's account (*Clin. Soc.*

Trans., vol. x., 1877, page 181). The patient was a girl of sixteen, and the loss of the nose was the result of an accident.

The Apparatus.—This is shown in Fig. 239. "A pair of ordinary stout well-fitting stays were first procured, to which were attached two perineal straps to prevent displacement upwards. A helmet, partly made of leather, was connected with the stays by a leather band running up the centre of the neck and back. A leather arm-piece, strengthened by a steel band, was moulded so as to extend from the wrist to the shoulder, where it was buckled to the stays. The wrist and hand were fastened to the helmet by a gauntlet, while the elbow could be fixed steadily in any required position by straps running from it to the stays, and to the sides of the head-piece, so that there was nowhere any undue strain, the pressure being so evenly distributed that each strap was almost slack.

"This apparatus was kept applied for some days beforehand, so that any point of undue pressure might be discovered and remedied."

The Operation. — "The first part of the operation was performed on Feb. 12th, 1877. A flap was mapped out on the inner aspect of the left upper arm, more than double the

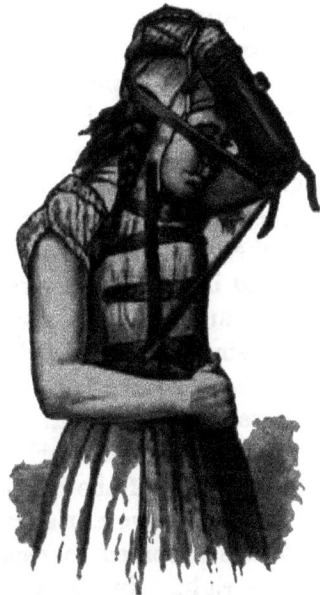

Fig. 239.—RHINOPLASTY BY THE ITALIAN METHOD : THE APPARATUS IN POSITION. (*MacCormac.*)

actual size of the estimated deficiency. The left arm was the one chosen to supply the flap, and the right side of the nose the one first operated upon, the septum being fashioned at the same time. The flap was left attached at the upper part of the arm by a broad, long pedicle, and so arranged that there should be no traction whatever upon it, whilst the raw surface from which it was taken should be accessible for daily dressing. With the flap I dissected up the subcutaneous fat down to the muscular sheath. Immediate retraction, both of the flap and of the denuded part of the arm, took place to a large extent, so that the raw surface on the latter was almost co-extensive with the whole inner aspect of the girl's arm, the flap appearing quite small in comparison.

"I now made a slightly-curved incision, nearly parallel to the free border of the nose on the right side, and about three lines above it—corresponding, in fact, to where the alar furrow should normally exist.

"This incision was prolonged some little distance into the cheek in the line of the cheek furrow, whilst the remains of the septum were split open in the median line. This nasal flap could now be turned down so as to become horizontal, or rather a little depressed beneath the horizontal line, to allow for retraction of the ingrafted piece. A triangular gap, the apex pointing towards the cheek, was thus left exposed on the right lateral aspect of the nose, and into this the triangular-shaped piece from the arm was inserted, and accurately attached by suture, the portion to form the septum being sutured in the groove already mentioned, formed by splitting the septum. In this way there was no paring of edges, nor was a single particle of the nose tissue sacrificed.

"The flap had a large line of attachment. Some suppuration followed on the eighth day. Sound healing of the flap did not take place for nearly three weeks. At the end of this time the base of the flap was detached from the arm. It was cut so as to have a triangular shape, and the left side of the nose was prepared to receive it in a manner precisely similar to the right. In the gap thus formed the detached portion was adjusted and sutured.

"Complete healing of this second part took place in fourteen days.

"The apparatus caused scarcely any inconvenience after the first forty-eight hours. The arm, when released, was stiff and painful, but soon recovered itself. The patient slept well during the treatment.

"The nostrils were kept dilated by short pieces of tubing. For the first three weeks after the completion of the operation much contraction took place in the new nose. Since then little change has ensued."

Woodcuts showing the state of the patient before and after the operation are given in Sir William MacCormac's paper. It may be a question with some whether the girl's appearance has been improved or not by the treatment.

In many accounts of the operation it is advised that the procedure be conducted by the following stages :—

1. The flap is dissected up as a bridge, and is allowed to granulate for fourteen days, a piece of oiled silk being inserted beneath it. (*See* Croft's operation, page 11.) This flap will measure about five inches by four inches, and will be attached at its extremities only.

2. The upper attachment of the flap is divided, and the flap itself is allowed to lie undisturbed for a few more days.

3. The margins of the defect are pared and are made ready to receive the flap. The apparatus is applied, and the arm is brought into contact with the face.

4. At the end of from ten to twenty days the lower attachment of the flap is severed, the apparatus is left off, and the arm set free.

5. A columna is fashioned from the lower lip (*see* page 22), and such other steps are taken as are needed to complete the new nose.

This measure has certain distinct advantages over the operation already described as carried out by Sir William MacCormac. It is more in conformity with the recent principles which have guided plastic surgery, and from Sir William MacCormac's subsequent writings it is to be inferred that it is the method he would himself be disposed to favour in any further attempts to carry out this form of rhinoplasty.

3. The French Operation.

In this procedure rhinoplasty is performed by the transposition of lateral or facial flaps. The method is of great antiquity, and was described by Celsus. It has undergone extensive modifications in modern times, and has been especially favoured by French surgeons.

The operation is considered to be best suited for cases in which the upper part of the nose remains intact.

The frontal scar is avoided, but the tissues of the cheek

are found by experience to be but ill-adapted for the formation of a substantial flap which will not undergo exceptional shrinking.

The new nose is apt to be quite flat, and its vascular supply is feeble, since the arteries of the flap which are derived from the facial are cut in the operation.

Hæmorrhage is very free during the cutting of the flaps.

A cicatrix of a somewhat prominent character is left upon the cheek of either side, and a scar marks the median line of the new nose.

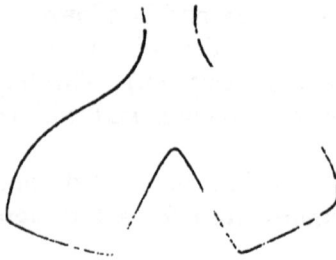

Fig. 240.—SYME'S METHOD OF RHINO-PLASTY: THE FLAP FROM THE CHEEK.

(A) *Syme's Operation.*—A large symmetrical flap of the shape shown in Fig. 240 is marked out on the cheeks. Its size is regulated by the rules already given (page 18), and by the dimensions required for the new organ. The pedicle of the flap is median, and is placed above at the root of the nose and between the two inner canthi.

The area to be covered having been freshened, the bilobar flap is freely dissected up, and when all bleeding has been checked, the two lobes of it are united in the median line, while its outer margins are sutured on either side to the raw surface at a proper distance from the nasal orifice.

The edges of the wounds left in the cheeks must be brought together, as far as is possible, by sutures; the triangular gap which will remain on each side close to the new nose being left to close by granulation aided by skin grafting (Fig. 241).

The contraction produced by the healing of these triangular gaps often enhances the apparent height and prominence of the new organ. The nostrils of the new nose must be supported for a time by a plug of gauze or by short pieces of drainage-tube.

Mr. Bell advises that if any part of the old septum remain, it may be made use of as a fixed point. A straight needle is thrust through one lobe of the flap close to its outer lower edge, is then passed through the septum, and is finally brought out at a corresponding point on the other lobe of the flap.

(B) *Nélaton's Operation.*—This surgeon marked out two thick trapezoidal flaps from the cheeks.

Each flap is intended to form the corresponding half of the new nose. The pedicles of the flaps are situated above near the lachrymal sac, while their bases are below. Each flap contains all the soft parts down to the bone, including the periosteum, which is stripped off the exposed portions of the ascending parts of the superior maxilla on either side.

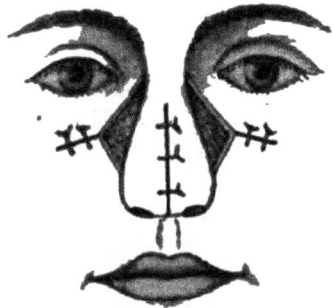

The flaps are sutured together along the median line, and are attached also by their outer margins as in Syme's procedure.

Fig. 241.—SYME'S METHOD OF RHINO-PLASTY: THE FLAPS IN POSITION.

The sides of the nose are supported and kept in contact by a hare-lip pin, which is passed through both alæ, while the parts transfixed are compressed by means of a pince-nez, which is steadied by the steel pin.

The results of these operations have not been very satisfactory.

4. Other Operations.

(A) *Ollier's Operation.*—A short account of this method is given by Dr. Joseph Bryant, in his " Manual of Operative Surgery," in the following words :—

"An operation was performed for a deformity caused by the loss of the alæ, columna, cartilages, lobe, and a portion of the septum, due to lupus. The nose was not more than an inch long, due to arrest of development of the ossa nasi, to which was attached a strip of cartilage. The integument of the lip and cheeks had been involved, and could not therefore be depended upon for flaps.

"Ollier commenced two diverging incisions in the median line of the forehead, two inches above the eyebrows, and carried them downward to within one-fourth of an inch from the outer side of the nasal orifice (Fig. 242).

".The upper portion of the triangular flap included the corresponding portion of periosteum down to the upper end of the nasal bones. The dissection was continued along the right nasal bone, omitting the periosteum, down to its lower end, from which the cartilage was separated; but it remained attached to the flap. The left nasal bone was separated from its bony connections with a chisel, leaving it attached to the flap by its anterior surface; the cartilaginous septum was then divided from before backwards and downwards with scissors, and left attached by its base to the cutaneous cartilage, that a central support might be provided for the new structure. The whole flap was then drawn downwards, until the upper border of the loosened nasal bone (left) came opposite to the lower border of the right one, when they were fastened together with a metallic suture. The sides of the flap were then united to the cheek, and the frontal incision closed above its apex."

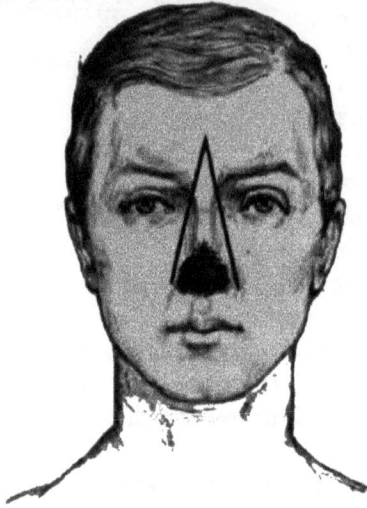

Fig. 242.—OLLIER'S METHOD OF RHINOPLASTY.

In this case it is said that the space left by the removal of the left nasal bone was filled by bone developed from the periosteum that had been slid down from the forehead.

(B) *Wood's Operation.*—In one case Mr. John Wood formed a new nose from a broad flap taken from the upper lip. The flap was freed of both its cutaneous and its mucous layers, and this separation extended as far as, but not through, the red margin of the lip. The flap was turned upwards, and was fixed by sutures to the upper margin of the defective area, which had been freshened to receive it. The raw surface thus presented was finally closed in by lateral flaps taken from the cheeks. It may be questioned in such a case whether the labial flap would really be of assistance, and whether it would in any material degree help to prevent the ultimate shrinking and flattening of the new nose.

(c) *Operations for Depressed Nose.*—In these instances the nose is perfectly flat. The integuments are probably sound, and no actual gap or defect marks the surface. The bones and cartilages, however, which support the organ are wanting to a greater or a lesser degree, and the resulting deformity is considerable.

Operative interference in this class of case has been attended with but unsatisfactory and disappointing results.

In some examples one of the above complete operations for the formation of a new nose has been carried out. In such instances the scanty tissues of the depressed nose have been made use of to form secondary flaps. The operative measures alluded to in the section on " operations to prevent depression of the new nose " (page 23) have been applied in these instances. In Verneuil's method, described below, the use of nasal flaps, aided by a much-modified frontal flap, is the conspicuous element in the operation.

It is at present a matter of question whether in these instances a better or less unsightly result cannot be obtained by the adjustment of an arti-ficial nose. As the operations in vogue cannot be considered to have been as yet entirely put aside in favour of mechanical appliances, the best known of them are here described.

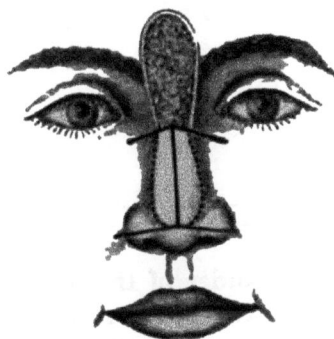

It is assumed that the tip and alæ of the nose are not wanting.

(a) *Verneuil's Operation.*— An incision is made vertically along the median line of the depressed organ.

Fig. 243.—VERNEUIL'S METHOD OF RHINOPLASTY: THE FLAPS IN POSITION.

At each end of this—*i.e.*, at the root of the nose and just above the alæ—a transverse cut is made. The two nasal flaps thus marked out (Fig. 243) are dissected up. A comparatively small oblong flap is now

d

raised from the middle of the forehead, its pedicle being placed between the two inner canthi.

It is turned downwards—without torsion of the pedicle—so that it closes the large opening made into the nasal fossæ by the dissection of the nasal flaps. The raw surface is anterior or external, the cutaneous surface looks towards the nasal fossæ.

This flap is fixed in position by a few sutures.

The two nasal or lateral flaps are now drawn over it, and are united together in the median line. The wound in the forehead is closed as far as possible by means of sutures and a hare-lip pin, and the granulating surface left is subsequently grafted. The pedicle of the frontal flap will, at a later period, require to be divided and trimmed. In Verneuil's case the new nose thus formed was raised one-third of an inch above the adjoining surface. The scars formed by the lateral incisions fade gradually into the naso-labial sulci and the folds beneath the eye.

Mr. Jacobson speaks well of this operation.

(b) *Dieffenbach's Operation.*—An incision is made with a narrow-bladed knife along the outer border of the depressed area on each side (a, Fig. 244). These two incisions mark out an intervening median strip of tissue, c, which should be three times broader at its lower or labial end than at its upper extremity. The upper part of this strip joins the forehead, the lower parts the lip.

At the outer side of each of these incisions another (b, Fig. 244) is made down to the bone. These lateral cuts commence a few lines below the first incision, are carried obliquely downwards, parallel with them, and, skirting the

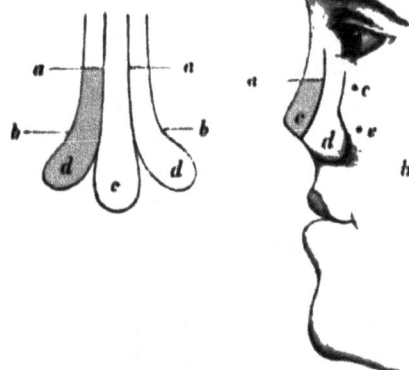

Fig. 244. — DIEFFENBACH'S OPERATION FOR DEPRESSED NOSE. (*After Dieffenbach.*)

outer limits of the nostril, serve to separate the alæ from the bones. The columna is elongated by means of short parallel transverse incisions made in the median part of the upper lip. The tissues of the cheek are sufficiently dissected up from the maxillæ through the lateral incisions to make them freely movable.

The three flaps (c, d, d) are then raised, and their lower borders pared obliquely, so that they have been compared to the stones of an arch.

The three strips are re-united with sutures, and are retained in position and made to project by drawing the detached portions of the cheek towards the median line of the nose. The cheek tissues are fixed in position by means of two long hare-lip pins, which are passed through their margins and beneath the nose. The points penetrated by the pins are indicated in Fig. 244 by the dots e e. The pins are fixed by being passed through two narrow strips of leather, and by means of these strips the new nose is compressed laterally, and its median part made to project.

Fig. 244 shows the result obtained by Dieffenbach and the appearance presented by the patient *after* the operation.

Fergusson advocated this operation, and carried it out in at least one case. He speaks of the result in this instance as being " as favourable as could reasonably have been desired."

Time has scarcely endorsed the opinion this great surgeon expressed of Dieffenbach's work. Of him he wrote:—"His skill in rhinoplastics seems to be such that he will repair or rear up this most important feature with all the genius of a Telford, and finish his handiwork with the Phidian touch of a Chantrey."

(e) *Dr. Weir*, of New York, in instances of undue shortness of the nose, advises that a cut be made across the nose in a transverse direction, that the tip be drawn down to the desired position, and that the wedge-shaped gap which results from such depression be filled in by transplanting flaps from the cheeks.

PARTIAL RHINOPLASTY.

The operations carried out for the relief of slighter deformities and partial defects of the nose are very numerous, and for the most part consist simply in the application of the common principles of plastic surgery to the part.

1. **Fistulous Openings** of small size, leading into the nasal cavities, may be closed by freshening the edges, by freeing the tissues of the margins, and approximating them by sutures.

Larger openings may be closed by one or other of the methods already described for dealing with defects of various sizes and shapes (page 4 *et seq.*).

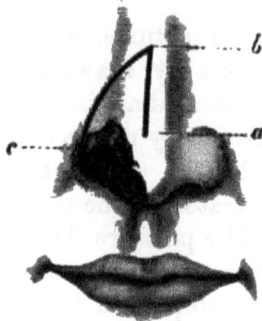

2. **Defects in the Central Part of the Nose**—the root and lower third being quite sound—may be remedied by the gliding method (page 4), or by means of definite lateral flaps derived from the tissues of the cheek.

3. **The Formation of a New Ala** may be accomplished in many ways.

Fig. 245. — DENONVILLIER'S OPERATION.

(A) *From the Nasal Tissues of the same Side — Denonvillier's Operation.*—A pedunculated triangular flap is cut from the sound tissues of the nose, just above the defective ala. The pedicle is placed internally at the tip (Fig. 245).

The incision is commenced near the tip on the sound side (*a*), and passes upwards (*a b*) nearly to the root of the nose. From the end of this a second cut (*b c*) descends obliquely to terminate at the upper and outer angle of the defect (*c*). This flap is dissected up, and its lower part should contain a strip of undestroyed cartilage. It is finally displaced downwards, and fixed in position by sutures—the margins of the defect having been already freshened to receive it.

(B) *From the Ala of the Opposite Side—Langenbeck's Operation.*—The most convenient shape to give the defect is a quadrilateral one. From the upper and inner angle of the defect an incision (*a b*, Fig. 246) is carried downwards along the dorsum of the nose, nearly to the apex on the sound side. A second incision (*c d*) is made, parallel to the first, and runs from just below the inner canthus to the junction of the ala with the cheek. The lower ends of the two incisions are united by a third cut (*b d*), which runs just along the free border of the ala.

The quadrilateral flap thus marked out is detached from the cartilage as far up as the line of its base (*a c*).

It is then drawn over to the other side, and is fixed by sutures to the freshened margins of the defective area.

It will be observed that a triangular piece of sound skin is left at the tip of the nose.

The defect left upon the sound side should be closed as far as possible, and, when granulating, should be vigorously grafted to prevent the contraction which would otherwise be inevitable.

(c) *From the Upper Lip—Weber's Operation.*—The margins of the defective ala having been freshened,

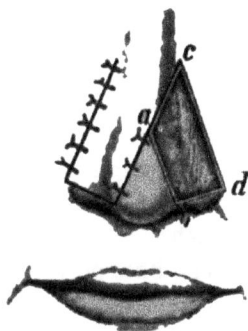

Fig. 246.—LANGENBECK'S PARTIAL RHINOPLASTY.

an oval flap is cut from the centre of the lip. The pedicle of this flap is attached alone to the columna, while its free margin reaches to the prolabium. Only a part of the thickness of the lip is concerned in the flap.

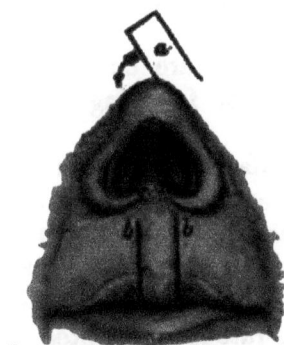

Fig. 247.—FORMATION OF A NEW COLUMNA.
b, c, From the lip; *a,* From the nose. Hueter's operation. (*Linhart.*)

It is turned upwards, and fixed into position by sutures. At the end of three or four weeks the pedicle is divided, and is applied to the inner surface of the flap, so as to give a thicker and rounder margin to the new ala.

4. The Formation of a New Columna is frequently called for.

(A) The columna may be formed from the tissues of the upper lip, in the manner already described (page 22).

(B) It may be derived from the dorsum of the nose—Hueter's operation. A quadrilateral flap (*a,* Fig. 247) is taken from the dorsum. The pedicle of the flap is placed near to the tip of

the nose, and its free border not far from one inner canthus.
The periosteum of the nasal bone is detached with the flap.

The flap is transplanted by twisting the pedicle.

OPERATIONS FOR HARE-LIP.

The Best Time for Operation.—Very different, and to some
extent quite irreconcilable, opinions have been expressed
upon this matter. The principal point of dispute has been
concerned with very early operations—operations undertaken
during the first few weeks, or even the first few days, of life.

The weight of evidence and of opinion is, I think, now
decidedly opposed to these early operations, and emphatically
opposed to operations undertaken within a few hours or days
of birth.

The best period for dealing with a hare-lip would appear
to be between the third and the sixth months.

In my own practice I prefer to operate in the later rather
than in the earlier part of this period.

It is well that the defect should be dealt with before
dentition commences. The first tooth to protrude (the lower
central incisor) makes its appearance about the seventh
month; the upper incisors are not usually "cut" until the
eighth month.

It is desirable, therefore, that the deformity should be
dealt with before the seventh month.

Against quite early operations, such as are undertaken
during the first or second month of life, the following objections may be urged :—

1. The vitality of the very young infant is low, and the
mortality of the first two months of life is remarkably high.
During the first four weeks after birth the death-rate is 571·32
per 1,000 ; during the next four weeks it is 218·37 per 1,000 ;
between two and three months of age it has fallen to 157·10 ;
and at the age of six months the death-rate is represented by
115·09 per 1,000 (Registrar-General's thirty-eighth Report).

2. In the very young infant the parts are small and
fragile, are difficult to handle, and are more readily damaged.
The tissues, moreover, afford a less firm hold for sutures.

3. The difficulty of feeding is soon got over with care and
attention, and the risk of marasmus, which is stated by some

to attend hare-lip, has not been shown to offer a valid reason for early operation. The child who has become wasted has probably been indifferently cared for, or is the subject of some intercurrent disease, and a hasty closure of a cleft in the lip can hardly be expected to remedy the one or to remove the other. The argument that the child has wasted is an argument for postponing rather than for hastening the operation. The marasmic infant is a wretched subject for plastic surgery; and if the feeding of the child has been properly and thoroughly carried out, the hare-lip can seldom be advanced as the cause of the mal-nutrition. If the palate be sound, many children with even severe hare-lip can suck admirably.

In order to ensure the success of the operation the child should be in good health, and its digestive functions in perfect order. It would be calamitous to discover, after the operation, that the infant was the subject of a cough or of severe coryza.

Another element necessary to success is a good nurse.

SINGLE HARE-LIP.—THE USUAL OPERATION.

The Form of the Hare-Lip will determine the details of the operation or the method selected. There may be merely a notch in the lip, or the cleft may extend into the nostril, or may end just short of it.

In the most favourable cases the edges of the cleft are equal, are of substantial thickness, and are not widely separated. The majority of the examples of hare-lip may, perhaps, be placed in this category.

In less favourable instances the margins of the split are unequal and widely divergent, and it may be that the tissues of the lip are scanty and adherent. Owing to the septum being turned over to one side, the ala of the nose of the opposite side may be flattened, and the nostril represented by a mere transverse slit.

The complication of cleft palate may exist.

The Instruments Required. — A fine, narrow, sharp-pointed scalpel or a small tenotome (for the less simple methods a slender double-edged knife is useful); slender-bladed dissecting forceps with toothed points; small sharp-pointed scissors curved on the flat; straight blunt-pointed scissors; artery forceps; sequestrum forceps with broad ends protected by india-rubber; needles and sutures; needle-holder; special "hare-lip forceps" to compress the lip; a gag and tongue forceps may be useful; properly-prepared plaster; small fine sponges.

The Operation.—The operation here described is that most usually carried out in Great Britain, and is the method adapted to the majority of the cases of single hare-lip.

The infant is wrapped up in a towel or sheet, so that the head alone projects. In this mummy-like guise it is easily handled, and the movements of its limbs are restrained.

The patient lies supine, with the head well raised and supported upon a sand-bag or firm cushion.

The surgeon faces the patient, or stands to the right-hand side. An assistant places himself behind the child, and steadies the head, while at the same time he compresses the facial arteries against the lower jaw. The administrator of chloroform will stand upon the left of the table.

First Step.—Grasping the upper lip, the surgeon proceeds to separate it—upon each side of the gap—from the maxilla. This can best be effected by means of small sharp-pointed scissors curved on the flat. The scissors must be kept close to the bone. It may be necessary to detach one ala of the nose from the maxilla. In any case the detachment should be sufficiently free to allow of the margins of the cleft coming together readily and without the least tension.

If the maxilla of one side project inconveniently beyond its fellow, it should be forcibly bent back with sequestrum forceps, the blades of which are protected by india-rubber. "The bone," writes Mr. Jacobson, "should be felt to crack when this is done, otherwise, if merely bent back, it springs forward again, and causes tension of the flaps."

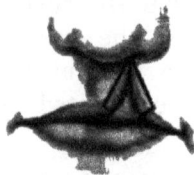

Fig. 248. — OPERATION FOR SINGLE HARE-LIP.

Second Step.—The edges of the cleft are pared. The lower angle of one flap of the lip is seized with fine-toothed dissecting forceps, is drawn upon, and the margin is then pared with the narrow scalpel. The incision for paring the edge should commence above, at the upper angle of the gap, and descending obliquely, should curve inwards, when the red margin or lower angle of the flap is nearly reached (Fig. 246).

When one side has been treated, the other is dealt with.

Or the lip on one side having been made tense, it may be transfixed in its whole thickness from before backwards, by the narrow scalpel. The point is entered just above the lower angle of the flap, and, the edge being directed upwards, the knife is made to cut towards the upper angle of the gap, to follow that angle, and finally to descend upon the other side. The knife is then withdrawn, and is not allowed to cut its way out. The piece isolated by paring will still be attached to the lip at both ends, and its detachment may be left until some of the sutures have been introduced, and until the amount of tissue required for the formation of a good free margin to the new lip has been ascertained.

In any case the paring must be freely, liberally, and evenly, carried out. The raw surface should be as wide as possible, especially below.

During this step there may be much bleeding, which must be checked either by pressure upon the facial arteries, or by the compression of each coronary artery at the angle of the mouth, between the thumb and finger of an assistant. The latter procedure is the more efficacious, but the operation area is encroached upon and disturbed, and in the place of an assistant's fingers some form of hare-lip compression forceps may be used.

Third Step.—The gap is now closed. The assistant who holds the head presses the cheeks together with his fingers, so that the two raw surfaces are approximated. The approximation must be exact. The margins are then united by means of silkworm-gut sutures carried on straight needles.

The first suture should involve the middle of the lip, the next the lower portion, and the third, the segment near the nostril. These are the three main sutures. They should include the whole thickness of the lip, excluding the mucous membrane only; and the first or median suture, if properly introduced, should command the coronary arteries when it is finally drawn tight.

It is well to pass the three needles one after the other, and to leave them in the tissues until it has been ascertained

that the best possible approximation of the raw edges has
been obtained. From the manner in which the cheeks are
held, the relations between the two sides of the cleft may
be disturbed. The three needles act as three temporary
hare-lip pins.

After the surgeon is satisfied that the best possible adjustment has been obtained (and one or more of the needles
may have to be re-introduced before it is obtained), the
sutures are drawn through, tied in the usual way (page 44,
vol. i.), and cut moderately short.

The three stitches are introduced about one-third of an
inch from each side of the cleft.

Two, three. or more sutures are now inserted at the free
margin of the new lip, especially upon its inner or alveolar
aspect. These are composed of fine catgut or fine silk, and
are passed by means of slender curved needles held in a
needle-holder.

Some of these fine stitches may be required along the
main wound, and one will usually be needed for the margin
of the nostril.

Dressing and After-treatment.—The wound having been
well dried with small pieces of fine sponge, the surface is
dusted with iodoform, and is covered with a strip of soft
gauze. The gauze may consist of several layers, and the
component strip must be cut to exactly fit the part, and
should not extend on to the cheek. It is well that the wound
be supported with strips of Seabury and Johnson's strapping.
Each strip is the width of the lip. One piece is divided for
half its length into two narrow limbs; the other piece is
narrowed for one-half its extent into a single limb. The undivided parts having been made fast to the checks, the free
strips are interlaced, and are made to draw the cheeks
together and to prevent tension upon the wound.

In the nursing of the case every care must be taken to
keep the area of the wound as dry as possible, to keep the
nostrils free from mucus so far as can be managed, and to so
feed the patient that no strain falls upon the wound.

Young infants can be kept perfectly quiet for many days
after the operation by the administration of repeated minute
doses of chloral. Children so treated remain remarkably still,

do not cry, and appear not to suffer the least harm from the use of the drug. In my own cases it is given regularly, and I have never seen anything but good result from its employment.

In patients a little older than the average of those who are subjected to this operation, steps must be taken to prevent the child from meddling with the dressing.

The wound should be inspected on the second, or at the latest the third, day. The child's head must be firmly held by the nurse, and the cheeks should be grasped and pushed forwards while the strapping is being removed and re-applied, so that the parts upon each side of the wound may be quite relaxed.

The wound must be carefully cleaned with cotton wool, and again dressed with a dry dressing.

As a rule no suture need be removed until the sixth or seventh day. They may be removed on successive days.

The strapping may be employed until healing is sound, or in a favourable case until about the tenth day.

At a later period a further plastic operation may be needed to improve the appearance of the parts, and especially to remove any notching which may occur at the free margin of the new lip.

Should the wound break down, the case should not be regarded as hopeless. The raw edges should still be kept approximated, and every assistance given to the process of granulation.

Comment.—The operation cannot be so well carried out, nor can the head be kept so steady, if the infant be held in the nurse's lap, as is not infrequently advised.

It is most essential that the lip should be well freed on both sides of the gap. If this be effectually done, there is no tension put upon the wound, and even in quite large clefts the pared margins are brought readily into contact.

The paring should be accomplished with a knife, and not with scissors.

The recommendation that as little as possible should be cut away is not one that should be followed. In paring the edges, there must be no stinting. The fault of the young operator consists usually in removing too little, rather than too much.

If the lips are pared as advised—the incisions terminating abruptly below—there is little risk of a notch forming when 'the scar contracts. The possibility of such notching has been urged as an objection to this operation.

Fenestrated artery forceps are not well adapted for seizing the margins of the flaps. The forceps used should have no "catch."

Hare-lip pins are very seldom needed. If the separation of the lip from the maxilla is as free as it ought to be, the use of the pin can but rarely be called for.

If the pin be used, some sloughing of that part of the wound which lies beneath the figure of eight ligature is not uncommon. Imperfect healing in that situation is frequent enough, and the cicatrices left by the pin are often unsightly and permanent.

If pins are called for in an exceptional case, they should be very slender, be made of fine steel, and should be removed in forty-eight hours.

The old-fashioned hare-lip pin was of large size, was made of such soft metal that it could be easily bent, and was amongst the most uncouth of surgical appliances.

Some surgeons use silver wire for the median suture (*i.e.*, the suture which commands the coronary arteries), employing gut or horsehair or silk for the other stitches.

Silkworm gut, if tied in the manner already described (page 44, vol. i.), answers admirably. There is no knot to press into the tissues, the ends of the suture lie flat, and it can be tightened or loosened while *in situ.*

Hainsby's truss is a very ingenious contrivance, but it cannot claim to be of practical value. It may well be dispensed with.

Louis's bandage is of service to support the tissues of the lip, and to keep the cheeks pressed a little forwards. Mr. Mason describes it as follows:—A double-headed roller, less than an inch in width, and a yard and a half long, is placed with its centre over the middle of the forehead, and the two ends are then carried behind the head over the ears to the occiput, where they are made to cross and are brought forward again.

Two slits are now made in one end, while the other end is divided into two tails. The two tails are passed through the two slits, and then, by making traction upon the ends of the bandage so treated, the edges of the lip are brought together. The ends are carried back again to the nape of the neck, and there fastened.

Mr. Jacobson calls attention to the fact ("Operations of Surgery," page 332) that "in some cases of hare-lip death from dyspnœa may take place very soon after the operation. Thus, where the cleft has been a large one, and the upper lip when restored is tight, when it overhangs the lower, if the nostrils are flattened and partially closed by the operation, owing to the tension of the parts, so little breathing-space may be left that temporary interference with respiration may occur, with grave and even fatal results before the breathing can be accommodated to the altered circumstances, and before the parts dilate and stretch."

OTHER OPERATIONS FOR SINGLE HARE-LIP.

Nélaton's Operation.—When there is only a slight notch in the lip, as shown in Fig. 249, this operation is very useful. Such a notch may be due to congenital defect, or may more frequently depend upon undue contraction at the site of a previous operation for hare-lip.

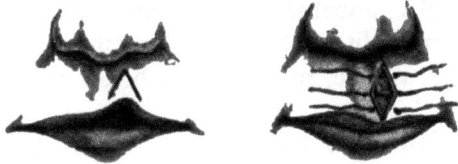

Fig. 249.—NÉLATON'S OPERATION.

The notch is circumscribed by a ∧-shaped incision, which does not, however, involve the border of the lip. With fine-pointed forceps the piece so isolated is drawn downwards, so that a diamond-shaped wound is produced. The opposite sides of the wound are united by sutures (Fig. 249).

The slight projection which is left at the edge of the lip will shrink and disappear in the course of time.

Malgaigne's or Clemot's Operation.—In single hare-lip of moderate degree, in which the margins of the cleft are equal, or nearly so, and in which there is but little divergence, this method is advised by some in the place of the usual operation.

It is claimed for it that the possibility of a notch being left at the edge of the lip is removed.

The edges of the cleft are freshened by detaching a flap on either side. Each flap is attached below, but free above, and they meet at the upper angle of the cleft.

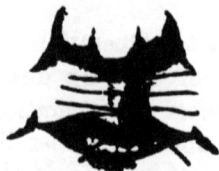

Fig. 250.—MALGAIGNE'S OPERATION.

The manner in which these flaps are cut is illustrated by the lateral flaps shown in Fig. 255.

These flaps are seized with toothed forceps, are drawn downwards, and are kept out of the cleft (Fig. 250). The upper part of the cleft is then united by sutures, while the projecting portions of the flaps are shortened to the extent required, and are then joined together by a few fine stitches (Fig. 250).

In the place of a notch a considerable prominence is left on the margin of the lip, and this may need a little paring down if it persists at the end of six months.

If the margins of the cleft are unequal, as is so commonly the case, a perfect apposition of the wound is very difficult when this method is carried out.

Mr. Jacobson also notes that "unless great care is taken, a little skin, imperceptible at first, but showing white after a time, may remain below the red line, or as a break in it."

Mirault's Operation.—When the edges of the flap are very unsymmetrical, and when they diverge considerably, the following operation gives admirable results :—

A flap is cut from the shorter or more vertical margin of the cleft. It is free above, and is attached below near to the red border of the lip (Fig. 251, *a*). It is most conveniently fashioned by transfixing the lip just above this border, and by allowing the knife to cut its way out at the upper angle of the cleft. This flap must be composed of the entire thickness of the lip, must be large and substantial, and not a mere paring from the edge of the cleft.

The longer or more oblique margin of the gap is now freshened by paring, and care must be taken that the raw surface is as wide as possible.

The flap is now drawn down and placed in position, and the wound closed by sutures (Fig. 251).

In this operation it is especially important that the separation of the lip, which has already been insisted upon (page 40), should be very freely carried out. It may be necessary to detach one or both alæ. The edges of the gap must be approximated without tension. A common fault in this procedure consists in making the flap too small and scanty.

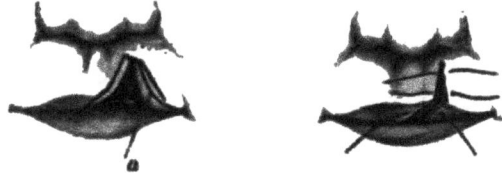

Fig. 251.—MIRAULT'S OPERATION.

Giraldès' Operation.—This is adapted for severe forms of single hare-lip, where the margins are very unequal and divergent, and especially where the cleft enters by a large gap into the nostril.

The tissues on each side of the cleft must be well and extensively freed from the maxilla. From the shorter and less oblique margin of the cleft a flap (Fig. 252, *a*) is cut, as in Mirault's operation. From the upper end of the incision terminating this flap a second cut (*b*) is carried outwards, just below the border of the nasal aperture.

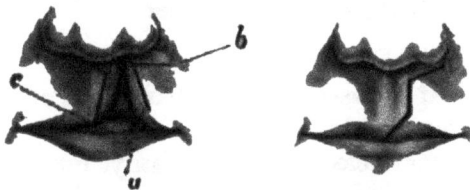

Fig. 252.—GIRALDÈS' OPERATION.

From the more oblique or longer side of the cleft another flap is fashioned with its apex or free end (*c*) downwards. The first flap (*a*) is drawn downwards, and forms the new margin of the lip. The other flap is drawn upwards, so that its apex (*c*) is fixed to the extremity of the incision (*b*), and this strip of tissue serves to form the lower boundary of the new nostril.

The somewhat complicated wound produced by the transposition of these flaps is closed by sutures, and the flaps themselves securely fixed in place.

Hagedorn's Operation.—With a sharp-pointed knife the incision 3-4-2 (Fig. 253) is made on the lateral side of the cleft,

and the incision 4-3-2 on the median margin. Finally, with a
pair of sharp scissors, the incisions 5-1-4 are made upon each
side of the defect. The margins of the gap thus isolated are
removed, *i.e.*, the whole of the margin from 5 to 2. The raw
surfaces are then adjusted as shown in the middle diagram
in Fig. 253. By this it will be seen that the points which
were before on each side of the cleft, and which are indicated by corresponding figures, are brought together—*i.e.*, the
point marked 3 on the right side is united to the point marked
3 on the left side, and so on. Or the incisions may be dis-

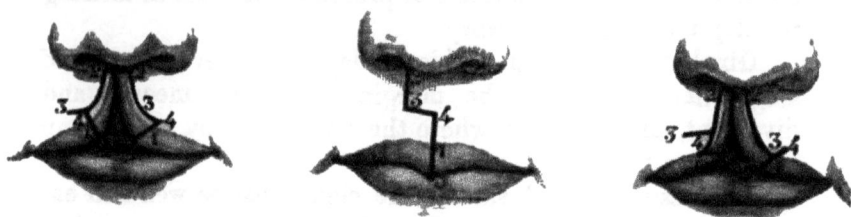

Fig. 253.—HAGEDORN'S OPERATION.

posed as shown in the right-hand side diagram in Fig. 253,
the points upon each side of the cleft, which are indicated
by corresponding figures, being brought together.

DOUBLE HARE-LIP.

The operation required in cases of double hare-lip is of the
same character as that already described.

In many instances the defect is more easily remedied
when it is double than when merely a single gap exists. In
the most favourable forms of double hare-lip the sides of the
cleft are symmetrical, and are, moreover, more nearly parallel
than is the case in single hare-lip.

A malplaced pre-maxillary bone is the most troublesome
complication met with in dealing with this deformity.

The Form of the Hare-Lip.—From the point of view of
operation, Mr. T. Smith (*Lancet*, 1867, vol. ii.) divides double
hare-lip into the three following varieties :—

1. When the pre-maxillary bone is *in situ*, and the two
clefts are simple and fairly bilateral.

2. When the pre-maxillary bone is separated from the
rest of the jaw, and projects forwards, in some cases slightly,

in others being attached to the vomer, and hanging from the tip of the nose.

3. When the pre-maxillary bone is small and ill-developed, and when the clefts are widely gaping.

The following are the operations adapted for the three varieties :—

First Variety.—In this simple form the skin over the pre-maxillary bone is freed from its deep attachments behind, and its edges are pared so that it receives a U- or V-shaped outline. The margins of the lip on each side are then pared in the manner already described (page 40).· The portions of the lip may or may not need to be freed from their attachments (Fig. 254). The raw edges are finally united with silkworm-gut sutures. Owing to the small size, and the shape of the central piece, the resulting wound is more or less Y-shaped.

In order to avoid the notching which not infrequently occurs in the median line, when cicatrisation has taken place after this operation, thick flaps with square ends may be cut from each

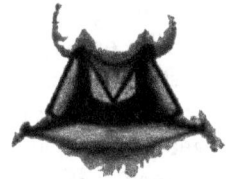

Fig. 254. — OPERATION FOR DOUBLE HARE-LIP.

margin of the main cleft, as shown in Fig. 255. These flaps have their attached ends downwards. They are united to the raw margins of the central segment above, and to one another along, what is now the new margin of the lip. The segments of the lip will need to be freed from their deep connections on each side of the cleft.

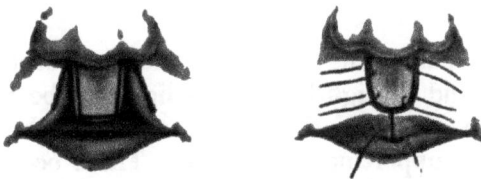

Fig. 255.—OPERATION FOR DOUBLE HARE-LIP.

Hagedorn's Modification of the usual operation is illustrated in Fig. 256, and can be best understood by a study of the diagram. The soft parts covering the pre-maxillary bone are pared liberally. The raw margin produced is bounded by the incision 4-*a*-1-*o*-4. The margins of the cleft are pared in the manner shown.

The part actually removed in the freshening process is left un-shaded in the diagram, and is bounded by the incision 4-2-3. The lateral cuts $a'1$ and $o'1'$ are nearly parallel with the free margin of the lip.

The raw edges are united in such a way that points marked in the figure by corresponding numbers are brought together by sutures (Fig. 256).

Second Variety.—In this variety the projecting pre-max-illary bone offers a serious obstacle to the proper closure of the cleft by operation.

Many very different plans have been proposed for dealing with this unfortunately-placed piece of bone.

It is needless to consider these various methods in detail : many are obsolete, many differ from one another in but the most insignificant feature.

The experience of the past and the expressed opinion of most living authors are practically unanimous upon one point, viz., that the pre-maxillary bone should be preserved when-ever possible, and that its excision is a procedure to be con-demned. If this little piece of bone be removed, a permanent

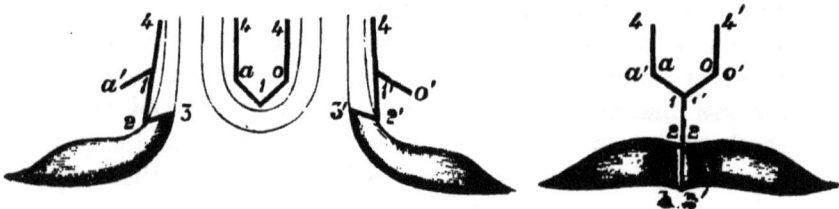

Fig. 256.—HAGEDORN'S OPERATION FOR DOUBLE HARE-LIP.

gap is left in the hard palate, the upper lip tends to become flattened, malplaced, and unsightly, and is liable to be re-tracted on inspiration. The patient loses a point which might prove useful in supporting false teeth. There occurs in time a want of correspondence between the upper and lower dental arches, and the patient is said to be "under-hung."

The following courses might be recommended in dealing with this bone :—

(*a*) In the simplest cases the pre-maxillary bone may be

forced back into line with the rest of the jaw. This may be done either with the thumbs or by using necrosis forceps with smooth blades protected by india-rubber.

This fracture can be effected when the attachment of the os incisivum is slender, and when there is room between the maxillæ to receive the displaced fragment.

If it tends to protrude after such fracture, the bone may be held in place by catgut sutures attached to the upper jaw.

If the maxillæ offer no space to receive the fractured fragment, a bed for the bone may be made by removing small portions of the maxillæ with the chisel, and then fixing the fragment in position with sutures.

(*b*) Very usually the bending back of the bone is resisted by the cartilaginous vomer of children, and the elasticity of that structure causes the fragment to be again protruded when the pressure is removed.

In such a case a portion of the vomer may be excised subperiosteally, as advised by Bardeleben, Guérin, and others. An incision is made along the free border of the septum, leaving its arteries intact; the periosteum and mucous membrane are then elevated on either side, and a triangular segment is excised from the vomer. The os incisivum may now be pushed into place, and may be retained, if needed, by one or more sutures.

The bleeding in this operation is apt to be free, unless the subperiosteal method be closely adhered to.

(*c*) Should a case occur in which by no method yet named the little bone can be reduced, then the mucous membrane covering it may be incised, and the main part of the bone, together with the temporary incisors, scooped out with a gouge. After such a measure, which was advised by Sir William Fergusson, little but periosteum and a thin plate of bone would remain.

After the reduction of the bone, the gap is closed by one of the methods already advised.

Third Variety.—In the last of the three varieties named, the two margins of the lip have merely to be brought together and united to one another, and to any portion of the central segment which may be available. To effect this, an extensive separation of the lip, and possibly of the cheek, on either side,

e 2

will have to be carried out, for until the soft parts have been
well freed from the underlying bones, no approximation is
possible.

It is in these cases that the use of the fine steel hare-lip
pins may be of service, and in any instance the lip must be well
supported, and the cheeks kept pressed forward. Strapping
applied as described (page 42), and Louis's bandage (page 44)
will serve to effect these ends.

An excellent series of woodcuts, illustrating almost every
known form of operation upon hare-lip, will be found in
Gerhardt's *Chirurg. Erkank. des Kindesalters*, vol. ii., page 132,
Tübingen, 1889.

CHAPTER IV.

Plastic Operations to Remedy Certain Defects of the Lips.

The defects here dealt with are, for the most part, such as result from the removal of epitheliomatous growths by operation, and losses of tissue due to destructive ulceration, to lupus, to burns and to injuries, and notably to gunshot wounds.

The defects will be mostly of triangular or quadrilateral outline.

The operations proposed, or actually carried out, in these cases are very numerous, and, in many instances, very complex. No one operation, nor even one method of operating, can meet the requirements of every case. Every individual example must be taken upon its merits, and much must be left to the judgment and ingenuity of the operator.

A very large number of methods for restoring the lips are depicted in Serre's Atlas (*Traité sur l'art de restaurer les Difformités de la Face*, Montpellier, 1842), and also in Szymanowski's *Handbuch der operativen Chirurgie*, 1870. Dr. Buck's work upon the subject is described in his "Contributions to Reparative Surgery," New York, 1876. In the following account of the most usual operations, I have drawn largely upon the excellent description of cheiloplastic methods given in Karl Löbker's *Chirurgische Operationslehre* (Wien, 1885).

General Observations.—In all these operations great care must be bestowed upon the sutures, and especially upon those which fix the new margin of the lip. The sutures should include all the tissues except the mucous membrane.

A few fine silk sutures involving the mucous membrane

only may be inserted along the free margin of the lip. The best material for the main stitches is silkworm-gut. Hare-lip pins will be required in many instances. They must be fine, and made of good steel, so that they cannot be bent out of a straight line. The thread fixing the pin should be of silk applied in a figure of 8, and as short a length as possible should be applied. The great mass of silk ligature sometimes twisted about hare-lip pins is capable of producing some sloughing from pressure, and of interfering with the healing of the wound at the most important part.

Hare-lip pins should be avoided whenever possible, and if the tissues upon each side of the gap to be closed are well freed their employment may be less often imperative.

A large proportion of these operations are performed upon old persons, in whom the tissues are lax and extensile.

The bleeding during the operation is arrested by compressing the coronary arteries, which is done either by the finger and thumb of an assistant or by special forceps or clamps.

One of the sutures or one hare-lip pin must be so introduced as to command the coronary arteries when the wound is adjusted.

Supporting strapping will very seldom be required.

Any carious teeth in the jaw, and especially diseased incisors, should be removed before the operation, and the mouth placed in as healthy a condition as possible.

In adult males the parts must be carefully shaved.

A dry dressing of the simplest character should be employed. Iodoform answers well, and the bandage of Louis already described (page 44) is of service.

Hare-lip pins should be removed on the third day, if not before.

It is important that the mouth be kept well and frequently washed out. Discharge—which the patient has no power to expel—is apt to accumulate between the cheeks and the lower jaw, and behind the lower lip. It is retained, and decomposes. The mouth should be frequently flushed out with an irrigator, and still more frequently rinsed out by the patient. One of the best solutions, both for the irrigator and as a mouth-wash, is a one in sixty or a one in eighty solution of carbolic acid.

THE LOWER LIP.

1. The Closure of Wedge-shaped Defects by the Method of Gliding or Lateral Displacement.

So long as the base of the triangular defect is less than half the normal width of the lip the surgeon may bring the edges of the freshened wound together and unite them by sutures. Even if the defect involve more than half the width of the lip, direct union by sutures may often be carried out, especially in old subjects with relaxed tissues and possibly edentulous jaws. If the defect be median, no loss of symmetry will be observed; but if—as is often the case—one lateral portion of the lip be involved more than the other, then some traction upon one corner of the mouth will follow, and the aperture will tend to become rounded on the affected side. The form of the mouth may be left considerably distorted, and the aperture be too small.

It is assumed that in the adult the normal oral aperture should admit three fingers placed side by side.

In such cases the *Method of Hueter* may be carried out. After the margins of the defect have been brought together, or the large growth excised, an incision is made in the cheek, starting from the oral angle and directed horizontally outwards. This cut involves the whole thickness of the cheek upon the distorted side. The mucous membrane upon each side of this new wound is reflected a little, and is then united to the skin by sutures, so that the raw surfaces are covered. In order that the new angle of the mouth should also be lined by mucous membrane an oblique incision running upwards and outwards is made in that membrane, and the little triangular flap thus marked out is drawn into the angular recess and secured there.

The entire incision in the mucous membrane will therefore have the outline of the letter ＜ placed horizontally.

This procedure is very similar to that known by French surgeons as *Serre's Method*.

In dealing with defects of considerable size and of triangular outline, one or other of the methods of gliding already described (page 4) may be employed. In the lower lip, the most convenient operation among these is that known as *Jaesche's*. (See page 5.)

In the case of a large median defect the incisions made
would be symmetrical, *i.e.,* a curved incision, starting from
the angle of the mouth and ending at the lower border of the
jaw, would be made upon either side. The flaps thus marked
out would be joined in the median line after they had been
well freed from the parts beneath.

2. **The Closure of Quadrilateral Defects, and the Restoration of the Lower Lip by means of Flaps.**

(A) *Langenbeck's Operation.*—The lower horizontal margin
of the defect is prolonged on either side by incisions, which pass
along the remainder of the lower lip, round the angles of the

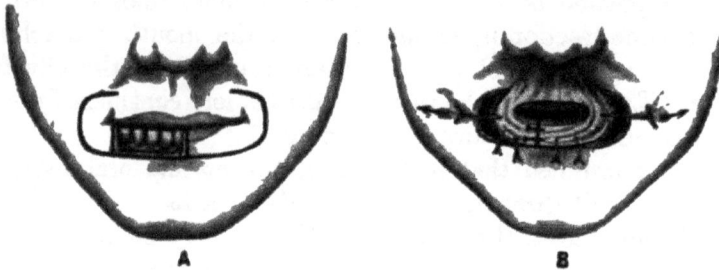

Fig. 257.—RESTORATION OF THE LOWER LIP : LANGENBECK'S OPERATION.
(After Löbker.)

mouth, and into the upper lip, in the manner shown in Fig.
257, A. The broader the defect to be closed in, the nearer
must the incisions approach the median segment of the upper
lip.

This segment, however, must always be left intact, so that
the communications between the coronary vessels and the
arteries of the septum may not be disturbed.

The portions of the lips thus marked out are mobilised,
and are drawn together towards the symphysis of the lower
jaw, and are there united by sutures. Sutures must always
be placed at the new angles of the mouth, in order to preserve
the normal outlines. The rest of the wound is finally closed
(Fig. 257, B).

This method is not adapted for cases in which the loss of
substance extends downwards beyond the movable part of
the lower lip. In such instances it would be impossible to
detach the upper lip sufficiently, and even if that could be
carried out the oral aperture would be too small.

(B) *Esthlander's Operation.*—This method may be employed when the loss of substance in the lip is partial, and on one

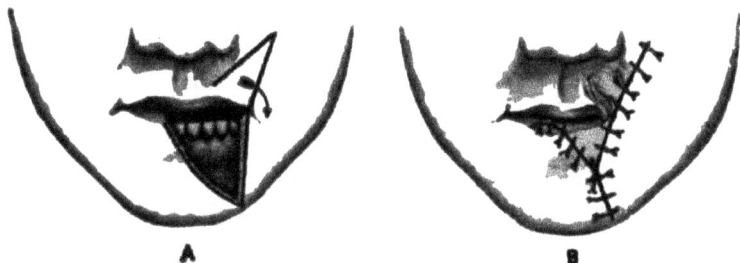

Fig. 258.—RESTORATION OF THE LOWER LIP: ESTHLANDER'S OPERATION.
(*After Löbker.*)

side, and when the defect extends downwards to the skin over the chin.

A triangular flap is so fashioned from the upper lip, that its pedicle or base contains the coronary artery, while its apex is situated on the cheek (Fig. 258, A).

This flap is then turned downwards, so that its apex comes to occupy the lower angle of the defect.

It is here fixed by sutures. The gap left in the upper lip is closed by suitable stitches (Fig. 258, B).

Both in this and in the preceding measure a lining of mucous membrane is obtained for the new lip edge.

(c) *Bruns' Operation.*—Bruns' method may be carried out when the whole breadth of the lower lip has to be restored, as shown in Fig. 259.

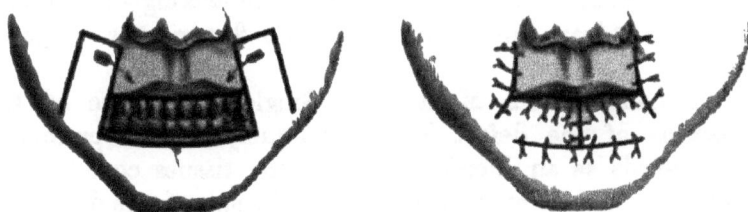

Fig. 259.—RESTORATION OF THE LOWER LIP: BRUNS' OPERATION. (*After Löbker.*)

Here two quadrilateral flaps are fashioned out of the whole thickness of the cheek and upper lip, and are placed one on each side of the mouth.

They will receive a liberal blood supply from the facial arteries. After having been mobilised, they are so turned downwards that their upper borders can be sutured together in the median line.

It may be possible to adjust the mucous membrane lining these flaps in such a way as to provide a mucous covering for the margin of the new lip (Fig. 259).

The wounds on the cheeks are finally closed by sutures.

(D) *Operations by Flaps derived from the Chin.*—When the tissues of the cheek or of the upper lip are unsuited or unavailable for flap formation, use may be made of the integuments of the chin.

The skin of this part is well adapted to form a sound flap, but in these operations a lining of mucous membrane is want-

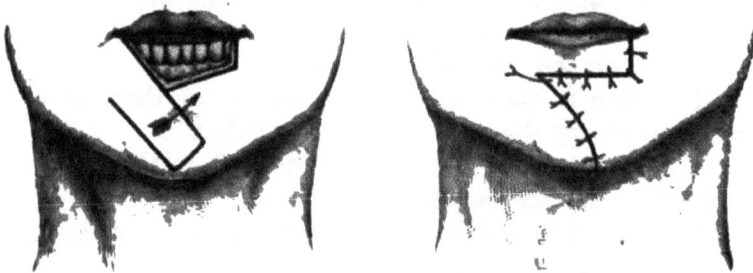

Fig. 260.—RESTORATION OF THE LOWER LIP: LANGENBECK'S OPERATION.
(*After Löbker.*)

ing in the flap, and consequently must be lacking—in the first instance at least—in the new lip. The flap may be single or double.

1. **Langenbeck's Method by Single Flap.**—One of the margins of the defect is cut obliquely, and is prolonged downwards as an incision through the tissues covering the chin. Its length must depend upon the size of the deficiency in the lip.

Between this incision and the lower border of the defect, a triangular piece of skin remains, which serves subsequently to support the flap. By means of two other incisions, which meet at right angles, a flap is formed with its base or pedicle upwards and outwards (Fig. 260). This flap is detached, is displaced upwards, and is secured in place by sutures. The wound in the chin is closed in like manner.

2. The Method of Syme and Buchanan by Double Flaps. —Each flap is made to correspond to one-half of the new lip, and is formed by prolonging the edges of the defect downwards by two incisions which meet and cross obliquely (*a b c′, a′ b c*, Fig. 261). Their length will depend upon the size of the gap to be closed after due allowance has been made for shrinking. From their lower ends two other incisions are made at right angles (*b c, b c′*, Fig. 261), and the flaps are completed by two final incisions, *c d, c′ d′*. These flaps are liberated, and are turned upwards, so that they may be united in the median line along the lines *b c, b c′*. The broad support for the flap which is provided by Langenbeck's method is wanting in this

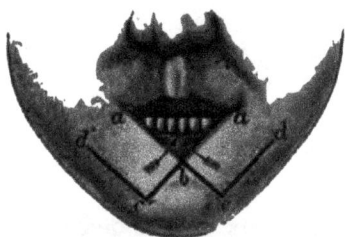

Fig. 261.—RESTORATION OF THE LOWER LIP: SYME AND BUCHANAN'S OPERA-TION. (*After Löbker.*)

operation. Two small triangular raw surfaces may be left below, and will be allowed to close by granulation. The central and prominent part of the chin is left undisturbed.

Only in extreme cases is it advisable to make use of the skin below the chin, or that of the neck, in forming a new lip. A flap with a narrow pedicle has been obtained from the front of the neck, and has been transplanted upwards by twisting the pedicle (Delpech).

The tissues over the chin have also been detached from their deep connections. Two broad lateral pedicles having been thus provided, the whole of the separated tissues have been displaced upwards *en masse* (Zeiss).

THE UPPER LIP.

Plastic operations are less frequently called for in the upper lip than in the lower.

Defects of small size may be closed by certain of the general methods already described (page 4), and in a few instances by operations akin to those above detailed, as performed upon the lower lip (page 55). The following special operations represent the most typical of the very numerous plastic measures which have been advised or carried out in this part.

1. For Partial Defects.

(A) *The Central Part of the Lip is Deficient.—Dieffenbach's Operation.*—The central part of the upper lip may be deficient, and an obtuse-angled triangular defect exist, with its apex below the nose, and with its edges covered with mucous membrane.

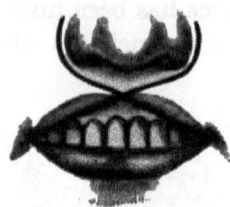

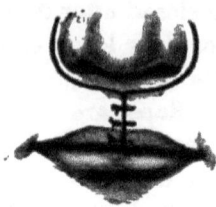

Fig. 262.—RESTORATION OF THE UPPER LIP: DIEFFENBACH'S OPERATION.

Two curved incisions start from the apex of the defect, and are carried round the alæ of the nose in the manner shown in Fig. 262. These incisions, together with the margins of the defect, mark out two flaps. These are detached from the subjacent parts, and are brought together in the median line (Fig. 262). The mucous membrane, which marked the borders of the defect, is preserved, and serves to form the free margin of the new lip.

(B) *One Side of the Lip is Deficient.—Buck's Operation.*—In the case cited one-half of the upper lip and a portion of the cheek had been lost.

The lower lip is divided where it joins the cheek by a vertical cut (*a b*, Fig. 263) at right angles to the margin of the lip, and one inch in length.

A second cut (*b c*), about one inch and a half long, starts

Fig. 263.—BUCK'S OPERATION FOR RESTORATION OF THE UPPER LIP. (*Buck.*)

from the lower end of the first incision, and runs forwards parallel to the margin of the lip. An oblique incision (half an

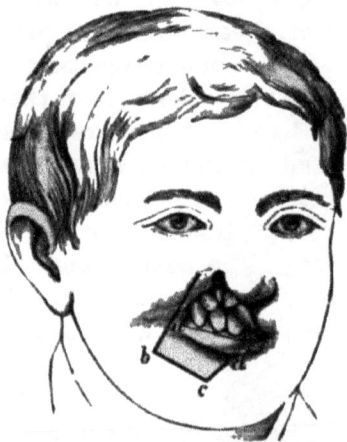

inch in length, c d) runs upwards from the second incision nearly to the lip. The attachment of the flap is at this point, and therefore the cut c d must not approach too close to the lip.

The edges of the defect are now pared, and the sound part of the upper lip freely detached from the bone beneath. The lower-lip flap is then twisted upwards, and its upper extremity is connected by sutures with the freshened edge of the upper lip.

The gap left by the removal of the flap is closed by sutures.

The result of the operation in Buck's reported case is shown in Fig. 264.

(c) *The Angle of the Mouth is Deformed or Contracted.*—*Buck's Operation.*—In the preceding case the mouth was left contracted, and the commissure of circular outline. Such a result may follow upon destructive disease or burn.

Buck's method in such cases is as follows :—

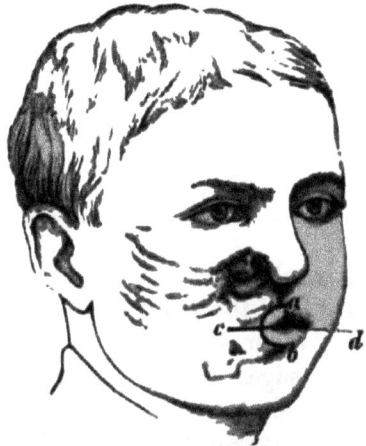

Fig. 264.—BUCK'S OPERATION FOR RESTORATION OF THE ANGLE OF THE MOUTH. (*Buck.*)

An incision (a b, Fig. 264) is made along the red border of the lip, and extends to an equal distance into both the upper and the lower lips, skirting the deformed angle.

This cut involves the skin only, not the mucous membrane. A sharp-pointed double-edged knife is inserted at the middle of the curved incision, and is directed flatwise towards the cheek between the skin and the mucous membrane, so as to separate them from each other, as far as the new angle of the mouth requires to be extended.

The skin alone is next divided outwards on a line with the commissure of the mouth (d c).

The underlying mucous membrane is now divided in the same line, but not so far outwards. The angles at the outer ends of the two incisions are accurately united by fine sutures. The freshly-cut edges of skin and mucous membrane, above and below, that are to form the new lip-borders, are shaped by paring (first the skin and then the mucous membrane) in such a manner that the latter shall overlap the former, after they have been united by fine sutures.

Serre's Operation.—The angle of the mouth is distorted by cicatricial contraction, or is occupied by a growth.

Incisions are so made (Fig. 265) as to mark out two

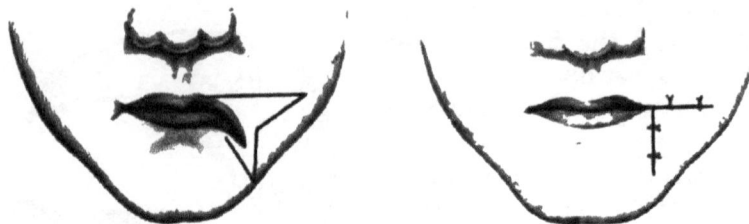

Fig. 265.—SERRE'S OPERATION FOR RESTORATION OF THE ANGLE OF THE MOUTH.

triangles, which meet by their bases at the site of the new angle of the mouth.

When the tissues thus circumscribed have been excised the edges of the wounds are united as shown in Fig. 265. The adjacent integuments are drawn together, a vertical and a transverse incision resulting.

2. The Whole of the Upper Lip requires to be Restored.

(1) *Operation by Lateral Flaps (Szymanowski's Method).* --Lateral flaps of the full breadth of the lip are cut from the cheek on each side. Their outer extremities are curved

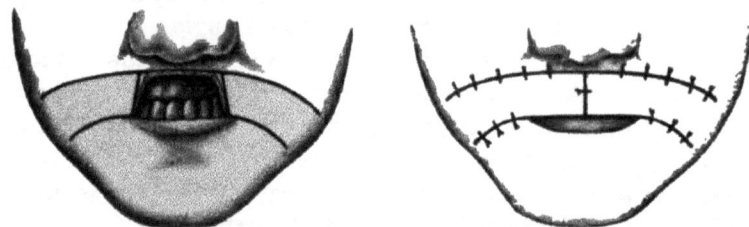

Fig. 266.—RESTORATION OF THE UPPER LIP: SZYMANOWSKI'S OPERATION.

downwards, so as to relieve them from tension. After they have been detached their inner extremities are brought together, and united in the median line (Fig. 266).

(2) *Operation by Vertical Flaps (Sédillot's Method)*—

Flaps of quadrilateral outline are raised by the use of the following incisions:—An internal one (a b, Fig. 267) starts from a point midway between the angle of the mouth and the lower eyelid, and ends a little above the prominence of the chin. An inferior horizontal incision (b c) passes outwards from the lower end of the internal incision for a distance of about one inch and a half. An external incision (c d) runs upwards from the outer end of the last wound to a point on a level with the ala of the nose. The two flaps comprise the whole thickness of the cheeks, and after detachment are dis-

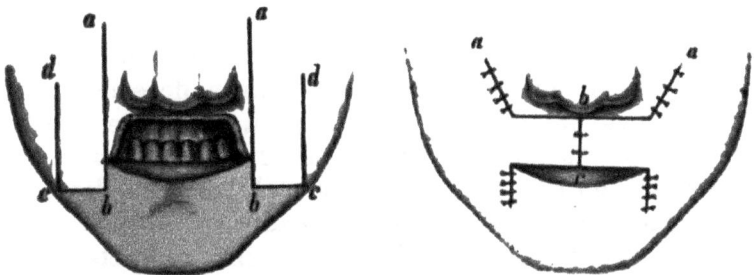

Fig. 267.—RESTORATION OF THE UPPER LIP: SÉDILLOT'S OPERATION.

placed inwards, so that their lower extremities (b c) meet in the median line (Fig. 267).

Dieffenbach's Method.—In this operation the flaps have their free ends directed upwards instead of downwards. A vertical incision (a b, Fig. 268) is made upwards from the angle of the mouth to a point above the level of the nostril; then a horizontal cut (b c) extends outwards more than equal in width to the defect to be remedied. The quadrilateral flap is completed by a vertical incision (c d) parallel to the first and ending beyond the angle of the mouth.

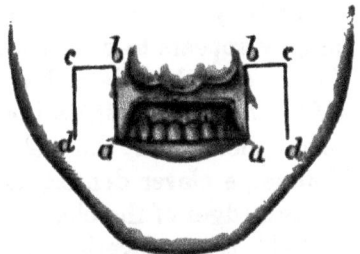

Fig. 268.—RESTORATION OF THE UPPER LIP: DIEFFENBACH'S OPERATION.

The flaps are detached, and are united by their upper extremities (b c) in the median line, after the manner of the previous operation.

CHAPTER V.

OPERATIONS FOR CLEFT PALATE.

THESE operations are among the most brilliant of those
which belong to plastic surgery. They are concerned with
the closure of clefts of all kinds in the palate, but are for the
most part limited to the congenital cleft. Perforations in the
palate, when due to disease, are usually dependent upon
syphilis, and are not suited for operation unless the health of
the patient be sound at the time. In selected cases large
defects in the soft palate, due to syphilis, may be closed, and
the same may be said of small perforations of the hard palate.
Large clefts in the hard palate in syphilitic subjects are not
well adapted for operation, and are usually best treated by the
introduction of an obturator. In any case, it is well that an
anti-syphilitic treatment be carried out for some little time
before the operation.

The term *staphyloraphy* is applied to the operations upon
the soft palate; the term *uranoplasty* to those upon the hard
palate.

History of the Operation. — The operation of staphyloraphy appears to have been first performed by Le Monnier.
The case is thus described by Robert, in his *Mémoires sur
différents objets de Médecine* (Paris, 1764):—"A child had the
palate cleft from the velum to the incisor teeth. M. Le
Monnier, a clever dentist, attempted, with success, to re-unite
the two edges of the cleft, first making several points of suture
to hold them together, and then refreshing them with a
cutting instrument. Inflammation ensued, terminated in
suppuration, and was followed by union of the two lips of the
artificial wound. The child was perfectly cured."

The modern operation, as now practised, was gradually
evolved by Graefe, Roux, Dieffenbach, and others during the
early years of the nineteenth century.

With regard to uranoplasty, the operative treatment of clefts in the hard palate is of much later date.

Dr. John Mettauer (*American Journal of Medical Sciences*, 1837) attempted to close clefts in the hard palate by what was termed the granulation process. Several incisions were made, and the separation of flaps was foreshadowed. Dr. Mason Warren (*American Journal of Medical Sciences*, 1848), however, was the originator of the method of closing these clefts by flaps composed of the soft parts. He commenced the detachment at the edge of the cleft, and proceeded outwards, using rectangular knives. Langenbeck elaborated the method. He commenced the detachment from the side of the alveolus, insisted upon the importance of separating the periosteum with the mucous membrane, and used raspatories (*Weitere Erfahrungen im Gebiete der Uranoplastik mittelst Ablösung des mücosperiostalen gaumenüberzuges*, Berlin, 1863).

Mr. Avery, of Charing Cross Hospital, is said to have been the first surgeon in England to close a cleft in the hard palate by operation (Holmes's "System of Surgery," 3rd edition, vol. ii., page 508).

Mr. Thomas Smith showed the possibility of operating upon children under chloroform. To this surgeon is due the credit of having brought this once complicated and unsatisfactory operation to its present position of perfection and comparative simplicity.

Extent of the Cleft.—The extent of the defect may vary from a bifid uvula to a cleft involving the whole of the soft and the hard palate, and which, passing through the alveolus on one or either side of the os incisivum, ends in a hare-lip. The cleft may be limited to the soft palate, and if the velum be entirely divided there is usually some want of union at the same time between the palate bones. Clefts limited to the hard palate are almost unknown, and when existing are represented usually by certain congenital holes.

The defect in the hard palate may be limited to the palate bones, or may extend as far forwards as the apex of the intermaxillary bone, or may be completed by the division of the alveolus.

The defect is usually somewhat to the left of the median

septum nasi—when the hard palate is involved—
adherent to the margin of the palate process of
xilla. In severe cases the bony septum may be
low from connection with any part of the palate.
ances affecting the Operation.—The severity of
ase (from the point of view of operation), and
y that may attend an attempt at closure, will
so much upon the length of the cleft as upon its
.tion to the amount of tissue available for closing
oft palate the velum on either side of the cleft
he one hand, of considerable width and substance,
, on the other, shrunken, small, and attenuated.

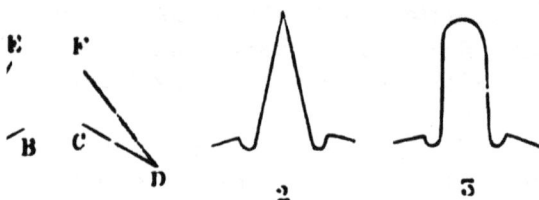

Fig. 269.

ird palate a great deal depends upon the height
he vault.

of highly arched palates which on transverse
d resemble a Gothic arch, the dissecting up of the
)aratively easy, and their approximation a matter
culty. If, on the other hand, the palate be but
ed, so that it would resemble on section a Norman
iere is difficulty in obtaining substantial flaps, and
fficulty in bringing them together. Mr. Howard
k'et, July 7th, 1888) well illustrates this by a
). "Supposing that in each of two cases the cleft
inch wide, and that in one the arch takes the
B C D, and in the other the direction A E F D
. When the soft parts are brought together the
id C D will be too short to bridge over the gap;
he much longer flaps A E and F D are brought
will meet easily, and even overlap." The manner
ə cleft of the hard palate terminates anteriorly is
'great moment. If it ends in a point like a thin

wedge (Fig. 269, 2), the shape is favourable. But if the anterior end is rounded "like the bow of a hair-pin" (Fig. 269, 3), as Mr. Howard Marsh expresses it, a great difficulty is introduced in the operation. The union of the septum nasi with one maxilla is a favourable condition, since there will be furnished for one side of the cleft at least an abundant flap.

Not a little of the difficulty of the operation will depend upon the size of the mouth.

The factors which influence the operation are the health of the patient, his intelligence, his amenability to treatment, and his age.

On this last point the observations of Mr. Thomas Smith, who must be regarded as the chief authority on palate operations, may be quoted.

Mr. Smith condemns very early operations. "Doubtless," he writes, "the deformity can be cured in very early infancy, but regard being had to the difficulty and even danger of the proceeding, and the many possible causes of failure at this period of life, it is prudent to postpone operative treatment. In the first three or four years of life clefts of the bony palate generally diminish greatly in width, especially at their anterior extremity, where in the process of growth fissures in the alveolar arch may be observed to close altogether by coalescence of their opposite edges. Thus with the lapse of time the operation becomes less difficult of performance, and no longer dangerous. . . . In deciding the question as to the best time for operating, the difficulty of the operation, and the constitutional condition of the patient, must be taken into consideration.

"In healthy children, clefts involving the velum only, without deficiency of the soft parts, may generally be cured in the third year of life. Fissures which affect the soft palate and more or less of the hard, may, as a rule, be closed before the end of the sixth year, if the cleft be not very wide, and there is a sufficiency of material for flaps.

"In cases of unusual local difficulty, or where the general health is feeble, or there is considerable infirmity of temper, the operation may need to be still longer postponed; but, if the case be curable at all, it is rare that this cannot be accomplished before the patient is twelve years of age.

ƒ 2

"When, from one cause or another, the operation has been long delayed, though a successful union may be more easily obtained, the results as regards articulation will be less satisfactory."

As another writer expresses it, the simpler the cleft, and the healthier the child, the earlier the operation.

Order of Operation.—In cases of complete cleft it was at one time advised that the defect in the velum should be first closed, and that the hard palate should be dealt with at a later period. Mr. Smith, however, advocates that the union of both parts of the palate should be attempted at one operation.

This practice I have always followed, and the results have shown that the recommendation is sound.

Mr. Smith makes one proviso. "When the bringing together of the whole cleft in one operation would necessitate so free a division of the soft parts as to endanger the vitality of the flaps, it is advisable to close first that part of the cleft that can be most easily approximated, whether it be the hard or the soft palate. This, if successful, will secure for the remaining portion a large supply of blood in the subsequent operation."

Instruments and **Suture Material.**—Probably for no operation have more numerous, more elaborate, or more remarkable instruments been devised, than for the treatment of cleft palate. A great variety and complexity of instruments means not only a difficult operation, but also that succeeding surgeons have made attempts to assist clumsy or unskilled fingers by mechanical means. The various plugs, gags, forceps, knives, and needles, invented by one man or another are legion, and to them must be added a medley of lip-holders, palate-holders, suture-twisters, and the like. The majority of these instruments are now fortunately obsolete. The surgeon should be able to work with simple instruments, and if he be unable to suture a cleft palate without an armoury of complex tools he had probably better leave the operation undone.

The following are the *instruments* required. Two sharp-pointed tenotomy knives in long and slender handles for paring the edges of the cleft. A blunt-pointed knife of the same kind for making lateral incisions to relieve tension. Fergusson's rectangular knife for tracing flaps when one has to be brought down from the septum nasi (Fig. 270). Two

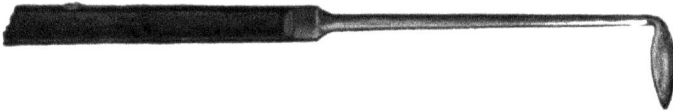

Fig. 270.—FERGUSSON'S CLEFT PALATE KNIFE.

pairs of long slender-bladed forceps, one serrated, and one with tenaculum points. A fine hook (Fig. 271). A pair of

Fig. 271.—CLEFT PALATE HOOK.

small sharp-pointed scissors curved to a quarter circle, for dividing the connection of the soft palate with the nasal mucous membrane at the posterior margin of the hard palate.

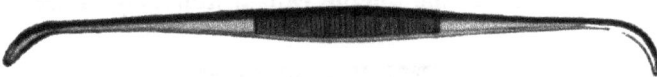

Fig. 272.—SMITH'S RASPATORY.

Small blunt-pointed scissors, curved on the flat, for the sutures, etc. Palate raspatories curved as an aneurysm needle, and another raspatory very slightly curved. Smith's raspatories (Fig. 272), or Ollier's instrument (Fig. 273), are admirably

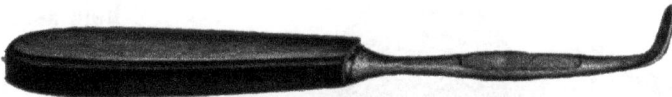

Fig. 273.—OLLIER'S CURVED RUGINE FOR THE PALATE.

suited for the purpose. Two needles on long handles, and with eyes at the point (Fig. 274. Smith's pattern), for the fine sutures. Smith's instrument for catching the sutures at the eye of the needle (Fig. 275). A tubular needle with a reel at the base for the wire sutures. A wire twister (Fig. 276). Ordinary torsion forceps make fair wire twisters. Many surgeons find needles twisted like a ram's horn, set in a handle, and with an eye near the point, most convenient. Some

Fig. 274.—SMITH'S CLEFT PALATE NEEDLE.

simple curved needles, and a plain needle-holder, may be useful.

A gag is needed, and Smith's well-known instrument answers in most cases admirably. It is most important that it

Fig. 275.—SMITH'S CLEFT PALATE SUTURE CATCHER.

should fit the patient, and that it should be carefully adjusted. Mr. Smith points out that cases are met with where the continued depression of the tongue causes difficulty in breathing.

Fig. 276.—WIRE TWISTER.

In such instances Mason's gag may be used, and the tongue be held down by a rectangular spatula.

Whitehead's speculum is shown in Fig. 277. It it be necessary to hold aside the cheek, the square rectangular retractors used in nephrectomy answer admirably.

A number of small Turkey sponges

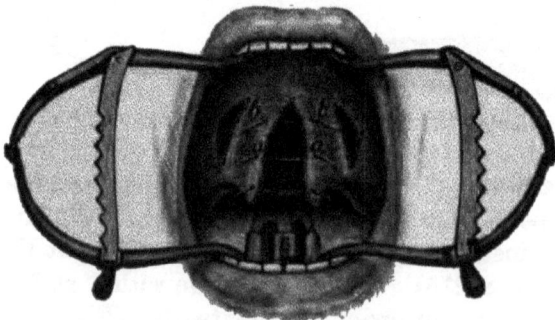

Fig. 277.—STAPHYLORRHAPHY. (*Löbker.*)

in sponge-holders are required, and the necessary material for the various sutures.

With regard to the suture material much must depend upon the custom of the individual surgeon. Horsehair answers admirably for the uvula, and for the lower and flaccid part of the velum. It is distinctly not suited for any part where there is tension. The sutures should be of full length, should be carefully selected, and should be softened before the operation by immersion in warm carbolised water. Horsehair sutures should be tied in three knots.

For the principal sutures, for those that have to bear strain, well-annealed silver wire or silkworm gut answers admirably. The latter causes apparently less irritation ; but as sutures of this material must necessarily be in short lengths, they are not so easily introduced, and are not so readily secured. The silkworm gut must be prepared by immersion in a hot solution of carbolic acid. The wire is secured by twisting; the gut by making a knot.

Position of the Patient.—The upper part of the body must be well raised, and the head be placed sufficiently high to prevent the surgeon from stooping. The head should rest upon a hard cushion, or be received in a depression in a sand bag. It must be thrown well back. The table should be narrow. The surgeon stands on the right facing the patient. The anæsthetist takes his place on the left. One assistant, standing at the end of the table, fixes the patient's head and attends to the gag. A second assistant, at the surgeon's side, assists in the operation.

Professor E. Rose advises that the head be so far thrown back that the vertex points towards the ground. By such means the palate is rendered horizontal and is under the surgeon's hands. Blood also cannot run down into the trachea. This posture is not so convenient as it may appear, is apt to cause great engorgement of the head, and will be found in practice to have little to recommend it.

Chloroform should be the anæsthetic selected.

THE OPERATION ON THE SOFT PALATE.

The gag having been introduced, the first step is to pare the edges of the cleft. The tip of one half of the uvula is seized with the tenaculum forceps, and is drawn upon so as to make the palate tense. With a sharp-pointed knife the edge is now pared from below upwards, *i.e.*, from the free margin of the velum towards the hard palate. The knife may follow the anterior angle of the cleft (assuming the hard palate to be sound), and may return in the opposite direction along the other margin of the cleft, that side of the velum being made tense in turn.

The whole of each side of the cleft must be well and liberally freshened. The anterior angle of the cleft and the tip of the uvula are especially apt to escape the knife. The raw surface should be wide, and of even width throughout.

Scissors should never be used to freshen the edges.

There will probably be no need for the flaps to be again touched with the forceps when this stage has been completed.

The next step is the passing of the sutures. They should be introduced from below upwards. The first suture is passed through the halves of the uvula, and after it has been tied, it is left uncut so that it may be used to make the edges tense, and thus avoid any handling of the palate with forceps. When the next suture has been introduced the one below (in this case the first suture) may be cut short.

Throughout this stage of the operation the suture last passed is always left uncut, so that it may be used to draw upon the margins of the cleft and steady them while the next stitch is being introduced.

The sutures must be placed at a sufficient distance from the margin of the gap to secure a good hold, and their number and arrangement must depend upon the degree of tension at any particular point.

The sutures should, whenever possible, be passed through both sides of the palate at one transit of the needle. The finer sutures (those for the uvula for example) are passed by means of the rectangular needle (Fig. 274), the others by one of the needles in handles used for carrying wire or silkworm gut. If the edges of the cleft will come together, the sutures should be fastened off at once by tying or twisting, as the case may be.

If the cleft be narrow, the sutures can be passed without difficulty. If it be wide, some especial method may have to be adopted.

The following is the most convenient:—A very long suture has a needle threaded at either end of it. One needle is passed through the left flap of the palate from behind forwards, and the other through the right flap in the same direction. The first needle passed must be held by an assistant while the other is being introduced. This is practically the method usually adopted in closing an abdominal incision. The needles employed should be small and curved, and must be passed by means of a simple needle-holder. Needles of various curves should be at hand. In no operation is a complex needle-holder more out of place than in this.

Avery's method for passing the sutures may be employed in these cases. It is executed as follows:—

A needle in a handle carrying a long suture is passed through one flap of the palate (say the left) from before backwards. The loop is caught when the point of the needle is in the cleft, and is drawn out of the mouth. The needle is then withdrawn, leaving the loop *in situ*. A long suture is in like manner passed through the other flap (the right) of the palate. It is in like manner drawn through the cleft and out of the mouth, not in the form of a loop but as a single thread. The needle is withdrawn. The left half of the velum will therefore be pierced from before backward by a loop of suture, the right half by a single thread. The single suture is passed through the loop. The loop is withdrawn, dragging the single suture with it. This suture therefore will have passed through the right half of the palate from before backwards, and through the left half from behind forwards.

" When there is too much tension to admit of the sutures being tied at once, they should all be passed, and being loosely twisted, the long ends may be cut off, and longitudinal incisions may be made on either side parallel to the cleft, and just internal to the hamular process (Fig. 277), avoiding the immediate neighbourhood of the posterior palatine foramen. It is well to make this incision with a blunt-ended knife, after puncturing the palate with a sharp-pointed knife. Sufficient relaxation being obtained, the remaining sutures should be quickly fastened off by twisting with torsion forceps" (T. Smith).

If after the lateral incisions have been made the tension is not amply relieved, it is well to introduce a slender-pointed raspatory through the incision, and with it to detach the muscular and tendinous structures from the hamular process. I have found such a step always to answer its purpose completely.

Sir William Fergusson divided the levator palati muscle by means of a rectangular knife, which was passed through the cleft and was made to sever the muscle by a transverse incision on the posterior aspect of the palate. Mr. Pollock divided both the levator and tensor palati muscles by means of a fine tenotome passed from before backwards through the velum just in front and to the inner side of the hamular process. Neither of these measures for the relief of tension has proved satisfactory in practice, and both have been for the most part abandoned.

The lateral incision is said to have originated with Dieffenbach.

Throughout the operation, bleeding must be checked by gentle pressure with a sponge in a holder. The sponge should, however, be used as little as possible. The indiscriminate and persistent dabbing of the palate with a sponge tends to excite movement of the palatal and pharyngeal muscles, to produce vomiting and coughing, and to greatly increase the flow of saliva.

In the adult the saliva from the parotid may sometimes be seen to squirt in a jet into the mouth, after a vigorous sponging.

The operation may have to be suspended from time to time to give opportunities to the anæsthetist.

THE OPERATION ON THE HARD PALATE.

The following is Mr. T. Smith's description of the operation. The procedure, although somewhat modified, is usually known as Langenbeck's Operation. (*See* page 65.)

"If there is sufficient material for closing the palate, the mucous edges of the cleft may be pared. If there is any doubt about this, the proceeding must be dispensed with, as involving a waste of flap. To bring down the muco-periosteum from the bones, a mere puncture should be made down to the bone with a scalpel, midway between the teeth and the margin of the cleft, and opposite the middle of the cleft (*i.e.*, midway between the anterior angle of the cleft, and the posterior margin of the hard palate.) Through this puncture the least curved of the raspatories should be thrust between the periosteum and the bone, and be pushed onwards towards the middle line until its point appears in the cleft. At this spot one of the more curved raspatories should be inserted, the instrument first used being withdrawn.

"The curved raspatory should now be used to separate the muco-periosteum from the bone, and this is best accomplished by to-and-fro movements, and by careful traction. The periosteum is easily detached until the posterior margin of the hard palate is reached, where the soft palate is firmly attached by fascia, and by its connection with the mucous membrane on the floor of the nose.

"Curved scissors should be used to divide this attachment, the palate being drawn forward with a hook to put it on the stretch while the scissors are passed behind it.

"The scissors may now be used with closed blades, as a raspatory, to draw forward the soft parts at the junction of the hard and soft palate, and complete their separation from the bone. When the hard palate is cleft up to the incisor teeth, there is often difficulty in completely separating the periosteum at the anterior angle of the fissure. Should this be the case, a small rectangular knife can be used to free the soft parts.

"The muco-periosteum being completely separated from one side of the palate, the assistant should thrust a sponge into the cleft, and press the flap firmly against the bone. This will restrain all hæmorrhage, give an opportunity for cleansing the fauces from blood, and allow of the re-adminis-tration of chloroform.

"The soft parts being separated from the bone on the opposite side of the cleft in the same manner, the sutures may be passed as in the soft palate, silver wire being used, and each suture being twisted up as far as practicable without risk of breaking, and cut short, so as to leave about a sixth of an inch projecting.

"Tension should be relieved by prolonging the small incisions made for the introduction of the raspatory forwards or backwards, as the circumstances of the case may require.

"The incisions should go quite through the palate, and they are best made with a probe-pointed knife. All slack sutures should now be twisted up with torsion forceps until the edges of the cleft are in exact apposition. In bringing together this part of the palate, care must be taken to evert the edges of the cleft with a small double hook in passing and twisting up the sutures; this secures the apposition of the raw surfaces of the flaps, and it is especially necessary when the edges of the cleft have not been pared" (Heath's "Dictionary of Surgery").

If the edges of the two flaps be sufficiently everted to bring their raw (superior) surfaces into apposition, it is a question whether the tissues are not encroached upon to an extent equivalent to the loss they would sustain had the margins been freshened. Many surgeons therefore pare the edges in every instance.

It is often more convenient to make the lateral incisions at once, and to detach the muco-periosteal flap by working from those incisions towards the free margin of the gap, instead of effecting the detachment in the opposite direction.

The gaps left by the dragging of the flaps towards the median line are allowed to close by granulation.

The detachment of the tissues about the hamular process may be very conveniently effected by a raspatory of small size made after Ollier's pattern.

Langenbeck used a special blunt-ended knife to effect this difficult separation.

The Dieffenbach-Fergusson Operation.—This operation, originally devised by Dieffenbach, was introduced to British surgeons by Sir William Fergusson, in 1874 (*Brit. Med. Journ.*, April, 1874).

The edges of the cleft having been pared, an incision is made in the palate about half-way between the gap and the alveolus, and parallel with the margin of the gap (A, Fig. 278). This incision is carried well down to the bone.

The bone exposed along this line is now divided with a chisel to the full extent of the incision. The passage of the chisel may be assisted by a series of preliminary holes made with a bradawl (B, Fig. 278). The blade of the chisel having been passed into the nose through the gap, each lateral portion of the palate is prised towards the middle line until the pared edges meet. Sutures—if not already introduced—are now inserted into the soft parts bounding the freshened margins, and the cleft is closed.

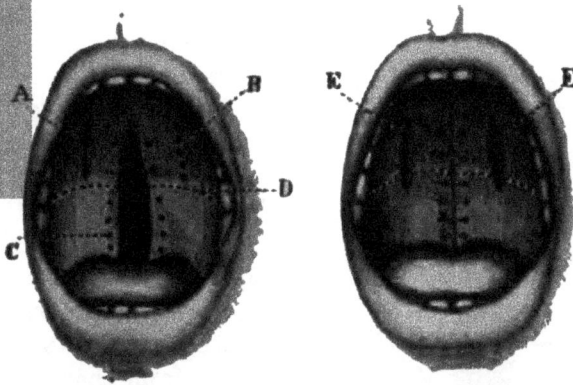

Fig. 278.—THE DIEFFENBACH-FERGUSSON OPERATION FOR CLEFT PALATE.

A, Incision over the hard palate; B, Punctures to give line for the chisel; C, Suture holes in palate; D, Margin of hard palate; E, Incisions through the bone completed. (After Bryant.)

Sutures may also be passed through the lateral apertures right across the gap, and the two portions of the palate be thus tied together. The lateral gaps are lightly stuffed with a little antiseptic gauze.

Should the vomer be attached to one margin of the cleft the introduction of sutures would be attended with great difficulty.

Lannelongue's Operation by a Nasal Flap.—Lannelongue has in three cases closed a cleft limited to the hard palate by a rectangular flap obtained from the side of the nasal septum (Bull. de la Soc. de Chir., 1877, page 472).

The size of the flap must depend upon the size of the gap to be closed. It is limited by three incisions: one superior and horizontal, and two lateral and vertical. The base or pedicle of the flap is therefore at the lower border of the nasal septum. The flap is detached by a suitable rugine from above, downwards. The lateral border of the fissure is pared, and the flap is then drawn across the cleft and attached to the freshened margin by sutures.

This plan may be carried out when the septum is adherent to one margin of the cleft, and where the opening is—with reference to the nasal septum—unilateral.

The case must be exceptional in which this excellent procedure will alone suffice to effect a cure, but the operation may be of great value in supplementing the usual measure as described above.

Davies - Colley's Operation.—This operation is described in the *British Medical Journal* for Oct. 25, 1890 :

First Stage.—A triangular flap (Fig. 279, *a b* c), consisting of the whole of the soft parts covering the bone, should be cut from that side of the hard palate which is the wider ; or if, as usually happens, the septum of the nose is attached to the palatal process of one of the superior maxillæ, the flap should be taken from this side. The apex of this flap

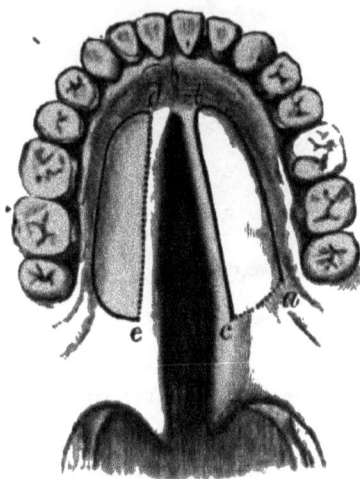

Fig. 279.—DAVIES-COLLEY'S OPERATION FOR CLEFT OF THE HARD PALATE.

The flaps (*a b* c and *d* e) marked out.

should reach nearly as far forwards as the insertion of the incisor teeth (*b*, Fig. 279). The outer border of the flap should begin just internal to the back part of the alveolar process, and should run forwards parallel to the margin of that process. The inner side of the flap should run backwards one-eighth of an inch external to the margin of the cleft, and should terminate a short distance behind the posterior border of the hard palate. The base which is left attached will therefore extend from close to the inner border of the alveolus for the last molar teeth, inwards and slightly backwards to the edge of the cleft of the soft palate, near to its anterior attachment (*a c,* Fig. 279).

Second Stage.—An incision is made down to the bone upon the other side of the cleft, at least one-sixth of an inch external to its margin. The greater part of the incision runs from before backwards parallel to the cleft. It should begin at the level of the anterior extremity of the cleft, and should end at the back of the hard palate (*d e*, Fig. 279). At its anterior and posterior extremities this incision should be carried inwards to the margin of the cleft. A raspatory is now inserted, and by it the muco-periosteum internal to the incision is separated from the bone as far inwards as the margin of the cleft.

Third Stage. — The flap made in the second stage of the operation is now turned inwards upon the hinge, so to speak, formed by its attachment to the margin of the palatal processes of the superior maxilla and palate bone, and is fixed in this position (so as partly to bridge across the cleft) by two moderately fine catgut sutures passed through its edge, and the thin strip of mucous membrane which was left *in situ*

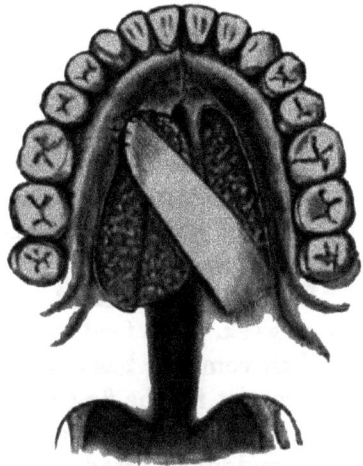

Fig. 280.—DAVIES-COLLEY'S OPERATION FOR CLEFT OF THE HARD PALATE.

The flaps in position.

on the opposite side of the cleft, internal to the triangular flap (Fig. 280).

Fourth Stage.—The apex of the triangular flap is now carried across the cleft, and the anterior part of its inner margin is attached by means of two or three silver sutures to the outer border of the incision upon the other side of the palate (Fig. 280). If there is any difficulty in carrying the triangular flap across the cleft, it may be necessary to detach its base more freely from the soft parts which connect it with the back of the hard palate. It will usually be found that the triangular flap lies very loosely in its new position, but no fear need be entertained that on this account it will fail to unite. The upward pressure of the tongue will constantly maintain the raw surface, which forms the upper portion of the flap, in close contact with the raw surface which, if the third stage has been properly carried out, is directed downwards so as to form a bed for its reception.

The subsequent treatment of the case is in no wise different from that after the ordinary operation.

The advantages claimed for this measure are these :—(1) There is less hæmorrhage ; (2) less bruising of the parts ; (3) less sacrifice of tissue ; (4) less tension upon the flaps ; and (5) the operation can be easily performed at a early age—*e.g.*, between the ages of one and two years.

The disadvantages are :—(1) The hard palate alone is united ; (2) a foramen is apt to be left in the front part of the cleft. (This can be closed later).

Mr. Davies-Colley recommends the operation in the cases of infants ; in cases where the usual operation has failed ; and where the gap is too wide to be bridged over by the usual operation.

The After-treatment.—The patient should remain in bed for a week. No food of any kind should be administered until all vomiting has ceased. The diet should be simple, and may consist for the first day of milk or milk-and-water only, and after that of beef-tea, broth, eggs, arrowroot, custard and sago puddings, bread-and-milk, stewed fruit, and the like. Porridge, pounded meat, or fish, may be given when a few days have elapsed. Two mistakes are frequently made in the after-treatment : one is to starve the patient, and the other is to feed him so frequently with small quantities of food, that the pharyngeal muscles are never at rest. One author, indeed, says that food should be administered " unceasingly."

The patient should be fed as an ordinary patient is fed, but the food must be fluid, or at least perfectly soft, and must be swallowed slowly and carefully. The pharyngeal muscles contract more completely around a small bolus than a large. This simple and almost fluid diet should be observed for two or three weeks, until, indeed, it is clear that the wound has healed, or has broken down hopelessly.

It is well to forbid much talking. For the first few days the less the patient speaks the better.

One important factor must not be overlooked—the mouth

must be kept clean. It is often rendered foul by decomposing milk and beef-tea, which remain in the recesses of the mouth, owing to the patient's exaggerated belief in the evils which attend swallowing. The best wash is a warm solution of carbolic acid (1 in 100 to 1 in 80). Boracic lotion also answers well.

The mouth should be rinsed out after every meal, and at other times as occasion suggests. I am in the habit of having the wound washed at least twice a day with a warm boracic solution, which is applied to the palate by means of a "scent spray." It is agreeable to the patient, and it keeps the part free from incrustation.

The advice that the palate in young children should not be inspected for one week after the operation is hardly consistent with the practice which obtains in the treatment of wounds elsewhere.

The sutures need not be removed until fourteen days or three weeks have elapsed. Sutures of silkworm gut and fine silver set up singularly little disturbance, and may be retained for weeks, but it is obvious that if firm union has not taken place in three weeks it will probably not take place in five.

Results.—The success of the operation may be compromised by severe vomiting, by the swallowing of solid food, by the development of whooping-cough, or an eruptive fever, or by the feebleness of the patient's health.

It must be remembered that the closure of the cleft does not remedy the defective articulation. The soft palate in those cases of congenital deformity is not only deficient in the median line, but deficient as a rule throughout. It is unduly short, and after the most successful operation it is doubtful if the palate is ever so completely restored that it is capable of shutting off the mouth from the nasal passage.

The operation, however, places the patient in a position to attain a normal articulation. It enables him to be educated to speak naturally. This education is tedious, and involves a great expenditure of time and trouble, but it is remarkable what excellent results may follow, even in cases which cannot be considered from a surgical point of view to be eminently successful.

CHAPTER VI.

PLASTIC OPERATIONS UPON THE BLADDER AND URETHRA.

THESE operations will be considered in the following order:—

1. Operations for Epispadias.
2. Operations for Hypospadias.
3. Operations for Ectopia Vesicæ.
4. Operations for acquired Urethral Fistula.

OPERATIONS FOR EPISPADIAS.

This condition is less common than hypospadias, but at the same time causes much more disturbance and greater inconvenience.

It often exists as an isolated deformity, and quite independent of extroversion of the bladder, but all examples of the latter malformation are associated with epispadias.

There are various grades of the deformity, but the commonest condition is that known as the "complete form." In this the penis is much shortened and flattened, and is curved upwards towards the abdomen. It is compressed against the abdomen, and usually turns also to the left side. The funnel-shaped opening into the bladder may be of sufficient size to admit the finger.

The prepuce is usually large and depends like an apron. In the completer forms there is incontinence of urine, and great distress is occasioned by the continual escape of urine, and by the chafing and excoriation that follow.

It is noteworthy that after a successful operation, and often after one which is partly successful, a control is obtained over the bladder. The affection was at one time regarded as quite incurable. Attempts to form a new roof to the urethra by means of flaps derived from the lateral parts of the penis failed. In 1852 Nélaton employed for the first time the

of the penis, one being placed on each side of the urethral
groove. These incisions are parallel to one another and to
the groove, and are placed a little external to the outer
margins of the groove.

They terminate at the corona glandis by one extremity,
and at the abdomen by the other. At each of these extremities of the two cuts two very short transverse incisions are
made at right angles,
and are directed out-
wards.

The minute and
almost linear flaps thus
marked out are dis-
sected up as far as the
lateral cuts will allow.

2. The proximal
ends of the two longi-
tudinal incisions are
now carried vertically
upwards on to the ab-
domen, and are united
superiorly by a trans-
verse wound. The
abdominal flap is
thus marked out. Its
breadth exceeds a little
the width of the inter-
val between the parallel
penile incisions, and

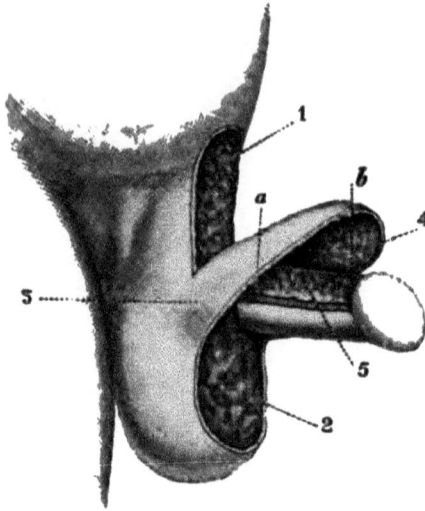

Fig. 281.—NÉLATON'S OPERATION FOR EPISPADIAS.

1, Raw surface left by abdominal flap; 2, Raw
surface left by scrotal flap; 3, Pedicle of scrotal
flap; 4, Scrotal flap; 5, Abdominal flap in
position; a b, Free edge of penile flap, beneath
which the margin of the abdominal flap has
been introduced.

its length is a little in excess of the length of the urethral
groove which is to be covered in (Fig. 281, 1).

This narrow flap, when separated from the parts beneath, is
turned down for the purpose of forming a roof to the urethra.
The skin surface lies towards the penis, while the raw surface
is uppermost or external (Fig. 281, 5). The edges are united
by sutures to the raw edges left by the dissecting up of the
minute penile flaps (a, b). The free, upper or transverse, border
forms the upper margin of the new meatus. The union of
this flap is so made that the edges which are brought together
overlap a little, the minute penile flaps overlapping the

margins of the abdominal flap. An extensive union is thus obtained.

It was found that if the operation were left at this stage the abdominal flap would by its contraction shorten the penis, curve it upwards, and gradually expose again more or less of the urethral groove.

To prevent this Nélaton made an additional flap from the scrotum as follows.

3. This flap is obtained from the anterior surface of the scrotum, and is limited by two curved incisions ; the upper one circumscribes the under half of the penis, and follows the groove between the penis and the scrotum ; the lower one is parallel to it, and is so placed that the length of the scrotal flap shall a little exceed the length of the penis. Both incisions are concave upwards.

The flap is liberated except at the sides, where is a wide pedicle (3, Fig. 281). The penis is then slipped under

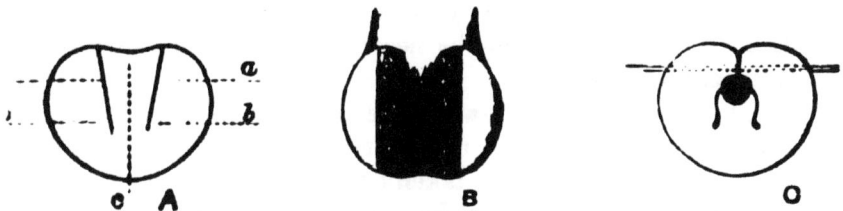

Fig. 282.—THIERSON'S OPERATION FOR EPISPADIAS (FIRST STAGE).

the flap, and its raw surface is attached by sutures to the raw surface of the abdominal flap which is already in position (5, Fig. 281).

The edges of the scrotal flap are united to the edges of the two penile flaps (*a b*, Fig. 281), and the operation is completed by closing in the raw surfaces (1 and 2, Fig. 281) left respectively upon the abdomen and scrotum.

After-Treatment.—An india-rubber tube well oiled is placed in the new urethra and passed well into the bladder. It must be held in place by a couple of sutures.

The wound surfaces should be well dusted with iodoform and covered with a light dry dressing.

Dry and infrequent dressings are best suited for this class of case.

It may be possible to attach a long indiarubber pipe to the tube already in the urethra, and to allow the urine to drain away into a vessel under the bed.

If this be attempted, a loop of the pipe must be attached to the bed cradle, so that the urethral tube cannot be drawn upon should the patient move in his sleep or turn over. The loop should give it sufficient play.

If this cannot be arranged, the patient must sit as nearly upright as possible, and a macintosh should be so arranged beneath him that the urine can easily drain away.

Constant care must be devoted to keeping the patient dry.

The bowels may be kep-at rest for a few days.

In the case of a young child chloral may be cautiously given after the operation to keep the patient quiet.

A simple nutritious diet should be advised, and plenty of fluid allowed, so that the urine may be as little irritating as possible.

The sutures will probably not be touched for eight or ten days. An anæsthetic may be necessary in order to carry out their removal safely.

The tube in the urethra may be removed in five or seven days, or less. If it excite undue irritation, or if urine escape by the side of it, it may be taken out earlier.

Result.—This operation has been fairly successful. The patient's condition is much improved, but two objections have to be noted. First, the glans remain uncovered, and, second, the new urethra is abnormally large. By means of Thiersch's operation an attempt is made to close the urethra without leaving these defects.

Thiersch's Operation.—This operation was described by Thiersch in 1869 (*Archiv. of Heilkunde,* 1869, Hft. I.). It has been adopted by many surgeons with excellent results. The procedure is divided into four stages.

First Stage.—Formation of a meatus and that part of the urethra which occupies the glans.

A deep incision (*a a,* Fig. 282, A) is made in the glans along each side of the urethral groove. These two incisions converge a little below and involve about three-fourths of the thickness of the glans

They serve to separate the dorsal part of the glans into three parts—a median and two lateral (*c, b b*, Fig. 282, A).

The surface of the outer lip of each incision is pared for its entire length (Fig. 282, B), and while the median portion is depressed by means of a short length of catheter, which is introduced, the two lateral portions are brought together, and are united by means of fine needles and figure-of-eight sutures in the median line (Fig. 282, C).

The middle segment carries with it the whole of the mucous membrane, and its surface is, therefore, not disposed to unite with the raw surface, which at first forms the roof of the new urethra.

Second Stage.—The formation of the penile urethra. When the wound in the glans has healed, and the pins have been removed, and when the urethral canal in the glans has been well established, the second step in the operation is undertaken.

An incision is made through the skin and subcutaneous tissues on the dorsum of the penis, on both sides of the urethral groove. The incision on the right side (Fig. 283, B) is made close to the urethral groove. The incision on the left is placed about half an inch from the left margin of the groove (Fig. 283, A). The two cuts are parallel to one another. By means of the transverse incisions (*c c, d d*) two long narrow flaps are marked out. The right flap (B) has its free edge abutting on the

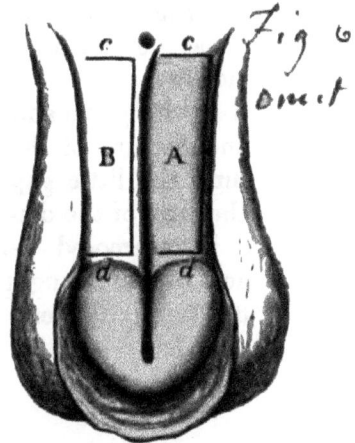

Fig. 283.—THIERSCH'S OPERA-TION FOR EPISPADIAS (SECOND STAGE).

urethral groove, while the left flap (A) has its base in that position. (See also Fig. 284, 1.)

The two flaps are then dissected up, and are made as thick as possible.

The left flap (Fig. 284, A) is now turned over to form the roof of the new channel, its raw surface being uppermost. A row of sutures is passed through it, near to its free margin in the manner shown in Fig. 284, 2 and Fig. 285, and are then made to pass through the base of the right flap (B). They are finally

, sutures, as shown in Fig. 284, 2 and Fig. 285.

lich has been already introduced along the
f the urethra, from the meatus to the bladder, is
essary, until the wounds have closed.

stage is completed, and the incisions have
, the third step is undertaken.

.—The covering-in of the small gap (Fig. 285, c)
of of the urethra
glans and the body

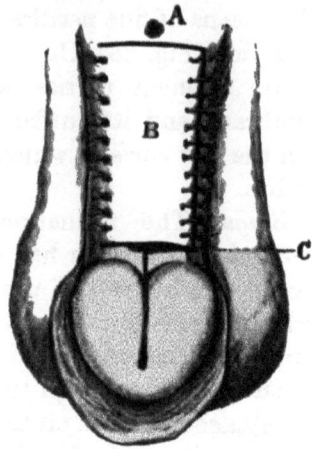

Fig. 285.—THIERSCH'S OPERATION
FOR EPISPADIAS (SECOND STAGE
COMPLETED).

his the apron-like
iperfect prepuce is
This piece of skin
and a transverse
cision is made in
this slit the glans

of the pendulous
was lowest now
most.

is of the glans and
the dorsum of the
ound the little gap
the ring of the dis-
e is interposed between them, and the raw
aces, thus brought together are united by
86). Another long interval is allowed for re-

Fourth Stage.—The closure of the funnel-shaped opening which leads into the bladder.

Two flaps are employed for this purpose, and one is taken from each inguinal region.

The flap taken from the left side is of triangular shape (Fig. 287, A), its base corresponding to the left half of the upper circumference of the bladder orifice. It is turned downwards, with the raw surface outermost, and is secured to the freshened margin of the skin forming the roof of the new penile urethra (Fig. 287). The right flap is long and quadrilateral, and has its base in the inguinal region, parallel to Poupart's ligament (Fig. 288, B).

It is placed over the raw surface of the left flap, and is fixed by sutures to this flap, to the skin to the left of the base of the same flap, and to the freshened area which

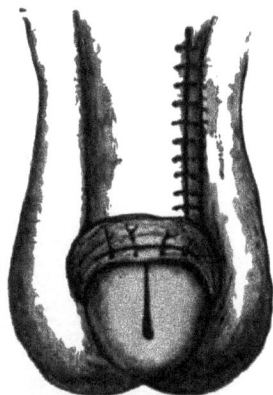

Fig. 286.—THIERSCH'S OPERATION FOR EPISPADIAS (THIRD STAGE).

surrounds the upper border of the bladder orifice (Fig. 288).

Comment.—If a proper interval be allowed between each stage of the operation, some months will elapse before the treatment has been completed.

The operation may fail at one stage, and may need to be repeated.

Thiersch first established a perineal fistula as a preliminary measure, in order that the course of the urine might be diverted during the period covered by the operations, but subsequent experience has shown that such a step is not necessary.

Duplay's Operation. — *First Stage.* — The penis is straightened (page 83).

Second Stage.—The urethra is formed. No flaps are used, but the new canal is formed almost exclusively at the expense of the corpus spongiosum and corpora cavernosa.

If the groove be shallow, a median incision is made along its whole length to render the adjustment easier.

The tissues on each side of the groove are now freshened,

the raw surfaces taking the form of strip-like quadrilateral areas, about half a centimetre wide, which traverse the whole length of the penis, and follow the margins of the median groove (*a b, a' b'*, Fig. 289). The freshened surfaces are now brought together in the median line by means of the quilled suture, which is introduced in the manner described in Duplay's operation for hypospadias (page 94).

Before the sutures are secured, a catheter is introduced into the groove, and is allowed to remain in the new canal.

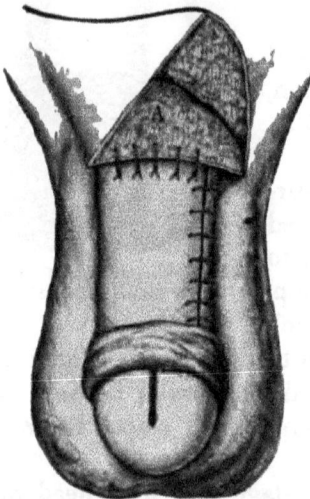

Fig. 287.—THIERSCH'S OPERATION FOR EPISPADIAS (FOURTH STAGE).

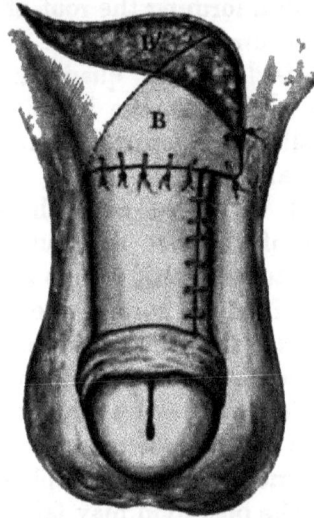

Fig. 288.—THIERSCH'S OPERATION FOR EPISPADIAS (FOURTH STAGE).

Its extremity enters the bladder, and it is employed until the wound has healed (Fig. 290).

Third Stage.—The treatment of the prepuce. The prepuce is treated as in Thiersch's operation, is pierced, and is brought on to the dorsum of the penis, where it is made— when sutured to a properly freshened surface—to provide a sounder covering of integument for the distal part of the dorsum of the penis.

By means of this flap of prepuce any little orifice which may remain open after the second stage of the operation is closed.

Fourth Stage.—The closure of the funnel-shaped opening

which leads into the bladder. This Duplay effects by freely freshening the opposed surfaces, and then approximating them and uniting them by shotted sutures.

In the *slightest forms of epispadias* there is no incontinence, and the deformity causes no trouble, but the appearance of the penis may be considerably improved by transplanting the redundant prepuce in the manner described in the third stage of Thiersch's operation.

OPERATIONS FOR HYPOSPADIAS.

This, the commonest of all the malformations of the urethra, has been the subject of a very large number of more or less complicated operations.

The varieties of the deformity are classified according to the position of the opening of the urethra. In front of the opening the urinary passage is either entirely absent or is represented by a groove, or by a partly pervious canal.

Fig. 289.—DUPLAY'S OPERATION FOR EPISPADIAS. (*Ashhurst.*)

1. **Balanitic.**—The opening is here at the site of the corona, the frænum is absent, and a hood-like prepuce exists.

2. **Penile.**—The urethra may open at any part of the undersurface of the penis, and if the opening be far back nearly the whole of the penile urethra will be wanting, so far as its floor is concerned.

3. **Scrotal.**—Here the opening is either at the junction of the penis and scrotum (peno-scrotal), or is on the perineal side of the scrotum (perineo-scrotal).

In all but the slighter cases the penis is small and deformed. It may be attached to the scrotum by a cutaneous web, or be held in a curved position by a fibrous band upon its under-surface, which represents the undeveloped urethra and the capsule of the corpora cavernosa. In extreme cases of curving of the penis the glans is forced against the scrotum, and only the dorsum of the shortened penis is visible.

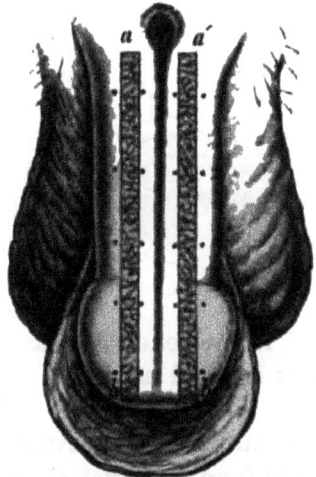

Purpose of Operative Treatment.—There is very rarely any incontinence with hypospadias, and in the majority of instances little inconvenience is complained of. The main difficulties depend upon the arching of the penis, and the existence of an opening far back. The curving of the penis renders micturition difficult and coitus impossible. Every time the patient makes water the scrotum and perineum are wetted with urine; and if care be not constantly taken, these parts may become eczematous. The urethral opening may also be so narrowed by the curving of the penis that micturition is impeded.

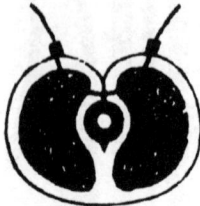

Fig. 290.

If any operation be carried out, it should be made without delay. If the deformity can be corrected early, the penis may, as growth proceeds, assume a very fair degree of development.

If the condition has been left untreated until the patient has reached adult life, it had better be left altogether. In such a case the man will have learnt how to overcome the difficulties of micturition. The penis, if it could be straightened (and it is not always possible at a late period) would be found to be short, wasted, and stunted. In these cases the testes are not uncommonly found to be small and atrophied, and the patient's sexual instincts are not so developed as to make him feel the impossibility of coitus.

In the balanitic form of hypospadias an operation can seldom be called for, and the deviation from the normal condition may be so slight, as not to cause any appreciable inconvenience.

Attempts to make a new urethra through the glans by perforating that structure by a trocar (Dupuytren) are quite unjustifiable.

The accepted operations for hypospadias have in view two objects: (1) the correction of the mal-position of the penis, and (2) the restoration of the canal of the deficient urethra.

1. The mal-position of the penis may be corrected by means of one or more transverse incisions which divide the band of contracted tissue passing between the glans and

the hypospadie opening. To overcome the curving of the penis completely it may be necessary to carry the incision deeply into the substance of the corpora cavernosa. It is usually better to effect this division through an open wound, the integumentary edges of which are united subsequently by sutures.

In the slighter cases a subcutaneous division may be possible.

Before proceeding further with the treatment of the case, some six or eight months should be allowed to elapse, in order that it may be made evident that the correction of the false position has been permanent.

2. The restoration of the canal may be effected by one or other of the following operations.

Duplay's Operation. — *First Stage.* — The penis is straightened.

Second Stage.—A new meatus is formed. This is effected by freshening at their lower parts the two lips (*b b'*, Fig. 291) of the depression which represents the meatus, and by placing between these two lips a small catheter tip (*c*), over which the freshened surfaces are united by several points of suture. If the depression be too shallow to permit the formation of a

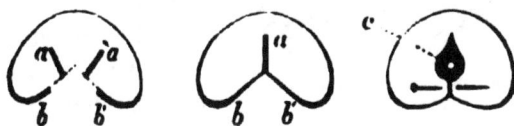

Fig. 291.—DUPLAY'S OPERATION FOR HYPOSPADIAS.

large enough meatus, two small lateral incisions (*a a'*, Fig. 291), or a median incision, *a*, made in the substance of the glans, will make it possible to introduce the tip of a catheter of proper size.

This part of the operation may be carried out at the same time that the penis is straightened, and the duration of the treatment be thus shortened.

Third Stage.—The new canal is formed.

On the lower surface of the penis, on each side of the median line, and some millimetres outside of this line, a longitudinal incision, *a b, a' b'*, is made, extending from the base of the glans to within 1 c.m. or even ½ c.m. of the hypospadic opening (*c*, Fig. 292).

The internal lip of the incision is now slightly dissected up, so that the narrow strip of skin between the wound and the median groove may be inclined inwards as a species of flap (the so-called inner flap) over the catheter, but without attempting to cover it entirely. On the other hand, the outer lip of each incision is to be dissected up freely, so as to draw towards the median line the skin of the lateral parts of the penis, *e d, e d'*. This skin is brought forward in the form of a loose flap (the so-called external flap). The cutaneous surface of the inner flaps is thus turned towards the cavity of the canal, whilst their raw surface is turned towards the outside, and is covered by the raw surface of the two external flaps. Although the catheter is thus not wholly covered by a cutaneous surface, Duplay has found no inconvenience to result from that circumstance.

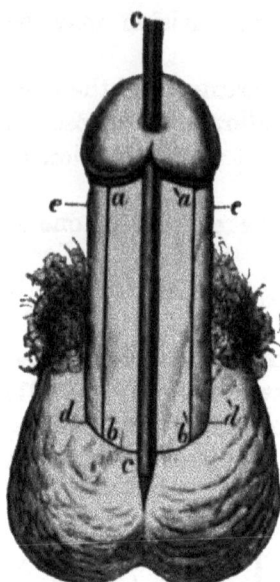

Fig. 292.—DUPLAY'S OPERATION FOR HYPOSPADIAS.

The displaced flaps are now united in the median line by means of a quilled suture. Very fine silver wire is used; each suture is made of a single wire, and is separated from its fellows by a distance of ½ c.m. The ends of each wire are passed through holes made in small leaden tubes, and are fastened by perforated shot (Fig. 293).

If the surfaces approximated by this suture leave a little separation externally, union is completed by a few superficial points of interrupted suture (Fig. 293).

Fourth Stage.—The two parts of the canal are united.

The margins of the openings to be approximated are freshened, and the raw edges are then drawn together and united—over a catheter—by means of a deep quilled suture and some interrupted superficial sutures.

The catheter is retained during all stages of the operation until healing is assured.

An interval of some months should be allowed to elapse between the third stage of the operation and the fourth.

Anger's Operation.—The operation, as here described, does not include the formation of a meatus. It is assumed that the penis has been straightened.

An incision (1 2, Fig. 294) is made on the right side of the penis from the glans to the scrotum, and half an inch from

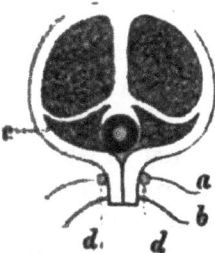

Fig. 293.— DUPLAY'S OP-ERATION FOR HYPO-SPADIAS.

a, Deep sutures; b, Sur-facesutures; c, Catheter; d, Leaden tubes or quills.

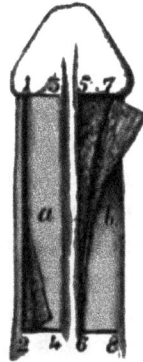

Fig. 294. — AN-GER'S OPER-ATION FOR HYPOSPADIAS.

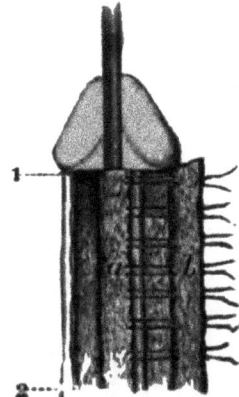

Fig. 295.—ANGER'S OPERA-TION FOR HYPOSPADIAS.

the median line. The transverse cuts, 1 3, 2 4, serve to mark out a flap (a, Fig. 294). This flap is dissected up and has its base along the median line. A second longitudinal incision, 5 6, is made to follow the left margin of the urethral groove. Two transverse cuts, 5 7, 6 8, about an inch in length, are made at each extremity of it. A flap (b, Fig. 294), with its free margin bounding the urethral groove, is thus marked out.

It is dissected up, and will possess at least double the width of the right flap (a).

A catheter having been introduced into the bladder, the first flap a is turned over so that its cutaneous surface covers the catheter (Fig. 295). Sutures are then passed as follows. Very fine silver or silkworm gut is used. To each end of the suture a slender needle is threaded. Each needle is made to transfix the free margin of the first flap a from the skin surface to the raw surface. The loop will be on the cutaneous surface. Both ends of each suture (*i.e.*, both needles) are then made

to transfix the base or outer part of the left flap (*b*, Fig. 295),
and in the cutaneous surface of that flap they are secured by
shot (Fig. 296, s).

The left flap (*b*) is drawn to the right so as to cover the
raw surface of the first flap (*a*), and the free edge of this more
superficial flap is then united by interrupted sutures (Fig.
296, w) to the raw border left by the incision 1 2, Figs. 294
and 295.

Other Operations have been devised, but they call for no
very full description. An account of *Szymanowski's* most
ingenious, but not very practical, operation will be found
conveniently summarised in Stephen Smith's "Operative
Surgery." *Professor Wood* and others have made use of the

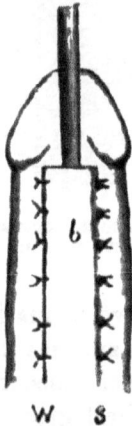

Fig. 296. — AN-
GER'S OPERA-
TION FOR HY-
POSPADIAS.

redundant prepuce (which is usually present in
hypospadias) to close in the canal in whole or
in part. This can be most conveniently carried
out when the urethra is wanting to the extent
of its anterior half only. When the deformity
extends as far back as the scrotum, Professor
Wood supplements the flap taken from the
prepuce by a flap cut from the front of the
scrotum.

Wood's method of arranging the preputial
flap is as follows :—A transverse buttonhole incision is made in the prepuce close to the coronal groove on the dorsum. The glans is slipped
through the aperture made. Two lateral flaps
are dissected up from the penis upon either
side of the urethral groove, and, being reversed,
are turned over, so that the skin surface is
towards the new canal. These flaps are united by a continuous suture of fine catgut. The transposed dorsal prepuce is then "split up into two layers at the cut edge,
which is opened and spread·out over the raw surface of
the reversed urethral flaps, and stitched to the edges by
closely applied sutures of fine silver wire" (Heath's "Dictionary of Surgery," vol. i., "Hypospadias").

In criticising this operation, it may be pointed out that
the integument of the prepuce and scrotum is not well
adapted to form the tissue of a primary flap. It is not

readily handled, and the lax subcutaneous layer renders œdema a troublesome complication. The prepuce may serve a useful purpose in assisting to close a small defect and in supplementing a more extensive operation, but it has not yielded satisfactory results when used to form the principal flap.

From Mr. Wood's account it is to be inferred that the lateral, or urethral, flaps are united in the median line, and to this practice also some exception may be taken.

h

CHAPTER VII.

OPERATIONS FOR ECTOPIA VESICÆ.

The Condition of the Patient.—Admirable descriptions of this deformity have been given by Mr. Wood (*Med.-Chir. Trans.*, vol. lii.; and Heath's " Dictionary of Surgery ").

It is only necessary here to allude to certain points bearing on the operation. Ectopia is more frequently met with in males than females, in the proportion of ten to one. It is invariably associated with epispadias. When the urine is ejected in a decided jet on coughing or crying some dilatation of the ureters is indicated. " Just on the upper margin of the red protruding mass (formed by the bare wall of the bladder) is a crescentric border of cicatricial tissue, which really represents the upper or omphalo-mesenteric part of the umbilicus. Above this will be seen and felt, in the median line—especially when the recti abdominis are put into action—a flat surface, hard and resisting, of from an inch to two or even three inches wide, bounded on each side by the recti muscles, and tapering upwards to the ensiform cartilage. This is the widened and expanded linea alba, and the structures covering the peritoneum here are sometimes very thin, although tough and resisting. The skin over this inter-rectal interval is smooth, and usually free from hairy growth. The recti are separated by the whole extent of the wide divergence of the superior rami of the pubes from the middle line " (Wood).

The scrotum is wide and shallow as 'a rule, and the testes are often in the groin. An oblique inguinal hernia often exists on one side or on both sides. The perineum is shorter and wider than normal, and the pubes are separated to the extent of from two to four inches.

The patients are often feeble and sickly. Renal disease, in the form of surgical kidney, is not uncommonly present especially in the older patients. It is a frequent cause of failure and of death after operation.

The ureters may be greatly dilated, and the kidneys cystic

Patients with ectopia have lived to reach old age without having undergone treatment of any kind.

The distress caused by this deformity is terrible. The urine is constantly dribbling away. The thighs, scrotum, perineum, and abdomen, are wet with urine and excoriated. The patient's clothes are soaked with urine, and the exposed portion of the bladder is commonly in a condition of cystitis.

Up to the present time no entirely satisfactory results have attended the use of the many forms of apparatus designed for ectopia. There is the difficulty of collecting the urine in all positions of the body without so pressing upon the integument as to produce excoriations or ulcers. The best apparatus is that by Wolfermann (Demme's model). A description of this appliance, with an illustration, will be found in Ultzmann's monograph on the bladder in the *Deutsche Chirurgie, Lief.*, 52, 1890.

For a consideration of the value of operative treatment in these cases, *see* the section which follows on the Results of Operation.

Age for Operation and Preparatory Treatment.—Operative treatment may be commenced when the patient is four or five years of age. It should in any case be undertaken and completed before puberty.

The treatment will extend over many months, and will usually occupy more than a year.

During this period the patient will be subjected to many operations. In a case quoted by Billroth the treatment occupied twenty-two months, during which time nineteen operations were performed. This experience is not exceptional.

Before the operation is commenced it is most important that the patient be in good health. There should be no cough, the bowels should be acting normally, the urine should be healthy and not irritating, and the skin as free from inflammation and eczema as is possible. The cystitis also must be dealt with. Much can be done by frequent bathing,

A 2

and by soaking up the urine by pads of compressed cotton-wool which have been impregnated with corrosive sublimate. To keep a patient dry by these means will require the unremitting attention of a nurse night and day.

Mr. Greig Smith, before performing Wood's operation in the case of a boy aged eight, carried out for fourteen days the following preparatory treatment:—" The patient was kept lying on his back in hopes that, by removing the weight of the abdominal contents, the tumour might diminish in size. The mucous membrane was covered with oiled silk coated with dextrine, over which was kept a double layer of boracic lint. The atmospheric air and other sources of irritation were thus excluded, and the deposition of phosphates, by prevention of evaporation, was much diminished. Bland and demulcent drinks were freely administered. Under this treatment the surface of the extroverted mucous membrane soon became less red and angry-looking ; and latterly, over its upper half, as low down as the orifice of the ureters, it became covered with true epidermis almost as white as that of the surrounding skin. The muco-purulent discharges diminished considerably in amount, and the excoriations on the contiguous skin entirely disappeared" (*British Medical Journal,* Feb. 7, 1880).

When a reversed flap is employed, and the integumentary surface is turned in towards the bladder, some trouble may result from the *growth of hair* from the displaced skin. The hair, if it attain any length, may block up the new urethra, and may lead to an accumulation of phosphatic concretions and other complications. Its growth is most likely to give trouble when well-developed hair is already growing upon the flap, as may be the case in an adult. When, however, the operation is carried out in very young subjects, the growth of hair seems to be subdued altogether. In other instances, in which the hair has continued to grow, it has been observed that the growth has declined in vigour as time went on, and that it has ultimately ceased entirely.

In cases where the hair at the time of the operation is unduly abundant, it is best to remove it by some depilatory. Mr. Wood recommends a drop of strong nitric acid applied at intervals, until all the hair is destroyed. When the acid is being applied, the skin and exposed mucous membrane must be carefully protected by a mixture of olive oil and chalk applied in a thick layer. No operation would be attempted until the skin thus treated has soundly healed.

Methods of Operating.—The very numerous operations advised or adopted in cases of ectopia vesicæ may be divided into three classes :—

1. Operations designed to divert the urinary passages.
2. Operations for closing in the defect by means of flaps.
3. Operations for narrowing the defective area by approximating the two innominate bones.

1. OPERATIONS DESIGNED TO DIVERT THE URINARY PASSAGES.

The procedures merely require to be enumerated. They have been up to the present time attended by great ill-success.

John Simon (*Lancet*, 1852, vol. ii., page 570) succeeded by means of threads passed from the ureters into the rectum in effecting a communication between the bladder and the bowel. Some urine passed per rectum, but much still escaped over the pubes, and the raw surface of the bladder was left uncovered.

Several operations, with the same object of diverting the urine into the rectum, have been carried out, but with no success, and with many deaths.

Mr. T. Smith's attempt to secure the ureters to the ascending and descending colon ended in failure (*St. Bartholomew's Hospital Reports*, vol. xv., page 9).

Sonnenburg (*Deutsche Chirurgie, Lief*, 52, 1890) succeeded in extirpating the bladder in a case of ectopia vesicæ in a boy aged nine, and in uniting the ureters to the dorsal groove of the penis. The bladder was separated without injuring the peritoneum. Catheters were introduced into the ureters, and tied there. The whole of the bladder was removed, and the ureters were cut free. The ureters were sutured to freshened surfaces on the dorsum of the penis. The gap in the abdominal wall was closed by flaps without difficulty. The ureters became fixed in their new situation, and healing is said to have been perfect.

2. OPERATIONS FOR CLOSING IN THE DEFECTS BY MEANS OF
FLAPS.

The early flap operations were more or less uniformly
unsuccessful. Attempts to close in the opening by definite
flaps were made as far back as 1844. The flaps were not
reversed, and failure followed.

Reversed flaps were first employed by Roux, Richard, and
Pancoast.

Roux (*L'Union Méd.*, 1853) dissected one flap from the
abdomen above, and another from the scrotum below, and
united them in a reversed manner over the exposed bladder,
so that the raw surfaces were turned outwards. Both flaps
sloughed.

Richard (*Gaz. Hebdom.*, vol. i., 1854), following the lines
of Nélaton's operation for epispadias, attempted a like operation a little later, but with a fatal result.

Dr. Ayres, of New York, operated upon an adult female in
1858 ("Congenital Exstrophy of the Urinary Bladder," New
York, 1859) by turning down a flap of skin from the abdomen
over the bladder. The cutaneous surface of this flap was
turned towards the bladder. Its raw surface was covered
by a process of gliding. The result was not very encouraging.

Dr. Pancoast, of Philadelphia (*North American Medical
and Chirurgical Review*, July, 1859), carried out an operation
in the same year (1858) which proved to be more successful.

Two lateral flaps were dissected up on either side of the
defect, and were turned over so as to cover the bladder (their
cutaneous surfaces being innermost). The flaps were reversed,
but not superimposed. Union took place between the edges
of the flaps.

Mr. Holmes first employed reversed and superimposed
flaps with success in England, in 1863 ("Surgical Treatment
of Children's Diseases," 2nd edition, page 149).

From these early operations the present more successful
procedures have been derived.

The two principal methods now in use are known as—

    A. **Wood's Operation.**

    B. **Thiersch's Operation.**

These may be regarded as two standard procedures,

founded upon different principles, and forming the bases for many modifications.

An account of Maury's operation will also be added.

A. Wood's Operation.

Here three flaps are formed—a reversed upper or umbilical flap, and two lateral transplanted flaps, which are made to cover over the upper flap. The following description is derived from Prof. Wood's account in Heath's "Dictionary of Surgery," 1887.

1. *The Cutting of the Flaps.*—The upper flap (Fig. 297, c) should be figured by a line extending along the side of the bladder surface vertically upwards as far as the measured distance from the root of the penis to the upper margin of the bladder, and then carried in a rounded curve across the "linea alba" at this point to join another vertical line of equal length on the opposite side of the bladder.

The two groin flaps (Fig. 297, A, B) for superposition are to be made of a rounded lancet shape, with the roots downwards and inwards at the base of the scrotum, and continued along the side of the urethral groove for

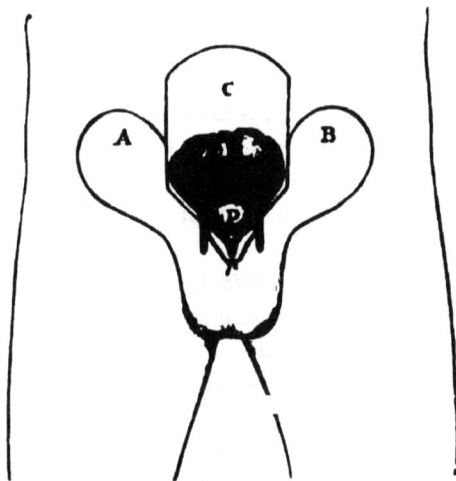

Fig. 297.— WOOD'S OPERATION FOR ECTOPIA VESICÆ.
A B, Lateral flaps ; C, Upper flap ; P, Prostate ; p, Penis.

about half its length. These flaps should be long enough and detached enough to meet in the median line for their whole length, and no sharp angles should be left in their outline. The incision for making them should join that of the lateral border of the first or umbilical flap at about its centre.

In raising the umbilical flap care must be taken not to make the skin too thin, which is apt to be done in the centre of its base near the upper margin of the bladder. The tissues are here so thin that there is danger of wounding the peritoneum.

The flaps should be handled with the fingers rather than with forceps. In raising the lateral flaps the superficial external pudic arteries are cut and may need to be ligatured. All bleeding must have been checked, and all clots removed, before the flaps are placed in position.

2. *The Adjusting of the Flaps.*—The upper flap is folded evenly down with its skin surface to the bladder, and is attached by sutures (Professor Wood uses silver wire) to the cut edge at the root of the penis on each side.

The groin flaps are then placed upon the raw surface of the umbilical flap. Their inner edges are united by sutures in the median line, and their bases should closely embrace the root of the penis. The raw surface left by the removal of the umbilical flap is closed by drawing the edges together with hare-lip pins. The surfaces left in the groin were in Professor Wood's first operation treated in the same way, but he now advises that the upper borders of the groin flaps be held upwards by one or two wire sutures, and that the raw surfaces which remain should be left to heal by granulation (Fig. 298).

In the Female the umbilical flap should be large, and the incision for the groin flaps on each side should be carried well down, so as to have their roots in great measure connected with the labia. When the flaps are finally sutured together, the vagina should be almost closed up by them, with but a small opening to allow the passage of the urine. (*See* Mr. Mayo Robson's modification of the operation, a page 106.)

3. *The Treatment of the Epispadias.*—This is effected by Nélaton's operation modified to meet the altered condition of the parts above the opening into the bladder. (*See* page 83.) In the place of the abdominal flap there described an incision is made parallel to and half an inch above the arched cicatrised urethral border of the covering of the bladder, and the integument thus marked out is then turned down in the form of a fold, with the skin surface directed towards the upper surface of the penis.

With this exception the operation follows the lines already indicated.

Comment.—This operation meets successfully with the two great difficulties which attended early procedures.

1. In these cases a sinus was left at the site of the umbilicus which it was found almost impossible to close.

Such a result may be certainly expected if lateral flaps are employed in the fresh state without reversion or without the addition of the umbilical flap.

2. The constant pressure upon the posterior wall of the bladder had in the early cases a tendency to cause a protrusion as the cicatrices contracted. As a result of this the opening above the penis became larger and larger. This difficulty is met partly by groin flaps of considerable size, which closely embrace the root of the penis, and partly by means of the scrotal flap, which prevents the tissues about the opening from being drawn up as cicatrisation and contraction proceed. The scrotal flap is an essential feature in dealing with the epispadias.

During the progress of the operation all the antiseptic washes or lotions used should be warm. In dissecting up the lateral flaps great care must be taken in cases where inguinal herniæ exist.

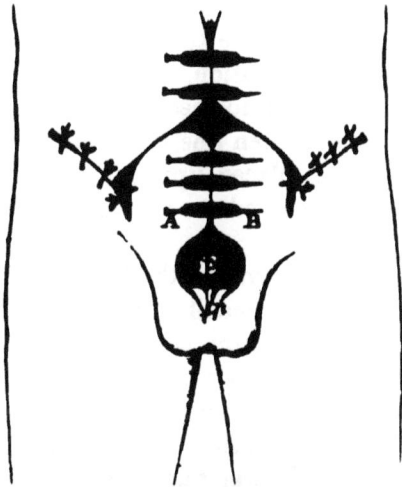

Fig. 298.—WOOD'S OPERATION FOR ECTOPIA VESICÆ.

A, B, Lateral flaps; C, Upper flap; P, Prostate; p, Penis.

If it be possible so to fashion the pedicles of the inguinal flaps that the external pudic arteries are not divided, a great point is gained.

Modifications of Wood's Operation.—Mr. Greig Smith, of Bristol (*Brit. Med. Journal*, Feb., 1880), makes the flaps of a little larger size. The umbilical flap is in shape like the wooden portion of a fire-bellows. The portion corresponding to the handle of the bellows is uppermost and in the median line, and when the flap is turned down this portion is used to cover in the urethra, and to afford a further attachment to the tissues dissected up from the penis and scrotum.

The umbilical flap and the lateral flaps are secured together by means of deep quilled sutures applied in a vertical line over about the middle of each lateral flap.

Mr. Smith reports two cases, in both of which an excellent result was obtained.

Mr. Mayo Robson (*Brit. Med. Journal*, Jan. 31st, 1885) reports a very successful case of Wood's operation carried out in a female child aged 8 years.

Allusion has been already made to the difficulty which arises in this procedure of preventing some reopening of the sinus, owing to the retraction of the flaps which cover in the bladder. In Mr. Robson's case this retraction caused the bladder surface to be once more exposed in part. To meet this complication, Mr. Robson so detached the folds of integument which formed the labia majora as to form on each side of the median line two triangular flaps which were capable of being displaced upwards. The upper margins of these flaps were attached to the lower margins of the flaps already in position.   ·

By this means the bladder surface was entirely covered in, and only a small slit was left for the escape of the urine. This procedure should be always carried out in operating upon the female subject by Wood's method. Some excellent drawings illustrate Mr. Robson's paper.

B. Thiersch's Operation.

Two lateral flaps are formed, one to cover the lower half of the defect, and the other the upper half (*Centralblatt für Chirurgie*, 1876, page 504). Each flap when first cut is large enough alone to cover the whole of the exposed area. From the nature of the method adopted, allowance has to be made for the shrinking of the flap. The flap first made is intended for the lower half of the bladder. It is marked out by two incisions. One commences at the upper margin of the defect, and proceeds vertically downwards to the root of the penis. The second is placed at a suitable distance to the outer side of the first, is parallel to it, and is continued down to Poupart's ligament. The flap is detached in the form of a strip or bridge, and is left connected with the body by its upper and its lower extremities. Beneath it is placed a plate of tinfoil or ivory, and for a period of three weeks its under surface is allowed to granulate. At the end of three weeks the upper attachment of the flap is divided, and it is laid transversely over the lower part of the defect. The margin of the defect will have been freshened, and to this raw border the flap is attached. The granulating surface of the flap is turned towards the bladder. (The use of granulating flaps in plastic surgery is dealt with on page 11.)

When this flap has soundly healed, and has become safely fixed in its new situation, the second flap is cut from the other side of the defect.

It is fashioned in exactly the same way, but the two parallel incisions do not extend so low down, but end at the place of attachment of the first flap. As this flap is to be of the same size as the first, the two incisions will have to be carried higher up on the belly. The bridge of skin thus marked out and separated is allowed, as before, to granulate for three weeks.

At the end of this time its upper end is divided, and it is placed transversely over the upper half of the defect.

Its granulating surface is turned towards the bladder.

Its margins are united to the margins of the defect, which will have been freshened to receive it.

The interval between the two flaps will now be indicated by a transverse line. When the second flap is securely united, the contiguous margins of the two flaps at this line are freshened, and are secured together by sutures.

Finally the upper margin of the second flap, and the adjacent (superior) margin of the defect are freshened, and are united by sutures. If the tissues of the abdominal wall at the upper margin of the defective area be too thin for sutures, then an attempt is made to secure the closure of this final gap by granulation.

When the bladder has been covered in, the epispadias is dealt with by Thiersch's method, the details of which have been already described.

The treatment involved by this method will extend over twelve or eighteen months, and will necessitate a great number of separate operations.

The results obtained by Thiersch have been very excellent.

Comment.—The especial points in this admirable operation are the following:—No umbilical flap is used, on the
grounds that its tissues are often so thin, scanty, and ill-
nourished, that some sloughing of the flap is not uncommon,
and also for the reason that in the dissection of this flap the
peritoneum may be injured, and a condition is provided for
the production of a ventral hernia.

The injurious action of urine upon raw surfaces is prevented by the system of granulating flaps. Upon the
granulating surface it seems to have no effect.

It would appear probable that a sinus would often be left
at the site of the umbilicus, but in practice this has not
proved to be the case.

The flaps are not used until their vitality has been tested,
until their capability of sustaining what may be termed a
partly independent existence has been proved, and until they
have undergone considerable contraction.

Thiersch's operation has on the whole decided advantages
over Wood's method, and in its principles it is more fully in
accord with those of modern plastic surgery.

Modifications of Thiersch's Operation.—Billroth adopts
the following method (*Clinical Surgery, Syd. Soc. Trans.*,
1881, page 285):—"I have come to the conclusion that the best
method is to dissect up two broad, lateral, doubly-peduncu-
lated flaps, whose narrow parts lie above and below. After
ten or fourteen days, when the under surface is granulating
well, I unite the two in the middle line without cutting
through the peduncles. If the flaps be sufficiently broad,
there is no need to unite them by their outer edges; these
lateral openings close spontaneously, in from five to six weeks.
The bladder is thus completely closed in, but an opening
should be left at the umbilicus through which the urine may
escape until the urethra below is completely formed; then the
umbilical opening is closed, and it heals up as the urine
escapes from the newly-formed passage. . . . The flaps
must be very broad—that is to say, in an adult they should be
at least 6 c.m. broad in the middle, and about 5 c.m. at the
upper and lower parts.

" The flaps should be so completely detached as to overlap each other for about half their width; a sheet of tin-foil is then laid underneath them in their whole length. In a few days they approximate so much that their curved shape becomes straight; later, notwithstanding a certain amount of rigidity, they will readily unite in the middle line. A broad surface must be made by scraping away the granulations and the superficial developing epidermis from the edges."

Maury's Operation.—This method must be included among the flap methods. It was considered by the late Professor Gross to be the method best adapted for the male subject. It is a modification of the original operation by Roux, and was described in 1871 (*Amer. Journ. of the Med. Sciences*, July, 1871):—

"A flap is taken from the perineum and scrotum by carrying a curvilinear incision from the outer third of Poupart's ligament across the middle of the perineum to a corresponding point on the opposite side. The flap is dissected up carefully, to avoid wounding the testicles or hernia, should the latter be present, until the root of the penis is reached, when that organ is slipped through a small opening made for it in the centre of the flap, by which means the urine issues without coming in contact with the wound. A curvilinear incision is then carried across the abdomen, and a short flap dissected up for about an inch; under this the scrotal flap, its cutaneous surface having been vivified, is slid and attached by several points of a modification of the tongue and groove suture of Professor Pancoast" (Gross).

This operation is simple, but little information is forthcoming as to the success which has attended it. It has been proved that the tissues of the scrotum are not well adapted to form the substance of a principal or primary flap.

3. OPERATIONS FOR NARROWING THE DEFECTIVE AREA BY APPROXIMATING THE TWO INNOMINATE BONES.

Professor Trendelenburg, of Bonn (*Centralblatt für Chirurgie*, Dec., 1885), is the originator of this method of treatment.

It is well known that in ectopia vesicæ the symphysis

pubis is deficient, and that a gap exists between the two pubic bones, which, according to Wood, may measure from two to four inches. Trendelenburg divides the sacro-iliac synchondrosis on either side, and finds that it is then possible to bring the two pubic bones together by quite slight pressure. The lateral margins of the defect are freshened, and are brought together when the bones are approximated. Immediate union of the wound is aimed at. The results obtained by this operation have been striking and very satisfactory.

Trendelenburg has performed the operation in at least five cases, four males and one female.

In one case failure occurred at the first operation, but success attended the second attempt at closure.

In two instances, immediate union of the lateral walls was obtained. In only one case had the formation of flaps to be resorted to.

An excellent account of the operation, with a successful case, has been given by Mr. Makins in the *Med.-Chir. Trans.* for 1888.

Best Age for the Operation.—Trendelenburg considers that the operation should be limited to a period between the ages of two and five years, and that the latter age is the most suitable.

In the case of failure above alluded to the patient was only fourteen months old.

The Operation.—The distances between the · anterior superior iliac spines and between the two pubic bones having been recorded, the patient is anæsthetised, and is turned upon the face.

An incision is made directly over each sacro-iliac synchondrosis. The average length of this incision will be about three inches.

The posterior sacro-iliac ligaments are exposed and freely divided. The knife is then passed into the cleft, and the interosseous and superior ligaments, together with the interarticular cartilage, are severed.

The bleeding is trifling. The anterior superior iliac spines are now approximated, and the joints will then be found to gape posteriorly to such an extent as to allow the introduction of the forefinger.

The two wounds are then closed, and a drain introduced, if necessary. A suitable dressing is applied.

Extension of the joints is provided for by Mr. Makins in the following way:—

The patient is placed in a cot, and a pelvic belt on which three loops of strong webbing have been sewn is applied to the anterior borders of the pelvis. These loops are crossed as a many-tailed bandage, and are carried over the opposite side of the cot, where weights are attached to them. These weights tend to draw the ilia together.

Very great care has to be taken to prevent urine from trickling down and reaching the wounds over the articulations.

When the wounds are healed, the attempt to close in the bladder may be made.

In Mr. Makins's case nearly two months were allowed to elapse between the division of the synchondrosis and the attempt to close the defect in the bladder. By this time the exposed surface of the bladder appeared at the bottom of a more or less narrow vertical groove.

The margins of the defect are freshened and dissected up, and are mobilised as far as is required. They are then approximated by sutures in the median line. A tube is introduced into the bladder, and is retained there.

Comment.—The advantages and disadvantages of the operation are fully dealt with in Mr. Makins's paper.

It is claimed for this measure that it is simple, that it effects a great saving of time, that it may possibly be completed in two operations, and that it is very satisfactory in its results. All these points must be allowed, and the operation must take a very high position among the methods available for ectopia vesicæ.

The main objection urged against the operation is that it tends to weaken the pelvis. It is well known that the pelvis in these cases is defective, and that the waddling gait of the patient is to some extent due to the deformity of this part of the skeleton. The symphysis pubis is wanting, the ossa innominata do not come into contact in front, and to divide the posterior and almost only remaining connections of the bones would appear to prepare the way for serious weakening of the pelvic girdle. Up to the present time, however, this theoretical objection has not been found to hold good in practice. The patients operated upon have walked well after the period of convalescence was passed.

It must be allowed that although the posterior synchondroses are opened up, yet that the anterior synchondrosis is to some extent restored, and that the rotation of the ilia, which is a feature in these cases, is overcome.

The value of the operation can only be tested by time.

It must be remembered that the operation can only be carried out in young patients, and in female subjects it is possible that an undesirable degree of narrowing of the pelvis may result. The extent to which the joints are freed must depend upon the needs of the case. The partial separation effected in Mr. Makins's case allowed the anterior superior iliac spines to be approximated one inch in a boy aged eight. With complete freeing of the joints Trendelenburg has lessened the distance between the two spines by two inches in a child aged two and a half years.

Such entire rupture of the connection between the ilium and the sacrum should be limited to extreme cases.

Neudörfer's Operation has been the outcome of a study of Trendelenburg's method.

Neudörfer does not separate the synchondroses, but he attempts to secure immediate union of the lateral margins of the defect—after they have been duly freshened—precisely as Trendelenburg does.

He relieves tension, and renders the approximation of the margins possible, by means of two lateral horseshoe-shaped incisions, which are carried through the whole thickness of the abdominal wall, down to the fascia transversalis. These incisions are convex outwards. Before bringing the cutaneous margins together, he detaches the mucous membrane of the bladder to a sufficient extent to allow of the two sides of the membrane being united by sutures in the median line. Over this cap of mucous membrane the skin is united as already described.

The penis and urethra are displaced backwards and downwards behind the symphysis.

The pubic bones on each side have their surfaces freshened, and are brought together by sutures.

THE AFTER-TREATMENT OF CASES OF ECTOPIA VESICÆ.

After any operation every care must be taken to prevent the urine from coming in contact with the wound.

To effect this end, the patient should be propped up in bed in a sitting posture, the shoulders must be well raised; a thick pillow must be placed under the knees, and the thighs should be kept drawn up by means of a bandage which passes under the knees, and across the shoulders and back.

The bed should be provided with a proper macintosh, and with such a mattress that the urine can escape through a funnel-shaped opening in the centre of the bed.

Troublesome erections may be controlled by the application of ice.

The bladder should be frequently washed out with a warm solution of boracic acid, and the tube placed in the urethra should be frequently changed.

Special care will be needed to prevent the formation of bed-sores.

Mr. Parker kept his patients in a hip bath of warm boracic lotion throughout the whole of the after-treatment, with the result that almost complete primary union followed a flap operation. With care the position of the patient in a hip bath may be made so comfortable that he will rest better in the bath than in the constrained and cramped position he must of necessity occupy in bed. The discomfort of lying upon a wet macintosh is also not inconsiderable.

It is needless to say that the lotion in the bath must be maintained at an even temperature, and be constantly changed.

Thiersch and others advise the use of a compressorium after the operation has been quite completed.

This instrument is intended to occlude the newly-made urethra, and to be removed when required.

It cannot be recommended, on these grounds:—In the first place, the capacity of the new bladder is very small; and in the second place, the constant pressure of the instrument is capable of producing a slough, or even a urinary fistula.

In the most successful cases a urinal cannot be dispensed with.

Results of the Operation Generally.—The results claimed

in the most successful cases are that the raw surface of the
bladder is protected and covered in, and that a urinal can be
worn which will keep the patient quite dry. Many patients
are free from the inconvenience of incontinence when they are
lying down, but in no instance can it be claimed that the
patient has acquired a control over the bladder.   These
results, however, are very satisfactory when the miserable
condition of the patients before operation is considered.

In placing the circumstances of operative treatment before
the patient's friends, the following facts must receive due consideration:—1. Patients with ectopia have reached old age,
and have had no operation performed.   2. It may still be
possible to secure an apparatus which will protect the bladder
and efficiently collect the urine.   3. The treatment is tedious
and painful, and may extend over many months, or over some
years.   In one case, as we have mentioned (page 99), treated
by Billroth no less than nineteen operations were performed.
4. The operative treatment is not without risk.   Ashhurst
states that he finds records of twenty deaths in 100 cases of
operation (" Encyclopædia of Surgery," vol. vi., page 339).

This average is probably below the actual death-rate, for
while all successful cases are almost sure to be reported, the
same publicity is not always accorded to the cases which die.
I should imagine that few operations in surgery are attended
with a larger percentage of partial or complete failures than
are the flap operations for extroversion of the bladder.

CHAPTER VIII.

OPERATIONS FOR ACQUIRED URETHRAL FISTULA.

THE remaining operations upon the urethra consist almost exclusively of various methods which have been adopted for the purpose of closing acquired urethral fistulæ. These operations involve no especial feature in plastic surgery, and will only be very briefly alluded to.

The principal difficulty in effecting a closure of these fistulæ depends upon the fact that the wound is apt to be saturated with urine every time the patient empties the bladder.

If this difficulty can be met, the treatment of these sinuses becomes comparatively simple.

It must be assumed, in the first place, that the cause of the fistula has been dealt with. In a very large proportion of cases the sinus has followed upon stricture, and it is needless to say that no treatment of the fistula will be of avail until the stricture has been cured.

Assuming, then, that the parts have been placed in the best possible condition for healing, the difficulty incident upon the passage of the urine can be most effectually met by establishing a perineal fistula through such an incision as would be made in median or lateral cystotomy.

Through such a wound the whole of the urinary current can be diverted if a suitable tube be retained in the bladder during the healing process. The ease with which such incisions close as soon as the urine is allowed to escape once more by the urethra is well known.

If there be any objection raised to the incurring of such small risks as attend a simple cut made into the bladder, then the surgeon must attempt to close the fistula while the urine is still passing by the natural passage.

In any such case a soft catheter must be introduced into

i 2

the bladder, and must be retained there until the wound has
healed.   To the end of this catheter must be attached a long
tube with a free lumen, whereby the urine as soon as it enters
the bladder can be conducted directly to a vessel placed
beneath the patient's bed.

If moderate good fortune attend the case, such a catheter
may be comfortably retained for a week, and at the end of
that time it may be withdrawn, the urethra washed out with
some mild antiseptic solution, and a fresh instrument, if
necessary, introduced.

In some instances, for one reason or another, the catheter
cannot be retained.   Very often it excites catarrh of the
bladder or urethra, and a muco-purulent discharge escapes at
the meatus.   In these cases it is of little avail to persist in
attempts to close the fistula, and the least risk and the least
inconvenience to the patient are involved in at once establishing a temporary opening at the neck of the bladder.

The skin of the penis is not very well adapted for plastic
measures.   It has the advantage of being mobile, but it is at
the same time very thin, and not capable of an active granulating process.

The operations which may be carried out in these cases
are the following :—

1. The margins of the fistula may be freshened, and
directly united by sutures.   Any tension upon the sutures
may be met either by means of lateral incisions or by freely
mobilising the integument all round the seat of the abnormal
opening.

2. The fistula may be closed by the process known as the
method by gliding or lateral displacement.   (*See* page 4.)

3. The closure may be effected by means of flaps, which
may be single or double, lateral or antero-posterior.

The formation of a pedunculated flap, and the adjusting of
the same by means of torsion, is not well adapted for this
part of the body.

The use of one reversed and two superimposed flaps has
been attended with considerable success.

The general plan of such an operation is identical with
that of Nélaton's operation for epispadias (page 83).

A long narrow median flap may be dissected up from the

tissues immediately behind or in front of the fistula. The base of the flap would correspond with the posterior or anterior margin of the fistula.

The flap is raised and is reversed, so that its skin surface is turned towards the urethra. It is attached to the freshened margins of the defect. Over it two lateral flaps are drawn, so as to cover its raw surface and to further strengthen the shield which is made to protect the breach. These lateral flaps will be united to one another in the median line.

It will be obvious that this last-mentioned measure is susceptible of considerable variation and modification. In connection with this subject the section on hypospadias (page 93) may be consulted.

CHAPTER IX.

OPERATIONS FOR RUPTURED PERINEUM.

Anatomical Points.—In the great majority of instances
the rupture for which an operation is required has occurred
during labour. If the laceration extend into the rectum, and
involve the sphincter ani, it is termed "complete." If it fall
short of the rectal tissues, it is described as "partial." In
carrying out the needed operation the surgeon must bear
in mind that he has not merely to form a bridge of skin

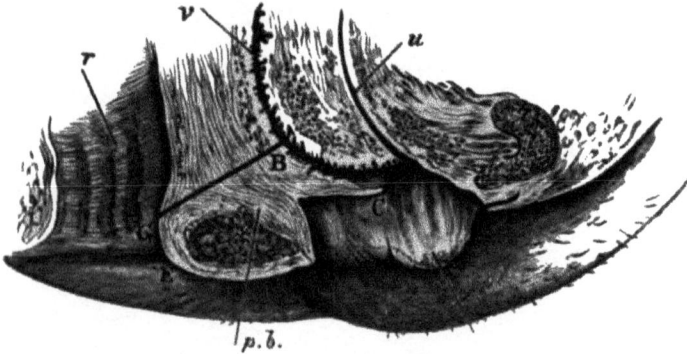

Fig. 299.—SAGITTAL SECTION OF FEMALE PERINEUM. (*Modified from Henle.*)
r, Rectum ; *v*, Vagina ; *u*, Urethra ; *n*, Nympha ; *p. b.*, Perineal body.

between the vagina and the rectum, but to restore the perineal
body. The term perineal body has been applied to the
pyramidal mass of tough elastic connective tissue which is
interposed between the lower ends of the rectum and vagina.
It is shown in part in the accompanying figure from Henle
(Fig. 299). The base of the pyramid corresponds to the skin
extending between the vagina and anus, which skin represents
the anatomical perineum. The apex is at some distance above
the orifices of the two canals. It may be roughly estimated
that the perineal body will measure about one inch and a

quarter in height, and one inch and a half in breadth. The complete restoration of this important supporting buttress is the main feature in operations for ruptured perineum.

In the anterior part of the base of the perineal body is the central point of the perineum, at which point the sphincter muscles of both the vagina and anus and the transverse perineal muscles meet.

When some weeks or months have elapsed after the laceration has occurred, and when the parts have well healed over, it is a little difficult at first to realise what has been the full extent of the injury, and what must be the full extent of the restoration. This is especially the case when the parts are patulous, when the mucous membrane is bulging downwards, and when the cicatrix is ill-marked.

The torn surfaces, which should be in contact, and vertically placed, are now widely separated, and are reduced to nearly the same horizontal plane. The position of the structures concerned can be best understood by comparing Fig. 299 with Fig. 301.

The raw surfaces C B G E and D B G F (Fig. 301) represent the perineal body split into two parts. The lines C E and D F were, before the accident, in the median line of the perineum. (*See* Henle, Fig. 299, C E.) They formed the raphé, and corresponded to the base of the perineal body. The apex of the perineal body is represented by the tissues along the line B G (Figs. 299 and 301); and the distance between B G on the one hand, and C E or D F on the other, will represent the "height" of the perineal body. It is not always easy at once to recognise that the central tissues about the line B G, which appear to continue the posterior median raphé of the vagina, and which are nearly on a level with the surrounding skin, should properly be placed at a point some inch and a quarter above the orifice of the anus and the skin of the perineum.

The pyramid forming the perineal body has been split into two, and has collapsed. The new raphé of the perineum will be formed when the lines C E and D F (Fig. 301) are brought together, the new vaginal raphé when C B and B D are approximated, and the new rectal raphé when G E and G F are united on the median line.

Preliminary Treatment.—It is always advisable to close the rent as soon as possible after the laceration has been produced. This may be attended with success, but the success will, as a rule, be partial only.

In the most usual circumstances the rupture will be of some weeks' standing when the case comes before the surgeon's notice, and the rent surfaces will have healed over.

It is desirable that the patient be in good health, and that there be no local complications. It is very important that the rectum should be empty, and that the intestinal canal should contain as little *débris* as possible. This is ensured by a few days' dieting, by the liberal use of aperients, and by the administration of an enema on the eve of the operation.

An existing vaginal discharge should be got rid of if possible. The condition is not infrequently complicated by piles; but unless these are of severe degree, they form no obstacle to the operation.

The parts must be very thoroughly cleansed before the operation, and any hair upon the perineum may be shaved off.

Operative Measures.—The treatment of ruptured perineum by operation dates from the time of Ambrose Paré. The procedures adopted by the older surgeons were simple enough. The torn surfaces were refreshed, and were united by sutures. In modern times innumerable modifications have been introduced. An essentially simple operation has been complicated by a number of intricate, and often ridiculous, methods. There is no form of suture designed by man that has not been tried upon the female perineum. The literature of the matter is voluminous and confusing, and is burdened with a perfect medley of ineffective terms. The subject has, in fact, been somewhat over-specialised, and the primary simplicity of the operation only becomes evident when it is freed of all such rags and tatters as do not belong to the bare elements of surgery. The operation below described is the simplest, and, so far as my own experience goes, the best. In Dr. Parvin's article in Ashhurst's "Encyclopædia of Surgery" (vol. vi., page 688) will be found an account of some of the many different methods which are carried out in this region. The description of the operation given by Dr. Galabin, in his work on

"Diseases of Women," is clear and admirable, and has been largely followed in the subjoined account. The two woodcuts which illustrate the operation have been derived from the same source.

OPERATION FOR PARTIAL RUPTURE.

The patient is placed in the lithotomy position, and the thighs are supported by means of Clover's crutch. The buttocks are brought well up to the end of the table. The

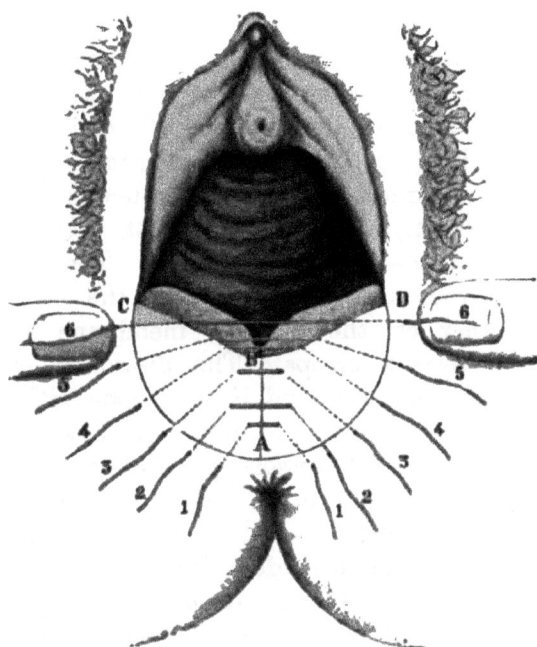

Fig. 300.—REPAIR OF RUPTURED PERINEUM. (*Galabin.*)

surgeon sits facing the perineum. Two assistants stand by the patient's pelvis, and each retracts the labium with one hand, while he sponges and otherwise assists the operator with the other. The extent of surface to be freshened is indicated, to some degree, by the cicatrix left by the laceration. "It is well, however, to go a little beyond the limits of this in all directions, especially up the median line of the vagina, and towards the lower halves of the labia majora, both in order

to secure, if possible, a perineal body somewhat larger and
deeper than the original one, and to allow some margin, in
case the surfaces do not unite completely up to the edges.
To put the mucous membrane on the stretch an assistant at
each side places one or two fingers on the skin of the thigh,
and draws the vulva outwards. The skin just beneath A
(Fig. 300), in front of the anus, may also be seized by a tenaculum, and drawn downwards. If still the mucous membrane is
not sufficiently on the stretch, from laxity of the vagina, the
posterior vaginal wall, some distance above B, should be
seized by long-handled tenaculum forceps, and pushed
upwards.

"Incisions are then made through the mucous membrane,
from B to A, in the median line of the vagina, and from
A to C and D, through the junction of the mucous membrane and skin (Fig. 300). These should not be extended in the direction of C and D further than the lower
extremity of the nymphæ at the utmost. There are then
two triangular flaps—A B C and A B D. These are to be
dissected up from the apex A towards the base B C and
B D, the corner of the mucous membrane at A being
seized with dissecting forceps. The dissection should not
be deeper than necessary, and if it is done with the knife
the surfaces are more ready to unite. If, however, there is
much tendency to bleed, scissors may be used. The apices
of the flaps are then cut off with scissors, leaving an
upturned border along B C and B D. When the surfaces
are drawn together, these borders form a slightly elevated
ridge towards the vagina; and if there be any failure of
union just along the edge, they fall over and cover it"
(Galabin).

Silkworm gut forms the best suture material. The
sutures may be most conveniently introduced, either by
means of a curved needle in a handle or by means of a
large Hagedorn's needle held in a holder. They should be
introduced as shown in Fig. 300, the dotted lines representing
the buried parts of the suture. The sutures 1, 2, and 3 may
be buried along the whole length of their course. "If, however," writes Dr. Galabin, "they are brought out in the centre
for spaces alternately short and long (Fig. 300), the surfaces are

more easily brought into contact at all levels without undue tension."

The sutures 4, 5, and 6 are brought out close to the margin along which the folds of mucous membrane, B C B D, are turned up from the vagina, and are not passed through the mucous membrane itself.

The sutures are tied in order from behind forwards—*i.e.*,

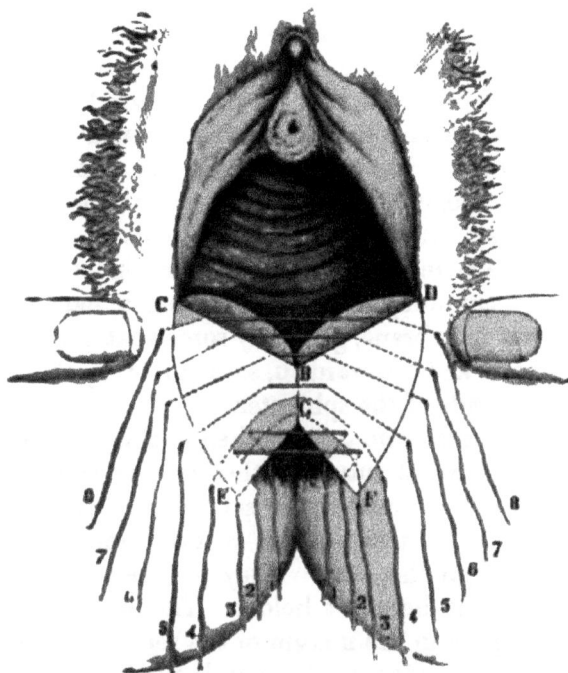

Fig. 301.—REPAIR OF RUPTURED PERINEUM.   (*Galabin.*)

from No. 1 to No. 6. As they are being secured a stream of some antiseptic solution from an irrigator should be allowed to play over the surface, in order that no blood clot may be enclosed in the depths of the wound.

OPERATION FOR COMPLETE RUPTURE.

The preliminary measures, already described, having been taken, the operation is proceeded with as follows :—

"A point (B, Fig. 301) in the median line of the vagina, a

sufficient distance above the apex of the rent in the septum, is taken, and an incision through the mucous membrane is made from B to G, and from G to E and F along the edges of the septum, between the rectal mucous membrane and the cicatrix. Incisions are also made through the skin from E to C, and F to D, so that the freshened surface may extend somewhat beyond the limits of the cicatrix, C or D not to be higher than the lower extremities of the nymphæ. The quadrilateral flap E G B C is then seized at E by dissecting forceps, and dissected up with the knife from the angle E, and afterwards from the angle G, towards the base B C. While this is done the parts are kept on the stretch by an assistant drawing down the skin below B with a tenaculum. The flap is then cut away with scissors, except an upturned border, which is left along B C. The flap F G B D is treated in a similar manner. If, as is usual, the ends of the sphincter at E and F have retracted from the margin of the cicatrix, it is well to cut away with the scissors a narrow strip of rectal mucous membrane, generally somewhat everted, a short distance from E and F towards G, so as to bring the freshened surface to the ends of the sphincter.

" Sutures of silkworm gut are then applied in the following manner :—First rectal sutures, either two or three, according to the extent of the rent in the septum, are applied. These are destined to be tied in the rectum, and the ends left projecting through the anus. They are best applied with a half-curved needle, held in a holder. The needle is passed in a little distance from the margin of the rent, and brought out almost at the very edge of the rectal mucous membrane, on the line G F. The needle is then threaded at the other end of the suture, and that is drawn through in the same way from without inwards on the margin E G. Next, two sutures at least are passed completely round through the remnant of the septum, by means of a curved needle, not too large, mounted in a handle. This is passed unthreaded, and draws the suture back with it on withdrawal. The first of these (3, Fig. 301) is passed in somewhat behind and below the angle F, so as to take up, if possible, or at least go quite close to, the end of the divided sphincter, and is brought out in a similar position near E. Thus, when tightened, it brings together the ends of the sphincter, drawing it into a circle; but it often brings into apposition, not so much the freshened surfaces above as the unfreshened rectal mucous membrane. This serves as a barrier to keep out fæcal matter, while the next suture (4) aids the rectal sutures in uniting the freshened surfaces. The remaining sutures (5 to 8) are passed, as shown in the figure, by a slightly-curved needle mounted in a handle, in the same way as in the operation for incomplete rupture" (Galabin).

When all the sutures are in position they are tied in the order of their numbers, and the operation is completed as in the previous account.

After-treatment of Cases of Ruptured Perineum.

After the operation the patient must lie in bed until the wound is sound and the sutures all removed. This will represent a period of from fourteen to twenty-one days.

The patient should be encouraged to lie upon the side. A cradle should be placed over the pelvis, the space under the bed-clothes should be ventilated, and every opportunity be taken to change the heated and close atmosphere with which the wound must of necessity be surrounded.

It is never necessary to tie the legs together, as was the barbarous and senseless custom at one period. No T-bandage is required. The wound is best dressed with iodoform. This may be liberally dusted over the part, the wound being left otherwise quite uncovered; or a "sanitary towel" well treated with iodoform may be worn, and the wound be supported by the soft pad of the "towel." The part should be kept throughout as dry as possible.

Opium and morphia should be avoided. Great difficulty with the bowels may result if these drugs are made use of. The following case, which came under my notice some years ago, serves to illustrate this point.

The patient was a young and nervous woman, and the rupture had occurred during her first confinement. It was complete. It was closed by operation six weeks after the birth of the child. The operation appeared to be quite successful. Silk sutures were employed. Opium was freely given. No attempt was made to bring about any action of the bowels until the eighth day, when an

enormous mass of hard fæcal matter was passed with intense
pain, and the wound was torn open from one extremity to the
other.

The urine should be drawn off as frequently as is
required during the first few days by means of a catheter.
The vulva must be kept scrupulously clean and dry. It may
be advisable to order a vaginal douche of some antiseptic
lotion to be employed every morning. The parts must be well
dried after its use.

The bowels should be opened by castor-oil on the morning
of the fourth day, assuming that they have not acted
naturally before then. The sutures may be removed between
the eighth and the fourteenth days.

In the case of the complete operation the perineal sutures
are removed first, and the rectal sutures at a later period.
The removal is in the reverse order to the introduction. A
small rectal speculum will probably be required when the
rectal stitches are taken out.

A note must be made at the time of the operation of the
number of sutures inserted, as it is not uncommon to find,
when weeks have elapsed, that one thread has been overlooked.

CHAPTER X.

OPERATIONS FOR THE RELIEF OF WEBBED FINGERS.

THIS somewhat common congenital deformity is usually symmetrical. The last two fingers are the ones which are most frequently found fused or joined together. If the web be but slightly developed, the usefulness of the hand may be little interfered with. If an operation be considered necessary, it should be carried out early—about the ages of six or eight. Operations much before this period are attended with risks and difficulties which it is unnecessary to encounter. The conditions of the operation depend upon the degree of the deformity. In the most favourable cases there is merely an extension forwards between the fingers of the normal web. This membrane may be comparatively thin and wide, and allow of considerable separation of the fingers (Fig. 302). In other instances the uniting material is thick, the fingers are joined closely together, and on a transverse section of the hand the "web" would be found to be almost as thick as the fingers themselves (Fig. 303). In the most severe cases the phalanges are actually fused together, and no separation can be effected by surgical means.

Many operations have been carried out in these cases. A useful summary of them, and an excellent bibliography, will be found in Beely's monograph in Gerhardt's "Handbuch der Kinderkrankheiten," 1880.

The Division of the Web after a Cicatrised Hole has been Established.—Rudtorffer's Operation.

A hole is made through the web at the root of the fingers, and about the spot where the natural web would cease. Through this hole a piece of thick silver wire, the size of a No. 5 to a No. 8 catheter, is passed. Its ends are bent back towards the wrist, and are secured there.

In the place of the wire a solid indiarubber cord of the

same or of larger size may be employed. Its ends also will be secured to a bracelet at the wrist.

The little wound suppurates and granulates, and in due course heals, just as does the hole made in the pinna for an earring. The process of healing is usually slow, and throughout the progress of the case the part must be treated with antiseptic care. As the child will probably be running about during the treatment, the wound may easily become septic, unless every precaution is taken. I have seen a very severe and extensive degree of inflammation follow this operation in a case in which the wound became septic.

When the wound has firmly healed, the wire or cord is removed, and after a few days have been allowed to elapse the web is divided down to the cicatrised spot. The two fingers are kept well covered up and well separated during the time required for the healing of the two lateral wounds.

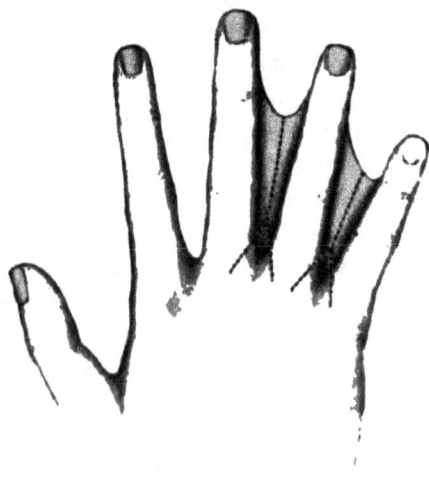

Fig. 302.—ZELLER'S OPERATION FOR WEBBED FINGERS.

This method answers very well in cases where the web is thin and comparatively wide.

It was first introduced by Rudtorffer, who used a leaden thread for the purpose ("Abhandlung über die Operation eingesperrter Brüche nebst einem Anhang," vol. ii., page 478, Wien, 1801).

Zeller's Operation.

This measure has undergone certain modifications since it was introduced by Zeller ("Über d. ersten Erscheinungen vener. Localkrankht.," page 109, Wien, 1810).

A triangular or V-shaped flap is raised on the dorsal aspect of the root of the web. Its base will correspond to the situation of the natural web. Its apex will reach about to the first inter-phalangeal joint.

The flap involves not only the tissues of the abnormal web, but also a little of the skin upon the dorsum of the adjacent phalanges (Fig. 302).

After it has been marked out and dissected up, the whole of the abnormal web is divided. The apex of the flap is then drawn down between the fingers, and it is attached by sutures to the skin of the palm, a suitable raw surface having been made to receive it.

The fingers must be fixed well apart during the healing process, lest the flap be unduly compressed.

A splint composed of two metal rings—one for each finger—with an adjustable bar between them, answers the purpose very well.

There is a tendency for the tip of the flap to slough, and to meet this it must be made of sufficient length. Dieffenbach made the flap of quadrilateral outline.

In any instance it must be narrow to avoid being compressed between the fingers.

Two triangular flaps have been cut, one on the dorsal and the other on the palmar aspect of the web, the dorsal flap being a little the longer of the two.

This operation, which seems to have fallen a little

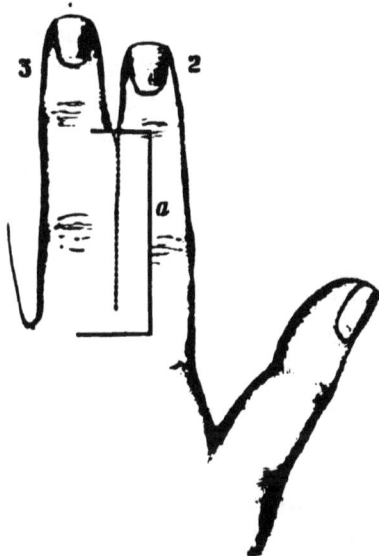

Fig. 303.—DIDAY'S OPERATION FOR WEBBED FINGERS.

into disuse in Great Britain, has been revived of late. (See paper by Mr. Norton, *British Medical Journal*, 1881, vol. ii., page 931.)

I have had only one opportunity of carrying out Zeller's operation, and in that one instance it answered admirably. It is best adapted for cases in which the uniting tissue between the fingers is not too thick—as measured from the dorsal to the palmar surface—and where the fingers are not brought into the closest contact.

j

Diday's Operation.—In this method two flaps are fashioned, the first from the dorsum of one finger, and the second from the palmar aspect of the other. The two flaps are adjusted after the fingers have been separated in the manner described below.

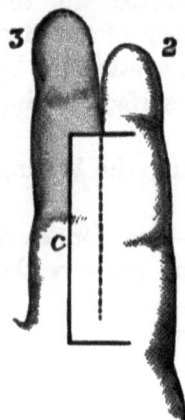

This operation is called by some Didot's operation, and by others Nélaton's operation.

A description of the procedure was furnished by Didot in 1850, but it would appear that Diday has a prior claim. I have not been able to obtain access to the original paper in the *Presse Méd. Belge*, but a full abstract of Diday's (or Diaday's) paper appears in the *Journal für Kinderkrankheiten*, xv., page 470, 1850.

Fig. 304. — DIDAY'S OPERATION FOR WEBBED FINGERS.

Two narrow quadrilateral flaps are fashioned, one on the dorsal aspect of one of the united fingers (*a*, Fig. 303), the other on the palmar aspect of the other finger (*c*, Fig. 304). These flaps must be carefully planned out. Their length will correspond to the length of the web, and their breadth to the breadth of the raw surface each flap has to cover. Each flap will be a little wider at its proximal than at its distal end.

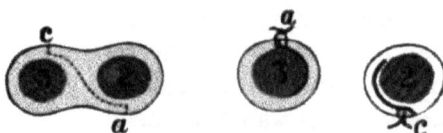

Fig. 305. — DIDAY'S OPERATION FOR WEBBED FINGERS.

The free edge of each flap will extend up to the median line of the finger at its distal end, but will extend beyond that line at its proximal end.

The two flaps are dissected up. They must not be too thin. If, on the other hand, they are too thick, they are difficult to adjust.

When they have been well separated, the remaining tissue which unites the two fingers is divided.

The dorsal flap from the one finger covers the raw surface on the palmar aspect of the other, while the palmar flap taken from this latter finger covers the raw surface left on the dorsum of the first-named finger. (*See* Fig. 305 ; the letters *a* and *c* and the figures 2 and 3 correspond throughout.) The flaps are fixed in position by fine sutures.

This operation may be carried out in cases in which neither of the former methods is applicable. The procedure is difficult, and requires infinite care in its performance. The most probable fault will be the fashioning of flaps, which prove when adjusted to be too narrow towards their proximal extremity.

Part IX.

OPERATIONS ON THE NECK.

CHAPTER I.

TRACHEOTOMY.

Anatomical Points.—The trachea in the adult is about four and a half inches in length. It is surrounded by an atmosphere of lax connective tissue, which allows a considerable degree of mobility to the tube. The mobility of the trachea is greater in children than in adults. The length of the trachea in the neck is not so considerable as may at first sight appear, and, according to Holden, not more than seven or eight of the tracheal rings (which number sixteen to twenty in all) are to be found above the manubrium sterni. The distance between the cricoid cartilage and the sternal notch varies greatly, and depends upon the length of the neck, the age of the patient, and the position of the head. If two inches of the trachea are exposed above the sternum when the head is erect, then in full extension three-quarters of an inch more of the windpipe will, as it were, be drawn up into the neck. According to Tillaux, the average full distance between the cricoid cartilage and the sternum is in the adult about two and three quarter inches (7 c.m.). The full distance in a child between three and five years is about one inch and a half (4 c.m.); in a child between six and seven, about two inches (5 c.m.); and in children between eight and ten years, about two inches and a quarter (6 c.m.). The effects of growth, and of the position of the head upon the position of the cricoid cartilage, have been shown by Symington in his work on the "Anatomy of the Child." In a child about two years of age the lower border of the cricoid cartilage is opposite the upper border of the sixth cervical vertebra when the head is acutely flexed, and opposite the upper border of the fifth vertebra when it is extended. At birth the lower border of the cricoid cartilage corresponds with the lower border of the fourth cervical vertebra, between the age of six and twelve months it is opposite to the upper border of the fifth vertebra, at five years it corresponds to the upper border of the sixth vertebra, and in the adult to the upper border of the seventh.

Symington confirms the statement by Allan Burns that in a child twelve months old the distance from the hyoid bone to the sternum is equal to the breadth of three fingers; and if these be placed in front of the neck, one finger would cover the larynx, half a finger the isthmus of the thyroid body, and a finger and a half the space between the thyroid body and the sternum; while if the head be extended, the latter space would be increased to the breadth of two fingers.

With regard to the diameter of the trachea, and the size of the tube, the following table is founded upon the observations of Symington and Guersant. (*See* Fig. 306.)

AGE.	DIAMETER OF TUBE.
Under 18 months . . .	4 m.m.
1½ year to 2 years . . .	5 m.m.
2 years to 4 years . . .	6 m.m.
4 years to 8 years . . .	8 m.m.
8 years to 12 years . . .	10 m.m.
12 years to 15 years . .	12 m.m.
Adults	12 m.m. to 15 m.m.

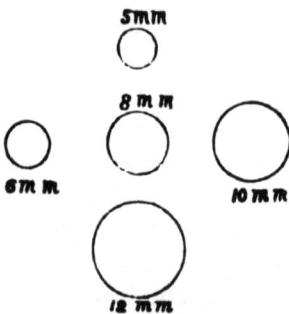

Fig. 306.—SECTIONS OF TRACHEOTOMY TUBES: SHOWING THE EXACT DIAMETERS, EXPRESSED IN MILLIMETRES.

The *relations of the trachea* are considered in the section which follows.

The Site of the Operation.— The operation is said to be " high " or " low," according as the trachea is opened above or below the isthmus of the thyroid body. In the adult the isthmus crosses the second and third rings of the trachea, and sometimes even the fourth. In the child the isthmus is narrow, and is usually somewhat higher up. It may even lie on the crico-tracheal membrane (Parker). The high operation is always to be preferred; it alone is described in the account which follows (V and VI, Fig. 308).

In cutting down upon the trachea in the middle line of the neck, from the cricoid cartilage to the sternum, the following parts are met with:—Beneath the integument lie the anterior jugular veins. As a rule these veins lie some little way apart on each side of the median line, and do not communicate, except by a large transverse branch which lies in the inter-fascial space at the upper border of the sternum. Sometimes there are many communicating branches in front of the tracheotomy district, or the veins may form almost a plexus in front of the trachea, or there may be a single vein which will follow the middle line. Then comes the cervical fascia, enclosing the sterno-hyoid and sterno-thyroid muscles. Above the isthmus a transverse communicating branch between the superior thyroid veins is sometimes found. Abnormal branches of the superior thyroid artery may cross the upper rings of the trachea. Over the isthmus is a small venous plexus, from which the inferior thyroid veins arise; while below the isthmus these veins lie in front of the trachea, together with the thyroidea ima artery (when it exists). The inferior thyroid vein may be represented by a single trunk occupying the middle line.

In the infant before the age of two years the thymus extends up for a variable distance in front of the trachea. At the very root of the neck the trachea is crossed by the innominate and left carotid arteries, and by the left innominate vein.

Advantages of the High Operation.—The anterior jugular veins are smaller here, and transverse branches are rare.

The muscles which are in close contact below diverge a little as they ascend. The great vessels are not in danger, the inferior thyroid vessels and the thyroidea ima are avoided.

The trachea is nearer the surface, is more fixed, and is much more readily exposed.

Disadvantages of the Low Operation.—The anterior jugular veins are larger, and transverse branches are common.

The muscles are in closer contact. The inferior thyroid veins and thyroidea ima are readily wounded. The great vessels and the thymus may be exposed to danger.

The trachea is much deeper, is more mobile, and is exposed with difficulty.

To these disadvantages Mr. Jacobson adds the following objections:—In the low operation (1) pus is more easily conducted into the mediastina; (2) broncho-pneumonia is more probable when the wound is low down in the trachea; (3) the suction action of the chest can more readily draw the tube into the wound when the incision is near to the thorax.

Instruments Required.—Scalpels; dissecting, artery, and pressure forceps; toothed forceps (Liston's artery forceps without the catch answer the purpose); sharp hook; blunt hook; scissors; needles; tracheotomy tubes and tapes. To these may be added a gag and tongue forceps, small wound retractors, and feathers to clear the tube, when first introduced.

A good tracheotomy tube should be of simple construction, should be easy to introduce, should be as large as the diameter of the trachea will admit, should lie exactly in the long axis of the windpipe without touching the tracheal wall with its extremity, should have a movable shield so that it is disturbed as little as possible, and the inner cannula should be capable of being easily inserted and removed.

Mr. Durham's well-known tubes are in all respects admirable; but care must be taken that no segment of the lobster-tail cannula is loose. Mr. Parker's tubes are spoken highly of by those who have used them, although it has been stated that they are somewhat difficult to introduce in little children.

THE OPERATION.

The patient is anæsthetised with chloroform.

1. **Position of the Patient.**—The child is enveloped in a thin macintosh sheet, and is placed close to the right edge of the table. The surgeon stands by the same side of the table. The neck is supported on a firm sand-bag of suitable size. When the child is ready the head should be drawn well over the upper end of the table, so that the vertex is turned nearly towards the ground.

The sand-bag will be placed close to the upper edge of the table, and over it the child's head is extended in this extreme manner.

This position renders the structures on the front of the neck tense, steadies the trachea, draws as much of that tube up into the neck as is possible, and brings it a little nearer to the surface. The superficial veins are, moreover, a little emptied of their blood by this attitude of over-extension.

The anæsthetist stands at the head of the table, and the important duty should be imposed upon him of holding the head steady, and of keeping the chin most rigidly in a line with the sternal notch. If the head be allowed to fall over to one or other side, the position of the middle line is lost.

An assistant stands by the side of the anæsthetist, and will, later, take charge of the sharp hook.

A second assistant, with sponges, etc., will take his place to the left of the table—*i.e.*, to the surgeon's right.

2. **The Exposing of the Trachea.**—An incision is made with a sharp scalpel very precisely in the median line of the neck. Its length will be about one inch or an inch and a half, and its upper extremity will be at the upper border of the cricoid cartilage. Before making this cut, the surgeon should have accurately defined the position of the thyroid and cricoid cartilages. The latter cartilage is often difficult to detect in stout subjects, and especially in young infants.

The skin and the trachea are steadied with the left hand while the cut is being made.

The right hand must be unsupported. If the operator rests his wrist upon the upper part of the child's chest, as he is tempted to do, he will find that the rapid movements of the thorax in laboured breathing render that part no proper place for support.

The surgeon, still fixing the trachea and soft parts with the left hand, cuts deliberately in the middle line through the subcutaneous fat and the anterior layer of the cervical fascia. The sterno-hyoid and sterno-thyroid muscles are reached, and the interval between them is opened up. All this is done by successive clean cuts.

The surgeon now separates the muscles, using the dissecting forceps and the handle of the scalpel for the purpose.

Keeping still to the middle line, and once more steadying the trachea, he divides cleanly, and by cautious cuts, the fascia covering that tube.

At this stage veins will probably be encountered, and may be displaced to one or other side by the handle of the scalpel. The isthmus of the thyroid will be seen, and is by a like means displaced downwards. If necessary, it may be drawn and held downwards by a small blunt hook.

The surgeon now feels for the tracheal rings with his left forefinger. He should be satisfied that the tube is well bared, and he should be able to see the white rings themselves.

3. **The Opening of the Trachea.**—A small sharp hook is now introduced into the cricoid cartilage, and is given to the assistant to hold who stands at the head of the table.

The hook is kept precisely in the middle line, and is used to fix and draw forwards the cricoid cartilage, and to render the trachea tense. The assistant must give a little play to the hook, as the larynx moves with each inspiration.

With the left forefinger the operator feels the upper rings of the trachea, and with a slender scalpel, held with the edge towards the patient's chin, he stabs the trachea in the median line some three rings below the cricoid, and cuts up on to the hook (v, Fig. 308).

The noisy rush of air entering and escaping through the wound, the coughing of the child, and the expulsion of mucus and membrane bring about a moment of confusion. The hook must not be removed. It remains as an easy guide to the median line of the trachea and the site of the opening therein. The opening must be free.

If the hook be not used, the operator may miss the slit in the trachea he has already made, and may, in his haste, proceed to make another one.

4. **The Introduction of the Tube.**—The right margin of the cut in the trachea should be lightly seized with the toothed forceps, which are held in the left hand ; and while the opening is thus for a moment demonstrated and fixed, the tube and pilot are slipped in. If the forceps be employed as directed, the tube can be introduced with certainty and ease.

If no such precaution be taken, much time may be wasted in driving the pilot hither and thither in search of the slit-like opening, which is very easily lost. The depth of the wound, the quantity of blood and mucus which may fill it, and the movements of the trachea, may readily cause the site of the opening to be lost, especially if the trachea has not been well exposed, and the fascia freely divided.

It will usually be found more convenient to restore the child's head to the erect position before the tube is introduced. When the tube is in place—and not before—the sharp hook is removed.

The tube is secured in place by tape, and the wound below the tube is brought together by a suture or two of silk-worm gut. A piece of lint properly shaped and smeared with a weak iodoform ointment is placed under the shield of the tube, and is made to cover and protect the wound.

Rapid and efficient sponging with small pieces of fine Turkey sponge is of great service throughout the operation.

5. The Detachment of Diphtheritic Membrane.—Mr. Parker advises that before the tube be inserted, an attempt should be made in all cases of diphtheria to rid the trachea of false membranes and retained secretions. This he accomplishes by means of a long feather which has been dipped in the following solution :—Bicarbonate of potash or soda, ʒij ; glycerine, ʒj ; water, ʒx. The feather is passed into the windpipe, and is twirled about so as to detach the membrane as completely as possible. Some is withdrawn, some is coughed up. The feather may be also passed up into the larynx and through the glottis.

This potash solution is said to dissolve and detach the secretions.

TRACHEOTOMY BY BOSE'S METHOD.

This method—often termed the bloodless method—is extensively practised in Germany.

A vertical incision is made in the median line. It commences opposite the centre of the thyroid cartilage, and is continued downwards for about one and a half or two inches. The incision is carried down to the lower part of the thyroid cartilage and the upper part of the cricoid. The soft parts being held aside by retractors, a transverse incision is made along the upper border of the cricoid cartilage in such a way as to divide the layer of the deep cervical fascia which lies in front of the trachea, and which holds the thyroid isthmus. A blunt director is now introduced through this transverse incision, and by its means the fascia and the isthmus, together with all the veins connected therewith, are fully separated from the trachea. A broad, curved hook (Fig. 307) is now

Fig. 307. — HOOK USED FOR DRAWING DOWNWARDS THE THYROID GLAND IN TRACHEOTOMY, ETC.

introduced, and the detached fascia, together with the other soft parts, is drawn downwards, leaving the trachea quite bare. The cricoid cartilage is now fixed by means of a double-pointed sharp hook, and the tracheal rings are incised in the usual way.

This method has much to commend it. It is simple and easy of performance. It involves some expenditure of time, and some damage may be done to adjacent structures by the director if care be not used. Veins are readily torn through by this instrument. If cautiously performed, the operation has distinct claims to be called " bloodless."

The procedure has been modified by Mr. Whitehead (*Lancet*, April 30, 1887), who carries out the tracheotomy as follows:—An incision is made in the usual situation, but of rather greater length than is common. The incision extends through the skin and fascia, as deep as the interval between the sterno-hyoid muscles. The scalpel is now laid aside, and the raspatory used, not only to separate the sterno-hyoids, but to split the strong fascia which runs down from the hyoid bone to enclose the isthmus of the thyroid gland. This fascia is split to a distance extending from the upper limit of the incision down to the isthmus below—that is, supposing it is desired to open the trachea above the isthmus. The split fascia is then pushed to right and left with the raspatory. Should there be any difficulty in doing this, the fascia is separated to some extent on each side from the upper border of the isthmus. Proceeding carefully, the isthmus itself can be pushed down and the trachea exposed to the necessary extent. If the trachea is to be opened below the isthmus, the procedure is similar—remembering that here, however, there is between the fascia and the trachea a quantity of areolar tissue, in which lies the inferior thyroid plexus of veins. The front of the trachea can in this way be cleared perfectly, and, since the method is bloodless, the rings of the tube are seen glistening white at the bottom of the wound. What is urged in favour of the operation is—firstly, the ease with which it can be performed; secondly, the small number of instruments required; and, thirdly, the manner in which it meets the four difficulties usually enumerated—viz., of reaching the trachea, of hæmorrhage, of opening the trachea, and of introducing the cannula. Again, it avoids in an especial manner those dangers met with when the operation is performed, as it too often is, practically in the dark—from the bleeding, and the not sufficient separation of the parts; thus it is impossible, in this operation, that the cannula should be pushed down between the trachea and the fascia lying in front of it, or that it should be thrust, as has actually happened, into the internal jugular vein.

Comment.—The operation, as here described, has been considered in connection with its most common surroundings—namely, with the operation urgent, and the patient a young child struggling against suffocation.

As an operation *quâ* operation, tracheotomy must be regarded as an easy and simple procedure. Those who have performed it only upon the dead subject must be at a loss to understand the terrible possibilities with which the introduction of a tracheotomy tube appears to be surrounded. In the adult, the operation is certainly but rarely in any way difficult or complicated; in an infant with a short stout neck, on the other hand, it may be attended with not inconsiderable difficulties.

For the accidents which so often occur during tracheotomy, the hurry and excitement of the operation, and the fear that the child is ceasing to breathe, are in the main answerable, and not the anatomical conditions of the operation itself.

Tracheotomy affords a striking illustration of the adage "the more haste the less speed." The surgeon who proceeds to open the trachea in a precise and deliberate way will have completed the operation before the frantic man who, with a palpitating heart and a trembling hand, cuts wildly towards the spine, and who appears to be actuated by the unsteady conviction that he must gash something or the child will perish. Artificial respiration may be relied upon to restore a patient who has ceased to breathe for some seconds, provided that the tube has been introduced without complication, and that the cessation of respiration does not depend upon uncontrollable conditions. The operation must be systematically done. The surgeon who seeks to be brilliant at this operation may be at once regarded as dangerous.

A child's trachea is very mobile, and it is marvellous to note the ease with which it may be made to collapse on pressure. To the finger roughly introduced the infant's trachea offers little resistance, and its mobility is such that it has been held aside unknowingly by retractors, while the operator is scoring the œsophagus (Durham).

The tracheal rings are very soft, and with a sharp scalpel little force is required to divide them.

I know an instance in which a young operator, in his anxious hurry, slit up the upper tracheal rings, together with the whole larynx, the knife only stopping at the hyoid bone.

The flimsiness of the infant's trachea cannot be too fully realised. I have seen a portion of the wall of the trachea bent upon itself, and forced by the pilot into the lumen of the windpipe. The opening in this instance was small, although it was found that the trachea had been incised in more than one place.

In young infants, and in children generally, care should be taken that the cricoid cartilage is not severed. If it be divided, the tube is found to be placed so near to the larynx as to produce undue irritation of it.

In children the isthmus of the thyroid body is small, may be disregarded, and may be safely divided if the section be in the median line. In adults it is readily recognised, and easily drawn downwards out of danger.

It must be expected that in almost every case there will be free venous bleeding. While it is well that the hæmorrhage should be checked before the tube is introduced, lest blood find its way into the lung, yet too long a time should not be devoted to attempting to secure the vessels. As soon as the tube is introduced, air enters the lung more freely, the right side of the heart is relieved, and venous bleeding, which before was very copious, ceases almost immediately.

The cervical fascia must be well and cleanly divided. The tube has many a time been introduced between the trachea and the imperfectly divided fascia, the operator being under the impression that it has been inserted into the windpipe. No air, however, escapes.

In cases where an extensive membrane exists, it may escape division when the trachea is opened, and the tube may then be inserted between the membrane and the tracheal wall. In this case, also, no air escapes from the instrument.

In most cases of tracheotomy performed by a novice, or carried out with undue haste, it will be observed that the time of the operation is more fully taken up by introducing the tube than by finding and incising the trachea.

If the hook and the toothed forceps be used as described, all bungling over the insertion of the tube may be avoided. Some time may be spent in endeavouring to find the slit which has been already made in the trachea.

No director is required in this operation, nor are the various dilators which have been devised really necessary, although they may be of use when much membrane has to be cleared away.

Some General Rules in Tracheotomy.—1. Let the chin be kept rigidly in a line with the sternal notch.

2. Cut only in the middle line.

3. Avoid anxious assistants with retractors.

4. See the white rings of the trachea, and feel them bare before plunging the knife into the windpipe.

5. Avoid hurry.

After-treatment.— This will obviously depend a great deal upon the nature of the case. The after-treatment of a case of tracheotomy performed for impacted foreign body will of necessity differ greatly from that performed for diphtheria. The period at which the tube has to be removed can never be decided in an arbitrary manner. It should be taken out at the earliest possible period. In a case of œdema of the glottis it may be possible to discontinue it at the end of a few days;

while when tracheotomy has been performed for a laryngeal growth, the tube may have to be worn during the remainder of the patient's life.

In a child, the sooner the rigid metallic cannula can be replaced by an indiarubber tube the better, especially if it be necessary to keep the tracheal sinus open for a prolonged period.

There is often much difficulty with children in getting them to take sufficient food; and if this difficulty be not readily overcome, it is well that the child should be fed, for a while, by means of a small Jacques' catheter passed down into the œsophagus through the nose.

With regard to the steam tent, or "croup bed," and the measures to be adopted to keep the tube clean, I cannot do better than quote the excellent and practical observations of Mr. Jacobson upon this head :—

"While fully aware of the need of moisture when the atmosphere is dry, when the membrane tends to crust and become fixed, I am of opinion that the unvarying rule of cot-tenting and use of steam is disadvantageous. The weakly condition of children with membranous laryngitis, and all they have gone through, must be remembered. Believing that such seclusion, and so little admission of air, tend to increase the asthenia, and any tendency to sepsis, I much prefer to be content to keep off draughts by a screen, which allows of the escape of vitiated air above, using steam, if needful, according to the size of the room, fireplace, etc., and according to the kind of expectoration, whether easily brought up by the cough or feathers, or viscid, quickly drying, and causing whistling breathing. If the temperature can be otherwise kept up to 60° or 65°, I much prefer to use a thin flat sponge, often wrung out in a warm solution of boracic acid. The inner tube must be frequently removed and cleansed, every hour or two at first. If the secretions dry on and cling to it, they are best removed by the soda solution mentioned below. At varying intervals between the removal of the tube, any membrane, etc., which is blocking it, appearing for a moment at its mouth and then sucked back, must be got rid of by inserting narrow pheasant feathers, and twisting them round before removing them. If the exudation is alight, moist, and easily brought up by cough or feather, sponging or brushing out the trachea is not called for, but should be made use of when there is much flapping, clicking, or whistling of the breathing; and if this is harsh, dry, or noisy, instead of moist and noiseless, two of the best solutions are sodæ bicarb., gr. v-xx to aq. ʒj, or a saturated one of borax with soda. These may be applied by a hand or steam spray over the cannula for five or ten minutes at a time, at intervals varying according to the relief which is given, or applied with a laryngeal brush, feather, or bit of sponge twisted securely into a loop of wire. When any of these are used, the risk of excoriation and bleeding, and the fact that only the trachea and large bronchi can be cleaned, must be borne in mind; and with regard to manipulations for cleansing the trachea and removing the inner tube, it is most important to remember that the caretaking may be overdone, and a weakly child still further exhausted by meddlesome interference."

LARYNGOTOMY.

Laryngotomy, or the artificial opening of the larynx through the crico-thyroid membrane, is occasionally performed as a substitute for tracheotomy. The operation has the advantage of being very rapidly and very easily carried out. It is quite inapplicable to children under thirteen years of age, owing to the narrowness of the crico-thyroid space. The great drawbacks of the operation are the proximity of the vocal cords and the difficulty of adjusting a suitable tube. Laryngotomy is totally unsuited for cases in which a tube has to be long worn.

The vertical height of the crico-thyroid space in the well-developed adult subject is only about half an inch.

The crico-thyroid arteries cross the space, but are usually of quite insignificant size. Occasionally they are large, and Mr. Durham states that "cases are recorded in which serious and even fatal hæmorrhage has occurred from these vessels."

For the general surroundings of the operation, the instruments required, the special precautions to be taken, and the after-treatment, the reader is referred to the sections on Tracheotomy.

k

The Operation.—The head is well extended over a sand-bag or hard cushion, and is kept fixed, with the chin in a line with the sternal notch. The anæsthetic selected is chloroform. The anatomical details of the part must be made out, and the crico-thyroid space defined (III, Fig. 308).

The larynx is lightly steadied with the left hand, while the surgeon makes a vertical median incision, about an inch and a quarter long, over the lower part of the thyroid cartilage, the crico-thyroid space, and the cricoid. The fascia having been divided, the interval between the sterno-thyroid and crico-thyroid muscles is appreciated, and is widened with the handle of the scalpel.

The crico - thyroid membrane is exposed, and is divided horizontally, just above the cricoid cartilage.

Care must be taken that the air-passage is well opened, as it is not difficult to pass the tube downwards between the crico-thyroid membrane and the mucous lining of the windpipe.

The laryngotomy tube is shorter than that used for tracheotomy, and is oval on section.

Some surgeons advise that the membrane be opened by a vertical incision, on the grounds that the operation

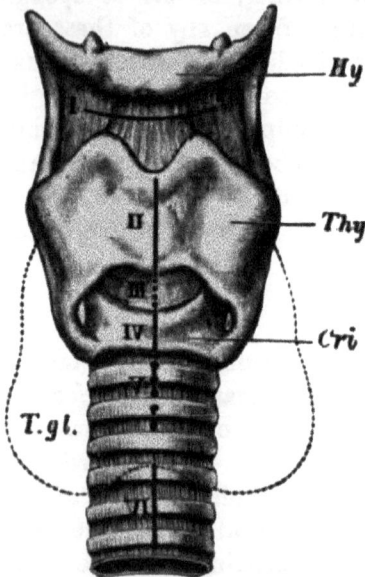

Fig. 308.—OPERATIONS ON THE LARYNX AND TRACHEA. (*Tillmann's.*)

I, Sub-hyoid Pharyngotomy; II, Thyrotomy; III, Laryngotomy; IV, Cricotomy; V and VI, High and low tracheotomy; *Hy*, Hyoid bone; *Thy*, Thyroid cart.; *Cri*, Cricoid cart.; *T. gl*, Thyroid gland.

can, if desired, be extended by dividing the cricoid cartilage, and that in the horizontal incision damage is usually inflicted upon the crico-thyroid muscles, and possibly also upon the lateral crico-arytenoid muscles.

Supra-thyroid Laryngotomy.—This operation, which is sometimes called sub-hyoid pharyngotomy, has been on a few occasions employed for the removal of growths situated at the upper opening of the larynx, and particularly of such as are connected with the epiglottis. The operation is simple, but even in the adult it rarely affords sufficient access for the efficient use of instruments (I, Fig. 308).

It was first suggested by Malgaigne (*Manuel de Méd. Opérat.*, Paris, 1835), and first carried out by M. Prat (*Gaz. des Hôpit.*, No. 103, page 849, 1859).

Solis-Cohen (Ashhurst's "Encyclopædia of Surgery," vol. v. page 735) has collected six examples of the operation for the removal of tumour. Three of these died within a few days of the operation.

A transverse incision is made through the thyro-hyoid membrane, parallel and close to the lower border of the hyoid bone. The skin, the fascia, the sterno-hyoid muscles (in whole or in part), the thyro-hyoid membrane, and the mucous membrane, are divided in order.

The epiglottis is at once exposed, and is drawn through the wound. The growth having been dealt with, and the bleeding checked, the wound is closed. The vessels wounded are few and insignificant, and the incision heals quickly.

Infra-thyroid Laryngotomy.—This operation has been carried out for the removal of growths situated on the under aspect of the cords or below the cords. Laryngotomy is performed some days before the attempted excision is made. Later, the crico-thyroid space is well opened up, and the cartilages separated to the utmost. Through the space thus obtained the growth is removed. Suitable forceps, etc., are required, and the site of the operation must be illumined by a mirror and a good concentrated light.

Thyrotomy.—By thyrotomy is understood the division of the thyroid cartilage in the median line, so as to gain access to the interior of the larynx. The operation is carried out for the purpose of removing certain laryngeal growths, and certain large or impacted foreign bodies, especially such as have found their way into the ventricles (II, Fig. 308).

The operation involves a great danger of permanently interfering with vocalisation, and in the treatment of morbid growths it is only employed when the intra-laryngeal method of removal cannot be effectually carried out.

Thyrotomy offers a rapid and ready means of entirely

eradicating laryngeal growths, and those advantages may be claimed for it which are ascribed to other radical operations.

The Operation.—The head is extended over a hard cushion or sand-bag, and is firmly held with the chin in a line with the sternal notch. The shoulders are raised. Chloroform is the anæsthetic administered. A preliminary laryngotomy or tracheotomy is carried out. The position of the opening for the tube will depend upon the nature of the case, the length of time the tube will probably have to be worn, and upon other circumstances. If the operation threatens to be extensive, as in dealing with large growths, a tracheotomy will be found to be the more convenient; but in such an operation as is carried out for the removal of a foreign body, a laryngotomy may be selected.

If much hæmorrhage is anticipated, as will be the case in dealing with extensive papillomata, the trachea must be plugged. This may be effected by a tampon, such as Trendelenburg's tracheotomy tampon, or by gently plugging the trachea on either side of the tube with a piece of fine sponge properly shaped, and attached to a long silk thread.

The incision is prolonged upwards in the median line, and the skin and subcutaneous tissues are divided down to the cartilage. The incision will extend over the cricoid and thyroid cartilages, the crico-thyroid space, and some part of the thyro-hyoid space.

The thyroid cartilage is divided accurately and carefully in the median line, the thyro-hyoid and crico-thyroid membranes being also cut if needed.

The division of the cartilage should be effected from above downwards, and from without inwards. In young subjects, and in females who have not passed middle life, the section may be accomplished by a small but stout knife. In aged subjects, in whom the cartilage will be calcified, a fine saw may be needed to effect a division. Bone forceps should never be employed.

In one case, in a woman about forty or forty-five, I had a difficulty in severing the cartilage with a knife, but found the division to be easily and precisely effected by using a pair of Salmon's pile scissors.

By means of two small sharp hooks the two alæ are now

drawn aside, and the interior of the larynx is exposed. In old subjects it may be necessary to make transverse incisions in the crico-thyroid and thyro-hyoid membranes, close to their respective cartilages, before the fullest view desired can be obtained.

The foreign body may now be extracted or the growth removed.

In dealing with papillomatous masses, the bulk of the growth may be crushed off with broad forceps, and the remainder removed with scissors, aided by Volkmann's spoon. The surface left by the removal of the tumour may then be touched with a saturated solution of chromic acid.

Finally, the two portions of the thyroid cartilage are united by two or three fine silver wire sutures, and the wound in the skin is closed.

The after-treatment will, with obvious modifications, be conducted upon the lines observed in dealing with cases of tracheotomy.

The results of thyrotomy in malignant disease are alluded to in the section (page 159) on the Results of Excision of the Larynx.

CHAPTER II.

EXCISION OF THE LARYNX.

THE term Laryngectomy has been applied to this operation. It involves the removal of either the whole of the larynx (complete excision), or of a considerable portion of it—usually one-half (partial excision).

The first complete excision of the larynx was performed by Dr. Patrick H. Watson in 1866, for stenosis of the larynx, due to syphilis. The patient, a man aged thirty-six, died in three weeks (*Trans. Internat. Med. Congress*, vol. iii., page 255, 1881).

The first complete excision for carcinoma, and the second operation in point of time, was carried out by Billroth in 1873 (*Archiv. of klin. Chirurg.*, bd. xvii., page 343). Death took place from recurrence in seven months.

The first unilateral or partial excision was performed by Billroth in 1878, for carcinoma of the left side of the larynx.

Excisions of the larynx have since these dates been very frequently carried out, principally by German surgeons.

Solis-Cohen ("Ashhurst's Encyclopædia of Surgery," vol. v., page 757, 1884) has collected ninety cases of complete excision of the larynx. Eighty were performed for carcinoma, four for sarcoma, one for lympho-sarcoma, two for papilloma, one for lupus, one for perichondritis, and one for cicatricial stenosis.

It will be seen that these operations are practically limited to cases of malignant disease.

One of the most complete and practical papers upon the operation is that by Hahn (Volkmann's *Sammlung*, No. 260, 1885).

COMPLETE EXCISION.

Preliminary Tracheotomy.—This should be carried out at least one or two weeks before the excision is attempted.

The advantages of such a step are these :—The patient will

get accustomed to breathing through an artificial opening. He will breathe more freely. The lungs, having become accustomed to air received through an artificial opening, will be less likely to become the seat of pneumonia after the operation. He can be more conveniently anæsthetised. The trachea will become adherent to the integument, and will need no artificial support to prevent its descent when the larynx is severed from it. A little of the time of the operation will be saved.

A tracheotomy carried out some time before the excision is especially called for when the patient has much dyspnœa or dysphagia, and has suffered much loss of strength.

The Plugging of the Trachea.—After the patient is anæsthetised, and before the actual excision is commenced, some means must be taken to prevent the entrance of blood into the air-passages. This is most surely effected by some form of tampon.

The well-known tampon of Trendelenburg is the one usually employed. Semon's modification of this tampon

Fig. 309.—SEMON'S MODIFICATION OF TRENDELENBURG'S TAMPON-CANNULA.

has some advantages over the original instrument (Fig. 309).

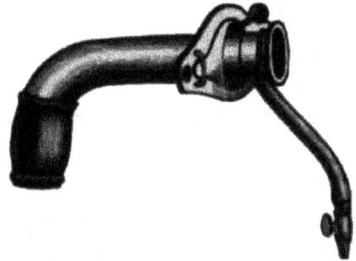

Certain objections have been urged against these cannulæ.

It is said that the sac may give way; that the indiarubber of which it is made, becoming slippery, may cause the tube to slide up in the trachea; and that the windpipe is not always efficiently plugged. The first objection cannot be sustained if care be taken to test the air sac, if the indiarubber employed be new, and if it be freshly applied for every operation. With regard to the two other objections, I have personally never met with the inconveniences named in using this tampon in the ordinary run of surgical cases. I have had no experience of excision of the larynx in the living subject. The air sac must fill the trachea well. Mackenzie states that if the sac or air b t be too fully or too suddenly distended, an asthmatic paroxysm may be produced. In a case published by Mr. Henry Morris (*Clin. Soc. Trans.*, vol. **xx.**) the tampon had to be given up on this account.

Hahn's tampon-cannula is preferred by many (Fig. 310). It is thus described by Mr. Butlin :—" It consists of an inner and an outer tube. The inner is much longer than the outer, so as to project for one inch or one inch and a half in front of the shield. Blood is thus very unlikely to find its way into the mouth of the tube. And in order to prevent this projecting piece of metal from inconveniencing the operator, it is made to bend down parallel with the trachea for about an inch before it stands out at right angles to the neck. The lower end of the outer tube is provided with a raised rim about 2 m.m. in height, and from this rim up to the shield is covered with a layer of compressed sponge, which has been, previously to the pressing, soaked in a solution of iodoform and ether (1 in 7). . . Shortly—*i.e.,* in ten minutes or a quarter of an hour—after the tube has been introduced, the sponge swells up from the absorption of moisture, and an absolute obstruction to the entrance of liquids into the trachea is provided."

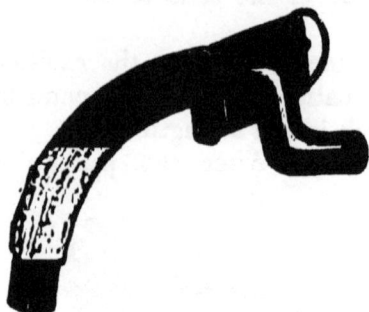

Fig. 310.—HAHN'S TAMPON-CANNULA.

An account of the preparation of the sponge will be found in a paper by Dr. Semon (*Clin. Soc. Trans.*, vol. **xx.**, page 47).

More than one surgeon—*e.g.,* Billroth and Gussenbauer—discard all special apparatus and use a simple cannula around which a piece of sponge is so inserted that it acts as a plug.

The Operation.—The patient lies upon the back, close to the right border of the table. The shoulders are raised, and the head is well extended over a hard cushion or sand-bag. The surgeon stands on the patient's right. The chief assistant takes his place at the head of the couch, and close to the surgeon's left. An incision is made in the median line from the centre of the thyro-hyoid membrane to the second or third ring of the trachea. At the upper end of this incision a transverse cut is made which is carried outwards on either side sufficiently far to reach the sterno-mastoid muscles.

The flaps thus marked out are turned back. Some division of the fibres of the sterno-mastoid muscles may be necessary. The vertical incision should go down to the thyroid and cricoid cartilages and the trachea.

The superior thyroid arteries may, if thought fit, be dealt with at this stage. They should be secured by two ligatures, and then divided between them. The vessels would be sought for at the posterior margin of the thyro-hyoid muscle, close to the upper border of the thyroid cartilage.

The inferior thyroid arteries may be exposed and dealt with in the same manner as they turn forwards at the lower margin of the larynx. They should be sought beneath the posterior edge of the sterno-thyroid muscle.

The fascia having been well divided in the middle line, a broad periosteal elevator or a rugine is introduced, and by means of it the soft parts can be separated from the laryngeal cartilages without employing the knife.

The crico-thyroid, sterno-thyroid, and thyro-hyoid muscles are detached on one side, and are, together with the other soft parts, held with a retractor while the larynx is, by means of a sharp double hook, drawn over to the other side. The attachment of the inferior constrictor muscle to the thyroid cartilage can now be severed, partly by detachment with the elevator or rugine, and partly by cutting it with curved blunt-pointed scissors, which are kept very close to the cartilage. The larynx is now pulled forwards as well as to the opposite side, and the tissues are divided about the gap which intervenes between the cut and now separated ends of the superior thyroid artery. The superior laryngeal nerve is also now divided. The thyroid gland is pushed aside with the soft parts.

If the larynx be now well drawn over to the other side, the other half of the organ can be stripped of its coverings in precisely the same manner.

The next step is to divide the thyro-hyoid ligaments and membrane, and to cut the extra-laryngeal connections of the epiglottis. This structure may be conveniently drawn forwards while its attachments are being freed.

The entire larynx is now pulled forwards by means of sharp hooks introduced into its upper part, and the organ is separated from its remaining connections with the pharynx and œsophagus—at first laterally, and then from above downwards.

If proper care be taken, the œsophagus should be nowhere "button-holed." Special care is required to separate the cricoid cartilage from the commencement of the gullet.

The trachea is now secured (unless already adherent) by means of two ligatures, which are held by an assistant, and the excision is completed by dividing the membrane between the cricoid cartilage and the trachea from behind forwards.

One or more rings of the trachea may be removed at the same time if it be considered necessary.

The upper end of the divided trachea, which has been prevented from slipping down by the two ligatures, is now secured to the integument by several points of interrupted suture.

Three or four deep sutures of silver wire are passed beneath the uppermost ring, and are made to attach the windpipe securely to the skin; a further series of fine superficial sutures unite the mucous membrane of the trachea to the cut margin of the skin.

The bleeding throughout the operation will be free, and each small vessel should be ligatured as soon as it is divided. The limited space does not favour the use of many pressure forceps.

Modifications of the Operation.—*The Preliminary Tracheotomy.*—Gussenbauer is opposed to the practice of performing a tracheotomy some time before the excision is carried out. He thinks that it leads to infiltration of the tissues about the trachea, to matting together of the parts around the wound, and thus to unnecessary complications when the trachea is approached in the major operation.

He believes that a high tracheotomy carried out as an initial step in the actual excision is the best practice in the majority of cases.

Excision of the Larynx from below upwards.—This order of proceeding is advised by some. The vertical skin incision having been made, the soft parts are detached from the front and sides of the larynx, and the trachea is exposed.

It is divided below the cricoid cartilage, is raised out of the wound, and is secured to the skin. A cannula is introduced into its lumen, and the tube around is closed by a plug of sponge, to which—as a precaution—a long silk thread is attached.

The larynx is now detached from below upwards.

This method is claimed to be the easier of the two, but it is not recommended by those who are most competent to advise upon the point.

Splitting the Larynx.—In cases where any doubt exists as to the extent of the disease, it is advised that the thyroid cartilage be split open in the median line, and the interior examined before it is decided that the whole of the larynx must be sacrificed.

The Epiglottis.—Few arguments have been advanced in favour of retaining the epiglottis in cases in which it has been found to be sound. The arguments in favour of removing it are these:—It is of no functional value, it may become the seat of a rapidly-recurring growth, and it interferes with the introduction of an artificial larynx.

The Cricoid Cartilage.—This structure is in most cases removed. When sound, it is advised by some that it be retained, on the ground that it affords an important additional support for an artificial larynx. Hahn, on the other hand, declares that if left, it interferes seriously with the act of swallowing, and that it should in every case be removed with the rest of the larynx.

General Observations.—In clearing the larynx, it is most important that the surgeon should keep throughout as close as possible to the cartilages, and that, if a knife be used, he should cut upon the cartilages.

It may sometimes be necessary to divide the isthmus of the thyroid between two ligatures when it is found that there is a difficulty in displacing that body from the larynx.

If any enlarged cervical glands be discovered, they should be removed.

If, after the skin has been reflected, it is found that the carcinoma has extended beyond the larynx, and has invaded the surrounding muscles and connective tissue, the operation should be abandoned.

The After-treatment.—The wound is well cleansed with an antiseptic solution, and is then filled with a light packing of carbolic or iodoform gauze. Before this is applied, the wound may be dusted with iodoform or other antiseptic powder. No sutures are introduced, except in the transverse part of the skin wound, the edges of which may be brought together by a few points of silkworm gut. A soft indiarubber tube is introduced into the stomach through the wound, and is secured in position by a suture. Through this tube the patient is fed. This mode of feeding must be supplemented by nutrient enemata. The tampon cannula used in the operation is left undisturbed.

The patient must be placed in a warm and well-ventilated room; and, if it be considered desirable, a steam spray may be used to render the inspired air moister.

The gauze dressings should be changed twice or three times in the twenty-four hours, and every care be taken to prevent decomposition from occurring in the wound, and to allow all discharges and secretions to escape.

The tampon-cannula may be removed at the end of twenty-four or forty-eight hours, and replaced by a tracheotomy tube of the largest size. Some surgeons retain the tampon for eight or ten days, as a precaution against the somewhat unlikely accident of secondary hæmorrhage. The tracheotomy tube must be kept scrupulously clean.

As soon as the wound is becoming firm, and the healing has advanced satisfactorily, the œsophageal tube may be removed, and the patient either be encouraged to swallow, or the tube be introduced from time to time as circumstances suggest. The feeding-tube has been left off as early as the fifth day, but it may, on the other hand, have to be worn for some weeks.

It must be borne in mind that it will be easier to swallow solid than liquid food in these cases, and that not a few deaths have been due to pneumonia, consequent upon the decomposition of food which has found its way into the air-passages.

Other elements in the treatment of the case will depend upon ordinary surgical principles.

The Artificial Larynx.—This instrument should not be introduced until the parts are satisfactorily healed, and from three to five weeks will usually elapse after the operation before any attempts to make use of the artificial larynx will be considered advisable.

The apparatus that appears to be the most satisfactory is Irvine's modification of Gussenbauer's instrument.

It consists of two tubes, a pharyngeal tube (Fig. 311, A), and a tracheal tube (Fig. 311, B). The pharyngeal tube is introduced first, and the tracheal tube is then passed through it. Fenestræ are so cut in these two tubes as to allow of the free passage of air throughout them (Fig. 311). Lodged in a groove in the pharyngeal tube is a plate carrying a reed (Fig. 311, C). This plate can be pushed in and drawn out after the manner of a table-drawer. It can therefore be readily freed from mucus, and cleaned. The expiratory current produces vibration of the reed, and the tone evolved serves as a basis for articulate speech. The sound is, of course, absolutely monotonous.

Dr. Solis-Cohen comments as follows upon this instrument:—"Great difference is presented in the toleration of these appliances. In some instances they give little trouble, and are used with great comfort. Some subjects bear the naked apparatus well, but cannot tolerate the phonal reed, which may impede respiration, may become obstructed with desiccated mucus, and may yield a tone to every breath of expiration. Some abandon them altogether, and stick to the simple tracheal cannula. In some instances saliva, mucus, and aliment will get into the tubes, and descend into the trachea. Some patients prevent the escape of food by plugging the upper orifice with cotton when they eat."

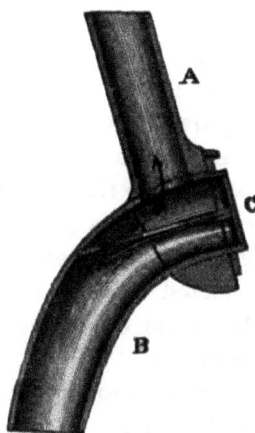

Fig. 311.—IRVINE'S MODI-FICATION OF GUSSEN-BAUER'S ARTIFICIAL LARYNX.

A, Upper tube; B, Lower tube; C, The reed.

PARTIAL EXCISION.

This operation is carried out upon the same lines as the complete excision. One-half only of the larynx or of the thyroid cartilage is removed.

The details of the operation are practically the same.

A preliminary low tracheotomy may be carried out some little time before the excision is attempted.

The incision is the same, save that the transverse portion need occupy only the diseased side. A tampon-cannula is introduced.

The larynx is laid bare in the middle line, and the thyroid cartilage is divided so that the interior of the larynx may be inspected. Preliminary ligature of the thyroid arteries is unnecessary.

The thyroid cartilage is now removed. It is cautiously bared of the soft parts which cover its outer surface by means of an elevator or a rugine. The surgeon must keep close to the cartilage. The attachments of the pharynx are separated by like means. The thyro-hyoid and crico-thyroid membranes are divided upon the affected side as close as possible to the margin of the thyroid cartilage. The superior cornu of this cartilage is divided at its base by pliers. The epiglottis is left, and the aryteno-epiglottic fold of the affected side is divided close to the cartilage of Wrisberg. In some cases the epiglottis has been split, and one half removed.

Every care must be taken to avoid opening the pharyngeal cavity. In clearing the cartilage, the elevator and the handle of the scalpel may be now and then assisted by a few snips from blunt-pointed scissors curved on the flat. Bleeding vessels must be taken up and tied as divided.

Mr. Butlin states that in partial excision for intrinsic disease " there is usually not the least necessity to remove the cricoid cartilage." It has, however, in most of the cases been split in the middle line, and one half of the ring has been removed with the half of the thyroid cartilage.

Mr. Butlin is in favour of leaving the thyroid cartilage also, whenever this is possible. He would split the cartilage in the middle line, open the larynx, and then scoop out, as it were, the contents of one half of the thyroid cartilage. The removal should be free, and when completed the ala should be restored in place. Mr. Butlin points out that cancer of the larynx far more often causes the death of the cartilage piece by piece than infiltrates it; and even if the surface of the thyroid has been encroached upon, he would be disposed to scrape away the affected part rather than sacrifice the whole ala.

The after-treatment is the same as in cases of complete excision. The treatment of the wound is the same. The patient will probably be able to take semi-solid food by the mouth in three or four days after the operation, and the cannula may often be dispensed with in the same time.

Results of Excision of the Larynx.—The usual causes of death are shock and hæmorrhage, and, above all, pneumonia. The risk of death from pneumonia must be present for at least fourteen days after the operation. The failure of antiseptic precautions, the passage of food and discharges into the bronchi, and the development of bronchitis from the altered mode of breathing, are the usual factors in the production of this complication. In complete excision the mortality directly due to the operation itself is over thirty per cent. In partial excision it is less.

The relief afforded in complete excision has been, in the majority of the cases, of but short duration, early recurrence being the rule. The state of some of the patients after the operation has been very miserable. If it be true that a palliative tracheotomy in cancer of the larynx may allow life to be prolonged some two and a half years, there must be strong evidence adduced to justify the complete removal of the organ.

The immediate success which has attended partial excision of the larynx in suitable cases, has been more gratifying. The mortality has been lower, and the patient has been able to swallow with ease, and to speak with sufficient clearness to enable him to make himself quite distinct. With regard to complete excision, Mr. Butlin wrote in 1887:—"Complete excision of the larynx has hitherto been in every respect unsuccessful. . . . And were it not that better results may be hoped for in future—by better managament of the patients, and by much greater care in the selection of cases—the operation must be condemned as unsurgical " ("The Operative Surgery of Malignant Disease," 1887).

A later review of this question is given by Mr. Butlin in the *British Medical Journal* for August 23rd, 1890.

The following table is abstracted from that paper :—

	OPERATIONS FOR MALIGNANT DISEASE.	DEATHS DUE TO THE OPERATION.
Thyrotomy	28 cases	3 deaths
Partial excision of larynx . . .	23 „	7 „
Complete excision of larynx . .	51 „	16 „
	102 „	26 „

Out of the 28 cases of thyrotomy . .	3 are pronounced cured
„ 23 „ partial excision . .	4 „ „ „
„ 51 „ complete excision .	8 „ „ „
102 cases	15 cases of cure

[By "cure" it is meant that the patients were alive and free from disease at periods of from three to twenty years after the operation.]

A series of very complete statistics, based upon papers by M. Pinçonnat and Dr. Kraus, is given in the *Centralblatt für Chirurgie*, No. 51, 1890.

CHAPTER III.

Excision of the Thyroid Body.

Anatomical Points.—The normal relations of the thyroid gland or body must be clearly appreciated before any operation is attempted upon this very dangerously-placed structure.

Most important is it to note the relations of the gland to the trachea and gullet, to the recurrent laryngeal nerve, and to the sheath of the great vessels of the neck.

The thyroid gland has a very large blood supply. The superior thyroid arteries—from the carotids—descend to reach the apex or upper part of each lobe. They supply the front and inner parts of the body. The inferior thyroid arteries are larger than the superior, enter the lower extremity of each lobe, and supply the posterior, inferior, and outer parts of the body. Each vessel runs for some little distance on the posterior surface of the thyroid before it pierces it. The thyroidea ima may supplement deficiencies in the other arteries, and when present will enter the lower part of the gland near the median line.

The superior thyroid veins follow the arteries, and end in the internal jugular. The middle thyroid veins pass out transversely, and enter the internal jugular a little below the level of the cricoid cartilage. The inferior thyroid veins descend as an irregular plexus on the trachea, and end in the innominate veins.

The quantity of blood contained in the softer varieties of goitre is enormous, and the size and number of the veins which leave it are remarkable. Partial or complete excision of the thyroid gland is usually carried out in certain selected cases of non-malignant bronchocele, especially in such as are causing severe disturbance from pressure. In the treatment of malignant disease of the thyroid the experience of surgeons up to the present time has been so unsatisfactory as to render it a question as to whether the operation is justifiable.

l

It will be evident that in cases of bronchocele the relations of parts may be much modified, essential landmarks may be lost, and vessels and other structures displaced.

The bronchocele may extend to great depths, may surround the trachea, and may have so insinuated itself among the various structures of the neck as to render any attempt at excision either desperate or entirely unjustifiable.

Dangers of the Operation.—In some instances, when the bronchocele is small and well encapsuled, the excision of one-half or of the whole of the gland may be carried out without much difficulty. But these simple cases are not the ones which are selected for operation, inasmuch as they are not the ones which produce such symptoms as would justify this serious measure.

In the great majority of instances these excision operations are dangerous, tedious, and difficult, and demand the exercise of the highest qualities of a good surgeon. Sir William MacCormac, in describing a case of excision of a non-malignant goitre (*Brit. Med. Journal*, 1884, vol. ii., page 229) speaks of the operation as one of the most difficult and most serious he ever had occasion to perform. The operation lasted two hours, and no fewer than 100 ligatures were applied. Nor is this case by any means exceptional. The larger the mass, the less defined its capsule, the broader its base, and the more vascular its structure, the less easy is the operation. The following are the principal dangers :—

1. *Hæmorrhage.*—In the course of the excision there is no great difficulty in dealing with the arteries. It is the veins which are the source of the trouble. They are found to be numerous, to be very large, to be arranged according to no familiar anatomical lines, and to be usually thin-walled. The dyspnœa from which the patient suffers causes them to be abnormally distended, and to bleed furiously if they be accidentally divided.

In the softer and more vascular forms of bronchocele the splitting of the comparatively thin capsule exposes a soft pulpy tissue, from which blood pours as if it were being wrung out of a sponge. No form of bleeding is less easy to deal with than this.

In indistinctly-encapsuled and wide-spreading goitres the

carotid artery and the jugular vein are in danger, and the artery may be wounded or the vein torn.

**2. *Injury to the Recurrent Laryngeal Nerve.*—This nerve is in intimate relation with the inferior thyroid artery, and in securing that vessel—or, rather, the series of vessels which represent it—it is by no means difficult to damage this important nerve. The accident has happened many times. The nerve has been in some instances cut, in others it has been included in a ligature, and in a third series of instances it has been torn or severely stretched.

**3. *Cellulitis.*—So extensive a tract of the connective tissue of the neck is opened up that if the wound become septic, there is little to prevent a diffused form of suppurative cellulitis, which will almost inevitably lead to death.

COMPLETE EXCISION.

The method of operating here described is that known as Kocher's. The patient lies upon the right-hand side of the table, with the shoulders well raised, and the head extended over a large sand-bag or hard cushion.

The chin should be kept in a line with the sternal notch, and the head be well fixed. The anæsthetist stands at the head of the table, and the chief assistant to the surgeon's right. Every preparation must be made for extensive hæmorrhage. The anæsthetic should be chloroform, or at least the A. C. E. mixture should chloroform be distinctly contra-indicated.

Ether increases to its utmost the engorgement of the veins of the head and neck.

An incision is made in the median line from the sternal notch to the upper limit of the bronchocele. From this point two lateral incisions are made upwards and outwards, one on each side. They are directed towards a point a little below the angle of the jaw, and when the cutaneous cut is complete it will have the outline of the letter Y. If the tumour be much more extensively developed on one side than on the other, the upper or oblique incision may be limited to the affected side. In any case the incision must not be spared. A primary requirement is that the tumour be very freely exposed. The lateral or oblique cuts will usually pass over the anterior borders of the sterno-mastoid muscles.

The platysma and fascia are divided. Any veins which are met with are secured between two ligatures of chromicised catgut, and divided. The sterno-hyoid and sterno-thyroid muscles will be found to be stretched over the goitre. These structures will probably be much thinned and very altered in appearance.

The surgeon must make his way down to the gland, and must convince himself that he has opened up the plane of connective tissue beneath these muscles, and is not wandering aimlessly over the outer surface.

The sterno-hyoid, sterno-thyroid, and omo-hyoid muscles will need to be divided in whole or in part.

It may be necessary even to cut one or both of the sterno-mastoid muscles. The operator must trust but little to retractors, but must rather aim at obtaining the fullest view of the bronchocele by dissection.

The muscles named will very often be closely adherent to the tumour, and in clearing them away the scalpel must be used very sparingly.

No instrument is more serviceable in this stage of the operation than a broad periosteal elevator. Its point is so blunt that it can do little damage, and its configuration is admirably suited to peel the tissues away from the capsule. This must be done with great care. The elevator is made to work its way beneath the muscles and the fascia, and when the precise relations are clear the tissues are divided over the elevator as over a director. In effecting this exposure of the goitre a pair of blunt-pointed scissors curved on the flat is more useful than a scalpel, and the handle of the scalpel is of more service than the blade. The elevator must not be vigorously thrust here and there, but must be made to find an easy path. No tissue should be cut until it has been well examined, and any especially-resisting structure must be exposed before it is torn across or cut.

A plexus of large, thin-walled veins will usually be found covering the tumour. They must be separately treated, and must be individually divided between two ligatures. These vessels are easily torn across, and are very apt to be adherent.

If the head be in the position of extension, the structures on the front of the neck, and especially those over the face of the tumour, are apt to be stretched, and a vein so stretched may be quite unrecognisable. It is well, therefore, to have the head lifted now and then, so that the veins to be dealt with may be brought well into view.

Step by step the surgeon clears the whole of the front surface of the swelling, dealing with every bleeding point as it is met with, and not trusting either to the pressure of fingers or of sponges, or to artery forceps.

When the anterior surface is cleared, the next step is to approach the lateral margins of the growth, and to secure the thyroid vessels. It must be remembered that the thyroid body touches the carotid sheath. The position of that vessel should be made out as early as possible, and the utmost care taken to avoid it. If the bronchocele is in close contact with the main vessels, some special care may be required in separating the huge internal jugular vein from the capsule. The superior thyroid artery is then sought for at the upper extremity of the tumour. It may not be made out without some difficulty. If the vessels cannot be individually isolated, a double ligature may be passed by means of an aneurysm needle, and the vascular pedicle ligatured in two places and divided between. The vessels embraced by these ligatures may be separately secured at a later period if thought necessary. The inferior thyroid artery is less easy to deal with. It is more deeply placed, has more numerous veins in relation with it, and is closely connected with the recurrent laryngeal nerve. No pains should be spared to expose it well. Baumgartner recommends that the ligatures be applied at some distance from the lower border of the tumour, and that the branches of the artery be cut through just as they enter the bronchocele. In this way there is less danger of including the recurrent nerves.

The whole of the lateral border of the tumour is now separated. The same precautions are observed. The blunt dissector is the chief instrument. The scissors are used as required, and the vessels encountered are all ligatured and divided in the manner described.

The mass is turned over towards the opposite side, and the posterior surface of the tumour cleared as far as the posterior median line:

The other lateral lobe is dealt with in precisely the same manner, and in due course the whole tumour is removed, with its capsule still unbroken.

The huge wound is now examined, and any remaining bleeding vessels secured. It is well flushed out with a weak antiseptic solution, to remove all clots. The less it is rubbed with a sponge the better. The margins of the skin incisions are united with silkworm-gut sutures, which are not too closely applied; and a large-sized drain is introduced at the lower part of the wound.

The best dressing consists of large sponges, well dusted with iodoform, which are surrounded with cotton-wool, and are bandaged in position with as much pressure as it is considered safe to apply.

When the patient is placed in bed, the shoulders and head must be kept well raised, and the head may be fixed in the hollow of a loosely-filled sand-bag.

PARTIAL EXCISION.

Excision of one-half of the thyroid, with division of the isthmus, is conducted in precisely the same manner as the above operation.

The incision is vertical, and is placed laterally over the most prominent part of the tumour.

The front of the bronchocele is cleared, and the superior thyroid artery is then secured.

After this vessel has been dealt with, the isthmus is severed. The fascia around it is divided, and the isthmus is then separated from the trachea by an elevator or director, and is well isolated. It may be then transfixed by a needle in a handle—such as is used in ovariotomy—and secured by a double set of ligatures, which are placed upon each side of the spot at which it is intended to divide it. It is treated somewhat like the ovarian pedicle. In cases of very large isthmus more ligatures may be called for. In some instances the isthmus may be more conveniently divided with a scalpel, and ligatures applied as required.

The tumour is now almost completely isolated, and the last step consists in ligaturing the inferior thyroid artery.

Tracheotomy in these Operations.—If there be much

dyspnœa in these cases of excision of the thyroid, the mass should be relieved from its tense surroundings as soon as possible, and the pressure removed from the trachea. Some assistance in this direction may be afforded by altering the position of the head, and by having the mass, as far as possible, withdrawn from the windpipe.

More immediate relief may be obtained probably by dividing the isthmus.

Tracheotomy is most emphatically to be avoided. The operation, if performed, would be carried out under the greatest difficulties, and the gravity of the whole procedure much increased.

Tracheotomy in these cases nearly always leads to a fatal issue. It is impossible to prevent the huge wound from becoming septic, and the patient soon dies of septic pneumonia or suppurative cellulitis. An excision of the thyroid, accompanied by tracheotomy, is so desperate an operation that it must be regarded as quite unjustifiable as a deliberately-planned procedure. In most of the cases the tracheotomy was called for unexpectedly after the excision had been commenced; but to complete an excision after a tracheotomy has been performed is a forlorn hope indeed.

After-treatment.—This calls for no especial notice. The drainage-tubes should be removed in twenty-four or thirty-six hours.

The shoulders should be kept raised, and the head well fixed, by being buried in a sand-bag.

In applying the dressings the bandages must be passed under the axilla, across the front of the chest, across the scapular region, and over the head, in order to secure a firm and tight covering for the wound.

Food is given by the mouth.

The treatment is, indeed, that merely of a deep and extensive wound in the neck.

At a later period healing, if delayed, may be promoted by fixing the head in a jury-mast, or by applying the cap used in the treatment of cases of cut-throat.

Results.—These operations, besides involving the ordinary surgical issues, involve also, in the cases of complete excision, the possibility of cachexia strumipriva. The matter has been carefully investigated by the committee of the Clinical Society on Myxœdema (*Clin. Soc. Trans.*, Supplement to vol. xxi, 1888, pages 162, 197).

The results are given as follows:—

" In a total of about 408 intentionally complete thyroidectomies, performed by fifty-six different surgeons, there were fifty-nine deaths in consequence of, or shortly after, the operation.

" In twenty cases the operation was performed for malignant disease of the thyroid gland.

" Deducting the cases of death from, or shortly after, the operation, the cases in which there was malignant disease of the thyroid gland, and the cases which were lost from observation almost immediately after the operation, there remain 298 cases in which total thyroidectomy was performed for simple goitre, and in which the patients are known to have fully recovered. Of these, in 277 instances the further fate of the patients could be followed up, with the result that in twenty-two cases either recurrence of goitre, or development of accessory thyroid glands, appear to have taken place; that in 186 cases the patients appear to have remained free from cachexia strumipriva, without recurrence or development of accessory thyroids having taken place; and that in sixty-nine cachexia strumipriva of a more or less severe type developed."

CHAPTER IV.

The Removal of Tumours of the Neck.

THE somewhat wide and varied series of operations which could be included under the above title may be very conveniently represented by the operation for the removal of scrofulous glands in the neck. The previous chapter, on Removal of the Thyroid Body, affords an example of a special operation for the excision of a large cervical tumour.

THE REMOVAL OF SCROFULOUS GLANDS.

These scrofulous tumours exhibit such infinite variety as regards number, position, relations, and physical characteristics, that their removal will involve a series of surgical procedures which extend from an operation of the very simplest character to one which is both complex and difficult. With Mr. Treves, of Margate, must rest the credit of first systematically treating all scrofulous glands of a certain grade by excision.

The trouble to be dealt with may be limited to a single gland, which is well-defined, well-encapsuled, firm, superficial, and more or less free from adhesions to surrounding parts.

Such a tumour, when exposed, "shells out" with the greatest ease, and the operation involved is of the most rudimentary description.

More usually, however, the surgical position lies within less simple lines. The glands are numerous, and are matted together. The more superficial tumours are connected with a string of others which are more deeply placed, and which may extend even to the anterior surface of the spine. These glands are of varying consistence; while some are firm, others are soft, and possessed of so thin a capsule that little force is required to tear them open and allow their creamy and caseous contents to escape.

Not only are they matted together, but they are wedged in among the tissues of the neck, and are fixed by adhesions which, for extent, for toughness, and for their capacity to obliterate the anatomical details of the part, have few equals in other regions of the body. The surgeon who commences to remove a large collection of scrofulous masses in the neck is setting forth upon no light undertaking, and must at first remain uncertain as to the direction in which he will be led, and as to the limit which he may reach.

The number of the tumours is often considerable, and no sooner is one string or cluster removed, than another comes into view.

The Dangers of the Operation.—The chief dangers in the operation consist in (1) the possible wounding or tearing of nerves and other structures, (2) hæmorrhage, and (3) the entrance of air into wounded veins.

An operation of this kind should never be undertaken unless the surgeon has perfect confidence in his practical knowledge of the anatomy of the neck.

Scarcely an instance can be cited in the range of operative surgery where a knowledge of structure and of relations is more essential than in these excisions.

1. *The Possible Wounding of Nerves and other Structures.*—The nerves, as a rule, give comparatively little trouble. They stand out well upon the matted tissues, and their isolation is seldom a matter of difficulty.

A nerve may be actually lost in a malignant growth of the neck, but a nerve passing through a coherent mass of scrofulous glands can nearly always be recognised, followed, and isolated. The nerves which usually come in the way of the operation are the ascending and descending branches of the cervical plexus, the superficial cervical being the one most commonly exposed. These nerves may be divided when such division appears inevitable, and no ill will follow. Indeed, in some instances of pain in the course of these nerves, produced by the pressure of the tumour, the section of one or more of them may now and then be deliberately carried out. The rule, of course, should be to isolate them, and to draw them aside with retractors.

Of larger and more important nerves, the one which

most frequently comes across the operator's path is the spinal accessory in the posterior triangle. An accidental division of that nerve is very readily effected. One author states that, in removing glands from the neck, he has divided this nerve more than fifty times (*St. Thomas's Hospital Reports*, vol. xviii., page 218). He adds that, "although most careful search was made for symptoms due to its division, none could ever be found." From this observation, it must be gathered that the nerve divided was the supra-acromial or the outer supra-clavicular, and not the spinal accessory. These cutaneous nerves are large, and can readily be mistaken for the motor trunk. If the latter nerve—when exposed—be scratched with the point of the knife, a twitching in the trapezius will always be noticed, no matter how deeply the patient is anæsthetised ; and division of the nerve will certainly lead to partial paralysis of the muscle.

The next nerves of primary importance are the phrenic, the vagus, and the recurrent laryngeal. It is very rare indeed for these nerve-cords to enter the field of the operation during the excision of scrofulous glands. Their division or injury in these operations is inexcusable. More than one case has, however, been recorded.

The pneumo-gastric has been divided without a fatal result. The descendens noni is not infrequently severed. The cervical sympathetic has been wounded in removing a deep-seated tumour which pressed upon the pharynx (*Clin. Soc. Trans.*, vol. xix., page 321). Sarcomata and other tumours have been dissected off the phrenic, the vagus, and the cords of the brachial plexus.

In every case the surgeon must make a most careful examination before operating, with the purpose of ascertaining if any symptoms are present which indicate pressure upon the nerves in the neck ; and if such symptoms exist, he must take especial care to isolate the nerve or nerves thus individualised.

In removing enlarged glands or other growths—such as lympho-sarcomata—from the root of the neck, two structures must be particularly respected—one is the dome of the pleura, which ascends some distance into the neck, and the

other is the thoracic duct. The pleura is readily torn in
dealing with a deeply-seated and adherent mass.

One surgeon, from whose work a quotation has already
been made (*St. Thomas's Hosp. Reports*, vol. xviii., page
219), states that he removed the extreme tip of the lung
in the course of one operation for strumous glands. He
states, very properly, that it was a " most remarkable case."

Mr. Jacobson cites an instance in which the left thoracic
duct was opened during the removal of enlarged glands from
the neck. Chyle escaped deep down in the wound, and the
case soon ended fatally.

In dealing with gland cases, it is quite possible that the
submaxillary salivary gland may be mistaken for a lymphatic
tumour, and that its true character may not be discovered
until the mass has been cleared for removal.

The parotid salivary gland could scarcely be the subject
of such a mistake.

2. *Hæmorrhage.*—The bleeding in these cases may be
very free, but it will be nearly always venous.

There is no difficulty in dealing with the arteries; their
position is known, and when they are cut a sharp spurt of
blood directs the surgeon at once to the bleeding point. The
vessel is readily picked up.

It is the venous bleeding that is troublesome. The wound
is deep, and its depths are not easily illuminated; the blood
wells úp in a steady and often copious stream, and the
details of the operation area are lost.

The inflammatory process spreads readily along the loose
connective tissue around the veins, and the manner in which
strumous glands follow venous trunks, and attach themselves,
as it were, to them, is very remarkable.

If the glands are fixed in any given cases, it may be taken for
granted that they have acquired an extensive hold of the veins
of the part, if of no other structures. The lymphatic vessels run
mainly with the veins, and this intimate association of the lymphatic tumours and the blood-channels is readily explained.

The veins so involved are found to be enlarged, and tortuous
and devious. Sometimes they are stretched over the gland,
and are more to be compared to bands of tape than to tubes.

Very often they have been so drawn upon and so extended

that they cease to look like veins, and are cut across under the impression that the knife is dealing with a band of connective tissue.

In many cases it is impossible to isolate the vein from the lymphatic tumour, and the vein, if small, has to be sacrificed. In more than one instance I have had to determine whether I should leave a portion of the tumour behind, or remove an inch or so of the internal jugular vein, in cases in which the growth had attached itself to that great trunk. In dealing with scrofulous glands, it is better to spare the vein, to excise as much of the mass as can be removed, and then to pare down what remains with a Volkmann's spoon, until nothing but a fragment of capsule is left clinging to the vein. In dealing with malignant tumours the vein must be sacrificed. I have accidentally wounded this vein on two occasions in removing strumous glands, and have then isolated the wounded part between two ligatures. I have seen no harm arise from this undesirable complication.

In other cases, as in removing cancerous glands from the neck, I have excised an inch or so of the internal jugular vein, and have in these cases also seen no evil follow from the practice. I might here add that if a malignant growth has acquired such a hold upon the part as to have completely buried the internal jugular vein in its substance, the circumstances must be very pronounced which would justify a persistent and determined attempt at excision. Early recurrence would be inevitable.

In some cases of extensive strumous disease I have found certain of the minor veins, such as the superior thyroid, lingual, or facial, of such enormous size as to be for the moment mistaken for the jugular.

In dealing with the lower part of the posterior triangle, the external jugular vein will nearly always require to be divided between two ligatures.

3. *Air in Veins.* — In these operations there is some danger of the entrance of air into the divided veins.

I have recorded certain examples of this terrible accident (*British Medical Journal*, June 30, 1883), and have dealt with the subject at some length in Heath's "Dictionary of Surgery," vol. i, page 27.

It is only necessary here to point out that the accident can only occur in what may be termed dry wounds—wounds cleared of all blood by sponging, etc. The injured vein must either be exposed to the air, or be separated from the air by only a thin layer of blood before it is possible for air to be drawn into the vein during the act of inspiration. If the wound be full of blood, the accident is impossible. It occurs most usually when a tumour is being dragged from its attachments, or just after a deep incision has been sponged out.

The treatment of the complication is as follows:—The moment the hissing sound is heard, the wound should be filled with water squeezed from a sponge. This at once prevents the entrance of more air. It is useless at the first to attempt to tie the vein. The damaged vessel is not easy to find, and to apply a ligature involves time. Moreover, if the ligature be applied during an inspiration, it would certainly prevent the entrance of more air; but if applied during an expiration, it would merely prevent the escape of such air as had already entered.

The second step is to endeavour to remove the air that has already entered the chest. This can be best effected by waiting until the next expiratory movement, and then bringing forcible pressure to bear upon the front of the thorax.

The ease with which a large quantity of air can be thus expressed is remarkable, and especially in children.

When all air has been expressed, the vein should be seized with pressure forceps and ligatured. The suggestion that air should be sucked out of the right auricle through a catheter passed into the heart through one of the main veins is preposterous. The advice given in nearly every text-book, that artificial respiration should be resorted to, is almost as silly. There is not too little air in the thorax, but too much.

The Operation.—The patient lies upon the back, with the shoulders very well raised, and with the face turned towards the sound side. The forearm of the affected side is placed behind the back. Sponges are wedged in under the nape of the neck, to absorb any blood which may run down in that direction. It is important that the general pose of the part should be such that blood can escape rapidly from the wound and not obscure the movements of the operator. A good light, and at least one good assistant, are necessary.

The anæsthetic should be chloroform or the A. C. E. mixture. The incision must depend upon the site and size of the masses, and must be subject to infinite variation.

In dealing with glands in the upper part of the anterior triangle, the best position for the incision is along the almost transverse skin crease which crosses the neck about the level of the hyoid bone. A fine cicatrix, following this natural fold, may in time become almost invisible. In the lower part of the posterior triangle a transverse incision is also to be advised. Elsewhere the incision may be oblique, and may follow the general line of the sterno-mastoid muscle.

On the ground of the after-appearance an absolutely vertical incision at right angles to the clavicle cannot be advised. Through a superior transverse incision, and an inferior oblique one, nearly every gland in the anterior triangle can be reached, and in most instances these two incisions are better than a single vertical one of considerable length.

The skin incision must be free, and the success of the operation should never be compromised by attempts to reduce the scar to the minutest possible limits.

The skin, and platysma, and deep fascia are divided.

The sterno-mastoid, when exposed, must be well freed and held aside by retractors. It may be necessary in rare instances to divide a few fibres of the muscle. This should, however, be always regarded as a most exceptional proceeding. A free division of the muscle may lead to a pronounced form of wry-neck. Glands buried beneath the muscle can be exposed by retractors, or reached through incisions placed on either side of the muscle.

The deep fascia must be divided along the full length of the wound.

When the mass of glands is reached, they may be found to be non-adherent, and to be capable of being "shelled out" with perfect ease.

As a rule, however, these glands are adherent, and the surgeon's first care must be to find out the least adherent side of the tumour or tumours.

He must take care that his dissection has extended down

to the very capsule of the gland, and the rule repeatedly insisted upon by Mr. W. Knight Treves, in his many papers upon this subject (*Lancet*, 1888 and 1889), that throughout the whole operation the surgeon must keep close to the capsule, cannot be too accurately observed.

As soon as a little clearing has been effected, the surgeon introduces his finger and seeks for the least fixed part or parts of the tumour. It is from these less adherent sides that the growth is attacked.

It is well that it should be approached from more sides than one. In digging out, as it were, the fixed gland, the scalpel is considerably assisted by blunt-pointed scissors curved on the flat.

The most useful instrument, however, in this part of the operation, is a simple old-fashioned periosteal elevator.

By means of this instrument the tissues over the gland may be peeled off, adhesions may be separated, and the gland be lifted out of its bed. Another useful instrument at this

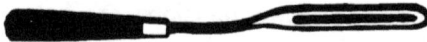

Fig. 312.—COOPER'S HERNIA DIRECTOR.

stage is Cooper's hernia director (Fig. 312), which is round-pointed and more slender than the elevator, but which is, however, used rather as an elevator than as a director.

The clearing of the gland must be carried out gradually and the process is tedious enough.

It is unwise to attempt to tear the mass out. If such be done, the gland will either break up and its softened contents escape, or a nerve to which it is adherent may be ruptured. or a part of the wall of a large vein be torn right away. Before a strand or bridge of tissue is divided, it should be relaxed a little, so that its true nature may be perceived. A vein put much upon the stretch may look like a band of connective tissue. If a layer of tissue, to be divided, be drawn up from the depths of the wound, it is well not to cut it at once while it is on the stretch, but to first relax it a little, so that its character may be better appreciated. In this stage of the excision the main axioms should be—keep close to the capsule ; make no cut in the dark ; be chary of cutting tissues which are only seen when put fully upon the stretch.

In process of time a kind of pedicle will be formed to the once adherent glands, and when this has been reduced to its smallest limits, it should be held by two fenestrated artery forceps, and divided close to the glands. It may or may not contain vessels which require a ligature. In any case the forceps will prevent the stump from dropping out of view, and in general terms it may be said that the inclusion of a large pedicle of uncertain composition within one ligature is to be condemned.

Every care must be taken to avoid wounding veins unnecessarily. Many have to be cut, and should in all cases be at once secured with a ligature, or with pressure forceps. I make considerable use of the latter means, for I notice that veins which bled furiously at one stage of the operation are found to be void of blood at the end of the procedure, and the application of unnecessary ligatures is thus avoided.

The greatest difficulty occurs when a large adherent vein has been opened by tearing. In such a case an inch or more of one side of the vein may have been removed. Pressure forceps avail little. The vein must be isolated and secured above and below the rent.

Care must be taken not to tear or wound the gland capsule. If this has been done the purulent or caseous contents escape, or the soft gland substance is squeezed out. The firm tumour becomes a flabby bag, the depths of the wound are obscured, and the removal of the collapsed gland is difficult. In such a case the capsule must be carefully dissected away, piece by piece, after the gland has been evacuated, and the wound well cleared out.

Now and then it may be found to be impossible, or at least very unwise, to complete the excision of a deep-seated gland. The surgeon must have good grounds for coming to this conclusion. The glands which have to be abandoned are exceedingly few, and neither lack of knowledge nor lack of perseverance should form bases for this determination. The gland so placed must be evacuated and cleaned well out with the sharp spoon. The capsule must then be dissected away as completely as is possible, and what tissue remains must be reduced to the smallest possible proportions by a further diligent application of the sharp spoon. I have found this

measure to answer well, to place no obstacle in the way of
primary union, and usually to lead to nq further trouble.

The removal of the gland, however, with its capsule entire,
is the only completely satisfactory measure.

The deep wound left by the operation must be well flushed
out with some weak antiseptic solution, and every trace of
bleeding must be checked.

Pressure with a sponge is the most effectual measure for
minor hæmorrhages.

The wound may now be closed.   Blunt hooks are introduced in the manner already described (page 59, vol. i.) in
order to ensure accurate approximation of the edges.

Silkworm gut is by far the best suture material.   The
threads are all introduced, and before the first one is tied
the surgeon must satisfy himself that the wound is still clear
of clots.   The highest sutures are secured first, and as they
are tied the assistant follows the closing wound with a sponge,
which should be so firmly pressed upon the part as to
obliterate the wound cavity.   In all cases in which the operation has been extensive, and the wound deep, or in which
there has been much bleeding, or portions of tissue left
behind, it is well to introduce a drainage-tube.   This tube
must be removed at the end of twenty-four hours.   I have
tried to dispense with drainage-tubes, but with less satisfactory results.

The best dressing for these cases is a large sponge or a
pad of Tillmann's linen dusted with iodoform, and packed
round with cotton wool.   The pressure applied while the
sutures are being secured must never be relaxed, and the
dressing must be made to press very firmly upon the part.
The bandage, to obtain a good hold of the neck, must
usually be carried beneath the axillæ, and possibly over the
head.

The pressure brought to bear upon the wound is considerable, and often causes some blueness of the face until the
effects of the anæsthetic have passed off.   I think, also, that
this interference with the venous current from the head may
possibly delay the recovery from chloroform.

If the patient have very enlarged tonsils the operation
should not be attempted until the tonsils have been removed,

because a properly firm dressing can seldom be applied in such a case without producing symptoms of suffocation.

Primary union can only be depended on when the wound cavity has been obliterated by pressure.

The After-treatment of these cases calls for little comment. The tight dressing, the collar of cotton-wool, and the elaborate bandaging, keep the neck stiff. In children the part may be maintained more completely at rest by fixing the head in a loosely filled sand-bag, as Mr. William Knight Treves advises. Absolute rest of the part is most essential, and should be observed with the utmost rigour for seven to fourteen days—that is to say, if primary healing with the minimum amount of scarring is desired. The child should not be allowed to talk, and all its food should be fluid, so that the muscles of mastication may not be used. The drain should be removed at the end of twenty-four hours, and the sutures between the fifth and the eighth day.

CHAPTER V.

EXCISION OF THE TONGUE.

EXCISION of the whole or of part of the tongue is carried out for the relief of many conditions. The great majority of the operations, however, are performed for malignant disease.

Cancer of the tongue is most usually situated on the dorsal aspect, and is especially common at the margin of the organ. It is comparatively rare on the under-surface or at the tip.

An excellent epitome of the history of the operation has been furnished by Woelfler, and elaborated by Mr. Barker ("Holmes's System of Surgery, third edition, vol. ii., page 597. 1883). From this it appears that Pimpernelle, who died in 1658, was probably the first to excise the tongue with success. Guthrie (in 1756) is stated to have been the first English surgeon to excise a cancer of the tongue, using the knife and cautery.

The Various Methods of Operating.—The following facts are derived from Woelfler and Barker's epitome :—

The Ligature.—The removal of the tongue by strangulation with a ligature was carried out by Inglis (1803) and others. The organ was usually split, and a ligature applied to each half. Cloquet (1827) introduced the ligature through a supra-hyoid incision.

The Écraseur. — This instrument was introduced by Chassaignac in 1854, and has been extensively employed. It has been used through the mouth, or introduced through a supra-hyoid incision after Cloquet's method. Both the cold wire and the galvanic écraseur have been made use of.

Preliminary Ligature of the Lingual Artery was introduced by Mirault in 1833. The method has been employed by Roux and Roser, and has been within more recent times revived by Billroth.

Division of the Cheek.—This was carried out by Jaeger in 1831, in order to obtain freer access to the tongue. Maisonneuve (1858) and Collis (1867) advocated and employed this method.

Division of the Lower Jaw has been effected to obtain a ready access to the tongue and the floor of the mouth. The method was introduced by Roux in 1836, and has been carried out and modified by Sédillot (1844), Syme (1857), and Billroth (1862).

The Infra-Maxillary Incision was first employed by Regnoli in 1838. The tongue was reached by an incision along the border of the lower jaw.

The method has been employed and developed by Czerny (1870), Billroth (1871-6), and Kocher (1880).

The Circumstances of the Operation and the Question of Hæmorrhage.—The main difficulties encountered in attempting to remove the entire tongue are dependent upon the narrow space in which the operation has to be performed and upon hæmorrhage.

To get over the first difficulty ingenious gags have been invented, and various cheek retractors employed, or the cheek itself has been slit up, or the jaw divided, or the mouth entered by an incision in the supra-hyoid or infra-maxillary region. It is recognised that the excision, to be satisfactory, must be complete, and to effect this the surgeon's movements must not be hampered.

To cope with the bleeding, the actual cautery, the ligature, and the écraseur, have been used, or the lingual arteries have been secured in the neck by a preliminary operation.

The Hæmorrhage cannot be said to be great in amount. It proceeds mainly from the two lingual arteries which are divided in the floor of the mouth. The lingual artery is small. The average calibre of the main trunk is only about 3 m.m. The artery is usually cut beyond the hyo-glossus muscle, and when it has received the name ranine. The two ranine arteries anastomose by a small loop near the tip of the tongue, but with this exception the right and left linguals only communicate by capillary branches. It is not the extent of the hæmorrhage that troubles the surgeon so much as the locality of the bleeding

The blood is poured into the mouth, and when even quite small in amount may entirely obscure the area of the operation. The operation is carried on, as it were, in a small cup, and this is soon filled. The blood is apt, moreover, to run back into the pharynx, and find its way into the air-passages. The narrow space within which the surgeon's operations are confined renders the securing of the bleeding-point often a matter of difficulty.

The lingual arteries follow a somewhat upward course in passing from the region of the great cornu of the hyoid bone to the frænum linguæ.

When the tongue has been removed, and these vessels are exposed in the floor of the mouth, it will be found that if the mouth be kept well open the stream of blood which issues from the cut vessels will be directed out of the mouth. The blood, as it spurts from the divided artery, is directed upwards and forwards, and thus under what may be termed natural conditions it is poured out of the mouth rather than into it. Very often, indeed, the jet of blood strikes the surgeon in the face as he is looking for the severed vessel.

The lingual arteries, especially in patients of the age at which cancer operations are usually undertaken, are often brittle, and are a little difficult to secure.

Unless a good view be obtained of the bleeding-point it is not easy to grasp the artery with forceps, without at the same time picking up much muscular tissue.

It must be remembered that when the tongue has been removed a very deep cavity is left in the mouth, and the floor of this cavity may appear far removed.

If all the fingers of one hand be placed on the skin between the lower jaw and the hyoid bone, and if the floor of the mouth be pressed vigorously upwards by the fingers so placed, not only is the cut surface brought well into view, but the hæmorrhage is, for the time being, controlled.

Or an assistant, placing both his thumbs in the same position, may take hold of the lower jaw with the fingers and force the floor of the mouth up with the thumbs.

To attempt to pick up the bleeding vessels, without first forcing upwards and fixing the floor of the mouth, is to make the attempt unnecessarily difficult.

Mr. Christopher Heath effects the same end by hooking the finger round the base of the tongue in the pharynx, and drawing the bleeding stump forwards. In this way, also, the cut surface is fixed, and is brought better into view, while the bleeding is for the time controlled. The objection to this plan, however, is that the finger must occupy the mouth, the hand is in the way, and the field of the operation is curtailed.

While bleeding is taking place into the oral cavity, care should be observed in maintaining a certain position of the head. If the head be thrown back, and the chin be in the median line, all the blood must gravitate backwards to the pharynx and air-passages. This is the position in which the head is not infrequently found after the excision has been effected. To minimise the evils of haemorrhage the shoulders should be well raised, the head should be pushed a little forwards, and should incline to one side, so that the cheek rests upon the table, or is at least the most dependent part. If this be done, all the blood will at first run into the flaccid hollow of the cheek. In old subjects, with tissues relaxed by the anaesthetic, the capacity of this cheek pouch is considerable. The blood can be readily removed from the pouch by sponges in holders, and is often found to have already coagulated.

The position described is not the most convenient for the operator, but it is certainly the safest for the patient.

Extent of the Operation.—Small innocent growths of the tongue or small portions of the organ can be readily excised with the scalpel or with suitable scissors. If convenient, the edges of the wound may be brought together with sutures. Sutures, however, are seldom necessary, and the wounds do well enough without them. The bleeding may be checked by sponge pressure, or by pressure forceps, or by torsion.

When the extreme tip of the tongue is involved, the part may be excised by a V-shaped incision, the base of the V including the tip of the organ, the apex being at the middle line, some distance from the tip.

The margins of the triangular gap thus left may be approximated by sutures.

In most cases of cancer it is better to remove the entire tongue. It is true that none but capillary anastomoses are effected between the right and left halves of the tongue, and it is true also that the disease may be very strictly limited to one half. It may also be added that in cases in which one half of the tongue only has been removed, it has not been shown that recurrence in the stump is peculiarly frequent. These points favour a partial excision. In favour of complete removal, it must be said that the larger operation involves no more risk; that it allows of a much more complete removal of the tissues upon the diseased side; that the after-trouble to the patient is less when the whole organ has been sacrificed than when one-half has been left. There is, I think, more after-pain in the partial excisions, more watering of the mouth, and more general inconvenience. As time goes on, the patient can neither speak nor swallow better, although one-half of the tongue has been saved.

The half that is left curls towards the diseased side, and forms an uncouth-looking mass in the mouth, as cumbrous in appearance as a parrot's tongue. It is like a foreign body, and is rolled aimlessly about as the patient is attempting to speak. I have repeatedly compared the results of these two operations, and so far the evidence is decidedly in favour of complete excisions.

This operation cannot be used to illustrate the proverb that "half a loaf is better than no bread."

Preliminary Measures.—For a day or so before the operation every attempt should be made, in cancer cases, to overcome the foul state of the mouth. For this purpose, a wash of carbolic lotion (1 in 80) may be used hourly, and especially after any food has been taken. Male patients should be shaved, and this is most necessary when the linguals are to be tied, or the supra-hyoid region opened up.

When the patient is under the anæsthetic, any quite loose teeth should be removed. The incisor teeth in cancer cases are often loose, uncovered by the gum, and foul with tartar. The cleaner the mouth can be made the better. It is often possible to scrape putrid particles of food soaked in discharge from between the teeth. The passage of a coarse brush along the teeth will usually bring away a quantity of indescribably offensive matter.

Better results would be obtained if a moderate amount of

care were taken to render the mouth less septic. It is unwise to deliberately carry out any excision in an atmosphere of putrefaction.

Instruments required:

1. When the operation is through the mouth—

Mouth gag. Curved needle in handle. Stout waxed silk. Tongue forceps. Mouth retractor. Tenaculum. Blunt-pointed scissors, straight and curved. Volsella. Artery, pressure, and dissecting forceps. Sponges in holders. Ligatures, &c.

2. If the lingual is tied in the neck, or glands are removed—

In addition: Scalpel. Retractors. Blunt hooks. Aneurysm needle. Needles and sutures. (*See* Ligature of Lingual artery, page 163, vol. i.)

3. If the cheek is split—

In addition: Hare-lip pins.

4. If the jaw is divided—

In addition: Keyhole saw. Hey's saw. Bone forceps. Bone drill. Stout wire. Wire nippers.

The following instruments may be needed in some cases: Paquelin's cautery. Tracheotomy tubes. Trendelenburg's tampon.

The best gag is Mason's or Coleman's. It must be strong, and the blades be capable of wide separation. The "catch" fixing the gag when open must be secure. A "catch" is better than a screw.

The best cheek retractor is the broad rectangular retractor used in nephrectomy operations. It is in every way excellent.

The scissors used for cutting out the tongue should be quite straight, and quite flat and strong. They should be longer than the usual pattern, and should end in square blunt points. The cutting edge should extend up to the very tip. Curved scissors should never be used to effect the actual excision.

The Anæsthetic.—Chloroform should be selected, and it is best administered by means of Dr. Hewitt's most ingenious and admirable gag. This consists of a Mason's gag, along the bars of which two small metal tubes run. These open at the mouth end of the gag, and at the handle end are connected with tubes from Junker's chloroform apparatus. The anæsthetic can be given without the very least inconvenience to the surgeon, and without the area of the operation being encroached upon. I have found Dr. Hewitt's method most satisfactory.

Position.—The patient lies close to the right-hand side of the table. The head and shoulders are well raised, and the arms are folded behind the back. The surgeon stands to the right and the chief assistant to the left. The anæsthetist stands at the head of the table, and by him an assistant who holds the gag and steadies the head. The gag is introduced on the left side of the mouth, is very firmly held, and, with a Mason's gag, it is a good rule to keep the handle of the gag always against the patient's ear.

A good light is essential.

The **operations** will be considered in the following order—

1. Whitehead's operation.
2. Excision after ligature of the linguals in the neck.
3. Kocher's operation.
4. Other operations.

These will include—

A. Excision after division of the lower jaw.
B. Excision after division of the cheek.
C. Regnoli's operation.
D. Removal by the écraseur.

1. WHITEHEAD'S OPERATION.

This method was described in the *British Medical Journal*, Dec. 8, 1877, in the *Transactions of the International Medical Congress*, vol. ii., page 401, and in later pamphlets.

The following description is derived from Mr. Whitehead's latest account of the operation (*Brit. Med. Journal*, May 2, 1891).

Chloroform is the anæsthetic selected. The patient is put completely under during the first stage of the operation, but afterwards only partial insensibility is maintained. The mouth is well gagged. The head is so supported that blood tends to gravitate out of the mouth rather than backwards into the pharynx. The patient's mouth ought to, roughly speaking, be on a level with the surgeon's axilla. The head is firmly held erect, with a slight inclination forwards. Steps must be taken to prevent the patient from slipping down on the table.

A firm ligature is passed through the anterior portion of the tongue for the purpose of traction. Much depends upon the care of the assistant to make the traction in the right direction and at the right time.

The first step in the actual operation consists in the separation of the tongue from its attachment to the floor of the mouth and the anterior pillars of the fauces. The ease with which the operation is continued depends largely upon the freedom with which this separation is carried out. The two structures principally responsible for the retention of the tongue within the mouth are the frænum and the anterior pillars of the fauces; and, if these are completely divided in the first instance, the tongue may be so freely drawn from the mouth that the operation is practically converted into an extra-oral excision. "Extended practice," writes Mr. Whitehead, "has made me conduct this part of the operation with less deliberation and more rapidity than was my habit in my earlier cases. Instead of the cautious snipping I originally advocated, I now boldly cut until I get close to the vicinity of the main arteries, disregarding all bleeding, unless an artery distinctly spurts, when I twist it and proceed. The more profuse the general oozing the more rapidly I proceed, my object being to get as quickly as possible to the main arteries, as I have confidence that all subsidiary bleeding will cease immediately after their division. There is, in reality, no difficulty in determining the actual position of the lingual arteries, as they are practically invariably found in the same situation, and it requires very little experience to seize them with a pair of forceps before dividing them; if this be done there need not be the slightest hæmorrhage from this source. When once the vessels are effectually twisted, the rest of the tongue may be removed without any further anxiety about hæmorrhage; but it is desirable, before finally severing the last attachments, to pass a loop of silk through the glosso-epiglottidean fold, as a provisional measure of security, in case it may become necessary to make traction on the posterior floor of the mouth either to assist respiration, or to arrest any possible consecutive hæmorrhage. Traction on this ligature of itself arrests hæmorrhage, and makes it an easy matter to secure any bleeding vessel. As the retention of this ligature is a source of some annoyance to the patient, I always remove it at the end of twenty-four hours." Strong straight blunt-ended scissors are employed.

After the tongue is removed, the floor of the mouth is washed with a solution of biniodide of mercury (1 in 1,000), is well dried, and is then painted with an antiseptic "varnish" introduced by Mr. Whitehead. This varnish contains the ordinary ingredients of friar's balsam, and differs from it in the fact that for the rectified spirit is substituted a saturated solution of iodoform in ether. With the ether is mixed one volume in ten of turpentine. This varnish dries immediately, and leaves a firm coating on the wound which lasts for twenty-four hours, and produces no irritation. It also acts as an admirable styptic.

Some surgeons simply dust the floor of the mouth with iodoform. Others resort to the objectionable practice of stuffing the mouth, or at least the lower segment of it, with gauze. I have dispensed with applications of any kind. The mouth is well washed out with an antiseptic lotion, and is left. It must be remembered that the discharge of saliva is fairly copious, and renders any "dressing" almost immediately ineffective.

Comment.—I think that the ligature left in the glosso-epiglottic tissues may well be dispensed with. As has been already pointed out (page 182), there is no difficulty in bringing the floor of the mouth into view in case of secondary bleeding.

When the disease involves the frænum, it is well—as Mr. Jacobson points out—to extract two or three of the lower incisors. If this be not done, it is very difficult to obtain a clear field for the scissors, and a complete excision of the implicated tissues may be found to be almost impossible.

Mr. Jacobson ("The Operations of Surgery," page 300) modifies the operation in the following manner :—

He splits the tongue in the median line and draws out the diseased half, which he proceeds to remove in the manner already described. He cuts the lateral connections of the tongue and the muscular layers entering the under-surface "as far back as is needful."

The tongue having been freed horizontally up to a point well behind the disease, it remains to make a transverse section of its root. This is effected in the following way :—
Instead of cutting straight across the isolated half of the tongue, and trusting to being able to secure the lingual on the face of the stump, Mr. Jacobson cuts a deep groove through the mucous membrane on the side and dorsum, and tears through the soft muscular tissue with a steel director until the lingual nerve and artery are seen. The latter structure is secured with torsion forceps, and the excision is completed.

If needful the surgeon then proceeds to remove the other half of the tongue. Mr. Jacobson is, however, in favour of partial excisions.

2. EXCISION AFTER LIGATURE OF THE LINGUALS IN THE NECK.

Ligature of the lingual artery as a preliminary measure to excision of the tongue was introduced by Mirault in 1833. The operation has been revived of late years by Billroth ("Clinical Surgery Syd. Soc.," page 113) and others.

I believe that the removal of the tongue with scissors after the linguals have been ligatured in the neck provides the best method of excising the organ.

The preliminary measures already alluded to (page 184) having been carried out, the surgeon proceeds to ligature the two linguals in the neck.

This operation has been fully described (page 163, vol. i.). The vessel is ligatured as it lies beneath the hyo-glossus muscle. Reasons for selecting this situation have been given.

The surgeon may begin with the right artery, as it is a little more easy to secure than the left.

The wound on each side is closed by a few points of silk-worm-gut suture. The closure is not allowed to be very complete, so that any blood which may ooze into the wound can readily escape through the gaps between the sutures.

The incisions are dusted with iodoform and covered with a

mass of cotton-wool, which is secured in place by a bandage passed round the neck.

After the tongue has been excised, the wool pads are removed from the wounds. The cavity of each wound is syringed out with a weak carbolic lotion: the fluid escaping in the gaps between the sutures. The parts are then well cleaned, and the wounds, which should now show no sign of oozing, are finally dressed with sponges dusted with iodoform, and firmly secured *in situ* by a flannel bandage.

After the arteries have been secured the gag is introduced and the tongue is removed with scissors in the manner already described.

The operator may ignore the trifling bleeding which takes place, and may complete the excision without let or hindrance. No time is occupied in securing vessels, or in arresting slight hæmorrhage by sponge pressure. The surgeon's whole attention can be devoted to effecting the excision in the best possible manner: the area of the operation is not occupied by a pool of blood, and the attention is not withdrawn from the primary operation by a vigorous bleeding at a critical period.

No excision could be simpler or easier, nor more free from disturbing circumstances. It may, if thought desirable, be carried out with remarkable rapidity.

There is no need to insert a ligature through the tissues at the base of the epiglottis.

After the tongue has been removed a piece of Turkey sponge of suitable size is introduced into the mouth, and is pressed against the floor of the cavity.

While it is held in place with the left hand, the right hand is occupied in removing any clots from the pharynx or from the hollow of the cheek by a sponge in a holder. The only bleeding is from the posterior part of the tongue, from the dorsalis linguæ vessels. The pressure of the sponge is usually sufficient to check it. I have never known the bleeding from this source to cause any notable trouble. In one or two instances I have grasped the bleeding-points with pressure forceps, and have allowed the instruments to remain attached until the patient is nearly ready to leave the operating-room.

This excision may be said in many cases to be practically bloodless. In no instance does the hæmorrhage amount to more than an unimportant oozing: and this in most instances ceases spontaneously.

3. KOCHER'S OPERATION.

This method was first described by Kocher in 1880 ("Deutsche Zeitschr. f. klin. Chir.," Bd. 13, page 147), and has been especially advocated in England by Mr. Barker.

The patient having been placed in position, a preliminary tracheotomy is performed.

An ordinary cannula is employed, and the pharynx is plugged with a clean sponge, which has been wrung out in carbolic lotion, and to which, as a security, a long silk thread is attached.

The mouth will have been already as well cleansed as is possible, and should have been very frequently rinsed out with some antiseptic solution.

Chloroform is administered through the tracheal tube.

An incision is made in the neck. It commences just below the lobule of the ear, and runs along the anterior border of the sterno-mastoid muscle.

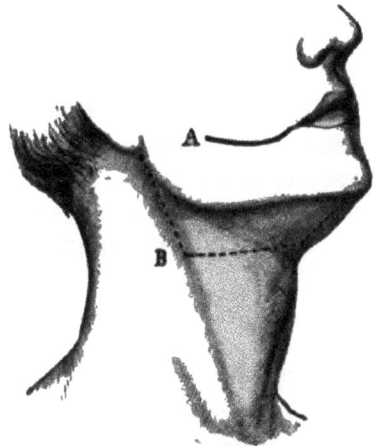

Fig. 313.—REMOVAL OF THE TONGUE.
A, Incision for splitting the cheek.
B, Kocher's incision.

When the middle of this border of the muscle has been reached, the incision is carried forwards to the hyoid bone, and thence to the symphysis along the anterior belly of the digastric muscle (Fig. 313, B.)

The flap thus marked out is turned upon the cheek. The facial vessels are ligatured, as is also the lingual artery before it passes beneath the hyoglossus muscle. The submaxillary fossa is now evacuated, the surgeon working from behind forwards. All the lymphatic glands of the region are removed. and also the sublingual and submaxillary salivary glands should the diseased tissue be in near association with them. The mylo-hyoid muscle having been cut through as far as is needed, the mucous membrane is divided close to the jaw, and the tongue drawn out through the opening.

The tongue may now be slit in the middle line, and one half removed with scissors.

If the whole tongue need to be removed, the lingual artery of the opposite side must be ligatured through a separate incision.

Kocher carried out the operation under the spray, and adopted " antiseptic measures " which are not now in vogue.

The skin incision is not closed by sutures, but the whole wound is left open, and its cavity is plugged with gauze or with a sponge wrung out in carbolic lotion.

The wound is allowed therefore to close by granulation, while the freest possible vent is provided for the escape of all discharges.

The tracheotomy tube is retained until the wound is granulating healthily. It thus happens that the patient breathes fresh air throughout the most important period of the after-treatment, or at least, the air inspired has not passed through the mouth and over the wound surface.

4. OTHER OPERATIONS.

A. **Excision after Division of the Lower Jaw.**—The operation of Roux, Sédillot, or Syme.

The soft parts are divided in the median line by an incision which bisects the lower lip, traverses the chin, and ends at the hyoid bone (Fig. 314, A). All bleeding having been arrested, one of the lower central incisors is extracted, and two holes are drilled through the jaw below the level of the teeth, each hole being about a quarter of an inch on either side of the median line.

The jaw is now divided as near to the middle line as possible. The section may be vertical, or may be slightly serrated, so that after the excision the two portions of the jaw may be to some extent interlocked.

The two halves of the jaw are held asunder by assistants while a stout silk ligature is passed through the tongue—in the manner already described (page 187)—and by means of this thread the organ is drawn well forwards and upwards.

The floor of the mouth is opened up. The mucous membrane between the tongue and the alveolus is divided with scissors; the genio-hyoid and genio-hyo-glossi muscles are then cut with the same instrument.

The excision of the tongue is carried out with the scissors. The tissues entering the under-surface of the tongue are divided in order from before backwards, and all bleeding vessels are at once secured. The operator should endeavour to ascertain the position of the lingual arteries, and each artery may be grasped with pressure forceps before the section is carried beyond the vessel. It is well that one artery should be secured before the other is cut. It is better to conduct the operation slowly, and to proceed step by step, rather than to attempt to slash the tongue away boldly by one or two vigorous cuts with a bistoury.

A very convenient plan is to split the tongue, and remove one half at a time. While the first lingual is being dealt with the tongue is held forwards by means of the intact half; and while the second artery is being dealt with, the stump may be drawn forwards by the forefinger, which is hooked, as it were, in the pharynx.

As much of the tissues in the floor of the mouth as appears to be involved must be removed.

Bleeding arteries should be secured by torsion rather than by ligature.

The two halves of the jaw are wired together by a stout silver wire passed through the two holes.

The wound is closed by sutures, and a drain is introduced into its lower angle.

A gutta-percha cap may be fitted to the chin to prevent displacement of the divided bone.

Precautions should be taken to prevent the falling back of the stump, which is apt to occur when the attachments of the hyoid bone to the jaw have been extensively divided. This complication may be met by securing the tissues of the stump to the tissues at the sides of the mouth by two or more silkworm-gut sutures. These sutures may be allowed to cut their way out in the course of time.

In certain cases, in order to effect a more complete removal of the cancerous parts, portions of the jaw have been excised together with the tongue. In these instances the implication of the floor of the mouth has been very decided. These operations are extensive and serious, and before a surgeon undertakes so grave a measure he should be quite convinced that the disease has not yet become so far extending as to render a complete and satisfactory excision almost impossible.

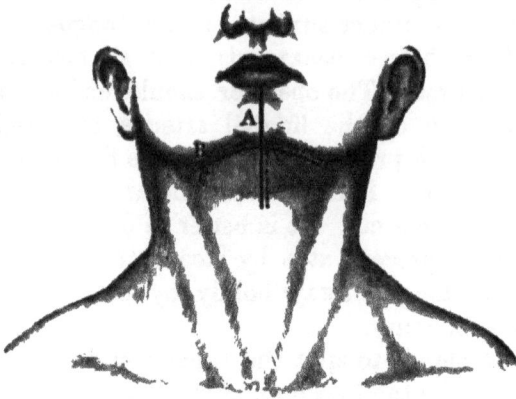

Fig. 314.—REMOVAL OF THE TONGUE.
A, Incision of Syme, Roux, Sédillot; B, Regnoli's incision; c, Billroth's incision.

B. **Excision after Division of the Cheek.**—This method has been employed by Jaeger (1857), Maisonneuve (1858), Collis (1867), Sir William Stokes, Furneaux Jordan, Gant, and others.

The incision made in the cheek is a curved one, and extends from the angle of the mouth to the anterior edge of the masseter muscle (Fig. 313, A). It has been modified in many unimportant ways.

A straight blunt-pointed bistoury is used in the making of the incision. While the cut is being made, an assistant grasps the tissues of the cheek above and below the line of the incision with the thumb and forefinger of each hand. In this way the bleeding, which is disposed to be very free, is controlled. All the divided vessels must be well secured before the operation is proceeded with.

The two flaps of the cheek are now held well aside, and a gag having been introduced the excision of the tongue is carried out through the large opening which has been obtained.

c. **Regnoli's Operation.**—Regnoli's account appeared in 1838 (" Bull. delle Scienze Med. di Bologna ").

An incision is made in the median line of the neck from the lower margin of the symphysis to the centre of the hyoid bone. Two lateral incisions extend outwards from the upper end of the median cut, and follow the lower border of the jaw as far as the anterior border of the masseter muscle (Fig. 314, B). The facial artery is not divided. The two flaps thus marked out are dissected up, and contain skin, cellular tissue, and platysma. A straight sharp-pointed bistoury is thrust from below upwards behind the symphysis, and into the mouth so that the point appears behind the incisor teeth. It is withdrawn, and a straight blunt-pointed bistoury is introduced in its place. The insertions of the genio-hyoid and genio-hyoglossal muscles are severed.

The knife is then made to divide the anterior insertions of the digastric and mylo-hyoid muscles, and the mucous membrane of the mouth as far back as the anterior pillars of the fauces. Such vessels as are divided are secured. The tongue is now seized, and is dragged forcibly through the opening, and is then excised by means of scissors, the same precautions being observed with regard to the lingual arteries as are described in the account of Syme's operation (page 193). It may be necessary to take steps to prevent the falling back of the stump. These have been already alluded to (page 187).

A drain having been introduced, the wound is closed.

This operation has been modified in many ways. Billroth omitted the vertical part of the cut, and carried the curved submental incision much further backwards on both sides, so as to be able to ligature one or both lingual arteries before extirpating the tongue and any affected glands that may exist (Fig. 314. C).

D. **Removal by the Écraseur.**—The écraseur has been applied to the tongue in several ways. It has been introduced through the mouth or through an incision made between the symphysis and the hyoid bone. It has been employed as a sole means of dividing the tongue, and has been used as a supplementary means, a part of the excision having been effected by the scissors or the bistoury.

n 2

The only method of using the écraseur that will be dealt with
is that advocated by Mr. Morrant Baker, and described by him
in the *British Medical Journal* for 1883 (vol. ii., page 765):—

"A gag having been introduced, two threads are passed
through the tongue, about one inch behind the tip, and half
an inch on each side of the middle line. One of these looped
threads is now given to an assistant to hold tightly ; and the
operator holding the other, scores the dorsum of the tongue with
a blunt-pointed scalpel, exactly in the middle line, extending
the cut well through the mucous membrane into the surface
of the muscular substance, and dividing the tip freely down to
and through the middle line of the frænum. The cut may be
extended back as far as the operator deems necessary, say, for
one inch beyond the level of the posterior edge of the cancer.
He then takes both threads, one in each hand, and, using the
forefingers much in the same way that he would for tightening
a ligature on a deep vessel, he splits the tongue into two
halves. At this stage of the operation the hæmorrhage is
usually very trifling if the operator has taken care to cut
along the middle line ; and even if he is a little to one side or
the other, the divided vessels are small and easily ligatured.
The thread which tethers the diseased half of the tongue is
now pulled quite taut either by the operator or his assistant ;
while the former, with blunt-pointed scissors, snips, as far as
he considers necessary, the mucous membrane and muscular
fibres which connect the tongue with the anterior part of the
lower jaw behind the symphysis. He then runs the scissors
along the floor of the mouth, immediately beneath the mucous
membrane, keeping close to the ramus of the jaw until he has
cut, if possible, to a point beyond the posterior edge of the
cancer. Then, with his forefinger and occasional snips with
the scissors, he frees the tongue as completely as may be
requisite from its attachments in front and at the sides and in
the floor of the mouth. The chief point aimed at, at this
stage of the operation, is to free the diseased half of the tongue
in such a manner that it may be surrounded by the loop of
the écraseur at some distance behind the disease, and without
danger of the cord slipping forward so as to embrace the
neighbourhood of the cancer, and much less the cancer itself.

"This is by far the most important part of the operation ;

and should the surgeon be in doubt about his having sufficiently freed the tongue with his finger, he should again introduce the scissors, and cautiously divide any muscle or other structure which prevents the due loosening of the tongue. Having now freed the tongue sufficiently, one, and sometimes two, blunt curved needles are made to perforate it at some distance, an inch, or more if possible, behind the cancerous mass; and the loop of the écraseur is now slipped over the diseased half of the tongue, and adjusted behind the needles. With the screwing-up of the écraseur this part of the operation is now completed, with the exception that, very commonly, at least when whipcord is employed, the main vessel and some other tissue, perhaps nerve fibres, are pulled through the end of the écraseur after the softer substance of the tongue has been crushed through. Under these circumstances a double ligature should be passed with an aneurysm needle, and the strand of vessels and nerves divided between the two knots, when the écraseur will, of course, at once come away, and the main vessels will be left on the face of the stump securely ligatured.

"In the event of both sides of the tongue requiring removal, an écraseur should now be slipped over the other half after it has been sufficiently freed from its attachments, and the diseased part guarded by a blunt-pointed needle."

Mr. Baker uses an écraseur of moderate size, which is curved a little on the flat near the end.

Both ends of the looped cord are shortened at the same time, and the material of the loop is a thick whipcord.

It will be seen from the above account that the écraseur is used only as a supplementary means. Its use is for the most part restricted to that segment of the tongue which contains the lingual arteries, at the intended point of division.

Mr. Baker's operation must be excluded from the ordinary category of écraseur operations. In these the loop is placed round the tongue in such a way that the excision is accomplished by the instrument alone. If Mr. Baker's method be adopted, certain of the very defined objections to the écraseur are removed.

THE CHOICE OF AN OPERATION.

Many decided and yet very opposite views have been

expressed upon the question as to which is the best means of excising the tongue.

Each surgeon will commend the operation of which he has personally most experience, and with which he is most familiar. This somewhat conservative attitude is not weakened by the fact that it is difficult to show by statistics that one particular method—among the more modern operations—is pre-eminently the most satisfactory and the most successful. Whitehead's operation, in the hands of Mr. Whitehead, has been attended with very admirable results, and it would be unfair to consider this particular excision as of slight value simply because another surgeon obtains less satisfactory results in his few attempts at removing the tongue with scissors. It would appear that in Kocher's operation better results have been obtained by the author of the method than by any other surgeon who has followed him.

In choosing a method of excising the tongue it is obvious that much must be left to the training and inclination of the individual surgeon, and that in giving advice to the student it may be excused if the advice is a little biassed by a personal and possibly somewhat restricted experience.

The three principal methods of operating are those first considered in the above account.

The operations dealt with in Section 4 have little to commend them.

I would venture to urge the following propositions in connection with the operation of excision of the tongue :—

1. The organ should be removed by cutting, i.e., either with scissors or with the bistoury.

2. The removal should, as a general rule, be effected through the mouth.

3. Every means should be taken to reduce the hæmorrhage to a minimum.

4. When the floor of the mouth is involved, or the glands are extensively involved, the excision should be carried out through the neck.

The wound made by a surgeon should be a clean cut—an incised wound. Such a wound accomplishes its end with the least possible amount of injury to the parts involved, and such a wound is made with the scissors or the scalpel.

The use of the écraseur, except in the modified manner advised by Mr. Baker, is to be condemned.

The instrument is barbarous and obsolete, and is not in conformity with the principles of modern surgery. It represents the most slovenly and the least efficient method of removing a part. It has the one advantage that its employment involves neither skill, judgment, nerve, nor education.

As a surgical undertaking *excision by the écraseur* has about it a distinct air of senility.

In the place of the clean cut it leaves a wound of almost the worst kind, viz., a lacerated and contused wound ; and inasmuch as septic pneumonia represents the chief risk after these operations, a needlessly evil element is introduced into the measure. The loop, as usually applied, is difficult to direct and difficult to maintain in place. The diseased tissue cannot be removed in any way that is desired. It must be removed upon a stereotyped plan. The loop directs the excision line. It must be a regular line, and the surgeon cannot depart from it. It is easy for the loop, under the great tension placed upon it, to encroach upon the cancerous district and leave some of the implicated tissue behind. The écraseur can but feebly imitate the deliberate and intelligent and exact excision which can be accomplished with the scissors or the scalpel.

The use of this uncouth instrument is excused upon the ground that it renders the operation bloodless. In the Middle Ages the écraseur would have been a useful apparatus, but since that period certain methods of checking bleeding have been introduced, and these can be as well applied to the cavity of the mouth as to the palm of the hand.

Even an exaggerated terror of hæmorrhage, and a sense of incompetency in dealing with it, afford no excuse for leaving in the mouth a wound that must in a few days exhibit a sloughing surface.

The objections here raised do not apply to the method of operating described on page 196. In that procedure the main portion of the raw surface left is represented by an incised wound, and only a comparatively small area would show the tract of the écraseur. Mr. Baker's method differs almost *in toto* from the operations which are usually

associated with the use of the écraseur, and in which the whole
tongue is, with little or no preparation, included in the looped
cord. Mr. Baker has applied his method to forty cases, with
only five deaths, one of which was due to diphtheria.

The galvanic écraseur has been so generally condemned
in these operations, that it only remains to regret that it is
still occasionally employed. It has all the disadvantges of
the simple écraseur, with the additional evils that it leaves
a still fouler wound, and is peculiarly prone to be followed
by secondary hæmorrhage. In six cases of removal of
the tongue by the galvanic écraseur, mentioned in the last
report of the London Hospital (1889), secondary bleeding
occurred in three. Mr. Barker states that out of sixteen
excisions with the galvanic loop at University College
Hospital, eight patients died.

Removal through the mouth involves no wound beyond
that made in the tongue. I have not yet met with a case
in which *splitting of the cheek* appeared to be called for.
Mr. Butlin states that division of the cheek is of immense
advantage in cases of extensive disease. More room is obtained, a better light is afforded, as well as a better command
over the stump of the tongue. It is open to question whether
these advantages may not be obtained in other and more
satisfactory ways.

Syme's Operation is quite needlessly severe, and needlessly
complicated. The after-treatment is of long duration, and
trouble often arises from the divided bone. As the attachments of the tongue to the hyoid bone are extensively divided,
the stump is apt to fall back, and the control over the larynx
may be so modified that the patient is less well able to prevent discharges from running into the air-passages.

The last-named of these objections may apply to *Regnoli's
Operation*. It gives good access to the floor of the mouth,
and may be employed when the tip of the tongue and the
anterior part of the floor of the mouth are involved. It fails,
however, to provide an equally free access to the base and
lateral parts of the tongue. Billroth's modification of this
operation has distinct advantages over the parent method.

Of the *three selected methods of excision* (viz., Whitehead's operation, excision after ligature of the linguals, and

Kocher's operation), I would venture to think that the excision of the tongue after securing the linguals at the neck is the best operation in the usual run of cases, and that Kocher's operation may be with advantage employed when the glands are much involved, and especially when one side of the floor of the mouth has been invaded. Of the value of Whitehead's operation there is, however, no question.

The possible advantages of the method *of excision after securing the linguals* over Whitehead's method are these :—

In the former operation, the excision can be conducted very safely and easily. There is no pool of blood on the floor of the mouth to obscure the surgeon's movements, and the excision can be carried out with great accuracy and precision. In *Whitehead's operation*, the bleeding may be copious and sufficiently free to hamper the surgeon's movements, and to complicate the operation. To an inexperienced operator the bleeding may be alarming, and may lead to hurried and incoherent action. The fact that the hæmorrhage is readily controlled does not render it the less troublesome or a less serious complication during the actual excision.

The advantages of the method by securing the linguals are not limited to the one feature of rendering the operation almost bloodless, and relieving the surgeon of all anxiety as to hæmorrhage. In cutting down upon the arteries the submaxillary lymphatic glands are exposed, and may be removed if found to be enlarged. I have often excised glands which were discovered during the operation, but which were not to be felt through the skin before the operation was commenced. If necessary, also the floor of the mouth can be opened up and the submaxillary salivary gland, which is not infrequently adherent to the diseased tissues, can be removed with the greatest readiness.

It has been said (1) that the preliminary ligature of the linguals adds to the dangers of the excision; (2) that it involves a difficult operation which consumes a great deal of time, and (3) that the bleeding may be as free after the linguals have been secured as it is when no such precaution is taken (Jacobson).

My answer to these objections is as follows:—

1. I find, from the Register of the London Hospital, that I have removed the entire tongue with scissors (after ligaturing both linguals in the neck) thirty-four times. Of these thirty-four patients two only died from the operation (one of pneumonia, the other of pyæmia). A third patient, with aortic and mitral disease, died suddenly very shortly after the operation, but it would be scarcely just to ascribe this death to this particular excision. These figures will show that the operation is not unduly dangerous. I might add, that I have had no death from this operation in private practice.

2. I have ligatured the lingual artery in considerably more than sixty-eight instances (*i.e.*, both arteries in the thirty-four cases). The operation is easy, and both linguals can be secured within fifteen to twenty minutes. Since attention was drawn to the length of time involved in this operation, I have noted that seven minutes represents a fair period of time within which the ligature of one vessel may be completed.

3. With regard to the third objection, I can only add that in no instance in which I have ligatured both arteries have I found any bleeding which caused the least inconvenience, and very little that called for any treatment.

I have known other structures to be ligatured in the place of the lingual artery, and the bleeding as a consequence to have been very free, "as free as in the usual operation with scissors." It is by no means difficult to make a mistake in securing this small and deeply placed vessel.

The anatomy of the tongue is simple, and is well known; the anastomoses of the lingual arteries have been thoroughly demonstrated, and my experience has distinctly taught me that if both lingual arteries are securely ligatured as they pass beneath the hyo-glossus muscle, the bleeding from the stump of the tongue will be arrested. Mr. Jacobson's position is, that after both linguals have been ligatured in the neck, the bleeding from the divided tongue may be as free as if the arteries had never been secured ("Operations of Surgery," page 362). No anatomical reasons are given to support this statement, which appears to be founded only upon an experience of three cases.

Kocher's Operation is severe, and involves a wide opening up of the connective tissue of the neck.

It appears to be somewhat too extensive for the ordinary case of excision of the tongue, and many surgeons may be inclined to dispense with the preliminary tracheotomy.

The incision can be carried out easily and completely, and the hæmorrhage can be kept well under control.

The operation is well suited for cases in which the tongue is affected far back, in which diseased glands exist, and in which the floor of the mouth is involved upon one side. The resulting wound can be kept clean, but the after-treatment is tedious. In one very successful case reported by Mr. Barker (*Lancet*, October 15, 1887), it is noted that the patient continued to be fed with a tube for sixteen days after the excision.

THE AFTER-TREATMENT.

In a case of excision of the tongue after ligature of the linguals in the neck, the following treatment is carried out:—

Nothing is applied to the mouth at the time of the operation. The slight oozing, and the salivation which continues for some hours after the excision, render an application of little avail. When the mouth is fairly dry, its floor is dusted over with iodoform.

The patient is encouraged to sit up in bed as soon as possible. Morphia should be avoided whenever it can be: it dulls the reflex sensibility of the patient, and may cause him to allow fluid to run down into the air-passages.

The man must be impressed with the importance of allowing all discharge to escape from the mouth, and of swallowing none of it.

The mouth must be kept constantly washed out. This rinsing of the mouth cannot be too frequently performed. Every half-hour in the day, and two or four times in the night, are not too often. The best wash is carbolic lotion (1 in 60 to 1 in 80).

After certain of the washings, say three or four times a day, the floor of the mouth is dried with a pledget of cotton-wool, and iodoform is dusted over the raw surface. It soon forms a more or less consistent pellicle over the stump. A watch must be kept for the symptoms of iodoform poisoning.

During the first twenty-four hours the patient should be fed per rectum, and ice only should be taken by the mouth. The use of ice should be very moderate, as it does little but fill the mouth with fluid, which gives the patient some trouble to get rid of. At the end of twenty-four, or at the latest forty-eight hours, the patient should swallow food. It is best given with an ordinary feeder, while the man sits upright, with his head inclined to one side.

The difficulty of swallowing is usually got over with a little patience and practice. Should the patient be quite unable to swallow, then he must be fed with an œsophageal tube.

One feature in the after-treatment of these cases must not be lost sight of. *The patient must be well fed.* As soon as enough nourishment is taken per os, the nutrient enemata may be discontinued. After every occasion upon which food is taken, the mouth must be well washed out.

Now and then the cavity may be flushed out with an irrigator. These operation cases demand the undivided attention of two nurses, one for day duty and one for night, for upon the careful nursing of the case as much of the snccess depends as upon the operation.

No drainage of the mouth cavity is needed in these cases. If the part becomes unduly offensive, a stronger solution of carbolic acid must be used, and the mere rinsing out of the mouth must be replaced by a flushing out of the cavity with the irrigator. The condition seems to be relieved also by allowing a carbolic steam spray to play about the head of the patient's bed.

These perpetual washings-out of the mouth involve considerable annoyance to the patient, but they are necessary only for a few days, and it must be borne in mind that the usual cause of death after these operations is septic pneumonia.

The wounds in the neck are treated in the usual way. They almost invariably heal up by first intention.

The patient may be allowed up on the fourth day, and in the majority of the cases I have treated at the London Hospital the patient has left the hospital between the seventh and the tenth day after the excision.

I have been very much disappointed with a solution of permanganate of potash as a wash, and have long since given it up. Boracic lotion is still more ineffective.

Some surgeons, notably Woelfler, have advised that the floor of the mouth be packed with iodoform gauze. I have tried this dressing, but cannot recommend it. It was employed by Mr. Butlin in one case, and the patient died of septic pneumonia. Mr. Whitehead tried it also in one case, and the patient swallowed the dressing.

Mr. Whitehead employs the varnish with which his name is associated (page 188). He does not encourage his patients to consider themselves invalids. They get up on the day after the operation, and may on that day take open-air exercise. Food is administered by the mouth on the day after the excision. In the matter of rapidity of recovery, Mr. Whitehead's cases stand pre-eminent.

Kocher and many others advise that the patient be fed with a tube to prevent any of the nutriment prescribed from lodging in the mouth and decomposing there. I would venture to think that the tube should only be employed in those few cases in which the patient appears to be really unable to swallow. Even in such instances the sooner it is abandoned the better.

The wholesale cauterisation of the wound immediately after the operation, with pure carbolic acid, a strong solution of chloride of zinc, or powdered permanganate of potash, cannot be other than condemned. It is purposeless, and attended with intense pain.

The after-treatment of these cases involves three great factors :—

1st, Let the patient be well fed.

2nd, Let all discharges escape from the mouth.

3rd, Keep the cavity of the mouth clean and sweet.

The After-results.—It is estimated that the duration of life in cases of cancer of the tongue, when no treatment is carried out, is twelve to eighteen months.

It has been clearly shown that even when recurrence occurs after excision, the patient's life has been prolonged, his more distressing symptoms relieved, and his comfort greatly added to.

Taking excision of the tongue generally, the mortality of the operation is now probably below 10 per cent.

Not many years ago the mortality was 30 per cent., and between the years 1860 and 1880, Billroth gives the mortality as 22·0 per cent.

Mr. Butlin thus analyses seventy cases of excision for cancer :—

   8 died of the operation.
  19 were lost sight of.
  32 died of early recurrence.
   5 were alive up to periods varying from some months to over two years.
   6 were alive more than three years after the operation.
   ——
   70

If the three years' test be applied to these cases, the number of patients " cured " out of the seventy would be represented by 8·5 per cent.

Individual statistics are of little value as means for comparison.

Whitehead has removed the tongue for cancer 139 times (in 104 of these the excision was effected with scissors), with 20 deaths. A mortality of 19·21 per cent.

Baker's operation with the écraseur, as performed by himself in forty cases, was attended by five deaths (one of these was a death from diphtheria). In a large, or possibly the larger, proportion of these cases only one-half of the tongue was removed.

Kocher has performed the operation known by his name sixteen times, with one death.

I have excised the entire tongue with scissors, after a preliminary ligature of the linguals in the neck, thirty-four times at the London Hospital. Three patients died, and of this number one died suddenly from heart-disease.

Nine cases of removal of the tongue with the wire écraseur performed at the London Hospital between the years 1885 and 1889 resulted in three deaths and one case of secondary hæmorrhage.

The most usual cause of death has been septic pneumonia, and after that pyæmia. A few have died of cellulitis, erysipelas, exhaustion, etc.

CHAPTER VI.

REMOVAL OF TUMOURS OF THE TONSIL.

THE growths concerned in these operations are usually either epithelioma·a, or round-celled sarcomata.

The malignancy of these tumours, their rapid growth, the early implication of the lymphatic glands, and the deep position of the tonsil, have rendered all attempts to remove them exceedingly unsatisfactory.

The operation may give relief.

The tonsil is in relation externally with the superior constrictor, and corresponds, as regards the surface, to the angle of the lower jaw. It is very vascular, receiving blood from the tonsillar and palatine branches of the facial artery, from the descending palatine branch of the internal maxillary, from the dorsalis linguæ of the lingual, and from the ascending pharyngeal. The internal carotid is about four-fifths of an inch to the outer and posterior aspect of the tonsil, but may be brought near to it when the vessel is tortuous. The facial artery, also when tortuous, may be brought close to the front border of the tonsil. Of important cervical structures the nearest to the tonsil is the glosso-pharyngeal nerve. The ascending pharyngeal artery is also in near relation with it.

A tumour of the tonsil may be removed through the mouth or through the neck (pharyngotomy).

1. OPERATION THROUGH THE MOUTH.

As a preliminary, a loop of soft catgut should be placed upon the common carotid artery. (*See* page 152, vol. i.) If this loop be drawn upon during the operation, the bleeding will be restrained, and in the event of any large branch being divided, the control of the hæmorrhage, which is effected by a temporary occlusion of the trunk, will give the surgeon the best opportunity of securing the vessel.

A tracheotomy should be performed, and the air-passage be blocked, either by means of Trendelenburg's tampon-cannula or by some other of the methods which have been already described (page 151).

The patient's head and shoulders must be well raised, and the best possible light obtained.

A Mason's gag is introduced upon the side opposite to the affected tonsil, and the mouth is as widely opened as is possible. The excision should be effected by long straight scissors, similar to those used for Whitehead's operation on the tongue. The growth may be fixed by long slender forceps of the dissecting-room pattern (but with toothed points), or by a tenaculum.

If it appears that sufficient room cannot be obtained through the mouth, the cheek must be slit up as far as is necessary. In effecting this division the facial artery will be severed.

The operator now proceeds to carry out the excision. In the case of a sarcoma, the growth (when the mucous membrane has been divided over it) may sometimes be shelled out with comparative ease, the surgeon using his forefinger, and supplementing its action with a broad periosteal elevator.

When the growth cannot be dealt with in this way, it must be removed by cutting with the scissors.

In carrying out the excision, the operator may encroach upon the palate or approach the tongue.

The mass should be drawn well into the mouth, and its excision should be effected deliberately and precisely, and without undue haste.

Bleeding may be checked by sponge pressure or by pressure forceps, or by torsion.

The use of the écraseur in such cases is to be condemned, and an attempt to remove the mass with the galvanic cautery or with Paquelin's cautery is needlessly dangerous. By using the cautery in this deep cavity, it is probable that the growth would be but imperfectly removed, while great risk would be incurred of producing eschars on the walls of adjacent blood-vessels, and of establishing conditions favourable for secondary hæmorrhage and for septic processes.

2. OPERATION THROUGH THE NECK (PHARYNGOTOMY).

A. **Cheever's Method.**—An incision some three or four inches in length is made along the anterior border of the sterno-mastoid muscle from the level of the lobule of the ear to below the level of the tumour. A second incision is made at an angle to the first along the body of the lower jaw.

The flaps of skin bounded by these incisions are drawn aside, and a dissection is carried down to the tumour.

In dividing the superficial structures, the commencement of the external jugular vein will probably be severed. The fascia must be well opened up. The lower branches of the facial nerve will be encountered. The stylo-hyoid, stylo-glossus, stylo-pharyngeus, and probably the digastric muscles, will need to be divided.

The facial artery and vein cross the area of the wound, and must be ligatured and divided.

The submaxillary gland is drawn forwards, the parotid upwards.

The internal jugular vein and internal carotid artery will be exposed, and must be drawn outwards with retractors.

The dissection terminates at the pharyngeal wall.

The tumour is now reached, and is removed with the scalpel or scissors, together with the portion of the pharyngeal wall to which it is attached.

The use of the actual cautery in these cases is to be condemned.

Any enlarged gland met with during the dissection may be removed. The skin-wound is closed and a drain inserted.

In the place of the incision along the ramus of the jaw, Mr. Golding Bird slit up the cheek, and was, in that way, enabled to approach the growth from both sides (*Clin. Soc. Trans.*, vol. xvi., page 9).

B. **Czerny's Method.**—A tracheotomy is performed, and the air-passage occluded by Trendelenburg's tampon-cannula, or by some other means. (*See* page 151.)

An incision is inclined downwards and outwards from the angle of the mouth to the anterior border of the masseter, and thence to the level of the hyoid bone.

The lower jaw is exposed, and is divided just in front of the last molar, the saw-cut following the same inclination as the skin incision. The two portions of bone are held well aside. The following muscles will need to be divided:— Buccinator, digastric, stylo-glossus, stylo-hyoid, stylo-pharyngeus ; and the following vessels will need to be secured:— The facial artery and vein, and probably the lingual and its vein. Care must be taken of the salivary glands, and of the lingual, hypoglossal, and glosso-pharyngeal nerves.

The tumour is removed with the scalpel or scissors. The two fragments of the jaw are adjusted by silver sutures. The skin wound is closed, and also the wound in the mucous membrane of the cheek.

A drainage-tube should be employed.

c. **Mickulics's Method.**—A preliminary tracheotomy is performed, and Trendelenburg's tube or some other tampon employed.

An incision is made from near the tip of the mastoid process to the level of the greater cornu of the hyoid bone.

The soft parts are then raised from the ascending ramus of the maxilla. Special care must be taken of the parotid gland, facial nerve, and external carotid artery. The raspatory is freely employed. With the rugine, the periosteum is separated from the inner and outer surfaces of the ascending ramus, near the angle. The bone is here divided, and the whole or part of the ascending ramus is excised. The body of the jaw is drawn forward and the growth exposed. The muscles in relation with the upper part of the outer wall of the pharynx will need to be divided (as in the previous operation).

The opening of the pharynx is delayed till the last moment.

The tumour is exposed and removed with scissors or the scalpel.

Comment.—These operations have, up to the present time, proved very unsatisfactory. There are the difficulties first, of treating the cases early enough ; and, secondly, of effecting a complete removal. A summary of the literature of the subject has been given by Dr. Benno Laquer (*Berlin. klin. Wochens.*, Oct. 27, 1890).

The intra-oral method should be attempted when the growth is quite small and easily defined. In all other instances, especially where there is any glandular implication, the pharynx should be opened from the neck. If there be extensive gland disease, any operation will probably be quite unjustifiable.

Mr. Butlin gives the following as the results of twenty-three operations for the removal of malignant tumours of the tonsil :—Three died from the operation ; three were lost sight of ; ten perished from rapid recurrence, and four from somewhat later recurrence; three only were alive at periods respectively of four, twelve, and twenty-four months after the operation.

The After-treatment of these cases resembles that carried out in the more extensive operations for the excision of the tongue (*e.g.*, Kocher's operation, page 191).

The mouth must be kept scrupulously clean, every facility must be afforded for free drainage, the wound must be frequently irrigated, and when the neck has been opened the patient should be fed through a tube for some days after the operation.

The head should be fixed after the manner adopted in treating cases of cut throat.

CHAPTER VII.

Operations on the Œsophagus.

ŒSOPHAGOTOMY.

Anatomical Points.—The gullet commences opposite the cricoid cartilage, and on a level with the sixth cervical vertebra.

The average diameter of its lumen is 20 m.m. (the width of a sixpenny piece); at the cricoid cartilage the width is only 14 m.m. The œsophagus in the neck follows the curve of the cervical spine, and also curves a little laterally (to the left), the sweep of the curve extending from the cricoid to the root of the neck. It is in close relation in the neck with the trachea, the thyroid body, the carotid arteries (especially the left), the inferior thyroid artery, the middle thyroid veins, and the recurrent laryngeal nerves.

The operation of œsophagotomy is carried out, as a rule, for the removal of foreign bodies which have become impacted in the cube. In one or two instances attempts have been made to dilate a simple structure of the gullet through an incision in the neck.

Instruments required.—Gag; tongue forceps; œsophageal bougie and forceps; scalpels; blunt-pointed bistoury; retractors; sharp hook; artery and pressure forceps; dissecting forceps; long-bladed, toothed dissecting forceps; scissors; needles; needle-holder; periosteal elevator to assist in removing the foreign body.

The Operation.—The general features of the operation are similar to those which attend a ligature of the common carotid. (*See* page 153, vol. i.) The gullet is approached from the *left* side of the neck, inasmuch as the tube inclines to that side. Should the foreign body be felt more distinctly upon the right side, then the incision may be made in that quarter.

The shoulders are well raised, the head is a little extended, and is turned to the right or opposite side.

Every attempt should have been made to define the exact position of the foreign body before the incision is begun. The situation of the cut will be influenced by the locality of the foreign body. Very usually it is the commencement of the œsophagus that is exposed.

The skin incision will commence opposite to the upper border of the thyroid cartilage, and will be continued downwards along the anterior border of the sterno-mastoid muscle for about three inches.

The first steps of the operation are identical with those for ligaturing the common carotid. (*See* page 153, vol. i.)

As soon as the skin and fascia have been divided, the finger should be introduced into the wound, and the position of the impacted substance be further defined.

The omo-hyoid muscle is drawn downwards, and must be divided if necessary. The sterno-hyoid and storno-thyroid muscles must be drawn a little aside, and, in cases where the foreign body is low down, may need to undergo some division of their fibres.

The sterno-mastoid and the large vessels are drawn outwards. The carotid sheath is not disturbed.

The trachea and larynx are drawn over, or rather tilted over, to the inner or opposite side.

The position of the gullet can now be readily made out.

It may be desirable at this stage to pass a bougie or a pair of œsophageal forceps, in order to accurately demonstrate the situation of the tube, and of the impacted body. It must be remembered that the œsophagus, when empty, is flat and tape-like, and does not exist as the well-rounded tube which figures in most anatomical text-books.

The inferior thyroid artery and the superior and middle thyroid veins must be carefully avoided. The last-named vessels will usually need to be ligatured and divided.

All bleeding having been arrested, the gullet is steadied by a pair of fine long-bladed toothed forceps, and is opened longitudinally over the site of the foreign body.

The recurrent laryngeal nerve runs in the groove between the œsophagus and the trachea. The gullet must be opened through its lateral wall, so as to avoid injury to this nerve.

In the actual operation it will appear that the œsophagus is being opened as far back as possible.

The opening in the tube must not be extended by tearing, or be dilated with dressing-forceps; it must be cautiously enlarged by a blunt-pointed bistoury.

The removal of the foreign body must be carried out with the greatest care, and a curved periosteal elevator will be found a most valuable instrument in freeing the substance and prising it into the wound.

When the body is of irregular shape, and has been long impacted, very great difficulty may be experienced in removing it. I was occupied in one case for more than twenty minutes in extracting from the gullet a hard-metal plate of teeth, which had been impacted for eleven months. If, when the gullet has been opened, the foreign body cannot be found, the thoracic part of the tube should be examined, with suitable sounds and probes introduced through the wound. The next narrow part of the gullet below the level of the cricoid is opposite to the fourth dorsal vertebra. By the introduction of forceps through the wound, foreign bodies have been extracted from the thoracic segment of the œsophagus.

If the wound in the gullet be a clean cut, if the case be recent, and the foreign body have been impacted for but a short space of time, then the œsophageal incision may be closed; and this more especially applies to the cases of children and young subjects. The sutures employed should be of very fine catgut, and they can be most conveniently introduced by means of a curved needle, held in a Hagedorn's holder.

If, however, the body has been long impacted, or if the wound in the gullet has been lacerated, and has been exposed to much bruising, then the use of sutures is to be avoided. In any case of doubt, sutures had better be dispensed with. The skin-wound may be narrowed above and below by a few suture points, but the median and main part of the wound must be left open. A good-sized drainage-tube should be passed to the bottom of the wound. In no case is it well to entirely close the superficial wound, even in instances where the incision in the œsophagus has been united. The wound in the gullet may yield, or may be torn open by violent vomiting, and the food-matters and mucus which find their way into the tissues of the neck should be permitted the very freest means of escape.

If in a case where the gullet wound has been closed no sign of extravasation occur for seven days or so after the operation, then the superficial wound may safely be closed.

An open wound is the great safeguard after œsophagotomy.

Even when the wound has been long open, and when food and mucus have escaped from the neck, and when much unhealthy suppuration has been induced, the parts at the end close well, and the resulting cicatrix is often wonderfully neat.

The wound is dusted with iodoform, and is dressed with light gauze, sal-alembroth, or other wool, or with sponge.

The After-treatment.—The after-treatment of these cases involves considerable care, and often not a few difficulties.

The patient should lie in bed, with the head and shoulders well raised.

The neck must be fixed and made rigid, and this can be effected by means of one of the simpler forms of apparatus employed in cases of cervical caries. It is essential that the part be kept at rest, and unless the head be fixed it will be found that the region of the wound is very frequently disturbed, especially when the patient is fed.

The longer the patient can be kept, immediately after the operation, without food per os, the better. The strength must be maintained by nutrient enemata. Ice may be allowed to dissolve in the mouth, but it is better if it be not swallowed. Thirst may be relieved by rectal injections of warm water.

The patient may be fed by a tube on the second or third day. The tube should be soft, and should be passed by the mouth. This method of feeding must be repeated until the parts are sound.

If the wound in the gullet has been closed, and has remained closed, the tube may be given up in seven or ten days. If the wound be left open, or if it re-open after it has been closed, the tube should be employed until the wound in the neck is granulating well, and has been reduced to small dimensions, and until it is evident that the cut in the gullet has healed.

When the aperture in the œsophagus remains free there is a great disposition for the cervical wound to become very foul in spite of ordinary attention. The mouth should be frequently rinsed out with a carbolic solution, and the wound, which should be dressed very lightly with gauze, should be irrigated with some antiseptic solution many times a day. When the patient is fed with the tube a little food is very apt to escape into the mouth, and also out of the wound. Both mouth and wound should, therefore, be well washed out after each act of feeding.

It is when milk is extensively employed that the parts tend to become most foul.

Iodoform forms a very suitable material for dusting upon the wound.

The chief cause of death in these cases is septicæmia, consequent upon the foul condition of the wound. Other elements in the mortality are erysipelas, cellulitis, pneumonia, and exhaustion.

Œsophagostomy and **Œsophagectomy.** — The former operation has been proposed as a substitute for gastrostomy in cases of cancer of the gullet. It is assumed that the stricture is high up, that the tube can be opened below it, and that the patient can be fed through the artificial opening thus established. The objections to this operation are, however, so numerous and so pertinent that it has not been adopted, and it cannot be considered to belong to the domain of practical surgery.

Œsophagectomy, or excision of portions of the gullet (for malignant disease), was first suggested by Billroth, and first carried out successfully by Czerny in 1877. Czerny's patient died of recurrence of the disease about a year after the operation. An account of the procedure is to be found in "Beiträge zur operativen Chururgie," s. 48, 1878. Mr. Butlin ("The Operative Surgery of Malignant Disease," 1887) has collected six examples of œsophagectomy. With the exception of Czerny's case these operations may all be classed as unsuccessful.

As Mr. Butlin points out, the operation has at present obtained no *locus standi*, and there is very little probability of its becoming a useful or even a justifiable method of treatment.

Part X.

OPERATIONS UPON THE ABDOMEN.

CHAPTER I.

ABDOMINAL SECTION.

THE term abdominal section is applied to the opening of the abdominal cavity either for purposes of exploration or with the object of operating upon the abdominal or pelvic viscera. The terms laparotomy and gastrotomy are frequently used in the same sense. Laparotomy implies an incision in the flank, and the word was originally employed in connection with such operations as herniotomy and colotomy. The term gastrotomy—which is very nearly the literal equivalent of "abdominal section"—is now by most writers restricted to an operation upon the stomach.

Abdominal section implies the opening of the cavity of the belly at any point on the parietes, although in the great majority of instances the incision is made in the median line. As an operation *per se* it has no very distinct individuality. It is obvious that little in the way of treatment can be accomplished by the mere opening of the peritoneal cavity. The section is employed for purposes of exploration and diagnosis, and in order that the fingers may be introduced so as to assist in certain extra-peritoneal operations. Owing to the very fortunate want of special names, however, the term abdominal section includes the incision made for the evacuation of pus within the peritoneal cavity, for the relief of peritonitis by irrigation and drainage, for the reduction of certain internal herniæ, and the liberation of snared or adherent bowel, for the unfolding of volvulus, for the reduction of intussusception, and for other purposes of like character. The majority of abdominal operations have special names, such as ovariotomy, gastrostomy, cholecystotomy, etc. It is important, however, to bear in mind that in all these procedures the major operation is the abdominal section. Abdominal surgery—in the sense in which the term is at present used—became possible as soon as it was shown by what means the peritoneal cavity could be opened with comparative safety, and the ordinary measures of surgical treatment applied to diseased conditions within its walls. The removal of a small ovarian tumour in an uncomplicated case is—as a surgical operation—a procedure of a comparatively trifling nature. The gravity of the case is represented by the fact that the excision must take place within the abdominal cavity. In the earlier periods of abdominal section the great shadow which haunted the operator was a deadly peritonitis, which at one time appeared to be almost inevitable, and which led to death after death.

It is well that it should be borne in mind that there is nothing especial in this particular branch of surgery, and that no exceptional principles are involved in the details of the many operations which it includes.

Abdominal surgery represents merely the application of the common principles of operative surgery to the treatment of parts within the cavity of the belly.

The progress of this branch of the surgeon's art has been impeded in its development by attempts to conduct operations within the abdomen upon principles which could not have found acceptance in the surgical treatment of allied conditions in other parts of the body.

The treatment of purulent peritonitis by incision and drainage involves no other than the ancient practice observed in the treatment of other retained inflammatory effusions. The removal of a pedunculated tumour by ligaturing the pedicle and cutting away the growth beyond the ligature is an illustration of one of the oldest principles in surgery. That such a mode of treatment could be safely applied to a tumour within the abdomen was a surgical revelation.

The art of removing a stone from the kidney is based upon the same elements which direct the surgeon's hand in dealing with a stone in the bladder. That the kidney could be freely cut into was the remarkable new thing.

What is phenomenal in the development of abdominal

surgery is the adaptation of a few common principles of treatment to parts with very varied anatomical features, to tissues of quite peculiar structure, and to organs of whose behaviour under direct surgical treatment nothing was known.

It would be out of place to attempt to deal here with the history of this brilliant branch of modern surgery. The facts and dates are known, but a critical history of this remarkable period in the development of medicine has yet to be written.

Without wishing to detract in the least from the distinguished part which McDowell, Nathan Smith, Atlee, Charles Clay, and other pioneers, have taken in the development of abdominal surgery, it may be safe to assume that in the future the history of this brilliant development will be associated mainly with the names of Sir Spencer Wells and Sir Joseph Lister. Spencer Wells developed the technical features, the method, the handicraftman's part. Ovariotomy, as a definite, well-founded surgical measure, grew under his hand. Among the numerous company who have devoted themselves especially to abdominal operations he stands forth, and always will stand forth, as the master surgeon. The work of Sir Joseph Lister rendered it possible that the common principles of operative surgery might be applied to the regions within the abdomen. It was he who explained the mystery of wound healing, the meaning of putrefaction in surgery, the lines of safety and the sources of danger in the treatment of operation wounds. The failure of this or that " antiseptic " drug, or this or that method of dressing an incision, affects in no way the value of Sir Joseph Lister's work. He laid bare the secrets of suppuration and pyæmia, and discovered the conditions which were essential to secure primary union.

Lister's work rendered abdominal surgery in its modern aspect a possibility, and it is under his ægis that this marvellous branch of the operator's art has advanced.

Anatomical Points.—The skin over the anterior abdominal parietes is movable, the subcutaneous tissue is lax, and the amount of fat in that tissue is often considerable. The surgeon can soon learn from experience to form a fairly correct idea of the thickness of the integuments in the specific case under notice, and the length of the incision will have to be regulated to a certain extent by the depth of the soft parts. It is impossible to give any data as to the thickness of the anterior abdominal muscles—should the opening be made away from the middle line. The beginner should remember that these muscles are much thinner than most text-books and anatomical plates would lead one to suppose.

There is no linea alba below the umbilicus, and it is scarcely possible, except in instances where the parietes have been much stretched, to avoid exposing one or both of the margins of the recti muscles. The precise construction of the rectus sheath, especially of that part that lies below the umbilicus, should be borne in mind. The pyramidalis muscle, when large, may entirely cover the median line, and section of the fleshy fibres cannot in such case be avoided. The muscle very seldom extends beyond the lower third of the interval between the pubes and the umbilicus.

The linea semilunaris may be represented by a slightly curved line drawn from about the tip of the ninth costal cartilage to the pubic spine. In the adult it would be placed about three inches from the navel. The outline of the rectus can be well seen when the muscle is in action. It presents three "lineæ transversæ," one usually opposite the xiphoid cartilage, one opposite the umbilicus, and a third between the two. The two upper of these lines are the best marked.

The site of the umbilicus varies with the obesity of the individual and the laxity of the abdomen. It is normally situated from three-quarters of an inch to one inch above a line drawn between the highest points of the two iliac crests.

The only arteries of any magnitude in the abdominal walls are the two epigastric arteries, some branches of the deep circumflex iliac, the last two intercostal vessels, the epigastric branch of the internal mammary, and the abdominal divisions of the lumbar arteries. Although all the superficial vessels are small, Verneuil has reported a case of fatal hæmorrhage from the superficial epigastric vessel.

Both the superficial and the deep epigastric arteries follow a line drawn from the middle of Poupart's ligament to the umbilicus.

The following landmarks may here be noted. The aorta

bifurcates about the level of the highest point of the iliac crest, and is therefore about three-quarters of an inch below and to the left of the navel. The cœliac axis comes off some four or five inches above the umbilicus. The superior mesenteric and suprarenal arteries are just below the axis. The renal vessels arise about half an inch below the superior mesenteric, opposite a spot some three and a half inches above the umbilicus, while the inferior mesenteric comes off from the aorta about one inch above the umbilicus.

It may be pointed out that in the female the respiration is more thoracic than abdominal. The converse holds good for the male in whom the anterior abdominal parietes are consequently less steady. In the larger number, however, of cases for which abdominal section is performed, the anterior belly wall is practically motionless.

The Preparation of the Patient.—Very many directions —some of them not a little remarkable and ridiculous—have been given under this head. The subject of abdominal section needs but the preparation that should precede any great surgical operation. (*See* page 22, vol. i.) There is very little that is especial to note. In not a few cases time for preparation is not forthcoming. If the patient be a female, the operation may be conveniently performed shortly after the complete cessation of a menstrual period. It is important that the condition of the kidneys should be investigated, and it is well that for a week before the operation the urine should be examined every day, and a note made of the precise amount passed in the twenty-four hours.

An aperient should be given over-night, and be followed by an enema early on the morning of the operation. When possible the patient should have a hot bath on the evening that precedes the operation. The anterior abdominal wall should be vigorously washed with soap and water shortly before the surgeon's arrival. The question of shaving off the pubic hair may be left until the patient is under the anæsthetic. The patient should empty the bladder just before being placed upon the operation table. If from nervousness or for any other reason the urine cannot be voluntarily passed, a catheter may be used. The details of the patient's dress have been already dealt with (page 24, vol. i.), as well as the preparation of the room in which the operation is to be performed (page 31, vol. i.).

The Instruments required.—Two stout scalpels, with a cutting edge of 1½ to 2 inches in length. Dissecting forceps (2 pairs). Straight probe-pointed bistoury. Pressure forceps (10 or more pairs). Large pressure forceps (4 or 5 pairs). Medium-sized pressure forceps. Artery forceps. 12 to 20 straight needles (3¼ inches in length). Hagedorn's needles (medium size) for the superficial sutures. Hagedorn's needle-holder. Two large blunt hooks. Scissors (straight and curved on the flat). Catgut and silk in various sizes. Silkworm-gut. Indiarubber and glass drainage-tubes. 20 sponges. Sponge-holders.

To these may be added—trays for instruments, macintosh sheets, the dressings and binder, an electric lamp or an ordinary lamp and hand mirror, and possibly Paquelin's cautery.

The pressure forceps.—The small pressure forceps are of the ordinary pattern (page 39, vol. i.). The large pressure forceps—designed by Sir Spencer Wells—are constructed upon the same lines, but are of much larger size. They measure about ten inches in length, the blades occupying about two and a half inches. Some are straight; others have the blades bent at an angle to the shanks (Fig. 315).

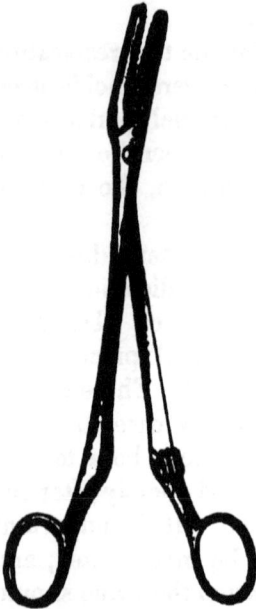

Fig. 315.—SPENCER WELLS'S LARGE COMPRESSION FORCEPS (CURVED BLADES).

They are extremely useful for seizing and holding a tumour or cyst wall, for grasping an extensive mass of adhesions, or for clamping omentum. They form, moreover, safe and convenient sponge-holders (page 224). Medium-sized pressure forceps with blades about one inch and a half in length, are occasionally useful.

The blunt hooks are used for the purpose of steadying the edges of the abdominal wound while the sutures are being applied (page 59, vol. i.).

The hook should be as thick as a No. 6 catheter, should have a perfectly blunt point, and should form the curve of half a circle with a diameter of not less than one inch. The hook is set in a substantial wooden handle.

The drainage-tubes best suited for draining the abdominal cavity are those made of glass. They are unyielding, and are uninfluenced by external pressure such as that exercised. by the intestines. The tubes are made of stout glass, and could not readily be broken by reasonable manipulation on the part of the surgeon, or moderate movements on the part of the patient. "During attacks of violent delirium or nervous agitation, when the patient tosses about, throws herself on her side, or even turns completely round, or jumps out of bed, the tube may become displaced, or may fall out, but it cannot readily be broken within the abdominal cavity" (Doran).

In the great majority of instances it is Douglas's pouch which has to be drained. Sometimes it is a cyst, the wall of which cannot be removed, or a cavity in the depths of the lumbar region. The tube must be long enough to reach to the bottom

Fig. 316.—KEITH'S GLASS DRAINAGE-TUBE.

of Douglas's pouch, and one about the size of the forefinger is the most convenient. Localised collections of pus near to the surface may be drained by indiarubber tubes in the usual way. Of the glass tubes that known as Keith's is undoubtedly the best (Fig. 316). It does not taper to a point. Its lower orifice is nearly as wide as its general calibre, and is very slightly inverted so that the edge should not be sharp enough to irritate the peritoneum. The perforations do not extend for more than about an inch above the extremity. Half an inch below the mouth or upper orifice is a broad rim, which not only prevents the tube from slipping into the abdominal cavity, but is also very convenient for the adjustment of an indiarubber sheet to protect the wound.

"This tube is constructed according to sound principles. The fluid which has to be removed tends to collect at the bottom of Douglas's pouch, and the tube accordingly is open at its lowest part, which is pressed into that pouch. The perforations counteract atmospheric pressure above sufficiently to allow the fluid to rise as it collects in the pouch. A tube perforated too high would interfere with the retention of fluid in and around the orifice of the tube" (Doran). The management of this tube is considered later (page 235).

The sponges should be selected with care. Supposing that twenty are employed, ten should be ordinary rounded sponges of medium size. Six should be small sponges, to be used with the sponge-holders, and the remaining four should be flat; two of them large, and two small. All should be of the finest Turkish sponge, and it is desirable that the flat sponges should be of very close texture.

The sponge-holders.—The ordinary sponge-holder is not very well adapted for abdominal operations. It consists, it is needless to say, of two or three slender metal bars, which are bent towards one another, are hooked at the point, and are kept in position in the substance of the sponge by means of a ring around the stem of the instrument. When there is much traction on the sponge, as in withdrawing it through a partly sutured abdominal wound, it is apt to tear away from the teeth that hold it. Moreover, it is possible for the ring to slip, and the sponge to become free. If this accident should happen while the holder is within the abdominal cavity, some damage may be done by manipulating this unprotected hooked instrument among the intestines.

Sponge forceps made upon the type of the largest pressure forceps, but much lighter, form the best sponge holders for abdominal operations. They hold the sponge evenly and very firmly, and are free from the objections just alluded to. They enable the surgeon also to retain perfect control over the sponge when it is traversing the depths of the peritoneal cavity.

A sponge-warmer is employed by some in abdominal operations. It consists of a large tin receptacle surrounded by a water-bath. The heat is maintained by means of a spirit-lamp. The receptacle is dry, and sponges dropped into it are soon warmed. The apparatus is of little use. The sponges used in become heated to too great a heat, and the temperature is not easily regulated. A simpler plan consists in the wringing of the sponges out in warm water, or a warm antiseptic solution.

Antiseptic solutions, etc.—The question of the use of the carbolic spray in abdominal operations has already been discussed (page 47, vol. i.).

The instruments should be kept in a 1 in 40 carbolic solution, and a like solution of the strength of 1 in 50, or 1 in 60 should be used for the sponges. For the external wound the solution used may be cold, but for all sponging within the abdominal cavity, and for the washing out of that cavity, a solution warmed to a temperature of 90° should be employed.

For the rinsing and washing of the sponges as they are used, a china foot-bath is much more convenient than several basins.

It may be once more stated that absolute cleanliness of hands, of macintoshes, of sponges, and of instruments, is of more importance than any antiseptic lotions. No surgeon would do well who would rely solely upon carbolic acid or corrosive sublimate. These substances can merely claim to ensure a cleanliness beyond that to be criticised by the eye.

The Position of the Patient.—The operation table should be of the usual height, and should be narrow. The patient should lie as near as possible to the right-hand side of it. The patient's right hand and forearm should be placed behind the back. The lower extremities are neatly enveloped in a small blanket, and around that a macintosh is tightly wrapped with equal care. No blanket is left exposed, and the macintosh reaches well up the thighs. Its object is to keep the blanket dry. The flannel jacket worn by the patient covers the chest and upper limbs. There is not the least need of straps or other means of securing the patient.

Before proceeding further the pubic hair should be shaved off. This is most essential in male subjects, in whom the hair often extends a considerable distance upwards along the median line.

The special waterproof sheet, with an oval aperture in the centre, which is used by some, and which is affixed to the body by adhesive plaster, is a useless encumbrance (Fig. 317).

Two large and scrupulously clean waterproof (macintosh) sheets are required—one to cover over the pelvis and the lower limbs, and one to cover the upper part of the trunk.

P

These should be so applied that only the area of the operation is exposed. No blanket is visible.

The surgeon's hands can only come in contact with macintosh; and should any instrument be laid down for a moment near to the wound, it will rest upon the same smooth and well-cleaned surface. The whole body indeed, with the exception of the face, left hand, and part of the

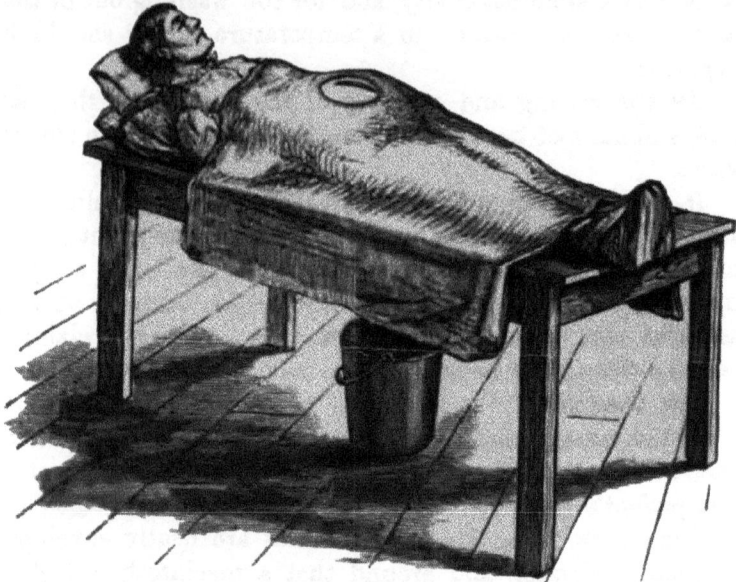

Fig. 317.—THE ARRANGEMENT OF THE PATIENT FOR ABDOMINAL SECTION.

abdomen, is covered with a waterproof sheet. The special macintosh sheet shown is not usually required. Before the sheets are finally settled in place, two large coarse sponges—not belonging to the operation set—should be forced in between the legs, and wedged up against the perineum. They will serve to collect any fluid which may find its way under the waterproof sheet, and save the delay of much sponging after the operation has been completed.

The table should be so placed that its foot is in front of a nurses are placed. A smaller table for the instruments stands close to the surgeon's right hand. Upon this table may also be kept a small bowl of warm antiseptic lotion, in which the surgeon can rinse his hand to remove blood clot, etc., from time to time during the operation (Fig. 1, vol. i.).

Two nurses at least are always required. Only one assistant is necessary for the operation. His duty is to sponge, to look after the forceps, to prevent intestine from protruding, to steady the wound edges while the stitches are being introduced, and to help in any other way. It is very convenient to have another assistant to attend to the instruments.

THE OPERATION.

1. **The Parietal Incision.**—The surgeon steadies the abdomen with the left hand, the thumb being on one side of the intended wound and the fingers on the other, and makes a clean cut in the median line from two to three inches in length.

The incision is usually placed midway between the umbilicus and the pubes, and should stop always some two inches above the pubes. In fat subjects the incision will have to be a little longer. The knife should make a clean cut through the skin and subcutaneous tissues down to the aponeurosis. Bleeding is checked by pressure forceps, which are left *in situ*. The operator need not trouble about the sheath of the rectus. There is no linea alba below the umbilicus, and the knife need only follow the median line, avoiding the cutting of muscle as far as possible. Unless the two recti are separated by distention, one or both of the rectus sheaths will as a rule be opened.

The transversalis fascia is now reached. It is possible to mistake it for the peritoneum, and the subperitoneal fat beyond for omentum. This fascia and the fat, if any, beneath should be divided by a clean cut of the knife. No director is required, nor should one be used. It is about this stage of the operation that some surgeons enlarge the area of the wound with the fingers, tearing up the fascia in a meaningless manner. All such handling of the wound is useless, and distinctly to be avoided. The advice that the peritoneum should be exposed by tearing is not sound.

p 2

It is important to clearly recognise the peritoneum. It is best identified by noting the tissues that have been cut through. The "blue colour," the "glistening surface," and the "arborescent vessels" belong to the department of fiction.

When adhesions exist, the peritoneum may not be demonstrable as a coherent membrane.

Before any attempt is made to open the abdominal cavity all bleeding should have been checked. Any pressure forceps that are attached need not be removed at the present stage. The peritoneum should be pinched up as a very minute fold with a good pair of dissecting forceps. Normal peritoneum can be so picked up. Thickened and adherent peritoneum cannot be thus dealt with, nor can the wall of the bowel be so minutely picked up, should a piece of gut be exposed and its surface mistaken for the lining membrane. The forceps that grasp the little fold of peritoneum should be moved to and fro and lifted up and down, to ascertain whether the membrane is free or not. The membrane is finally divided by cutting upon or close to the point of the forceps, while they are being drawn away or lifted up. No hook or other unusual instrument is required to pick up the peritoneum.

When adhesions exist, there is difficulty in ascertaining when the abdominal cavity has been really reached, and there is nothing to guide the operator but his surgical intelligence. Any doubtful layer of tissue should be picked up and gently rolled between the finger and thumb. Its character can in this way be at once estimated, and the existence of deeper attachments demonstrated. The operator who has the fear of adhesions before his eyes, and who has not noted the layers of tissue as they have been cut, may readily separate and strip off the undivided peritoneum with his fingers, under the impression that he is dealing with adhesions within the abdominal cavity. This is especially apt to occur when a large smooth tumour is pressed against the parietes.

The peritoneum should be divided by a clean even cut. It may conveniently be divided by scissors if preferred. I have seen the membrane rent open with the fingers—a practice that has nothing to commend it.

As soon as the abdomen is opened, two fingers can be introduced for purposes of exploration.

If the incision has to be enlarged, it is effected with a straight probe-pointed bistoury, the two fingers being used as a grooved director. If the wound be extended downwards, the position of the bladder must be defined before the knife is used.

If the hand has to be introduced, the incision must of necessity be increased. There is often a disposition not to make the wound large enough. More harm may be done by rough efforts to drag a solid growth through a small incision than by a liberal extension of the incision in the median line.

As soon as the wound has been completed, a large sponge should be at once introduced and forced into the pelvis. It is retained there during the operation, and by absorbing any blood that finds its way into Douglas's pouch saves much sponging at a later stage. The intestines must be prevented from protruding either by the introduction of sponges or by the fingers of an assistant. One of those present should be entrusted with the responsibility of taking count of all sponges introduced into the abdomen.

The omentum often gives much trouble, especially the fine thin omentum of young children, by clinging to the fingers and to sponges, and by becoming entangled in instruments. It may be necessary to keep it out of the way by means of a long narrow sponge.

2. The Treatment of Adhesions.—Adhesions must be dealt with according to common surgical principles. The lighter and more slender can be broken down by the finger or by a sponge in a holder.

The firmer must be clamped, divided, and tied—either with catgut or fine silk. Extensive strands of adhesions should be clamped in sections, cut, and the bleeding points picked up individually with artery forceps, and tied in the usual way.

Except in very especial circumstances, the use of the actual cautery is not to be commended for the arrest of bleeding from divided adhesions. The eschar produced is apt to be rubbed off in the subsequent sponging necessary to cleanse the peritoneal cavity.

sections. The adhesions may be peeled off with the finger.
Portions, of the thickness of the forefinger, may be included in
one ligature. It is more satisfactory, however, in dealing with
omentum, to ligature the individual vessels with catgut
whenever practicable. The method adopted must depend
upon the vascularity of the tissue. In some cases, where
much traction has been exercised upon the epiploon, its cut
surface will scarcely bleed at all. On the other hand, when an
ovarian cyst, with a twisted pedicle, is obtaining its chief or
sole blood supply from omental adhesions, the vascularity of
the tissue is often considerable.

Adhesions may in some cases be so dense, so close, and so
extensive that they cannot be dealt with, and may have to be
left. It must be borne in mind, however, that such adhesions
have sometimes but a slight vascularity, and that they can be
now and then divided without remarkable bleeding. Indeed,
I have observed that the hæmorrhage from a surface exposed
by such division is often not so considerable as that from the
area exposed by tearing down soft recent adhesions with the
finger. Still, these dense attachments must always be
regarded with the greatest respect; and to divide with scissors
or scalpel adhesions that can neither be clamped nor ligatured is probably bad surgery.

Assuming that the object for which the Abdominal Section
was performed has been carried out (*see* subsequent chapters),
the next step is the cleansing of the peritoneal cavity.

3. **The Toilet of the Peritoneum.**—The thorough cleansing
of the peritoneal cavity, well termed by Worms "*la toilette du
péritoine*," is a matter of primary importance in abdominal
section.

In the least extensive exploratory operation some little
blood must find its way into the peritoneal cavity. This
should be removed. In more complicated procedures not
only will much blood find its way into the pelvis and among
the intestines, but a collection of pus might possibly have discharged itself during the operation, or fæcal matter might
have escaped through a perforation of the bowel, or the
abdominal cavity might have been flooded with the fluid from
a torn cyst. It is needful to remark that the steps taken to
cleanse the peritoneum must be measured by the needs of the

individual case.* It is quite as possible to do too much as to do too little. After a perfectly simple laparotomy, without complication of any kind, it is unnecessary to flush out the quite clean cavity of the belly with water, and to scour equally clean coils of intestine with sponges. On the other hand, when a quantity of unwholesome fluid has escaped among the viscera, no trouble must be spared until the peritoneum has been cleansed of the impurity. I do not think that the presence of pure blood in the peritoneal cavity is quite so serious a thing as some would appear to suppose. There is reason to believe that it may be extensively absorbed. It is probably evil only in so far as it affords an excellent pabulum for the process of decomposition, should the elements of decomposition be present. I do not say that every possible care should not be taken to cleanse the peritoneum of such blood as has escaped during the operation; but in some procedures, where the patient is becoming exhausted, and where the operation has already lasted a considerable time, it may be a question whether a greater risk does not lie in indefinitely prolonging the anæsthesia in order that the very last speck of blood should be removed.

As to the actual process. The sponge which was placed in the depths of the pelvis at the commencement of the operation should be removed, and then all the soiled districts of the peritoneum are cleansed by small round sponges on holders (page 224). Such sponges must be passed in every direction where it is possible that blood or other extravasated fluid might lie.

It is especially, of course, in Douglas's pouch that fluid is apt to collect. Another district is the iliac fossa, and another part that particularly encourages the accumulation of fluid is the renal region. In extensive operations where a large parietal wound has been made, these districts may be sponged out with a larger sponge held in the hand. In dealing with intestine, sponges have to be gently passed among the coils many times and in many directions before the parts can be properly cleansed.

If the wound be large enough, the cavity should be frequently inspected, in order that any visible clots may be picked up and removed.

In cases where there has been a very extensive extravasation of fluid, it may be necessary to wash out the peritoneal cavity. For this purpose boracic lotion,* heated to blood heat, or a weak carbolic solution (1 in 100) of the same temperature, should be employed. Many surgeons use plain warm water, or water to which a small quantity of iodine has been added.

The assistant holds up the margins of the abdominal wound while the surgeon pours the water into the cavity. It is best poured from a common jug. Many quarts or gallons may be required. The fluid should be poured in until it escapes clear. The surgeon can assist matters by introducing his hand, or, if the wound be small, a sponge in a holder, and very gently rinsing the parts as the fluid is poured in. This flushing with water at blood heat has also the advantage of assisting to check capillary hæmorrhage, and is, perhaps, the only means whereby coagula can be washed out of deeply-placed hollows—such as may be found among extensive old adhesions—or from among intestinal coils. It undoubtedly saves time, and is certainly most efficacious. It avoids undue sponging of the parts, and after a long operation the introduction of a large quantity of hot water into the peritoneal cavity frequently acts most beneficially upon the pulse.

In cases where peritonitis exists, or where fæcal matter has escaped into the abdominal cavity, or where the extravasation consists of glairy cyst fluid, or of pus, or where much colloid or semi-solid matter has escaped, there is no doubt but that the thorough flushing out of the abdominal cavity with warm water is the only surgical means available for cleansing it.

As soon as the fluid poured in comes out clear, what remains may be taken up with a sponge. The patient's shoulders should be raised, so that the fluid lying among the intestines and in the hollows of the loins might drain down into the pelvis. By this change of posture enough fluid to fill Douglas's pouch will often run down, although before moving the patient the abdominal cavity might have appeared to be practically dry.

Before preparing to close the wound any spot suspected of

* A saturated solution of boric acid in cold water.

bleeding, or the site of any especial ligature or suture, may be inspected. If the tissue to be examined be deeply placed, it may be brought into view by means of two wide ivory spatulæ, so introduced as to press the viscera aside.

4. **Counting of Instruments.**—On completing the intra-abdominal operation, great care should be taken to ensure that no sponge or instrument has been left in the depths of the cavity. The sponges and clamp forceps should be formally counted. The leaving of a sponge or instrument within the peritoneal cavity is a catastrophe which no surgeon would feel greatly disposed to make public, and yet Dr. Wilson (*Trans. of Amer. Gynæc. Soc.*, vol. ix.) has collected no less than twenty-one instances of this unfortunate lack of care.

5. **The Drainage of the Peritoneum.** — In the great majority of cases of laparotomy the wound in the parietes may be at once closed, and no drainage-tube introduced. In the following circumstances, however, a tube may be inserted :— In cases of laparotomy attended with peritonitis with effusion ; in operations undertaken for the relief of peritonitis (the abdominal cavity having been previously washed out) ; in cases in which fæculent matter, or pus, or putrid fluid, has found its way into the serous chamber, and it seems probable that all traces of such fluid have not been removed by washing and sponging ; when colloid or semi-solid matter has escaped, and its complete removal is, for one reason or another, a matter of uncertainty ; when deep and extensive adhesions have been dealt with, and when, for this or other reasons, after-bleeding may be anticipated ; when an extensive raw surface has been left, from which oozing appears probable. The term drainage is possibly misapplied when employed in connection with an abdominal wound. The tube cannot drain the cavity by gravity unless the amount of fluid be considerable. In the majority of instances it can be claimed for the tube that it renders fluid within the peritoneum apparent and capable of being withdrawn.

It may be said of this drainage that more harm may often be done by neglecting it than by inserting a tube. The measure offers a comparatively harmless expedient to those who wish to be particularly cautious.

As a rule, the sooner the tube is removed the better. In

instances where it is inserted to meet anticipated bleeding, it may be removed at the end of twenty-four hours should no fluid be found to have escaped into the abdominal cavity. In other instances it may be retained so long as any discharge continues, and especially so long as that discharge remains offensive.

The best tube to employ is that known as Keith's glass tube (page 223). It is introduced between the two lowest parietal sutures; and when those sutures are tied, the apposed margins of the wound keep the glass in place. The end of the tube should reach the bottom of Douglas's pouch, and the rim on its upper end should lie nearly level with the skin. When the abdominal wound has been closed, a piece of india-rubber cloth—about ten inches square, and perforated in the centre—is slipped over the tube, so that the hole in the sheeting tightly embraces the tube immediately below the glass rim. This waterproof protects the wound from any discharge which may escape through the drain. Over the end of the tube a large round sponge, well dusted with iodoform, is placed. To the sponge the lower corners of the sheet and its lateral margins are pinned, in order that the sponge may be kept in place. It is undesirable to so adjust the sheeting that escaping fluid may be pent up within its folds. It is better, if the discharge be excessive, that it should escape from beneath the binder, and the fact be thus rendered evident that the sponge is saturated. Arrangements should be made to ensure the frequent changing of the sponge, should this be necessary. In some cases it may be required to be changed every hour or so for a while.

Whenever the sponge is changed, the tube should be emptied. This is effected by means of a glass syringe, to which a long piece of indiarubber tubing—about the size of a No. 15 catheter—is attached. The tube and syringe should be kept at hand, lying in a basin of carbolic lotion, and should be most carefully cleaned after using. The fluid in the tube is drawn up by the syringe, and before the evacuation is completed a little boracic or carbolic (1 to 50) lotion may be injected into the tube, in order that the passage may be washed clean.

The tube itself need not be disturbed until it is necessary

to remove it finally, or until it becomes desirable to introduce a drain of a different length.

6. **The Closing of the Abdominal Wound.**—A thin flat sponge of greater length than the parietal wound is placed upon the intestines under the opening. It is retained during the introduction of the sutures. It serves to protect the intestines and to absorb such blood as oozes from the suture points before the sutures are tied. Various suture materials may be used. The best are No. 2 Chinese twist, or a medium-sized silk braid, or silkworm gut. If the thread be too small and the parietes thick, the suture has a tendency to cut through the tissues. If it be too large, it acts as a species of seton. Large-sized threads of silkworm gut appear to be peculiarly well adapted for these wounds. They merely require care in tying (page 44, vol. i.).

Straight needles, three inches in length, should be used. The needles must be passed through the whole thickness of the parietes, and it is especially important that they should include the peritoneum. They are most conveniently introduced in the following manner :—

A large blunt hook is inserted into either extremity or angle of the incision, and by exercising traction upon the hooks in opposite directions (precisely in the median line) the edges of the wound are rendered straight and parallel to one another. The incision opening can be made, in fact, a mere chink. By the use of the hooks the most perfect adaptation of the edges of the wound is ensured (Fig. 15, vol. i.). If the abdomen be distended, the narrowing of the incision opening tends to prevent protrusion of the intestines. If the belly wall be flaccid, the hooks enable the assistant to make the skin tense, and at the same time to draw the part of the parietes about to be sutured away from the viscera, and thus render a wound of the latter less easy.

If silk be used, the suture is about twenty inches in length, and a straight needle is threaded to each end of it. One needle is passed through the right-hand margin of the wound ; the other through the left. Both should be passed from within outwards—*i.e.*, should be made to transfix the peritoneum first and the skin last. The surgeon holds the wound-edge between the finger and thumb as each needle is passed. He can evert the margin of the cut a little, and ensure the penetration of the whole thickness of the parietes. The sutures should be introduced about a quarter of an inch from the margin of the wound, and at intervals of half to three-quarters of an inch from one another.

After each suture has been passed, the two needles are removed, and the ends of the thread are carried out of the way of the operator. No suture should be tied until all the threads have been introduced, and until it is seen by traction upon the threads that a perfect adjustment of the edges can be effected.

If silkworm gut be employed, a single needle is used, and care should be taken to leave the ends of the threads long; if short, they are apt to become buried and lost in the folds of the skin.

The sutures should be tied in order from above downwards, traction being maintained all the while upon the blunt hooks. Care should be taken that the suture, as it is being tied, does not pick up and include a shred of the omentum. The peritoneal surface of the wound should be carefully examined with the finger from time to time. Before the last two, or possibly three, sutures are tied, the flat sponge should be seized with a pair of large pressure forceps and carefully dragged out, the blunt hooks being relaxed the while. By this means the peritoneal side of the incision is wiped dry. Omentum is more apt to be included in the last sutures tied than in any others. The hooks are not removed until all the deep sutures have been secured.

Before the last hook is withdrawn, the surgeon may, by gentle pressure of the hand, expel from the peritoneal cavity any air that might still occupy it.

Superficial sutures may now be introduced at any spot along the wound where the skin still gapes between the deep suture points. These are best introduced by a Hagedorn's needle of medium size held in the needle-holder.

I do not think that in any case it is necessary to support the wound with strapping; the sutures are sufficient.

ACCIDENTS DURING THE OPERATION.

The special accidents which may occur during the operation

almost entirely concern wounds and other injuries of viscera. Such accidents are scarcely possible in a simple
laparotomy, and could only result from inexcusable care-
lessness.

Accidents connected with the Parietal Wound.—In
not a few exceptional instances the intestine, and even the
bladder, have been incised in making the parietal wound.
The bowel may have become adherent to the parietal
peritoneum, or be very closely pressed against it in cases
where it is distended. Moreover, when enormous coils of
dilated bowel are lying tightly wedged against the anterior
parietes, it may be difficult to tell when the peritoneal cavity
has been opened. In such a case, the thinned bluish-
coloured wall of a coil of distended bowel may be mistaken
for the parietal peritoneum, and may be picked up with
forceps and incised. This is a more excusable accident when
the serous coat of the bowel has been dulled by commencing
peritonitis.

When extensive and complicated adhesions exist between
the intestines, and possibly also between them and the
parietal peritoneum—as in some instances of chronic peritonitis—it is very easy to wound the bowel in attempting to
demonstrate the peritoneal cavity.

The bladder has been wounded in making the parietal
wound, even when the viscus had been carefully emptied by
catheter before the operation. In such circumstances it has
usually been found that adhesions have prevented it from
contracting and from sinking into the pelvis. In all cases
extreme care should be exercised when, for any reason, the
incision in the abdominal parietes has been continued lower
down towards the pubes than usual.

Sir Spencer Wells records a case in which he cut into
a patent urachus, from which urine escaped. He closed the
opening by one of the sutures used to close the incision in the
abdominal wall, and no inconvenience followed.

**Accidents connected with the Intra-abdominal Opera-
tion.**—These include the accidental wounding of viscera
with the knife or scissors, but the great majority occur
in connection with the treatment of adhesions. It is in
attempting to remove ovarian tumours embedded in exten-

sive adhesions that the most numerous accidents have occurred. The anatomical outline and the aspect of a part may be greatly altered by serous adhesions, and a viscus so disguised may be wounded in dealing with the false membranes that cover it.

In attempting to break down adhesions, the intestine has been torn, and the same accident has happened to the bladder.

The rectum has been lacerated or divided during the separation of adhesions. The ureters have been cut accidentally, and have been included in ligatures attached to deep adhesions. "It is remarkable," writes Sir Spencer Wells, "that in cases of adhesions low down in the pelvis the ureters should escape injury so often as they do. I suspect that their condition has been overlooked in some post-mortem examinations, and it is probable that in some of the cases where suppression of urine has been a prominent symptom, one or both ureters may have been injured."

The liver has been lacerated during the separation of adhesions. In one of Sir Spencer Wells's cases some ounces of the lower edge and under-surface of both lobes of an enlarged liver were removed. The hæmorrhage was stopped by perchloride of iron. The patient recovered.

Mr. Greig Smith had to remove the vermiform appendix for injuries done to it during the separation of adhesions.

Treatment of Injuries to the Hollow Viscera.—Wounds of the intestine should be carefully cleaned, and at once closed by the Lembert or Czerny-Lembert suture.

During the remainder of the operation care should be taken to protect the coil so treated from pressure or further injury.

In cases of more extensive damage—as where a portion of the gut has been torn away—the bowel should be resected, and the divided ends at once united by suture or by Senn's plates. Should this accident occur during an operation that has been already of unusual duration, and should it seem unsafe to further prolong the operation in order to unite the bowel, the two ends of the intestine may be brought out together at the parietal wound and an artificial anus established. This can be closed by a subsequent resection procedure.

After wounds of the rectum have been closed by careful

suture, a rectum-tube should be continuously or very frequently used by the patient.

Wounds of the bladder must be adjusted by sutures in a double row—the first involving the mucous membrane only, the second the outer coats. After the operation a syphon catheter should be introduced, so that the bladder may be kept perfectly empty for four or five days. Twice a day the bladder should be gently washed out with a weak boric acid lotion.

Laceration of the gall bladder could not be safely treated by suture only. Either a biliary fistula should be established, or the entire gall bladder should be removed.

In cases of division of the ureter, the distal end should be secured by ligature, and the proximal end brought out of the wound and a fistula established. For the relief of the fistula a nephrectomy may subsequently be required. In one case (Nussbaum) communication between the kidney and the bladder was re-established.

Treatment of Injuries to the Solid Viscera.—The liver is the only solid organ that appears to have been injured during ovariotomy. Bleeding from a wound or laceration may be arrested by pressure with a sponge; and if that fails, by the application of the actual cautery.

Serious lacerations of the spleen or of the kidney may demand excision of the damaged structure. It is possible that small clean wounds of these viscera may be closed by fine sutures, and especially by uniting the peritoneum over them.

THE DRESSING OF THE WOUND.

This will depend, of course, upon the individual practice of the operator. Every possible form of dressing has been employed. For my own part, I adopt the following:—The wound and the skin around are well sponged and dried, and the parts then liberally dusted with iodoform. The principal dressing is a single sponge well dusted with iodoform, and sufficiently large to cover the whole wound. The whole area around the sponge is packed with loose carbolic gauze, from the costal cartilages down to the hollows of the groin. This gauze may be conveniently applied in long strands, arranged in concentric circles. It fills up all inequalities, and should be sufficient in amount to reach the level of the sponge. It also may be dusted with a little iodoform. Over the sponge and the gauze packing may be placed a large, but thin, pad of gauze, evenly folded. It serves to keep the whole dressing in place. Over all comes the binder.

The binder should be made of fine flannel. It should be " gored " in four places along its upper part, in order that it may fit closer to the waist (Fig. 318). This "fitting" of the binder is important in all cases, and especially in women, and in patients from whom a tumour of great size has been removed.

That portion of the binder which should come in contact with the patient's back is lined with lint, which has been carefully sewn on.

The binder is tightly and evenly applied, and secured by four large safety - pins, each two inches in length.

The weak part of all dressings applied to laparotomy wounds is the lowest part. It is here that the dressing or bandage " rucks up," and it is easy in this direction for tainted air to reach the wound on account of its comparatively close proximity to the genitals and anus. To obviate this defect two narrow strips of flannel bandage are so applied around the thigh as to keep the binder in place, and also in close contact with the skin.

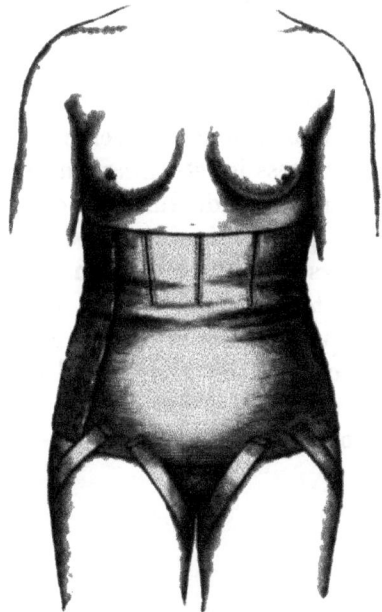

Fig. 318.—BINDER FOR USE AFTER ABDOMINAL SECTION.

Each strip is applied while the thigh is flexed, is pinned to the binder over the pubic region, is made to traverse the perineum, and is finally attached again to the binder over the region of the iliac crest (Fig. 318). When the thigh is brought upon the upper part of the binder.

General Measures.—The patient must lie absolutely upon the back, and the knees may be kept a little flexed by placing a pillow beneath them.

A large cradle is placed over the trunk. It protects the abdomen from the pressure of the bed-clothes, and helps to ventilate the bed. The patient's body is covered by a blanket, which is placed beneath the cradle, and in direct contact with the trunk. The rest of the bed-clothes are in two sets, so folded as to meet transversely in the centre of the bed. They are placed over or outside the cradle, overlapping at its summit. This arrangement permits of the wound being inspected and dressed, and enemata, etc., given without disturbing the bed-clothes that cover either the upper part of the body or the lower limbs.

The bed should be well warmed with hot bottles before the patient is placed in it, and hot bottles may be kept in contact with the feet and thorax for some time after the operation.

The patient's movements should be restrained while consciousness is returning, and the nurse may support the wound with the hands during the first attack of vomiting. The less the patient is interfered with during the first twenty-four hours after the operation the better. The practice of taking the temperature in the vagina, and of giving laudanum by frequent rectal injections is bad. The thermometer should be placed in the axilla; and opium, if given at all, should be given in the form of a hypodermic injection of morphia. Morphia should be avoided whenever it is possible, and hould never be given as a matter of routine. One-sixth of a grain is sufficient at a time. One injection only will probably be found to be sufficient.

The less taken by the mouth during the first twenty-four hours the better. Thirst may be relieved by sucking ice, or by an occasional teaspoonful of milk and soda-water. The nurse should be instructed to encourage the patient to take as little as possible. The reckless and immoderate sucking and bolting of lumps of ice, which is encouraged by the nurse who believes a patient is doing badly who is not constantly swallowing something, is most pernicious. The stomach becomes filled with cold fluid, and a sense of great faintness and discomfort persists until the melted ice is ejected by vomiting.

If really distressing thirst is experienced during the first twenty-four hours, it is best relieved by an enema of warm water. No other form of rectal injection should be allowed until the first day has been completed. It is a question whether the use of nutrient enemata within a few hours of the operation serves to do other than annoy the patient. During the second day the patient may take milk and soda-water or barley water in very small quantities, provided that such nourishment does not cause vomiting. In many instances in which cold fluid food is rejected, a little very warm tea is taken with great satisfaction and is retained.

A catheter should be passed when required. The sooner the patient can discontinue its use the better. The catheter should be kept very clean, and when not in use should lie in a weak carbolic solution (1 in 80). I think that I have traced cystitis in women in some instances to the practice of retaining the instrument in a too strong carbolic lotion. Some of the potent irritant is introduced into the bladder, and a catarrh of the mucous membrane follows. It is still more important that the external genitals—especially in the female—be kept scrupulously clean. If this care be neglected the catheter can readily convey septic matter into the bladder. The practice of passing a catheter by routine once in so many hours is most decidedly to be condemned. As a rule very little urine enters the bladder during the first twenty-four hours after the operation. After this time has elapsed, nutrient enemata may be given. Previous to the injection a rectum tube should be passed (page 245), and retained for some ten or fifteen minutes. The enema should be given by a glass syringe, and may consist of one ounce and a half of peptonised beef-tea with (if needed) half an ounce of brandy. The mixture should be heated to blood heat. These injections, if well borne, may be administered every three hours. It is claimed that nutrient suppositories act equally well.

In some instances—as in very brief and simple exploratory laparotomies, and in some operations for intestinal obstruction—these enemata are not indicated. They should be discontinued as soon as the patient can take a proper amount of nutriment by the mouth. In the majority of cases they are only employed for two or perhaps three days.

In a case that is doing well the diet from the third to the fifth day may consist of tea and toast, beef-tea, arrowroot, bread and milk. Milk in large amount is not usually well borne, and leads to the formation of scybala, while the indiscreet perseverance in a slop diet often causes nausea and flatulence. What food is given should be given often and in small quantities. A little fish may be given on the fifth day and meat on the seventh.

The bowels may possibly act spontaneously. As a rule however, they do not. In such circumstance an aperient followed by an enema should be administered on the fifth or sixth day.

This applies to an ordinary or uncomplicated case. It is seldom desirable, however, that the bowels should be left confined for longer than a week, or even for so long a period. The aperient selected should be that which the patient is accustomed to take. A simple saline aperient, or castor-oil, or the compound liquorice powder, are probably selected. The enema is most important for the purpose of clearing out the lower bowel. It may be repeated if there be any evidence that the rectum is not well emptied. The injection need not be copious; and in cases where extensive pelvic adhesions have been dealt with, even small enemata often cause distress.

Flatulence or distension of the belly is frequently complained of at an early period after the operation.

It may to a great extent be relieved by the use of the "rectum tube." This consists in the vaginal pipe of an ordinary Higginson's syringe. The tube is passed about two or three inches into the rectum, and may be left there for ten or fifteen minutes, or so long as it appears to afford the patient relief. A small soap-dish must be placed under the free end of the tube, to receive any particles of fæcal matter that may escape.

In these cases of flatulent distension minute doses of a carminative, notably of one of the aromatic oils, often have a very excellent effect, and the same may be said in a lesser degree of sal-volatile and spirits of chloroform.

Now and then it will be found that about or before the seventh day after the operation—often about the fourth or fifth—the abdomen is distended, the tongue is coated and foul, the belly is tender, and complaint is made of the tightness of the binder, while there may be a little vomiting or nausea. The temperature remains normal, the respiration unaffected, the complexion unaltered, and the pulse and general condition good. The symptoms in such a case may depend upon the fact that the bowels had not been well evacuated before the operation, or the intestine may have been paralysed by too much opium, or the diet since the operation may have been such as to lead to tympanitic distension. The patient who presents these symptoms is often greatly relieved by a saline or other aperient. The bowel is well cleared out, and the sickness, the pain, and the distension vanish.

It is possible that cases of this character, relieved in the manner indicated, may have been described as examples of acute peritonitis treated by saline aperients.

In ordinary cases of abdominal section the temperature rarely rises above 100° or 101° F. Whilst the skin is still dry for the first twelve hours after the operation a rise of must not be taken on and off, but kept on till the temperature has steadily gone down, remaining below 100° " (Doran).

The complications after abdominal section—among which may be mentioned internal hæmorrhage, peritonitis, septicæmia, intestinal obstruction, fæcal fistula, thrombosis, parotitis, pulmonary embolism, and tetanus — must be treated according to the measures advised in the treatises on surgery.

It may be mentioned that in some cases—without evident kidney disease—the urine becomes scanty and concentrated, the skin is dry, and the patient presents some of the symptoms of uræmia. Such a condition may be relieved by the hot-air bath, which can be employed without disturbing the patient, and by the administration (as Sir Spencer Wells advises) of a mixture of the citrates of potasa and lithia.

Thrombosis of the veins of the lower limb leading to phlegmasia is sometimes met with after abdominal section, but especially after ovariotomy. It is most apt to occur in patients who are allowed to stand or walk too soon. It should be treated in the usual manner.

Mr. Paget has collected no less than 101 cases of parotitis consequent upon disease or injury of the abdomen or pelvis.

The complication is rare after abdominal operations.

The trouble appears to be non-pyæmic, and very commonly ends in suppuration.

The After-treatment of the Wound.—The dressing may be removed on the fifth day, the wound well cleansed with carbolic lotion (1 in 40), and a new binder adjusted.

This early dressing adds greatly to the patient's comfort, and allows of the removal of any suture which has been applied too tightly and is cutting into the tissues.

The wound should be dried—especially in the fissures about the sutures—well dusted with iodoform, and then simply covered, together with the rest of the abdomen, with a substantial layer of loose gauze. The thigh pieces are once more adjusted as already described.

On the seventh day the part is again exposed, well washed and dried, and all the sutures removed.

If any sutural abscesses have formed, they must be treated in the usual way.

In the case of the smallest abdominal incision the wound

may be left, provided it has well healed; but in larger incisions, and in instances where any strain upon the wound may be anticipated, the cicatrix should be well supported with strapping.

I am in the habit of using Leslie's adhesive strapping on holland, cut in the way depicted in Fig. 319. The two pieces of plaster are so fashioned that when applied to the body the "tails" interlace; and by drawing the ends of one piece in one direction, and the ends of its fellow in the other, the margins of the cicatrix are drawn well together.

Each piece of this "gridiron" strapping should be sufficiently long to reach well into the loins on either side.

It should not exceed about four inches in width, and in the case of a very large wound, more than one set of two pieces will be required. Each little "tail" of the dressing is

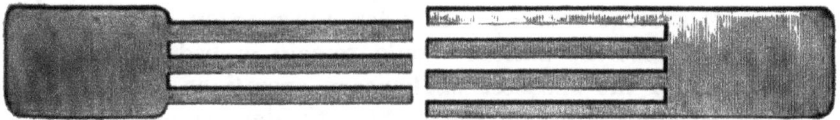

Fig. 319.—STRAPPING AS USED TO ADJUST AND SUPPORT THE WOUND.

penetrated, so that the wound is not covered up entirely when the strapping is applied, and any discharge that may exist—notably that from sutural abscesses—is able to escape.

Before the "tails" of the strapping are finally drawn tight and secured, a narrow strip of gauze about the width of the finger is laid along the whole length of the cicatrix, in order that the plaster may not adhere to the freshly-healed wound. The incision line is dusted with iodoform, and the part packed with loose gauze as before. The binder and thigh pieces are of course retained.

The wound may be inspected once or twice a week, and the strapping readjusted or reapplied when necessary.

The thigh pieces may be discontinued at the end of a fortnight. The strapping should be retained for a month, or even longer in cases of large or weak wounds, or of wounds that have not healed by first intention.

Throughout the whole period of convalescence the binder should be retained, and be always carefully applied.

In cases where the wound fails to heal, or where it has burst open after the removal of the sutures by reason of violent expiratory movements on the part of the patient, or where the incision has been deliberately opened up by the surgeon, the margins should be kept well adjusted by means of the " gridiron " strapping, which, in such cases, will require to be reapplied once, or possibly twice, in the twenty-four hours.

For the first fortnight after the operation the patient should lie upon the back, and be kept as still as possible. At the end of this time he or she may be allowed to be a little raised in bed, or to lie upon one side while the back is well supported with pillows.

Between the third and the fourth week the patient may be allowed to get up.

Such are the times which may be observed in an ordinary case of average severity. In a large proportion of instances it is well that the patient should remain in bed one month, whereas in the simplest exploratory operations the patient may be allowed up on the eighteenth day, or even before. Some surgeons will allow a woman convalescent from ovariotomy to leave the hospital on the eighteenth day. It is well, probably, to err in the direction of encouraging a longer period of rest after these operations. Some complications, notably that of phlegmasia, appear to be encouraged by too early movement.

Before the patient leaves the surgeon's care an abdominal belt should be ordered. This should be largely composed of elastic, and may be worn from six to twelve months. After the simplest procedures a flannel binder is all that is necessary ; but in cases of pendulous abdomen, and in instances where the healing of the wound has been imperfect or interrupted, or a very large tumour removed, a well-made and very carefully-fitted belt is required.

The primary object of a belt in these cases is to assist the cicatrix in resisting the weight of the viscera and the passive pressure from within, which is exercised when the bowels are distended with flatus. It is probable, as Mr. Doran says, that "distension of the cicatrix occurs not so much from frequent coughing or straining, as from passive pressure from within."

It must be remembered that the abdominal wall is made up of muscular and aponeurotic tissues. It is required that these tissues should not be weakened. Like tissues elsewhere, they atrophy from disuse, and are rendered strong by exercise. The very elaborate, rigid, and heavy belts which are sometimes worn after abdominal section, especially after ovariotomy, may possibly do harm by taking upon themselves too much of the function of the muscles and aponeuroses. The responsibility of supporting the viscera falls rather upon the belt than upon the muscle, and the latter is in consequence encouraged to waste.

I think, therefore, that while the belts worn after abdominal operations should be large enough to cover the whole of the belly, and should be quite rigid in the vicinity of the cicatrix, they should be as light as possible elsewhere, and contain a great deal of elastic.

In the case of any belt it is important that the lower margin be kept well in position, and be prevented from "rucking up," by means of suitable perineal bands.

CHAPTER II.

OVARIOTOMY.

History of the Operation. — Robert Houston, of Glasgow, treated an ovarian tumour by operation in 1701. The patient recovered, but the operation appears to have been represented merely by an incision into the cyst and the evacuation of its contents. The first complete and deliberate ovariotomy was carried out by Ephraim McDowell, of Kentucky, in 1809. The pedicle was secured by a ligature, the ends of which were brought out of the wound. The patient made an excellent recovery. In 1821 Nathan Smith, of Connecticut, who appears to have been ignorant of McDowell's work, performed a successful ovariotomy, in which he secured the pedicle with animal ligatures, which were cut short. The operation made great progress in America in the hands of Dunlap, Atlee, and others, and by the year 1850 at least thirty-six ovariotomies had been performed in that country, with twenty-one recoveries.

In Great Britain Lizars is reported as operating in 1824 and 1825, but his results were not encouraging. Granville operated in London in 1826 and 1827. In 1842 Charles Clay, of Manchester, commenced to perform ovariotomy. He carried out a large number of operations, and met with a fair degree of success. By the year 1850 ninety-one ovariotomies had been performed in Great Britain, with a mortality of 36·27 per cent. Spencer Wells performed his first complete ovariotomy in 1858, and Keith in 1862. For some years these surgeons were the two prominent figures in the development of ovariotomy, and it was under their hands mainly that the modern operation was evolved. Ovariotomy has now been shown to be one of the simplest and safest major operations in surgery, and there are very few surgeons who have not had a personal experience of this measure.

The history of the operation is associated to a large extent with an account of the different manner in which the ovarian pedicle has been treated at different times. McDowell used a single ligature, and left the ends outside. Nathan Smith carried out the now accepted method of securing the pedicle with ligatures, which were cut short, and of dropping the stump into the abdomen.

This procedure was unfortunately departed from, and the progress of the operation was seriously hindered by the use of the clamp, which was introduced by Mr. Hutchinson in 1850, and by other methods which were advocated for treating the pedicle by an extra-peritoneal method. The treatment of the pedicle outside the peritoneal cavity is ascribed to Stilling in 1848. In 1850 Atlee used the écraseur, and many followed him. Some surgeons employed the cautery, and in 1865 Koeberlé invented his serre-nœud.

Ovariotomy, the most frequently performed of abdominal operations, includes not only the procedure for the removal of ovarian tumours, but also of tumours of the parovarium, broad ligament, and Fallopian tubes.

Anatomical Points.—The following account of the surgical anatomy of the ovary, Fallopian tube, and broad ligament is taken from Doran's admirable work :—

Each *Fallopian tube* lies between the layers of the broad ligament, which are reflected over its upper surface, and meet along its lower surface, when they are continued downwards towards the ovary. The serous membrane is held on to the tube by connective tissue, generally a little tenser and firmer than that which lies between the layers of the broad ligament lower down. Still, it is easily stripped off from the tube whether by design or accident. The thin-walled cysts, so common in the folds of the broad ligament, are rare along this line of reflection over the tube ; and when they develop there they seldom, if ever, grow large.

The surgeon must not forget the fact that the ostium of the tube opens into the peritoneal cavity. Fortunately, inflammatory processes tend to close the ostium, and thus protect the peritoneum. If the tube be divided during an operation, care must be taken that the orifice on the proximal side is well closed. Each tube measures about four inches

in length when not stretched artificially. It is seldom or
never of the same length on the two sides. It becomes
extended to an extreme degree in cases of simple broad
ligament cysts which press against it.

The first inch from the fundus of the uterus outwards
is straight and narrow ; this is known as the isthmus. The
remainder is dilated, and is called the ampulla. This terminates externally in the conspicuous fimbriated extremity,
which surrounds the ostium, or opening of the tube into the
peritoneal cavity.

The canal of the tube is very narrow at the isthmus, barely
admitting a bristle, and is narrowest at its junction with the
uterine cavity. Along the ampulla the canal is wider.

There can be no doubt that the Fallopian tube is naturally
patent. Vaginal injections (as Dr. Matthews Duncan has
shown) may pass into the peritoneal cavity and set up
peritonitis.

Of the fimbriæ one is much longer and thinner than the
rest, and is known as the ovarian fimbria. It runs on to the
tissues of the ovary. It is a good guide when the parts are
altered by new growths—indeed, the fimbriæ altogether are
excellent landmarks. Unfortunately they are rapidly obliterated in inflammatory diseases of the tube itself, and this
may cause great confusion to the operator. The ovarian
fimbria is extremely elongated in cases of simple broad
ligament cyst.

The outer part of the Fallopian tube turns downwards
external to the ovary, so that its fimbriæ embrace to a certain
extent the outer part of that organ. The ovarian fimbria runs
upwards towards the ovary—not downwards to the ovary, as
usually represented. This relation of the tube to the ovary
accounts for the singular shape of a dropsical tube, which
curves outside and a little below the ovary, and also for the
position of the fœtal sac in cases of gestation in the outer part
of the Fallopian tube, the sac lying not above the ovary, but
outside, and often partly below it.

As the uterus always leans a little to one side, the ovary
on that side hangs more than its fellow, which is held almost
horizontally between the ovarian and the infundibulo-pelvic
ligaments.

The *ovary* is connected with the back of the broad ligament by its dense and tough hilum, which is invested by a plexus of veins, the bulb of the ovary. As the tissue of the hilum is continuous with the connective tissue between the folds of the broad ligament, morbid growths, developed in its substance, tend to burrow into these folds. The parenchyma,

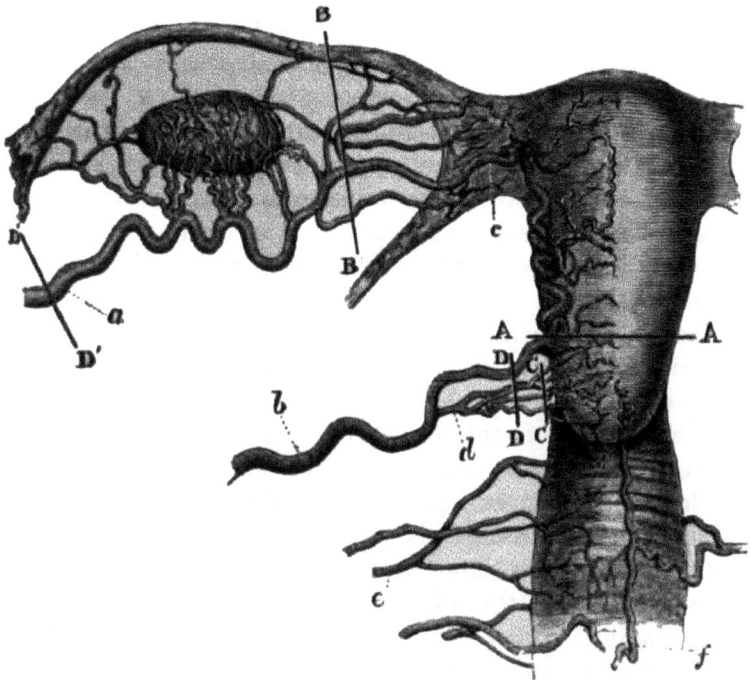

Fig. 320.—THE ARTERIES OF THE INTERNAL FEMALE ORGANS. (*Modified from Hyrtl.*)

a, Ovarian artery; *b*, uterine artery; *c*, anastomosis of ovarian and uterine arteries; *d*, artery to the cervix; *e*, vaginal arteries; *f*, azygos artery of vagina. A A, Line of amputation in supra-vaginal hysterectomy; B B and DD, vessels secured in hysterectomy; B B and D′D′, vessels secured in ovariotomy; C C, vessels divided in freeing the cervix.

or ovum-bearing part of the ovary, hangs behind the broad ligament. It is connected with the uterus by a prolongation of the muscular tissue of the latter, called the ovarian ligament, and invested by an elevation of the peritoneum.

This ligament is an important landmark when the surgeon is engaged in exploring the appendages during an operation : it is much stretched in cystic disease of the ovary, and generally hypertrophied in fibroid disease of the uterus.

The average weight of the normal ovary is at least 100 grains. Its long axis is a little over two inches, its short axis one inch, its thickness quite half an inch.

The reflection over the fundus uteri extends along each Fallopian tube, and outwards and backwards over the ovarian vessels. The layers of peritoneum meet, after investing the tube, to form the *broad ligament*. The fold over the ovarian vessels is slight, yet well marked, and is known as the in-fundibulo-pelvic ligament. It appears as a short fold of peritoneum, which runs from the brim of the pelvis to the ovary. It is described by Drs. Hart and Barbour as that part of the upper margin of the broad ligament unoccupied by the Fallopian tube. It is a structure of great importance, since it forms the outer border of the ovarian pedicle. It is easily recognised, on account of the pampiniform plexus of veins, which is con-spicuous even in the normal condition. In ovarian cystic disease this ligament becomes hypertrophied, and appears as a conspicuous fold running from the brim of the pelvis on to the pedicle.

The layers of the broad ligament are closely applied between the tube and the ovary. Below the level of the ovary the layers separate, and pass to the sides of the pelvis. The pelvic connective tissue fills the space formed by the parting of the layers. This tissue can be felt as a tense band, running from the uterus to the side of the pelvis, on digital exploration of the vagina. When the rectum is explored, the back of the broad ligament can be reached. This is an impossibility in vaginal examination.

The layers of the broad ligament are often separated by tumours, which push in between them, either from the direction of the ovary or from the uterus, as in fibroid tumours. In the former case there will be difficulty in making a good pedicle; in the latter oöphorectomy may be dangerous, as the broad ligament no longer forms a sheet-like structure, but often becomes a pyramidal body, with its base towards the uterus, highly unsuited for the safe application of the ligature.

The ovarian artery (Fig. 320) enters the broad ligament from the pelvic brim, and becomes very tortuous when it reaches the infundibulo-pelvic ligament; and this tortuousness increases as it passes between the layers of the broad ligament, below the level of the ovary, upwards and inwards to the upper part of the body of the uterus. Before reaching the uterus it divides into two branches; the upper supplies the fundus, the lower anastomoses with the uterine artery, which passes vertically upwards to meet it. The branches of this artery are numerous. Several small vessels run to the dilated outer end of the Fallopian tube, supplying the fimbriæ. Half-a-dozen short tortuous branches of wide calibre supply the ovary itself, entering that organ through the hilum. Two or three branches run across the broad ligament to the inner two-thirds of the Fallopian tube, and the round ligament receives a special branch.

In ovariotomy and allied operations on the uterine appendages, the ovarian artery is divided in two places. It must be cut through at the outer border of the pedicle, where it lies in the infundibulo-pelvic ligament, and also at the point where it crosses the line of ligature of the pedicle—that is, in the middle of its course towards the uterus, between the layers of the broad ligament. Hence a complete segment of the artery is cut away, and may be easily detected on examining the tumour after operation.

The liberal supply of arteries to the broad ligament, and the shortness of secondary branches, account for the free hæmorrhage which occurs when the ligament is wounded or split in an operation on the internal organs, especially through faulty tying of the ligature. It is evident that the main trunk of the ovarian artery will bleed as much from its distal as from its proximal end, if not secured. The ligature applied to the outer border of the pedicle secures the ovarian artery as it lies in the infundibulo-pelvic ligament. The ligature which secures the inner half of the pedicle will, or should, hold firm the distal part of the ovarian artery, which communicates freely with the uterine. The division of the ovarian artery into two large branches, between the layers of the broad ligament, close to the uterus, is a source of peril when the pedicle of an ovarian tumour is very short.

The ovarian vein has the same general course as the ovarian artery. It forms near the ovary a plexus—the pampiniform plexus—which lies in the broad ligament, and communicates freely with the uterine veins. The ovarian artery can be felt, or even seen, pulsating amidst the turgid mass of veins. The plexus is surrounded by much loose connective tissue, which may inflame, and even suppurate if damaged by careless handling in abdominal operations. The bulb of the ovary is a venous plexus surrounding the hilum, and extending to the ovarian ligament. It communicates with the pampiniform and uterine plexuses. It is very plainly seen in

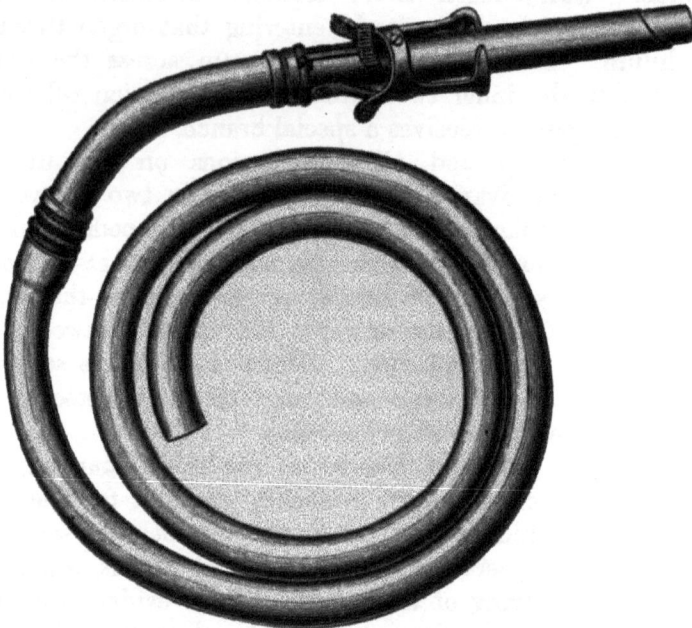

Fig. 321.—SPENCER WELLS'S OVARIOTOMY TROCAR.

cases of oöphorectomy, when the ligature is tightened above a diseased ovary.

The Preparation of the Patient.—This matter, together with the question of the position of the patient on the operation table, and the general disposition of the assistants, etc., has already been dealt with in the chapter on Abdominal Section (pages 221 and 225).

The Instruments Required.—The following special instruments are required, in addition to those already enumerated as needed for the operation of abdominal section (page 222).

Ovariotomy trocar and cannula with tubing, Nélaton's

volsella (two pairs), plain volsella, pedicle needle, simple trocar.

The Ovariotomy Trocar most generally used is that known as Sir Spencer Wells's syphon trocar (Fig. 321). The instrument is simple, and is admirably suited to its purpose. Its mechanism should be well understood before it is employed, and the surgeon should practise the movements necessary to withdraw and protrude the cannula. The spring hooks at the side of the trocar are for the purpose of holding the margins of the hole in the cyst against the instrument. It should be borne in mind that these hooks have seldom so firm a hold as to allow unusual traction to be exercised upon the whole mass of the tumour. The gutta-percha tube at the end of the instrument should be three feet in length.

Nélaton's Volsella is a powerful instrument, used for grasping and holding the cyst when required. It should measure about nine inches in length, and must be strongly made (Fig. 322).

Pedicle Needle.—That known as Sir Spencer Wells's blunt-ended needle is the best. The needle is fixed in a stout handle some four inches in length, while the shank is about six to eight inches long. The point is blunt, as are also the sides of the needle near the point. The eye is large and oval.

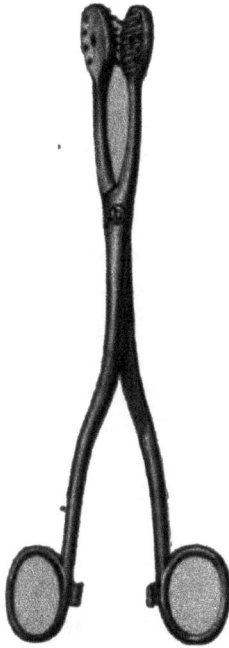

Fig. 322.—NÉLATON'S CYST FORCEPS.

Plain volsella forceps are occasionally useful in grasping the cyst wall, and also in picking up extensive bleeding points, as after the division of large adhesions, or the slipping of a ligature which has been applied to the same. A common trocar may be needed for the purpose of tapping secondary or deeply-placed cysts.

THE OPERATION.

1. **The Incision.**—The abdomen is opened after the manner already described. The incision should be of such

a length as to enable the surgeon to extract the tumour with ease. About three inches is the average length of the skin incision when first made. It may be commenced about three inches below the umbilicus.

2. **The Exposure and Examination of the Cyst.**—The cyst is exposed and is recognised by its white shining surface when free. Occasionally the peritoneum is found to be much thickened, or to be adherent to the cyst wall (page 259). In attempting to demonstrate the cyst under the latter condition, it should be remembered that to cut prematurely into the cyst is less serious than to strip the peritoneum from the parietes, under the impression that it is the wall of the cyst.

If any ascitic fluid be discovered, it should be allowed to escape, and should be pressed out of the flanks by the assistant. As soon as the peritoneal cavity is opened, a ruptured ovarian cyst may be discovered. "If the effused fluid be sweet," writes Doran, "it may be removed by sponging and pressure on the abdominal walls. If it be colloid, or otherwise semi-solid, it may be removed by the hands. When it is clearly fœtid, the hands must be scrupulously kept out of it." Such matter can be best got rid of by pouring in many jugs full of water or weak antiseptic lotion, at blood heat, and continuing the washing until the fluid flows out clear and sweet.

At the earliest possible opportunity the position and state of the uterus should be made out.

The possibility of pregnancy in cases of supposed ovarian disease should never be lost sight of.

It is possible also that the reputed ovarian tumour may be uterine.

"Uterine fibroids are of a pale brick-red colour, owing to the presence of plain muscular fibres and considerable vascularity. Sometimes the surface of a fibroid is very pale indeed, so as closely to resemble that of an ovarian cyst; and if the fibroid be cystic, there will be some difficulty in diagnosis at this stage. A fibroid bleeds violently, even if only slightly cut with the scalpel. In many ovarian or broad ligament tumours which have become invested anteriorly by a layer of the broad ligament, the surface also appears reddish in tint. The presence of the tube, stretched and elongated over the wall of the tumour, also indicates a tumour of this class, and may presage an easy operation, or else imply that some deeper complication exists; for tumours which burrow into the folds of the broad ligament often have very troublesome pelvic connections. The tube and broad ligament may happen to lie on the front of an ordinary multilocular cyst; in this case the exposed surface appears like a veil of thin red membrane covering deeper structures, and very vascular. The tube, generally below, can be recognised. On pushing this membrane aside, the characteristic surface of the cyst wall will be exposed. When uncertainty exists about the tumour being of ovarian or uterine origin, further exploration will be necessary, even for bare diagnosis.

" When secondary cysts bulge freely from the surface, the chances are that the tumour is an ordinary multilocular cyst. When the cyst wall is smooth and shiny, but greenish-grey and semi-transparent, the tumour probably contains a great quantity of adenomatous growth. Malignant ovarian tumours are usually dull-brown or yellow-coloured; sometimes they may be recognised at once as solid masses of sarcoma; but when they contain large cysts, their diagnosis before tapping is often uncertain, the cyst which presents at the wound possibly bearing no malignant characters. A cyst with a whitish surface, rather dull, and not very smooth, is probably an ovarian cyst with a twisted pedicle. A dull-white cystic tumour with orange or ochreous patches is very possibly dermoid " (Doran).

3. The Demonstration of Adhesions.—Assuming the case to be a straightforward one of ovarian cyst, the tumour should be allowed to project into the wound.

The fingers or hand may be passed round the cyst to ascertain if any adhesions exist, and to estimate their character.

During such examination the lighter forms of adhesion may readily be broken down as the fingers pass gently over the surface of the growth. If firmer adhesions are found to exist, they must be left undisturbed. Adhesions of all kinds are more readily to be dealt with after the tumour has been emptied by tapping. By attempting to break down adhesions before the cyst has been emptied, a portion of adherent bowel may be torn away, or bleeding may be occasioned.

"When a cyst is adherent," writes Sir Spencer Wells, "it is often extremely difficult to find out the exact limits or boundary between cyst and peritoneum; and rather than make any improper or dangerous separation, it is better to extend the incision upwards and downwards, until some point is reached where the cyst is not adherent."

4. The Tapping of the Cyst.—Before actually introducing the trocar, a sponge may be inserted between the cyst wall and the lower angle of the incision, in order to absorb any fluid which may escape.

The cyst is steadied by the surgeon's left hand while the trocar is driven into its wall. In order to bring the walls well up to the hooks on the trocar, the plain volsella may be used; or the assistant may drag the cyst wall up within the grasp of the hooks as the tumour becomes more flaccid. The volsella is apt to make holes in the cyst, through which fluid may escape. Traction upon the cyst should never be made through the hooks on the trocar alone. These hooks are more for the purpose of holding the cyst wall against the cannula. "After the first cavity has been emptied, a second, a third, and more, if necessary, may be tapped successively, without removing the cannula from its hold, merely by pushing the trocar forward and thrusting it through the septum which separates the emptied from the adjacent full cavity. In this manner the whole tumour may be emptied of its fluid contents, and its bulk so reduced that it may be drawn through the abdominal opening without undue force.

"In a case where there are several cysts, which cannot be tapped one through the other, they must be emptied singly, either by the same trocar or by another. Great care must be taken, if the same trocar be used, not to perforate the main cyst wall, lest some fluid should escape into the abdominal cavity" (Sir Spencer Wells).

5. The Removal of the Cyst.—As soon as the part of the cyst that has been pierced by the trocar is well free of the abdominal cavity, the cyst wall may be grasped by two Nélaton's volsellæ, and traction upon the main body of the tumour made by means of these instruments. At this time also the sponge introduced at the lower angle of the incision may be removed.

As the cyst is drawn from without the abdomen, the chief assistant follows it, as it were, from above.

By means of two large sponges—one held in each hand—he keeps the edges of the upper part of the wound together, exercises gentle pressure upon the escaping cyst, and prevents the protrusion of any coil of intestine or of the omentum. If the tumour be still of large size, any remaining secondary cysts may be tapped with a common trocar, or the supporting septa may be broken down with the fingers. When the secondary cysts are small and numerous, and the mass feels semi-solid, or when abundant glandular growths exist, the substance of the tumour may be broken up by the hand. To effect this the trocar puncture must be enlarged, and, the edges of the opening having been grasped by Nélaton's volsella, the hand can be introduced. Care must be taken that the forceps are so held that none of the broken-down contents can find their way into the abdominal cavity.

In manipulating the cyst, and especially when freeing it from adhesions, it is possible to tear the cyst wall, and to allow the cyst contents to escape into the peritoneal cavity. The accident is not a serious one. If the rent be small, it may be closed by being grasped with large pressure forceps; if larger, an attempt should be made to bring the opening without the abdominal wound, and, by means of wedging sponges around the tear, to conduct the escaping fluid out of the belly.

In this way the injured cyst may be entirely emptied, and little of the fluid have found its way into the serous cavity.

In the case of more solid tumours the abdominal incision must be enlarged. It is much less serious to increase the size of the wound than to run the risk of rupturing the tumour by endeavouring to drag it through too small an opening. Such endeavours, moreover, must lead to bruising of the margins of the wound, and may seriously interfere with healing by first intention. The escape of solid tumours is much assisted by judicious lateral pressure upon the abdomen, exercised by the hands of the assistants.

6. **The Treatment of Adhesions.**—This matter has already been dealt with (page 229).

7. **The Treatment of the Pedicle.**—The cyst having been drawn without the abdomen, and the edges of the parietal

wound having been approximated by sponges held by the assistant, nothing remains but to deal with the pedicle, which, in an uncomplicated case, now occupies the lower angle of the incision. In the majority of cases the pedicle is long, free, and tolerably broad. It is easily recognised by the Fallopian tube, which marks its upper or inner border.

"The ordinary pedicle will consist of a plane surface, two or three inches wide, and about the same length, representing the tube, the broad ligament, the ovarian ligament, which may or may not be readily detected, and, lastly, an elevated ridge running from the back and outer part of the plane,

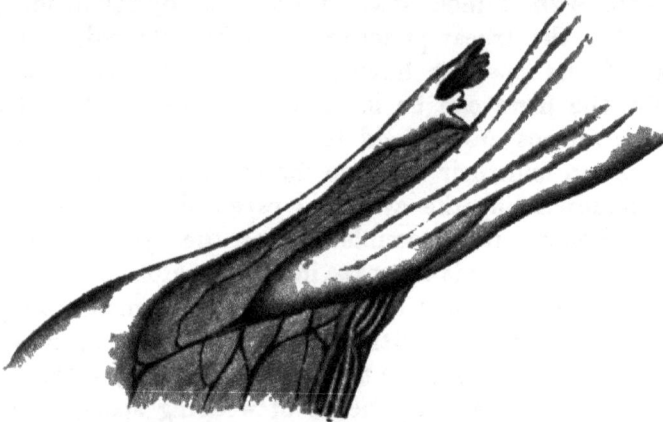

Fig. 323.—PEDICLE OF AN OVARIAN CYST.
The cyst has been tapped. The vessels in the outer border of the pedicle are indicated (semi-diagrammatic). (*Doran.*)

upwards, outwards, and backwards, towards the lumbar region.

"This ridge, which forms the outer border of the pedicle, is filled with the large veins forming the pampiniform plexus and the ovarian artery" (Doran). (*See* Fig. 323.)

The pedicle is secured by a ligature. It is never safe, as Sir Spencer Wells points out, to trust to a ligature which does not transfix the pedicle, unless this be very long and slender. It should be a rule, therefore, to transfix a pedicle, and, according to its size, to tie it in two or more portions, before the cyst is cut away.

The ligatures are introduced as follows :—The assistant so holds the cyst as to display the pedicle as clearly as possible

The surgeon with his left hand will, at the same time, so hold the margin of the pedicle as to expose its full width. In his right hand the surgeon holds the pedicle needle (page 257), armed with fine whipcord. The ligature should be about three feet in length, and should be tested, before it is passed, to ensure that it is of sufficient strength.

The needle is made to transfix the pedicle about its middle, care being taken that no blood-vessel is damaged in the process. The loop of the ligature is drawn through and cut, and the needle removed. The pedicle is now ligatured in two sections, one including the Fallopian tube, and the other the main vessels. The less tissue should be included in the section bearing the blood-vessels. The knot tied should be a double reef or surgeon's knot, and the threads should be drawn as tightly as possible. Sir Spencer Wells's advice upon this point may be endorsed. " I always tie the ligature as tightly as I can."

The exact point at which the pedicle is transfixed must be determined by common surgical sense. The ligatures should not be placed quite close to the uterus on the one hand, nor too near the cyst on the other.

The threads must be cut short, and the pedicle divided with scissors three-quarters of an inch beyond the line of the ligatures. It is not necessary to apply a second inclusive ligature around the pedicle on the proximal side of the original ligatures.

Before the stump of the pedicle is dropped back into the pelvis, two clamp forceps may be attached to either margin of it, so that at any time before the completion of the operation the divided surface may be drawn up for inspection.

There is nothing to commend the practice of clamping the pedicle before the ligatures are applied.

In examples of very broad pedicle the tissues may have to be ligatured in three or more sections.

A great deal has been written about the securing of the pedicle by ligature, and especially about the danger of splitting the pedicle. This accident is supposed to happen when the pedicle is secured by transfixion in the manner just described. I have never met with this trouble, and do not consider it possible if ordinary care is exercised. To avoid it, wound having been approximated by sponges held by the assistant, nothing remains but to deal with the pedicle, which, in an uncomplicated case, now occupies the lower angle of the incision. In the majority of cases the pedicle is long, free, and tolerably broad. It is easily recognised by the Fallopian tube, which marks its upper or inner border.

" The ordinary pedicle will consist of a plane surface, two or three inches wide, and about the same length, representing the tube, the broad ligament, the ovarian ligament, which may or may not be readily detected, and, lastly, an elevated ridge running from the back and outer part of the plane,

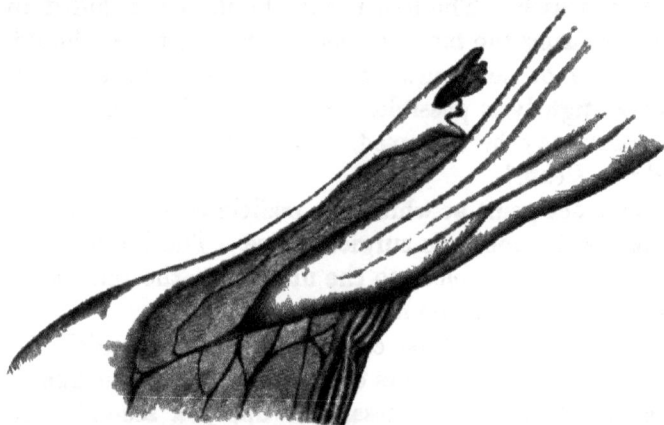

Fig. 323.—PEDICLE OF AN OVARIAN CYST.

The cyst has been tapped. The vessels in the outer border of the pedicle are indicated (semi-diagrammatic). (*Doran.*)

upwards, outwards, and backwards, towards the lumbar region.

" This ridge, which forms the outer border of the pedicle, is filled with the large veins forming the pampiniform plexus and the ovarian artery " (Doran). (*See* Fig. 323.)

The pedicle is secured by a ligature. It is never safe, as Sir Spencer Wells points out, to trust to a ligature which does not transfix the pedicle, unless this be very long and slender. It should be a rule, therefore, to transfix a pedicle, and, according to its size, to tie it in two or more portions, before the cyst is cut away.

The ligatures are introduced as follows :—The assistant so holds the cyst as to display the pedicle as clearly as possible although it is sometimes impossible to avoid this. The tissue of the uterus under all conditions affords an uncertain hold to a ligature, and all knots that concern this part must be very carefully and tightly tied.

(2) In other cases the pedicle is obscured by pelvic adhesions. These must be secured and divided one by one, or area by area, until a pedicle can be demonstrated. Mr. Doran points out that an atrophied second pedicle, in cases where the tumour consists of two cystic ovaries fused together, may be taken for an adhesion. When the pelvic adhesions are very short, broad, and tough, and a practicable pedicle exists, it is better to secure the pedicle first and deal with the adhesions later.

(3) The pedicle may have been twisted, and consequently reduced to a mere cord almost devoid of blood-vessels.

(4) There may be no pedicle at all. In such a case the original pedicle has been twisted, has atrophied and disappeared, the tumour receiving its sole blood supply through adhesions, such adhesions being very commonly with the omentum. " When the pedicle is missing, the nature of the case may be proved by passing the hand along the sides of the uterus. Then, if an entire appendage be wanting, the truth will be revealed. Sometimes in these cases the proximal end of the pedicle is reduced to a mass of fatty or fibrous tissue, ending in an irregular, cord-like structure, the sole relic of the tube and broad ligament" (Doran). (*See* also page 266.)

8. **The Completion of the Operation.** — All bleeding having been arrested, the opposite ovary may be reached by passing the fingers along the uterus, and may be drawn up and examined.

The peritoneum is now well sponged and cleansed in the manner already described. The stump of the pedicle should be drawn up by means of the forceps still attached to it, and, having been examined, the instruments may be removed. Sponges should be counted, and the greatest care taken that no sponge or instrument has been left within the abdominal cavity.

The question of possible drainage has already been considered (page 234). Nothing now remains but to close the abdominal wound after the method described in the previous chapter.

9. The After-treatment has already been detailed. The period for recovery in an ordinary case may be reckoned at one month. Some surgeons allow their patients to get up at an earlier period than that named in the account on the after-treatment (page 248). Thus Mr. Thornton writes :—" Hospital patients are generally quite well enough to go to a convalescent home from the eighteenth to the twenty-fourth day after operation." As a rule, a longer confinement is usually advisable.

The patient should be cautioned to keep quiet, and rest during the first menstrual period which follows the operation, as hæmatocele from the pedicle is occasionally met with.

THE TREATMENT OF ENCAPSULED OVARIAN CYSTS.—INCOMPLETE OVARIOTOMY.

The following account of the treatment of encapsuled cysts is derived from Mr. Doran's "Gynæcological Operations " :—

Encapsuled Ovarian Cyst.—On exposing or on tapping an ovarian cyst, it may be found that the cyst wall is invested in front by a capsule, generally of a very pale-red colour, and contrasting strongly with the white cyst wall behind it. The capsule is formed by the distended layers of the broad ligament into which the tumour has forced itself, and by peritoneum detached from adjacent parts of the pelvis. In extreme cases the inferior part of the cyst may lie below its serous capsule, touching the pelvic fascia, and in close proximity to large vessels, the ureters, and the adjacent viscera.

When a capsule is detected, the operator should draw it upwards with the cyst wall after the cyst has been tapped. He may then find that capsule and all can be removed entire, there being enough space between the uterus and the tumour to form a true pedicle. This, however, is rare. When, on drawing up the capsule, it is found to be deeply connected with other parts, the surgeon must not venture to take it out torn through, and must be secured with pressure forceps. Great care must be taken that the capsule be not perforated or lacerated. The process of enucleation often causes much shock.

The fundus uteri will be found as the deep part of the tumour is reached. It generally lies outside the capsule, and forms a valuable landmark.

The base of the cyst must be very carefully separated from its attachments, and several large vessels will require immediate ligature; they can generally be detached and secured before division.

The management of the empty capsule is most important.

In some cases its deeper part can be transfixed and ligatured, as though it were a normal pedicle. After ligature the capsule is cut short, and its free edges beyond the ligature can be sewn together by a continuous No. 1 silk suture. In many cases the base of the capsule lies very deep in the pelvis, and cannot be treated in this manner. As much of the capsule as possible must then be raised out of the abdominal wound, so that the greater part can be cut away, the remainder being left behind and drained. When the upper part of the capsule, or as much as can be safely pulled forwards, is cut away, all bleeding vessels in the cut edge must be secured with pressure forceps as they are divided. The free edge is then attached by suture to the borders of the lower part of the abdominal wall. Any holes or rents in the capsule must be sewn up from the outer or peritoneal side, and care must be taken that this remnant of the capsule is entirely cut off from the peritoneal cavity.

Lastly, a glass drainage-tube is passed into the capsule. The peritoneal cavity above the capsule is cleansed, and the upper part of the abdominal wound closed.

Irremovable Base of Cyst.—Sometimes the base of the cyst itself cannot be shelled out of its capsule. It must then be left behind and sutured, together with the remains of the capsule, to the edges of the abdominal wound, and drained. All solid growths must be cleared away from the piece of cyst left behind.

Incomplete Ovariotomy.—This term is applied to cases in which the operation has been commenced, but has not been completed, the major part of the tumour having been left behind.

In some instances—not included under this term—an abdominal section or exploratory incision alone has been performed.

The tumour is exposed, and is seen to be malignant and unremovable, or to be so intimately adherent to important viscera that its extraction during life would be impracticable. The abdominal wound is then closed again.

Incomplete ovariotomy, so called, concerns cases such as the following:—The tumour has been exposed and tapped, and it is afterwards found that the adhesions about its posterior surface and base are of such a nature that its removal is impossible. Or, before this discovery is made, the semi-solid contents of the cyst may have been broken down, and the whole cavity of the tumour thus opened up.

"If the difficulty is recognised early," writes Sir Spencer Wells, "and the cyst only exposed and emptied, the patient is scarcely in a worse condition than after tapping. Indeed, the incision leads to the avoidance of some of the dangers of tapping: the surgeon can see what vessels he wounds, and he can close the opening in the cyst if he pleases, while a short incision in the abdominal wall can, by itself, add little to the risk to the patient."

If, however, the surgeon has gone further than this, and has separated intimate adhesions and opened up the cyst cavity freely, his retreat will have to be more tedious.

All bleeding having been arrested and the peritoneal cavity cleaned, the margins of the rent in the cyst should be attached by sutures to the edges of the abdominal incision at its lower part. The sutures should be so applied as to bring the surface of the cyst in contact with the parietal peritoneum. The abdominal wound is then closed above the part involved in the attachment of the cyst, and care should be taken that the cyst cavity is entirely cut off from the peritoneal cavity.

The interior of the cyst should be as completely evacuated as possible, and an attempt made to reduce it to a simple cavity. Arrangements should then be made for its efficient drainage. For this purpose I employ a very large indiarubber drainage-tube, the lumen of which is one inch in diameter. This tube is passed to the bottom of the cyst, and the space between the sides of the tube and the edges of the opening in the cyst is lightly packed with gauze dusted with iodoform.

The cavity must be well washed out with a powerful irrigator several times in the day, a solution of boric acid being employed for the purpose.

The progress of these cases is as a rule not satisfactory. In some instances the cyst cavity has contracted well, and has attained such a size that it could be stuffed daily with gauze, and encouraged to close by healing up from the bottom. As a matter of fact, however, the tissues of the cyst wall are not of a character to exhibit a healthy healing process and develop healthy granulations.

The adhesions that exist do not allow of a ready contraction of the great cavity, and the portions of the growth left within the cyst are apt to slough and to give rise to a very offensive discharge.

I am not aware that the histories of any large number of these cases have been followed up, but my impression is that the majority die, after a more or less protracted interval, from the immediate or remote effects of suppuration.

RESULTS OF THE OPERATION.

The mortality of ovariotomy has been steadily reduced year by year since the operation was first introduced.

At the early periods of its development the death-rate was very high—so high that the procedure was condemned as unjustifiable by many. Up to 1876 Sir Spencer Wells had performed ovariotomy seven hundred and thirty-seven times, with a mortality on the whole series of about 26 per cent.

Sir Spencer Wells's analysis of one thousand cases of ovariotomy, published in the *Med.-Chir. Trans.* for 1881, is a contribution of great interest and of historical import.

The mortality is now represented by 5 per cent., or even, it is stated, by 3 per cent.

The conditions which influence the mortality of the operation are the same as those which affect the death-rate after other operations.

The special complication of *pregnancy*, however, requires notice. Ovariotomy has been performed with perfect success during all periods of pregnancy up to at least the seventh month.

In one instance (Pippingsköld) the operation was carried out at the commencement of labour, the patient recovering.

In some cases the patient has reached the full term, and has been delivered without complication of a living child. In other instances abortion has followed the operation at periods varying from a few hours to several days. Abortion directly due to ovariotomy has, according to Olshausen, occurred in less than 20 per cent. of all the recorded cases.

The same authority states that the operation has been performed during pregnancy in thirty-six cases, with only one death.

CHAPTER III.

REMOVAL OF THE UTERINE APPENDAGES.

THE operation conveniently described by this name has been defined as "the removal of one or both of the uterine appendages for any reason excepting the extirpation of what is generally known as an ovarian tumour" (Doran).

It is known also as "normal ovariotomy," as "Battey's operation," and as "oöphorectomy."

The last-named title, to which there are some few obvious objections, is one in very general use.

The operation has been carried out under the following varied conditions :—

1. To remove diseased uterine appendages. Under this heading are included chronic and subacute inflammation of the ovary, abscess of the ovary, displacement of that body, Fallopian pregnancy, and the various inflammatory and other affections of the Fallopian tubes.

2. To induce a premature menopause, in order to check hæmorrhage from the uterus, such as may be associated with uterine myoma.

3. To remove real or supposed cause of reflex disturbance in cases of mania, epilepsy, and severe hysteria.

The history of the operation is a little confused. Its development is especially associated with the names of Battey, Tait, and Hegar By Mr. Tait especially the operation has been wonderfully developed, and he has shown that in skilled hands the mortality of the operation is quite trifling. A short review of the evolution of the operation will be found in Mr. Greig Smith's "Abdominal Surgery."

The removal of the uterine appendages in cases where the structures are anatomically normal or practically so, is an exceedingly simple procedure. Such an operation would be illustrated by "oöphorectomy" carried out for the relief of some nervous condition.

When, however, the appendages are diseased, the surgeon who proposes to remove them embarks upon an enterprise the precise course and ending of which he cannot foretell. Some of these operations are difficult and complicated, and present a very uncertain and intricate series of conditions.

In not a few cases it has been found to be impossible to complete the intended excision.

When very large myomata exist, the procedure is complicated by the size and position of the tumour.

Every case must be considered upon its merits, and the surgeon must have clear notions as to the amount he intends to remove in various circumstances. In the majority of instances the operation involves, or should involve, the complete removal of the appendages upon the two sides. The parts excised will be represented by the ovary, the parovarium, the outer three-fourths of the Fallopian tube, together with the corresponding part of the ovarian artery, the pampiniform plexus, and the broad ligament.

The operation will be described as it would be carried out in a case in which the parts are practically normal. The treatment of the various complications which arise when the parts are not normal will be considered subsequently.

The Instruments Required.—The same as for ovariotomy with the exception of the trocar, the volsella, and the cyst forceps. Two long ivory spatulæ (paper-knives) may be found to be of use.

The Operation.—The patient having been prepared for abdominal section, a vertical incision about two and a half inches in length is made over the linea alba below the umbilicus. The centre of the cut will be nearer to the symphysis than to the umbilicus.

The cavity of the peritoneum is opened in the manner already described.

All bleeding having been checked, two fingers are introduced into the wound, and the fundus uteri is sought for. The fingers embrace the broad ligament as if they were the blades of very long dressing-forceps, and are carried outwards —one on each side of the Fallopian tube—until they are arrested by the ovary.

The ovary is now drawn out of the abdomen by the two fingers, which retain the same forceps-blade attitude.

In the simplest cases the fingers of the left hand may be used to draw forth the ovary, and between these fingers the parts to be removed may be held while the surgeon applies the ligature with the right hand.

Before applying the ligature the Fallopian tube is drawn out as far as is possible, and the exposed part of the broad ligament is well spread out.

It often happens, even when no adhesions exist, that there is some difficulty in dragging the ovary well out of the wound. This is notably so when there is a thick layer of fat upon the abdominal parietes. In such cases much strain falls upon the broad ligament, and the surgeon's fingers alone are not sufficient to hold the parts in place. In these instances it is necessary that the appendages should be seized by large-

Fig. 324.—OÖPHORECTOMY.
The appendages are grasped by large pressure forceps. The broad ligament is being pierced by the pedicle needle. (*Doran.*)

elbowed pressure-forceps (Fig. 324). This method of securing these somewhat slippery parts is the habitual practice of many, even when the appendages are easily drawn forth.

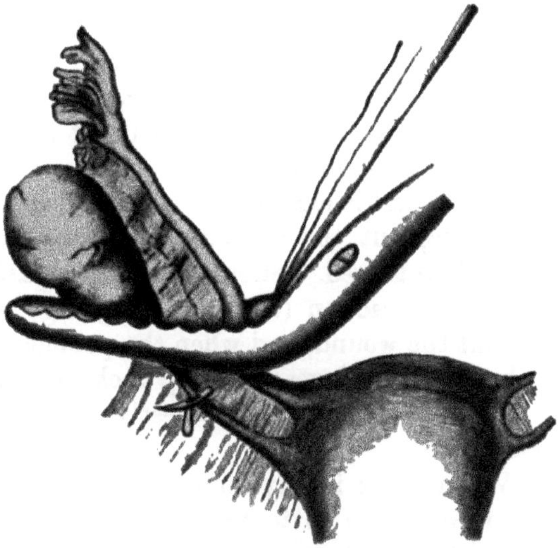

The ligature is applied by means of a blunt-pointed needle in a handle, which is made to transfix the pedicle. The pedicle in this operation is secured in precisely the same way as in ovariotomy (page 261). The silk employed for the ligature may be a little thinner.

The parts are cut away close to the retaining fingers or the retaining forceps, and at least a third of an inch from the ligature.

Before the division is made, it is well to fix one or possibly two pairs of artery forceps upon that part of the pedicle which lies between the ligature and the intended line of section. When the division is made, the forceps—which inflict no damage upon the part—prevent the stump from falling at once back into the pelvis, and allow it to be examined at leisure, and to be drawn forth should the ligature become loosened.

The appendages of the opposite side are sought for and dealt with in the same manner.

The surface of the peritoneum is freed of any blood by means of a small sponge in a holder.

A little oozing may result from trifling laceration of the tissues here and there, the result of the manipulations and the dragging upon the parts.

The wound is closed, and is dressed in the usual way.

Throughout the operation the anæsthetic must be carefully administered. Should the abdominal muscles undergo sudden contraction (as from coughing) when the ovary is without the wound, and when the pedicle is about to be dealt with, the appendages may slip back into the abdomen again if lightly held, or be needlessly dragged upon if rigidly grasped.

When there is any difficulty in drawing the appendages well forward, so as to expose the pedicle, the surgeon may be assisted by two ivory spatulæ which are placed transversely across the belly immediately above and below the protruded organ. By means of these spatulæ the abdominal parietes in the immediate vicinity of the wound can be depressed and flattened.

The Treatment of Complications.—1. *When the Appendages are Adherent or extensively Diseased.*

The omentum may be adherent to the appendages, and may at the same time also be attached to other parts of the surface of the peritoneum. As a result of these adhesions the anatomy of the part may be greatly confused, and a condition be induced which is at first peculiarly puzzling. In other instances the appendages may be bound down by adhesions, or be lost in a confused mass of cicatricial tissue. It may be impossible to identify the ovary by the touch. The surgeon may be quite unable to demonstrate any kind of pedicle. The structures to be removed may be adherent to the bowel, or to the bladder, or to the peritoneum lining the floor of the pelvis. They may be the seat of abscess or of some variety of cystic formation, and the removal of the diseased parts without rupturing the abscess wall may be attended with the greatest difficulty.

Each case must be considered on its merits. Omental adhesions can be dealt with with comparative ease, but the adhesions which fix the appendages may defy the most patient and most skilful operator. Until the adhesions have been dealt with it will be impossible to bring the appendages into view or into such a position as will enable the operator to apply the necessary ligature.

In such cases the wound must be enlarged; and by means of suitable retractors and a good light, aided by efficient sponging, the parts to be removed must be exposed, and the adhesions dealt with as the particular case requires.

There is little to commend the practice of attempting to effect the separation of the appendages with the fingers, only working through a small incision. Skilful fingers might effect much—and in few operations is a highly-educated touch of greater value—but there is nothing in this procedure to justify a direct departure from the sound principle that the surgeon should, whenever possible, be able to see what he is doing, and that manipulations in the dark are not worthy of encouragement. Of the two evils—a large incised wound in the median line of the abdomen, and the risk of tearing structures while breaking down adhesions which are hidden from view—the former is without doubt the less. In some of these cases the bleeding is described as being occasionally "truly alarming." If there be a risk of "alarming" bleeding from wounds and lacerations in the depths of the pelvis, let the external wound be large enough to allow the surgeon to deal with that hæmorrhage in a straightforward manner. This is more satisfactory than staunching the blood which wells up from a small external wound by sponge pressure, or by dabbing the parts with a solution of iodine.

s 2

The small incision in these cases involves a procedure which is unsafe and difficult, unsound and clumsy. It can appeal only to those who aim at a certain theatrical effect, and who test the greatness of an operator by the littleness of his incisions.

2. *When the Operation is Performed for Uterine Fibroids.*

When the myomata are small, the operation presents no difficulty; but when the growths are large, the removal of the appendages may be attended with the utmost difficulty.

The appendages are apt to be much displaced. The uterus is not infrequently rotated, so that while one ovary is brought near to the surface the other is out of reach in the pelvis.

One of the appendages may be buried in a deep groove between two outgrowths from the surface of the tumour, or may be wedged in between the tumour and the pelvic wall.

In any case, it is well not to remove one ovary until it has become evident that it is possible to remove both.

The parietal incision in these instances must be free, and the surgeon must expect to find parts displaced and distorted. Care must be taken not to tear off any of the outgrowths from the tumour.

"The most serious condition," writes Mr. Doran, "is that where, on raising the appendages on one side, the broad ligament is seen to form a pyramid with its base on the side of the tumour—that is to say, when its two folds have been widely parted along their line of reflection on to the uterus.

"Large vessels run behind each fold, lying far apart from each other towards the base of the pyramid. Now the apex of the pyramid is formed by the ovary and the outer part of the tube held up in the surgeon's hand, and the ligatures must be passed through the middle of the pyramid. . . . It is self-evident that the chances that the large and turgid vessels will slip must be great, for the broad ligament becomes very tense when its layers are pulled tight by the ligature." In such cases an attempt should be made to secure the vessels separately, picking up each one by means of an aneurysm needle, and securing it between two ligatures before it is divided. In some of these cases the hæmorrhage

CHAPTER IV.

HYSTERECTOMY.

HYSTERECTOMY, or removal of the uterus, is carried out for myoma, for incurable inversion, and for malignant disease.

In the first condition the excision is usually not complete, more or less of the cervix is allowed to remain behind, and the operation is carried out through an abdominal incision. For incurable inversion the removal may be partial or complete. In dealing with malignant disease the removal should be complete, and experience up to the present time teaches that the excision should be effected through the vagina. To this operation the name of vaginal hysterectomy is given.

History of the Operation.—Granville, in 1827, is reported to have removed a uterine myoma, but without success. A few isolated instances of the operation are recorded in succeeding years, but none of the patients recovered. The first successful operations were performed by two American surgeons—Burnham in 1853, and Kimball in 1855. In 1861 Sir Spencer Wells performed his first hysterectomy for myoma. Mr. Keith's first case was in 1874. The development of the operation owes much to the successful and brilliant operations of Keith, who may be said to have first turned the tide in the direction of success.

The first successful vaginal hysterectomy for cancer is ascribed to Sauter of Constance, who operated in 1822.

For many years the cases operated on were very few and the mortality very high. The operation was revived by Czerny in 1879, and was rapidly developed by Billroth, Schroeder, Mickulicz, and others.

Freund carried out the abdominal method of operating in these cases, and his procedure was extensively imitated. The results, however, were such—the mortality proving to be about 70 per cent.—that at the present time this method of extirpation in cases of cancer may be considered to be abandoned in favour of vaginal hysterectomy.

Anatomical Points.—The peritoneum which covers the uterus is closely adherent to the fundus, but is less firmly attached to the lower part of the organ, where it is reflected to form the utero-vesical and utero-rectal pouches. The reflection of the peritoneum from the uterus to the bladder is about the level of the internal os. On the posterior part of the uterus the serous membrane descends for nearly an inch over the posterior vaginal wall before it is reflected on to the rectum.

The median utero-vesical pouch is separated from the para-vesical pouch on either side by two slightly-marked folds, wherein are slight bands of unstriped muscle. Below these, and embedded in the subjacent veins, are the ureters. When the bladder is empty, and the uterus normal in position and size, a distance of nearly half an inch will separate the cervix from the point of entrance of the ureter into the bladder.

The lower third of the cervix projects into the cavity of the vagina; the middle third is connected with the base of the bladder in front, but projects behind into the vagina; the upper third is supra-vaginal, and is in direct relation with the bladder in front, but is covered by the peritoneum behind. The peritoneum can readily be detached from the posterior part of the vagina and cervix.

The ureter on entering the pelvis crosses the bifurcation of the common iliac arteries, and makes its way towards the cervix uteri. The uterine artery crosses it upon its inner side. The ureter will run parallel with the cervix, and at a distance of nearly half an inch from it, and will pass through the plexus of uterine veins, and beneath the broad ligament. Keeping close to the vagina, it enters the interval between the vagina and the bladder, and opens into the latter viscus about opposite to the middle of the anterior vaginal wall.

The ovarian artery and vein have been already described (page 254). The uterine artery is, under normal conditions, no larger than the posterior auricular. In its course forwards, it keeps near to the floor of the pelvis, and reaches the uterus at its junction with the vagina. It gives branches to the vagina. It runs upwards on the side of the uterus, between the layers of the broad ligament, and follows an exceedingly tortuous course.

It is crossed by the ureter about the level of the external os. It supplies the uterus by very numerous branches, and ends superiorly by joining with a branch of the ovarian artery (Fig. 320).

The uterine veins form an extensive plexus—the greater part of the blood from which is returned by the ovarian vein.

The following **operations** will now be described:—

　1. Supra-vaginal hysterectomy for myoma.
　　A. With extra-peritoneal treatment of the pedicle.
　　B. With intra-peritoneal treatment of the pedicle.
　2. Vaginal hysterectomy for cancer.

1. SUPRA-VAGINAL HYSTERECTOMY FOR MYOMA.

The Instruments Required.—The same as for ovariotomy, with the following modifications:—The trocar and cannula will be replaced by some form of serre-nœud. The surgeon must provide himself also with wire, and a pair of nippers and pliers, and with plenty of ligature material. He may also have at hand one or more large hooks in handles for the purpose of taking hold of the tumour and more easily manipulating it. A strong elastic ligature, or very stout whip-cord, will also be required, and likewise certain especial pins.

The best serre-nœud is that known as Koeberlé's. The steel cylinder is about four inches in length. The loop is usually made of stout, soft, flexible iron wire about one foot long. Piano-wire is strongly recommended by some. Care must be taken that the key of the serre-nœud is not wanting. Special pins for fixing and securing the uterine pedicle outside the peritoneal cavity are required. Each pin is over four inches in length, and is made of steel. It has an oval flattened handle, and a cap or button of like shape is used as a guard for the point after the pin has been passed.

The Preparations for the Operation.—These are the same as in other grave operations involving Abdominal Section (page 221). The position of the patient, the surgeon, the assistants, and the general disposition of the operating-room have been already considered (page 225).

A. **Hysterectomy with Extra-Peritoneal Treatment of the Pedicle.**—The following account is abridged from Mr. Doran's excellent description in his work on "Gynæcological Operations":—

1. The abdomen is opened in the median line, as in variotomy. Special care must be taken to avoid the bladder, which is more easily wounded in hysterectomy than in variotomy.

The tumour is usually of a pale brick-red colour.

The hand is introduced into the abdomen, and the tumour and its relations investigated. Especial attention is paid to the pelvic relations, to the condition of the broad ligaments, and to the situation and extent of any existing adhesions. The abdominal wound is enlarged to the extent necessary to remove the mass with readiness.

2. Adhesions must be dealt with as their circumstances require. Parietal adhesions are not so common in these as in ovarian cases. On the other hand, intimate connections between the omentum and the fibroid are very common. Adhesions to the intestines, to the bladder, and even to the stomach, may be met with.

These false membranes are dealt with in the manner already described. Active capillary hæmorrhage may follow the slight laceration of the uterine tissues which may attend the stripping-off of some adhesions, e.g., such as implicate the intestine.

3. When the adhesions have been dealt with, the tumour is pulled forward out of the wound. As it is delivered, the exposed viscera should be protected by warm sponges. If the abdominal incision be very large, a competent assistant may —at this stage—close the upper two or three inches of it with the usual sutures.

4. It behoves the surgeon now to carefully examine the lower part of the mass, in order to make sure of its relations to the uninvolved portion of the uterus, to the appendages, to the cervix, and to the bladder.

The appearance of the appendages may be greatly altered. A collection of sub-serous bullæ may be observed, the result of long-standing œdema of the broad ligaments.

The broad ligaments are seldom found to be symmetrical,

the natural axes of the pelvic organs may be entirely altered, and the search for the appendages may be attended with great difficulties. The ovaries may be found swollen, and full of blood ; or flattened out, or stretched into white ribbon-like cords.

5. The wire of Koeberlé's serre-nœud is now passed round the pedicle. The pedicle is simply the lower part of the uterus, or the upper part of the cervix. Whenever possible, the wire loop should surround the pedicle a little above the level of the os internum (Fig. 320, A A).

Mr. Doran observes that " the practice of applying large pressure forceps, elastic ligatures, or temporary clamps of any kind to the pedicle, cutting away the tumour, and then applying the serre-nœud, involves great dangers and difficulties. Hard as it may sometimes be to distinguish the relations of the pedicle before the removal of the tumour, the task becomes far harder afterwards, and the risk of damaging the bladder or a ureter will be greater. There may be cases where this practice of applying the serre-nœud to the pedicle after the removal of the tumour is justifiable, but such cases are exceedingly rare. . . . When the enlargement lies chiefly towards the fundus, and when, at the same time, the appendages proceed from the sides of the tumour symmetrically, so that it is evident that the wire can readily be passed round the lower part of the uterus, below them, there will be little difficulty in this stage of the operation. Often, however, the tumour invades the lower part of the uterus, or, what is still more frequent, small dense fibro-myomata are developed in its walls, at the level of the proposed pedicle. In these cases it may be necessary to shell the tumour out of its capsule. . . .

" The relations of the appendages to the proposed pedicle must also be ascertained. When they lie even, and high up on the sides of the tumour, the wire may be passed entirely under them ; that is to say, as the wire is slipped round the pedicle, the tubes, ovaries and greater part of the broad ligaments are held or pulled by the assistant well above the level of the loop of wire, which will grasp them, as experience has proved, with sufficient firmness. Sometimes, however, one or both appendages lie too low for this kind of treatment—

for the wire cannot be safely passed round the middle of the appendages, which are often tense, so that the proximal part will not be secure against hæmorrhage after the tumour has been cut away."

If an appendage be placed too low to be included in the loop, it should be removed, and its pedicle ligatured separately.

Before passing the wire round the tumour, the position of the bladder must be ascertained, and, if necessary, demonstrated by means of a catheter. Mr. Doran has twice seen the fundus of the bladder accidentally included in the wire, and cut across in dividing the pedicle. Both patients died.

6. The wire loop is tightened gradually. The two pins are then passed through the pedicle, close to the loop, and upon its distal side. They are introduced transversely, *i.e.*, at right angles to the line of the wound in the parietes.

There is usually some difficulty in so passing the pins that they are both quite extra-abdominal, and it will be necessary to depress the abdominal integuments below the level of the constricting wire with ivory spatulæ while these pins are being introduced.

7. The tumour is now cut away beyond the pins, the wire is still further tightened, the abdominal and pelvic cavities are cleared of all coagula, and the area of the operation thoroughly cleansed.

The stump of the pedicle is trimmed up, and reduced to its smallest limits. It is well drawn towards the lower angle of the abdominal wound, which is then closed in the usual way.

The wound and the stump of the pedicle are freely dusted with iodoform or some other suitable powder, and the part dressed according to the custom of the individual operator.

In any case, the dressing should be a dry one.

Other Forms of the Extra-Peritoneal Method. — Sir Spencer Wells transfixed the pedicle with two strong needles, below which he placed a ligature. The stump was fixed in the parietal wound. Keith uses a special clamp, by means of which the pedicle is fixed and strangulated.

Olshausen and others employ an elastic ligature. The pedicle is transfixed by the ligature, and secured in halves.

Many ingenious instruments have been devised to facilitate

the passage and the tightening of the ligature. Elastic ligatures are cut away usually about the tenth day.

The After-treatment. — The general after-treatment in cases of hysterectomy is conducted upon the same lines as are observed in other examples of abdominal section.

There is more pain after hysterectomy than after ovariotomy. There being little room for the bladder to expand, it needs to be emptied more frequently than usual.

The stump of the pedicle must be carefully watched. If any oozing take place from its surface, the wire of the serrenœud, or the bars of the clamp, must be tightened. It is advised that throughout the treatment the wire loop be tightened once a day, or oftener, in order to keep the surface of the stump dry and to hasten the necrosis of the constricted parts.

The stump is kept as dry as possible, and is best treated with iodoform powder and pads of absorbent wool.

When the exposed part of the pedicle is converted into a hard dry mass, the wire is removed.

The pins, however, must still be left in place. If prematurely withdrawn, the gangrenous stump will slip back into the abdominal cavity. It may even be necessary to re-introduce the pins a little lower down on the pedicle, if they appear disposed to cut their way out through the sloughing tissues.

Complete separation of the constricted part of the pedicle takes place usually in from seven to fifteen days. That part of the parietal wound which is occupied by the pedicle, ultimately heals by granulation.

Many weeks may elapse before this portion of the wound has entirely closed in.

B. **Hysterectomy with Intra-Peritoneal Treatment of the Pedicle.**—This method of removing the uterus as a complete and detailed operation was devised by Schroeder, and somewhat extensively employed by him. An account of his operation is furnished in the *British Medical Journal* (vol. ii., 1883, page 714).

Kaltenbach in 1874 proposed the intra-peritoneal treatment for small pedicles, with suture of the edges of the wound in the uterus and in the broad ligaments.

A little later than this, Hegar employed the same plan with success.

In 1878 Czerny surrounded the pedicle with an elastic ligature, and allowed the stump to fall back into the abdomen. Intra-peritoneal operations, in which the pedicle was somewhat roughly secured by many ligatures, have been carried out by many surgeons.

As already stated, the most precise—and at the same time, it may be said, the most scientific operation—is that elaborated by Schroeder, and to the consideration of that measure the following sections will be restricted.

The Instruments Required.—The instruments required in hysterectomy have already been enumerated (page 280).

In this method of performing the excision no serre-nœud or clamp is needed. Some means, however, must be adopted for securing the pedicle temporarily. This may be effected by an elastic ligature or a ligature of stout cord. A convenient instrument is a large old-fashioned écraseur carrying a strand of stout whip-cord. The loop of the instrument can be gently tightened and made to act as a temporary compressor.

The Operation.—I have adopted the following method of performing Schroeder's operation :—

1. The abdomen is opened in the median line, and the tumour is exposed. Any adhesions encountered are dealt with. The relations of the mass are investigated, and the possibility of forming a convenient pedicle is considered. Provided that the case admit of it, the growth is delivered, is drawn out of the abdomen, and is lifted vertically upwards by one or more assistants.

2. The next step is to secure the arteries which supply the myoma. These vessels are two in number on either side—the ovarian, and the uterine. Their position can be ascertained without difficulty, and they are subject to very little anatomical variation. They are no larger than are the arteries which may have to be dealt with in removing very large tumours from the surface of the body, and the vessels can be reached before the trunks are breaking up into many branches.

The ovarian vessels are defined in the broad ligament, are secured between two sets of ligatures, and divided. The surgeon proceeds to sever the broad ligament—when that structure is still present as a ligament—in a direction which would correspond to a line roughly drawn from the brim of the pelvis to the cervix uteri. It is throughout divided between two sets of ligatures. The veins of the pampiniform plexus are apt to be very voluminous, and may be as large as, or larger than, the thumb. The round ligament will need to be severed between ligatures. In due course the broad ligament upon either side will have been divided nearly to the uterus and all the vessels belonging to the ovarian set will have been secured.

The remains of the broad ligament and the appendages will be attached to the tumour. The former site of the ligament will be represented by a linear breach in the peritoneum along the floor of the pelvis, marked by many ligatures. The surgeon should endeavour in this part of the operation to render the broad ligament as flat as is practicable, and to have the tumour so held that it is as little in the way as is possible.

3. The uterine artery has now to be secured close to the neck of the uterus. Its position has been referred to, and is depicted in Fig. 320. It is best picked up by a large aneurysm needle, which is passed (unthreaded) close to the cervix, and which is then threaded and withdrawn, leaving the ligature in place. In this manœuvre very great care must be taken not to damage the ureter.

When these two arteries have been secured, there remains no known vessel to supply the growth.

4. As a precaution an elastic or cord ligature may be passed around the pedicle before it is divided.

This is intended to act as a temporary compressor, and, as already stated, the loop of an old-fashioned écraseur answers very well.

If the surgeon is assured that the vessels have been well ligatured, this temporary compression may be omitted.

The upper part of the pedicle—about the level of the internal os—is now severed with the scalpel.

The part is so cut as to leave a V-shaped surface; the apex of the V will be in the centre of the divided cervix, and will correspond to its divided canal.

If a temporary ligature be used, the stump must be grasped

ith velsella before the division is complete. If this be not ne, it will slip from the grasp of the ligature.

Blood runs freely from the great tumour, but it is blood hich is no longer circulating.

If the vessels have been properly secured, the face of the ump is pale, and the oozing from it is quite inconsiderable, nd not comparable to such as may take place from a surface rom which thick adhesions have been stripped.

5. The mucous membrane of the divided canal should now be united by a continuous catgut suture.

The divided surfaces of the cervix—the surfaces of the V—are brought together with deep catgut sutures, which take a good grasp of the tissues. The raw surface is in this way closed in. Finally, the peritoneum covering the part is, if possible, brought together by fine sutures, so as to cover the scam left on the stump. In one case I effected this easily, in another the serous membrane was only made to cover the deep scar partially. To ensure this protection to the deep wound, the compressing ligature might be conveniently avoided; and some peritoneum may be stripped off the mass before the section with the knife is made. None of the sutures are "buried," except the single one uniting the mucous membrane.

6. Nothing remains but to unite, as far as is possible, the breaches made in the peritoneum upon either side of the stump. Each breach will follow the line of the broad ligament. The pelvic cavity is carefully cleansed, and the abdominal wound is closed. No drainage-tube is required.

The operation as above described I have carried out in its entirety, and without difficulty. The cases were, however, simple and uncomplicated. In one instance the tumour was very large, weighing 21½ lbs.; but the size did not add to the difficulties. The patients recovered as perfectly as after an ovariotomy. Unfortunately, the surgeon cannot depend upon meeting with uncomplicated cases.

On this matter Schroeder writes as follows :—

'The difficulties of the case become very numerous when we have to remove a fibroid developed at the lower part of the uterus, and extending into the cellular tissue of the pelvis. The uterus is sometimes dragged upwards on one side so far that it is impossible to reach the os with the finger. In such cases I ligature the appendages, and I then enucleate the tumour out of the pelvic cellular tissue. This latter manipulation is generally very easy.

" Tumours firmly located in the pelvis are thus made free from the surrounding tissue, and appear attached only to the cervix. The india-rubber ligature is then applied around the cervix, the tumour is cut off above it, and the stump stitched up according to the principles described above.

" The cavity of the uterus or the cervical canal is cauterised with a ten per cent. solution of carbolic acid, in order to destroy any infectious germs that may be present. The denuded surfaces of the stump are first united in the depth near to the mucous membrane of the uterus; these sutures are covered up by several rows of other sutures, uniting the walls of the stump; finally, the peritoneum is pulled over the stump, and attached to it and to the peritoneum of the other side by a line of loose-ly-placed stitches.

" There remains, however, a cavity out of which the tumour has been enucleated. This can be treated in different ways. If I do not expect a very abundant secretion from it, I leave the walls of the cavity simply to close upon each other, and drop the whole into the abdomen. In other cases, I insert a drainage-tube from the cavity into the vagina, and close the wound towards the abdominal cavity by stitching the peritoneum over it."

The subject of complicated cases is further dealt with in the " Comment " which follows.

The question of covering the stump with one or more omental grafts has been raised. The matter is alluded to, in a subsequent chapter, on the use of omental grafts after suture of the intestine (page 315).

The After-treatment in these cases differs in no essential particular from the after-treatment in a case of ovariotomy.

Comment.—*The Extra-Abdominal* and *Intra-Abdominal Methods Compared.*—In comparing these two procedures it may at once be said that the intra-abdominal method is the better, is the more perfect, and is the one more completely in conformity with the soundest principles of operative surgery.

The main difficulty in these cases is bleeding. In the

early history of most excisions which involve exceptional hæmorrhage, there has been a period when the difficulty was met by strangulating the tissues by a ligature or cord. In the removal of tumours of exceptional size, and in the excision of such organs as the tongue and the thyroid body, this has been a feature in the development of surgery in the past.

In the earlier days of surgery the " mediate " ligature was employed in securing vessels, but nearly one hundred years have now elapsed since operators learnt to adopt the " immediate " ligature as the perfect method. (*See* page 100, vol. i.)

The screwing up of a bleeding stump in a wire noose takes us back to the old " mediate " ligature, and to the primitive methods which were adopted to meet the emergencies of hæmorrhage.

In removing a large goitre no surgeon would now think of including great tracts of tissue suspected to contain blood-vessels in a strangulating noose. It is true, it was the practice at one time; but the practice now is "immediate" ligature—the securing of the main vessels precisely and separately. And here it may be observed that the hysterectomy must be complex indeed which can compare in the matter of difficulty and danger, and in the demand for the highest operative skill, with the operation for the removal of a large thyroid tumour.

The following observations, which refer to the serre-nœud, would hardly appear to belong to the surgery of the nineteenth century:—" A mass as thick as the wrist can be squeezed into a loop an inch or three-quarters of an inch in diameter. The part of the pedicle beyond the wire or the ligature is removed by pressure necrosis. A sort of dry gangrene, which is not actively putrefactive, and which does not set loose foul discharges, is sought to be produced by various means."

The serre-nœud is not an instrument which is compatible with the accepted principles of modern surgery. In spite of the violent advocacy of those who use it, it will not survive. It will come to hold the same position with regard to hysterectomy that the clamp has occupied in the development of ovariotomy.

The serre-nœud has served an admirable purpose, and has played a distinguished part in the development of hysterectomy.

It has brought the operation into the region of practical surgery, and has rendered a great and difficult procedure possible. It may be safe, however, to infer that it will in due course yield to methods which are more in accord with the surgery of the time.

The intra-peritoneal method aims at securing all the arteries which supply the growth. These vessels, as main trunks, are only two in number, and are liable to but little variation.

The ovarian artery may in cases of difficulty be secured as high up almost as its origin from the aorta. The uterine artery may be secured by the side of the pedicle as soon as any pedicle can be demonstrated.

This method of Schroeder's has been vilified with that illogical and vulgar coarseness which has obtained for some writers on abdominal surgery a distinctive position in the literature of the time. The operation may, indeed, be said, as one writer observes (*Lancet*, Nov. 29th, 1890), to have been "universally condemned;" and it is to be regretted that a judicial criticism has been replaced by much virulent and personal abuse. It is urged by those who affect this method of discussing scientific questions that the intra-peritoneal operation cannot always be carried out. This may, at the present time, be true, but the assertion has not yet been demonstrated to be perfectly accurate.

It is satisfactory to note, however, that the greatest authority on hysterectomy, and the most brilliant operator in this department of surgery, is in favour of intra-peritoneal methods (*British Medical Journal*, Dec. 10th, 1887).

Those who have read the interesting accounts which Mr. Keith has furnished of his numerous daring and most remarkable operations, must acknowledge that hysterectomy may be attended with exceptional difficulties. Adhesions of the most complex kind have been met with. Extensive districts have been bared of peritoneum, and numerous vessels of great size have had to be dealt with. One writer met with "enormous coils of dilated veins, which looked as large as the small intestine." Such vessels would have had a diameter of from one inch and a quarter to one inch and a half, but even these gigantic blood-carrying cylinders are better dealt with a ligature than by a serre-nœud. I have not noticed a case in which there appears to have been an insuperable diffi-culty in ligaturing the ovarian artery and its companion veins; and if the pedicle can be so prepared that a serre-nœud or a clamp can be passed around it, then I cannot be induced to believe that it would have been impossible to secure the uterine arteries lying in this tract of tissue which has been pre-pared for treatment by strangulation and gangrene.

If the ovarian and uterine arteries on both sides have been secured, then, so far as the teaching of anatomy goes, the main blood supply, and apparently the sole blood supply, of the tumour has been cut off.

The intra-peritoneal method leaves a clean cut in the pedicle of the growth united by precise sutures; it leaves an incised wound in the place of an incoherent mass of gangrenous tissue; it allows the abdominal wound to be closed; it lessens the inconvenience and shortens the duration of the after-treatment; and it does not place the surgeon in the dilemma of dealing with cases "where the pedicle cannot be pulled outside the parietes without exerting dangerous tension on the parts."

Few can claim that there is much to admire in what is termed the "combined intra- and extra-peritoneal method of treating the pedicle."

Hysterectomy for Intractable Inversion comes rather in the category of those operations which are exclusively termed gynaecological.

2. VAGINAL HYSTERECTOMY FOR CANCER.

An admirable review of the position of this operation is given by Dr. John Williams in a recent paper (*Lancet*, Aug. 23rd, 1890). As I have no personal experience of this opera-tion, I have extracted the following account—a little condensed —from Mr. Doran's well-known work on "Gynæcological Operations" (page 318).

The Instruments Required.—Clover's crutch; Higginson's syringe; Sims's speculum; volsellæ; scalpels; small sponges in holders; two pairs of long-handled scissors curved on the flat; pressure forceps; broad metal retractor; pediclo needle; needle-holder; needles; ligatures; drainage-tube.

The Operation.—The patient is placed in lithotomy position, and the lower limbs are separated by a Clover's crutch. The buttocks are brought close to the edge of the table. The surgeon sits facing the perineum. The chief assistant stands on his right and the chief nurse on his left.

The vagina is washed out with carbolised water. The cancerous ulcer should have been previously plugged with iodoform wool, and the parts made as clean as possible.

A Sims's speculum is passed along the posterior vaginal wall. The anterior lip is seized by a volsella, and the uterus is drawn down as far as possible.

1. The assistant now takes charge of the volsella, and pulls the cervix backwards and downwards. The surgeon then cuts through the vaginal mucous membrane along its anterior reflection on to the cervix by means of the scissors, so that a semi-circular wound is made in the anterior fornix, with its convexity forwards.

The hæmorrhage must be kept in check by sponging.

A catheter is passed into the bladder. The anterior part of the uterus is then cut away, with scissors, from its cellular connections with the bladder. The blades of the instrument must be kept close to the uterus. The peritoneum should not be opened at this stage.

The speculum is now removed, and the cervix completely separated from the vaginal mucous membrane. To effect this the cervix is drawn forwards, so as to bring its posterior aspect into view. The mucous membrane along its posterior reflection on to the cervix is divided with the scissors. This semicircular incision forms, with the one already made in front, a complete ring around the cervix.

2. The cervix being thus detached, Douglas's pouch is now opened up. Care must be taken not to cut too much laterally, lest the broad ligaments be wounded.

At this stage the uterus will remain connected to the surrounding parts by the broad ligaments and the utero-vesical fold of peritoneum. This fold is at once divided.

In order to do so, the operator slips his left forefinger through the hole in Douglas's pouch over the fundus and front of the body of the uterus, till the point of the finger presses on the reflection of peritoneum from the bladder on to the uterus.

The peritoneum is then divided with scalpel or scissors, the operator cutting close to the uterus, and the finger behind the peritoneum serving as a guide. The catheter should remain in the bladder during this stage.

The broad ligaments now alone remain.

3. In order to secure the broad ligaments, the fundus is pulled through the posterior part of the wound with the aid of a strong volsella. This forcible retroflexion is never easy to effect. The right hand should be pressed on the hypogastrium, whilst the left forefinger is passed through the posterior part of the wound and hooked over the fundus.

When the body of the uterus is pulled down into the wound, the operator must grasp it with the volsella.

The most dangerous stage of the operation is now reached. It is desirable that the ovaries and tubes should, if possible, be removed entire; but this cannot, as a rule, be accomplished.

The surgeon will usually have to satisfy himself with dividing the ligament on the uterine side of the ovary.

The ligament is secured by ligatures, and then cut. The difficulties of even this step will be at once appreciated. The structures to be transfixed can never be brought well into view, and it is scarcely possible to relax the ligament sufficiently while the loop is being tied.

The usual procedure—that, namely, of dividing the broad ligaments upon the uterine side of the ovary—will now be described.

A pair of large straight-bladed pressure forceps is made to grasp the broad ligament close to the uterus. A strongly-curved pedicle needle armed with silk transfixes the broad ligament from behind, external to the forceps. The ligature is then secured as in ovariotomy. As the ends of the thread are being pulled tight the assistant must remove the large pressure forceps. The ends of the other thread are then tied round the opposite side of the broad ligament.

The broad ligament is now cut through between the ligature and the uterus. The ends of the ligature should be left uncut till the vaginal wound has been attended to later. The uterus is then drawn to the ligatured side, and the opposite broad ligament is secured in the same manner.

When the ovary and the fimbriated end of the Fallopian tube are removed, the process will be far more difficult.

The ligature is very hard to apply; the tissues transfixed are upon the stretch, and the possibility of the knot slipping after it has been tied is considerable.

4. The uterus now comes away. Any remaining bleeding points must be secured by ligature.

The vaginal wound may be closed by sutures, which are inserted with a curved needle held in a needle-holder.

Some surgeons leave the vaginal wound open, and trust to packing of the vagina to prevent the prolapse of bowel or omentum through the rent.

Drainage is advisable in most cases. The simplest form of tube is a long glass drainage-tube, which is passed about half an inch beyond the vaginal wound. The vagina is then packed with iodoform wool.

The After-treatment.—A thick pad of iodoform wool is laid over the vulva after the vagina has been dressed, and a sponge is placed over the mouth of the drainage-tube if that appliance has been employed. The iodoform wool plugs must be frequently inspected and changed.

When the drainage-tube is used, the pelvic cavity must be washed out, should the temperature rise high, or the discharge from the tube become fœtid. The sutures in the vaginal wound must be removed at the end of a fortnight, a Sims's speculum being passed along the posterior wall of the vagina after the patient has been placed on her back, so as to bring the wound well into view.

Comment.—The methods for performing vaginal hysterectomy are very numerous, and have been subjected to endless variation and modification.

The chief distinctive feature of each operation turns upon the method of securing the broad ligaments.

In this, the most difficult and important step of the operation, every device has been tried which has been carried out for the control of hæmorrhage.

Ligatures have been employed in various ways, the écraseur has been made use of, and the division has been effected by means of the actual cautery. Those who favour mechanical methods in operating, employ a clamp; and in spite of the objections that will naturally be raised against this clumsy method of controlling bleeding, the clamp appears to have been attended with no little success. In this particular operation the clamp is scarcely a more formidable foreign body than a glass drainage-pipe.

To readily control the bleeding, to effect a complete removal, and to take away with the uterus the ovaries and the tubes entire, it appears to me that it would be better to divide and secure the lateral attachments of the uterus through a median abdominal incision, and then to remove the organ through the vagina in the manner already described.

The uterus has been bisected from the os to the fundus, and has been removed in two segments after the broad ligament upon either side has been secured.

The bladder and the ureter have been wounded in this operation. It is also stated that an intestinal fistula has been caused by the pressure of a drainage-tube.

As will be apparent from what has been already stated, the great danger in the operation is from hæmorrhage.

THE RESULTS OF HYSTERECTOMY.

On this subject Mr. Keith's valuable paper in the *British Medical Journal* for December 10, 1887, should be consulted.

The general mortality of hysterectomy for myoma, as derived from a series of combined statistics, is given by Mr. Greig Smith as about 30 per cent. In the hands of a few operators it does not exceed 15 per cent., and Keith's mortality has reached the remarkable proportion in most unpromising cases of only 7·9 per cent.

Vaginal hysterectomy has been attended with a mortality of about 20 per cent. Mr. Greig Smith gives the more recent mortality as 10 per cent. Dr. John Williams states that it has in some instances been reduced to 5 per cent. The precise prospect of "cure" of the cancer in these cases has not yet been demonstrated.

It is apparent that in a very large proportion of the cases a comparatively early recurrence takes place.

The whole matter is well reviewed by Dr. John Williams in the paper already alluded to (*Lancet*, Aug. 23, 1890).

CHAPTER V.

Operations on the Intestines.

Anatomical Points.—In my Hunterian Lectures delivered at the Royal College of Surgeons in 1885, I gave an account of the disposition of the intestines, which was founded upon the examination of one hundred fresh bodies. These bodies were all examined within twenty-four hours of death.

From the published account of these Lectures ("The Anatomy of the Intestinal Canal and Peritoneum in Man," London, 1885), the following points, bearing upon the surgery of the bowel, are abstracted :—

The average *length* of the small intestine is about twenty-three feet, and of the colon about four feet six inches.

There is no systematic *arrangement of the coils* of the small intestine. There is a disposition for the bowel to follow an irregularly-curved course from left to right, but in the adult this disposition can never be relied upon. Such as it is, it may be expressed as follows. The gut, starting from the duodenum, will first occupy the contiguous parts of the left side of the epigastric and umbilical regions; the coils then fill some part of the left hypochondriac and lumbar regions; they now commonly descend into the pelvis, reappear in the left iliac quarter, and then occupy in order the hypogastric, lower umbilical, right lumbar, and right iliac regions. Before reaching the latter situation they commonly descend again into the pelvis.

The coils most usually found in the pelvis belong to the lower ileum, and to the bowel between two points respectively six feet and twelve feet from the duodenum.

In examining a coil of protruded small intestine, the following points may be made use of to *distinguish jejunum from ileum* :—

The jejunum is wider than the ileum, its coats are thicker and more vascular, and the valvulæ coniventes—as seen on holding the coil to the light—are large and well-marked. These folds are absent in the lower ileum, while it is in that part of the canal that Peyer's patches are most distinct.

With regard to the *mesentery*, its upper or right layer is continuous with the under layer of the transverse meso-colon, and with the peritoneum that invests the ascending colon. Its lower or left layer joins with the serous membrane that encloses the descending colon, that forms the sigmoid mesentery, and that descends over the lumbo-sacral eminence into the pelvis.

The parietal attachment of the mesentery is liable to considerable variation. It commences at the end of the duodenum, just to the left of the spine, and thence follows an oblique line which runs downwards and to the right, crossing the great vessels, and ending in a somewhat uncertain manner in some part of the iliac fossa. The mesentery becomes elongated in hernia, and is liable to many congenital variations.

With regard to the visceral attachment of the mesentery, attention must be drawn to the excellent and practical investigations of Mr. Wm. Anderson (" MacCormac on Abdominal Section," London, 1887, pages 25 and 80):—" Owing to the divergence of the two layers of the mesentery as they approach the bowel, a portion of the circumference of the jejunum and ileum is destitute of serous investment. The separation of the laminæ of the mesentery begins at a distance of about two-thirds or three-fourths of an inch from the intestine, and leaves a triangular space, the base of which, averaging about five-sixteenths of an inch in width, is formed by the uncovered muscular tunic. This interspace is occupied by fat, by the vessels and nerves of the gut, and by delicate fibres of connective tissue (Fig. 325).

" Unless this disposition of the peritoneum be taken into account, it is obvious that a suture applied in the manner of Lembert might fail to bring into contact the true wall of the intestine at the mesenteric attachment, and a leakage from the interior of the tube might take place into the inter-serous triangle and peritoneal cavity.

" The *disposition of the arteries* within the triangle is

ice. The last row of anastomatic loops, from
ιe direct branches of supply, is placed much
intestinal wall in the lower than in the upper
₂ bowel, and towards the termination of the
nly lies within one-third of an inch of the
canal. From these loops are given

off, at moderately regular intervals,
straight vessels, which do not inter-
communicate, but pass at once to the
muscular floor of the triangle, either
to pierce it on each side near the
lateral angles of the interspace, or
to run for a short distance between
the serous and muscular tunics before entering the latter. As each of
these vessels has a fairly well-defined
territory, it appears undesirable to
interfere with the loops from which
they spring, and it is hence safer to
divide the mesentery as close as
possible to the portion of bowel to
be resected, the cut edges of the
redundant part left after suture of the
intestine being folded and the edges
united by fine catgut sutures.

OF SMALL
ᴇsᴇɴᴛᴇʀʏ.
Triangular
f triangle;
m, Mus-
ι, Mucous
o bowel.

ortant to remember that the thickness of the
₂ of the small intestine varies within rather wide
₂rent subjects, and in all cases diminishes, to-
ᴉe calibre of the tube, from the upper towards
emity of the canal. In the jejunum, about two
commencement, the depth of the tissue ranges
ɳtieth to one-fortieth of an inch, while in the
the ileum, about two feet from the ileo-cæcal
ɩkness is reduced to about one-half or even one-
measurement. The difficulty and danger of
ill hence be greater the more remote the portion
from the stomach; but fewer sutures will be

mucous tissue has a considerable degree of
d is usually thick enough to bear a fine suture,

applied after Lembert's manner, without implicating the epithelial surface of the mucous membrane."

In connection with the last-mentioned point, it must be borne in mind that the glands of Lieberkühn penetrate the mucous membrane for some distance, and that if the suture pass through them, the lumen of the bowel is practically opened. The tough submucous tissue is air-tight and water-tight. It is much better marked in many animals used for experiments (*e.g.*, dogs and cats) than in man.

The *cæcum* is always entirely covered by peritoneum. In shape and in position it is liable to considerable variations, some of which may be congenital, while others are acquired. The cæcum usually lies upon the psoas muscle, its apex corresponding with a point a little to the inner side of the middle of Poupart's ligament.

The *appendix* is subject to very numerous variations, both as to shape and to situation. It commonly lies behind the end of the ileum. It is often in close relation with the iliac vessels and the ureter. It is not infrequently found in the pelvis.

The general disposition of the *colon* need not be here described.

I made a careful examination of the peritoneal investments of the ascending and descending parts of the colon in one hundred bodies, with the following result:—In fifty-two bodies there was neither an ascending nor a descending meso-colon. In twenty-two there was a descending meso-colon, but no corresponding fold on the other side. In fourteen subjects there was a meso-colon to both the ascending and the descending segments of the bowel; while in the remaining twelve bodies there was an ascending meso-colon, but no corresponding fold on the left side.

It follows, therefore, that in performing lumbar colotomy, a meso-colon may be expected upon the left side in thirty-six per cent. of all cases, and on the right side in twenty-six per cent.

The line of attachment of the left meso-colon is usually along the outer border of the kidney, and is vertical; that of the right is less vertical, and crosses the lower end of the kidney from right to left, to ascend along the inner margin of the gland. (*See* Fig. 353.)

The so-called *sigmoid flexure* forms, as I have pointed out in the Lectures alluded to, a loop which resembles a capital omega, but which cannot be called sigmoid (Fig. 326). This omega loop extends from the point of ending of the descending colon—at the outer border of the psoas—to the middle of the sacrum. It includes, therefore, what is known as the first part of the rectum. Its average length in the adult is seventeen and a half inches. The mobility of the loop is remarkable. Its meso-colon is quite distinctive. Its average length is as follows:—Over the psoas, one inch and a half; at the bifurcation of the common iliac vessels, three and a half inches; on the sacrum, one inch and three-quarters. (*See* Fig. 326.) The outline of the loop, when spread out, is much influenced by changes in the sigmoid meso-colon. Some notable variations in the outline of the omega loop are shown in Fig. 327. These matters are of concern in the operation of inguinal colotomy.

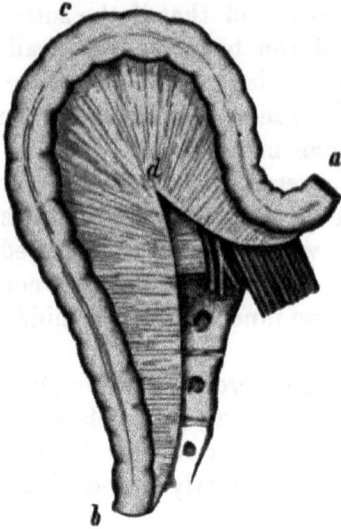

Fig. 326.—THE SIGMOID FLEXURE OR OMEGA LOOP.

a, End of descending colon ; *b*, Lower part of rectum ; *c*, Summit of the loop ; *d*, Neck of the sigmoid meso-colon.

The inter-sigmoid fossa is in this meso-colon. It is the seat of the inter-sigmoid hernia, and at its neck is the sigmoid artery.

SUTURE OF THE INTESTINE.

The first principles of intestinal surgery involve a consideration of the best method to be adopted for closing wounds and breaches in the bowel, and for bringing together the divided ends of the tube when a segment of the intestine has been resected.

The future of the most elaborate and the most fortuitous operation upon the intestinal canal may depend upon the integrity of a few sutures. If one stitch fail, the wound in the gut may gape, and fæcal matter may escape.

It may be said literally of some intestinal operations, that their success hangs upon a thread.

The history of the suture as applied to the intestine or the development of the operation of enteroraphy, as some term it, is full of interest.

No more valuable contribution to our knowledge of the subject has been provided than that afforded by Travers's

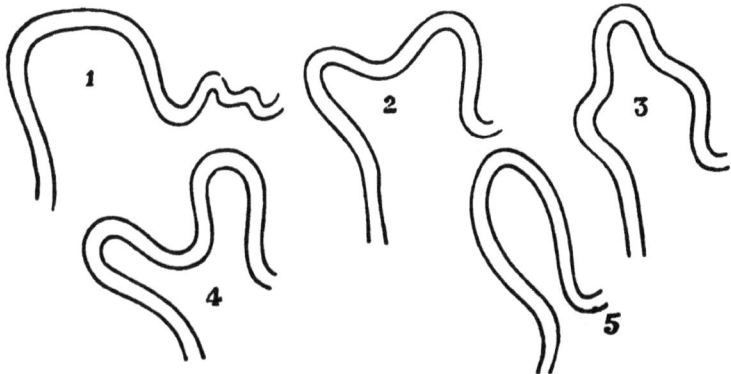

Fig. 327.—DIAGRAM TO SHOW THE OUTLINES OF THE SIGMOID FLEXURE OR OMEGA LOOP AS OCCASIONALLY MET WITH.

famous monograph, "An Enquiry into the Processes of Nature in Repairing Injuries of the Intestine," published in 1812. An excellent *précis* of the development of this branch of intestinal surgery is to be found in South's edition of "Chelius's Surgery" (vol. i., page 456).

To Ramdohr in 1780 (*Moebii Dissert. Obs. Misc. Helmst.,* 1780) is ascribed the honour of having been the first to successfully unite the bowel by suture after complete division.

Since this time invention has run riot among methods for uniting the intestine, and the forms of suture which have been considered as especially adapted to the bowel are now legion.

The methods devised have been not only very numerous, but also very varied. Some are imperfect, others are bizarre, not a few are merely curious, many are ingenious, the majority are elaborate.

It is possible, however, to arrange the greater number of the procedures that have been devised under the following divisions or plans :—

Methods. — 1. The divided bowel is brought into the abdominal wound and is retained there. No immediate attempt is made to close the breach in the intestine. An artificial anus is of necessity established. The closure of this fæcal fistula is left to a subsequent period.

This method was advised by John Bell.

2. A rigid cylinder of some kind is employed, and over this the two ends of the bowel are drawn, and are so united as to cover in the cylinder. Various materials have been used in this operation, such as the trachea of an animal, tubes of oiled cardboard, of decalcified bone and of dry gut, plugs of dough, tallow, and isinglass.

Allied to this method, although in execution it is quite distinct from it, is the method of uniting the bowel by means of bone plates, invented and successfully carried out by Dr. Senn. (See pages 327, 334, and 336.)

3. One end of the bowel is invaginated into the other. If possible, the upper end is introduced into the lower. This method was first practised by Ramdohr in 1780, and has been extensively modified. The earlier operators brought the outer serous coat of the inner or entering segment of the bowel into contact with the mucous lining of the outer or receiving segment. In 1827 Jobert so modified this procedure that the serous coats of both ends of the bowel were brought into contact with one another. To effect this, the free (divided) edge of the lower or receiving segment of the intestine was turned inwards.

4. The divided margins of the bowel to be treated are brought together by means of some form of suture. This is effected without employing any supporting foreign body, and without producing any invagination of the tube.

A great variety of *sutures* has been devised to effect this object.

The principal and most generally-accepted methods of uniting the divided intestine will now be described. These selected methods represent the chief modern procedures concerned in enteroraphy.

The Qualifications of a Good Suture.—An efficient intestinal suture should have the following qualifications :—

1. It should bring into contact two broad surfaces of peritoneum, these surfaces belonging respectively to the bowel above and below the breach to be closed.

2. It should effect a complete closure of the wound, the test being that the seam should be water-tight.

3. The mucous membrane should be excluded.

4. The suture should not strangulate the free margin of the intestine with which it is concerned.

5. The suture should not pass through both the mucous and the serous coats. Such a suture—especially when made of silk—would tend to act as a seton, and would be apt to conduct the intestinal fluids to the outer surface of the bowel by means of capillary attraction.

6. The suture should be simple, should be easily introduced, and should be capable of effecting a rapid closure of the wound.

7. The thread should take so firm a hold of the tissues that there is no danger of its "cutting out" when strain is put upon it, as may be the case if the viscus become distended.

The chief forms of intestinal suture will now be considered.

A. **The Continuous Suture.**

1. *Dupuytren's Method* (*Méd. Oper.*, vol. ii., page 138, Paris, 1822).—The edges of the wound are turned inwards, and the opposed folds of serous membrane are then brought together by means of the ordinary continuous suture (Fig. 328). The suture does not involve the

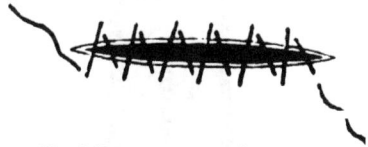

Fig. 328.—DUPUYTREN'S SUTURE.

mucous membrane. This suture may be very rapidly applied.

2. *Gély's Method* (*Nouv. Dict. de Méd. et de Chir.*, vol. xix., page 237).—A long thread is armed at either end with a simple straight round needle. One needle is introduced 4 to 5 m.m. behind, and to the outer side of one end of, the wound, and is made to traverse the outer coats of the bowel in a direction parallel to the edge of the wound for a

distance of 4 to 5 m.m. The same procedure is carried out
with the other needle upon the opposite side of the breach
(Fig. 329). The needles are then crossed, and precisely similar
stitches are taken on either side of the wound, care being

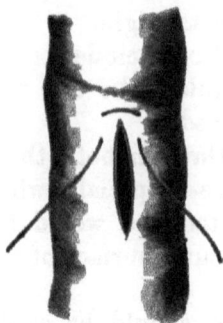

Fig. 329.—GÉLY'S SUTURE
—FIRST STAGE.

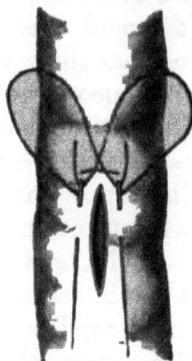

Fig. 330.—GÉLY'S SU-
TURE—SECOND STAGE.

taken that the needle enters the hole which has been already
made by the opposite needle in making the previous stitch
(Fig. 330).

Like stitches are taken along the whole length of the
wound (Fig. 331). In order to close the wound, each trans-

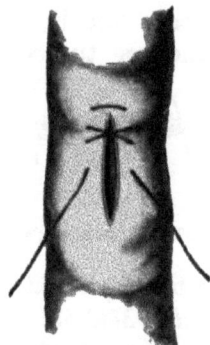

Fig. 33L—GÉLY'S SU-
TURE—THIRD STAGE.

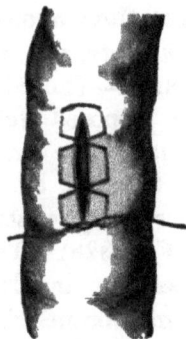

Fig. 332.—GÉLY'S SU-
TURE COMPLETE—
THREADS READY TO
BE DRAWN TIGHT

verse thread is drawn tight by dissecting forceps, the margins
of the wound being at the same time depressed. The opposed

serous surfaces are thus brought into close contact, and the threads are lost to view. The two threads are finally knotted at the end of the wound opposite to that at which the suture was commenced (Fig. 332).

3. *The Right Angle Continuous Suture.*—This is described and advocated by Dr. Cushing in a well-illustrated pamphlet published in Boston in 1889. The stitch is a modification of that known as Appolito's. The suture is com-

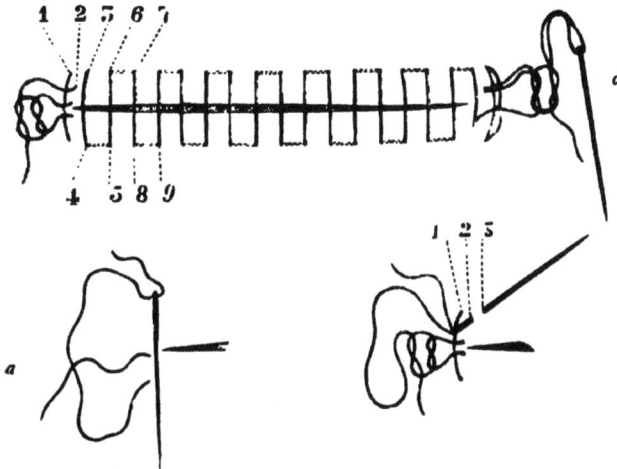

Fig. 333.—CUSHING'S RIGHT ANGLE CONTINUOUS INTESTINAL SUTURE.

a, Beginning of suture ; *b*, Knotting of the same ; *c*, The right angle suture applied. (The numbers 1, 2, and 3, in Figs. *b* and *c*, point to the same needle punctures ; the numbers 4 to 9 indicate, in order, the track of the needle.)

menced as shown in Fig. 333, *a.* It is knotted as soon as a hold upon the bowel has been obtained (Fig. 333, *b*), and the right angle stitches are now commenced.

The thread is then carried to and fro across the wound as shown in Fig. 333, *c*, and is finally knotted at the far extremity of the breach after the manner illustrated in the wood-cut.

The great feature of the suture consists in this—that the needle never enters the lumen of the bowel. The tissues are picked up by passing the needle parallel to the line of the wound. The needle passes through the serous and muscular coats, but avoids the mucous.

u

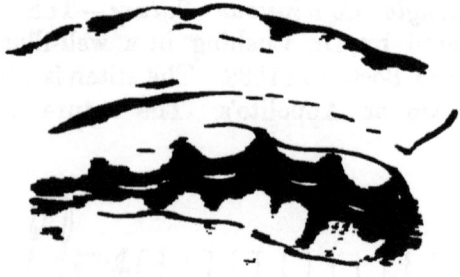

the needle after ... the wound. It then ... right angles to its course and also parallel to the wound). The thread is carried once more across the wound, and is made to pick up the tissues from 6 to 7, and so on.

When the suture is drawn ... shown in the right-... in Fig. 314.

... suture and is unnecessarily

... suture are employed. I ... the best. The suture

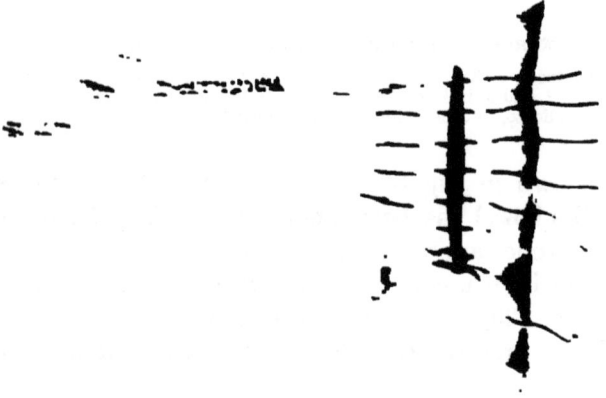

FIG. 315. LEMBERT'S SUTURE.

carried over to the corresponding spot on the other side of
the wound, where a precisely similar fold is picked up
(Fig. 335). The margins of the wound are
turned in, and the serous coats are brought
into close contact (Figs. 336 and 337). The
needle should pick up more than the serous
coat; it should include a part or the whole
of the muscular coat also. It must on no
account trespass beyond the limits of the
latter tunic (Fig. 337).

The width of the fold picked up will be
from one-tenth to one-twelfth of an inch.
The inner row of needle points will be from
one-twelfth of an inch to one-eighth of an
inch from the edge of the wound. In very
small and simple wounds of the intestine, the
needle may be brought out nearer to the free
border of the gap to be closed. The amount
of tissue picked up, *i.e.*, the width of the fold,
will depend upon the thickness of the tissues
involved, the amount of strain likely to be
brought upon the sutures, and the character
of the breach to be closed.

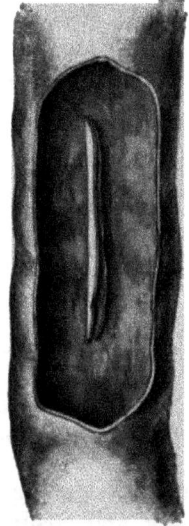

Fig. 336.—LEMBERT'S
SUTURE OF THE IN-
TESTINE (as seen
from the mucous
surface).

The closeness of the sutures to one another must vary
somewhat according to circumstances. They may be usually
estimated at about ten to the inch. It will rarely be safe to
apply them less closely than this.

The extremities of each suture are knotted together, and
the ends cut short. The knots need not be tied with the
utmost degree of tightness.

Much trouble is saved, and the inconvenience of a long, wet,
and sticky thread is avoided, if separate threaded needles are
prepared for each suture.

If the supply of needles be limited, the thread carried be
each needle may serve for two, or at the very utmost for three,
sutures.

In applying Lembert's suture after resection of the bowel
Mr. Greig Smith employs the following plan:—

"Four quilt-sutures are inserted on the opposite sides of
the divided gut, in the exact line in which the Lembert

sutures are to be placed; the two on each side are gathered together in the blades of catch forceps, and gentle and steady traction made on them by an assistant. This raises a well-defined fold along the edge of the bowel; into this fold the sutures are inserted.

"The insertion of these quilt-stitches makes certain that equal distances of the bowel are arranged for suturing, and

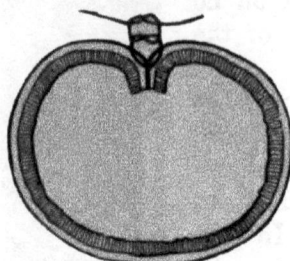

Fig. 337.—LEMBERT'S SUTURE.

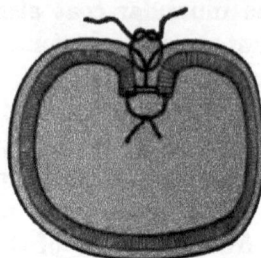

Fig. 338.—CZERNY-LEMBERT SUTURE.

also, by raising a fold, makes the insertion of stitches more easy, and ensures their being placed in a straight line."

2. *Czerny's Suture* (*Sammlung klin. Vortrage*, 1881. No. 201).—This is a Lembert's suture with the addition of an inner row of interrupted sutures which unite the mucous membrane only (Fig. 338). The knots of this inner row are turned inwards. Fig. 370 shows the method of introducing the first row of sutures, *i.e.*, those which implicate the mucous membrane only. In the case of small or limited wounds of the bowel, and in the case of the nearly-closed wound which results from suturing the divided ends of the bowel after resection, the knots of the inner layer of sutures must of necessity be tied towards the outer surface of the tube. The ends of the suture are cut short,

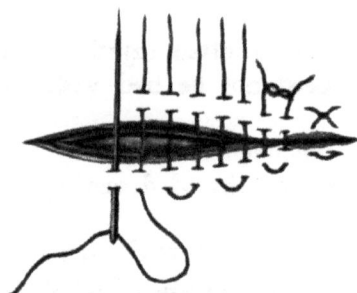

Fig. 339.—HALSTEAD'S PLAIN QUILT-SUTURE.

and the row of knots inverted as far as is possible. The row of knots is then covered in by the muscular coat when Lembert's suture is applied.

3. *Halstead's Plain Quilt-Suture* (*Internat. Journ. Med. Sci.*, Oct., 1887) is another modification of Lembert's method. The monograph in which this suture is described is a valuable contribution to the surgery of the intestine.

The details of the suture are shown in Fig. 339. Dr. Halstead insists that each stitch should include not only the whole muscular coat, but also a little of the tough submucous coat. All the stitches are applied before any one is tied. It is claimed for this suture, as compared with that of Lembert, that the stitches compress the tissues less, tear out less readily, and allow of a more accurate apposition of the peritoneal surfaces.

c. **The Invagination Method.**

This has been applied only in instances in which the whole circumference of the bowel has been divided.

Jobert's Method.—This was described in 1827 (*Mém. sur les Plaies du Canal Intestin.*, Paris, 1827).

The upper and lower ends of the gut having been identified, the mesentery is dissected away for one-third of an inch from each end of the bowel. A straight needle carrying a long thread is then made to transfix the upper segment about a third of an inch from the divided margin, and along the line of the mesenteric attachment. A like suture is introduced upon the opposite (free) margin of the bowel (Fig. 340).

The margin of the lower end of the gut · is now invaginated. This is a difficult manœuvre to effect.

The two ends of the thread hanging from the upper end of the bowel are both armed with needles, and the double fold of the intestinal wall produced by the invagination is transfixed by the two needles, which will pierce the gut at a little distance from one another. A like plan is adopted with both the sutures. The threads will pass through corresponding parts of the

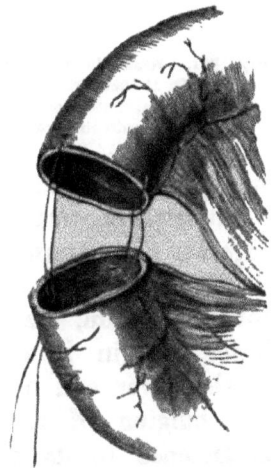

Fig. 340.—JOBERT'S SUTURE FOR THE INTESTINE (sutures placed preparatory to invagination).

two segments of the bowel. The upper end of the bowel
is now forced into the lower, partly by traction upon the
sutures, and partly by squeezing. The serous coats of both of
the ends of the gut are thus brought into contact (Fig. 341).
The ends of the sutures are finally knotted externally upon
the outer surface of the lower segment of the divided intestine.

Jobert himself did not knot the threads, but brought
them out through the surface
wound, and removed them at the
end of five days.

To make this method secure,
the two segments of the bowel
should be transfixed by at least
four sutures instead of two, and
the peritoneal surfaces on the
outer aspect of the tube at the
point where the two segments
meet should be brought together
by numerous points of Lembert's
suture.

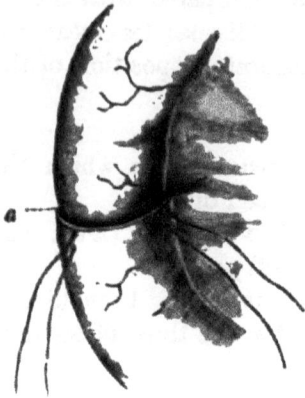

Fig. 341.—JOBERT'S SUTURE FOR
THE INTESTINE.
a, Line of invagination of the upper
segment into the lower.

*Senn's Modification of Jobert's
Method* is as follows :—

The upper end of the bowel
which is to become the intus-
susceptum is lined with a soft, pliable rubber ring, made of
a rubber band transformed into a ring by fastening the ends
together with catgut sutures.

This ring must correspond in width to the length of the
intussusceptum, viz., from one-third to half an inch. Its
lower margin is stitched by a continuous catgut suture
to the lower end of the bowel, which effectually prevents
the bulging of the mucous membrane. After the ring
is fastened in its place, the end of the bowel presents a
tapering appearance, which facilitates the process of invagination. Two fine catgut sutures are threaded each with two
needles. The needles are passed from within outwards, transfixing the upper portion of the rubber ring and the entire
thickness of the wall of the bowel. The two sutures are
equi-distant from one another, one being near the mesenteric

border, and the other at the opposite point (free border) of the intestine.

During this time an assistant keeps the opposite end of the bowel compressed, to prevent bulging of the mucous membrane.

The needles are next passed through the serous and muscular coats of the lower segment of the bowel, at points corresponding to those selected on the upper segment.

The actual place of puncture will be about one-third or half an inch from the divided margin of the bowel.

When the needles have been passed, equal traction is made by an assistant upon the four threads (each of the two sutures is double), and the surgeon assists the invagination by turning in the margins of the lower end of the bowel with a director, while he gently pushes the rubber ring into the intussuscipiens.

In time, the catgut holding the rubber ring gives way, and the ring is set free as a flat rubber band.

Senn does not advise superficial peritoneal sutures, and finds in animals that two invagination sutures are quite sufficient.

The rubber ring greatly facilitates the operation.

As the sutures pass through the ring, an efficient obstacle is offered to the conduction of the intestinal fluids along the sutures to the peritoneal surface.

The ring also protects the coats of the bowel from undue pressure and undue traction from the invagination sutures. It serves, moreover, to keep the lumen of the intestine patent during the stage of inflammatory swelling.

The Best Form of Intestinal Suture.—The methods of suturing the bowel above described have each their especial advantages, and all may be regarded as accepted and sound measures for uniting divided intestine.

The Invagination Method last described is more especially adapted for cases of resection of a portion of the bowel.

So far as experiments upon animals go, it appears to be an efficient, ready, and rapid method of uniting the bowel after complete division. In reading accounts of experiments with this method, it must not be forgotten that the intestine of the dog, and more especially of the cat, differs considerably from the human bowel.

For the *continuous sutures*, the following advantages are claimed :—The suture is readily and rapidly applied. Time is not lost in tying some twenty or thirty knots with very fine silk or catgut which is wet and sticky. The suture is strong, takes a firm hold of the parts, and can sustain considerable strain. It produces a very perfect apposition of the margins of the wound.

The objections to it are these :—A considerable length of ligature material is left in the coats of the intestine. It is not always easy to pull all parts of the suture evenly tight. Some part of the thread is apt to be loosened as the gut contracts ; some strangulation of the margins of the gut to be united is apt to follow when the suture is drawn tight.

The suture may well be employed in instances where speed is a matter of importance, where the bowel is already well contracted, and where an additional suture is needed in a dangerous part.

The simplest of the sutures described is Dupuytren's. It is readily introduced. It fails, however, to effect a very even apposition of surfaces, and is apt to produce strangulation of the margins of the wound.

Gély's suture brings the parts well together, but has the disadvantage of being complex and difficult of application. Large tracts of tissue are included within the grip of the thread.

The right angle continuous suture is, on the whole, the best of the three named. The apposition of the surfaces is very complete, and very neat. The suture is buried. The disposition to produce strangulation of the margin of the wound is scarcely more than is to be noted in the interrupted suture.

The interrupted sutures have many advantages. The strain upon the wound is distributed over many threads. The surfaces concerned are brought into very accurate contact. The vascular supply of the margin of the wound is not interfered with. The sutures are easily introduced, and the amount of suture material employed is reduced to a minimum. The securing of these sutures, however, involves considerable time ; and unless they are very closely placed together, there is some risk of leakage in the gaps between the threads.

Lembert's suture has stood the test of time, and it may be safely said of it that it is, on the whole, the *best form of suture* with which we are acquainted.

Its extreme simplicity, the rapidity with which each stitch can be inserted, and its undoubted efficiency, are points in its favour which all operators have recognised.

It may be supplemented by a second row of stitches, as Czerny advised.

Halstead's plain quilt-suture may be regarded as an ingenious compromise between two excellent methods—Lembert's suture on the one hand, and the right angle continuous suture on the other.

The Needles Employed.—The needles selected for suture of the intestine must depend upon the taste and custom of the individual operator. A straight, slender sewing-needle has appeared to me to be the best in most cases, and is especially suited for Lembert's suture. Sutures in the mucous membrane are perhaps more conveniently introduced by means of a curved needle. A curved needle is also used by many for the superficial sutures.

The straight needle should be about one inch and a quarter in length, and must have a round shaft. A common sewing-needle of this length is excellent, and is infinitely to be preferred to the lancet-pointed or triangular-pointed needles often found in use.

The curved needle should have a round shaft, should form a complete semicircle with a diameter of about five-eighths of an inch, and the extremity of the eye should not be larger than the rest of the shaft. It should not taper too much towards the point, but the full size of the shaft should be reached a short distance from the point. Many of the special "intestinal needles" are needlessly small.

The simplest possible form of needle-holder should be used. I have not found either Hagedorn's needle or his needle-holder convenient for suturing the intestine.

Possibly the worst form of intestinal needle is that known in instrument-makers' catalogues as the "half-curved."

The Sutures Employed.—I have found the best suture

material to be the very finest purse-silk, stained red, so that it can be easily seen. It is strong, is easily manipulated, is of close fibre, runs very easily, and ties in a very small and very firm knot. It does not twist up, and is even more easy to deal with when it is wet than when it is dry. It should, indeed, always be used wet.

Fine catgut is employed by many, but it has certain drawbacks. There is no catgut made which has so smooth a surface as purse-silk that has been dipped in water (carbolic solution). As a consequence catgut " runs " somewhat stiffly. The catgut thread, moreover, is a little rigid, and, when tied, forms a comparatively large and clumsy knot, which has, on more than one occasion, given way. In many intestinal operations it is felt that a suture of a somewhat more abiding nature than catgut is desirable.

The General Details of an Operation for Suturing Intestine.

It would be out of place to enter into any details as to the circumstances in which suture of the intestine is called for. A mere outline of the matter will suffice. The case may be imagined to be one of penetrating wound or of gunshot injury. The already-existing wound is enlarged, or the abdomen is opened in the median line. The damaged coil is at once drawn forward into the wound, and is so held there by an assistant that no more of the intestinal contents can escape. If there be reason to believe that there are other wounds of the bowel, a careful and detailed examination of the whole length of the intestine must be made. Any wounded loop which may be discovered is brought into the parietal incision.

The breaches in the gut having been for the time secured, the next care should be to flush out thoroughly and cleanse the peritoneal cavity of every trace of blood and extravasated matter. After this has been done, the treatment of the gut may be commenced.

The wounded loop is drawn out of the parietal wound, and is laid upon a fine sponge. The opening into the belly around the protruding loop is carefully plugged with sponges. The gut is held above and below the seat of the wound by the fingers of an assistant. The isolated segment is emptied of its contents, if necessary, and is, in any case, most thoroughly cleansed. The sutures are applied, and the gut is returned into the abdomen.

If the gut be extensively damaged, an artificial anus should be established which may be closed at a later period.

Before establishing such an artificial opening, a segment of the damaged bowel may be resected, should the circumstances call for such a measure.

When there has been much extravasation into the peritoneal cavity, a drainage-tube should be introduced before the parietal wound is sutured.

This subject has been dealt with in a number of very admirable monographs. Among them are the following:—Dr. Parkes' "Gunshot Wounds of the Small Intestines," Chicago, 1884; Sir William MacCormac's "Abdominal Section for Intra-Peritoneal Injury," London, 1887; and Dr. Morton's "Abdominal Section for Traumatism," Chicago, 1890. The last-named paper contains a very valuable series of tables which deal with 234 cases of intra-peritoneal injury treated by operation.

The Use of Omental Grafts after Suture of the Intestine.

After uniting the bowel by suture, Dr. Senn, in certain of his experiments, fixed a flap of the omentum over the seam left by the enteroraphy. These flaps soon became adherent, and proved an additional safeguard against perforation during the process of repair. The free or distal end of the flap was fixed in position by sutures; the proximal end remained connected with the omentum.

An obvious objection to this procedure in surgical practice is based upon the possibility of the attached omentum forming a band or bridge beneath which a loop of gut may be strangulated.

To meet this objection, Dr. Senn cut off portions of the omentum in the form of isolated grafts, and fixed them by stitches around the bowel at the suture line.

The grafts used were from one and a half to two inches in width, and were of sufficient length to completely encircle the bowel.

The experiments were carried out upon dogs.

In all instances the grafts retained their vitality, and in a few hours became adherent in their new positions. The intestinal peritoneum was lightly scarified before the graft was fixed in place.

From his experiments upon animals, Dr. Senn ventures to deduce the following conclusions ("Intestinal Surgery," Chicago, 1889, page 208) :—"After suturing a large wound of the stomach or intestines, a strip of omentum should be laid over the wound, and fastened in its place by a few catgut sutures. After circular enteroraphy the operation should be finished by covering the circular wound by an omental graft about two inches wide, which should be fixed in its place by two catgut sutures passed through both ends of the graft and the mesentery.

"Omental grafting should also be resorted to in repairing peritoneal defects in visceral injuries of the abdominal organs, and in covering large stumps after ovariotomy or hysterectomy when the pedicle is treated by the intra-abdominal method."

CHAPTER VI.

RESECTION OF THE INTESTINE.

UNDER this title are included operations which concern themselves in the removal of comparatively small portions of either the small or the large intestine.

Excision when applied to the lesser bowel is termed enterectomy, and when carried out in the colon colectomy. The somewhat pedantic title, cæcectomy, has been bestowed upon excision of the cæcum.

Indications.—Most of these operations have concerned the lesser bowel, and have been performed to remove gangrenous parts in strangulated hernia, or to restore the canal after a fæcal fistula has been produced. Enterectomy has also been performed for the relief of strictures of the bowel, both simple and epitheliomatous, for occlusion due to adhesions and certain neoplasms, for the relief of irreducible intussusceptions, and in certain examples of extensive injury, as after gunshot wounds.

The greater number of the cases of colectomy have been performed to effect the removal of a malignant growth, or to restore the bowel after an artificial anus.

History.—Accounts of the excision of portions of gangrenous bowel in hernia are to be found among the earlier annals of surgery. The operations were a little uncouthly performed, but were attended with some success.

In 1727 Ramdohr successfully removed two feet of gangrenous bowel from a hernia. (*See* paper by Dr. Ill, *New York Med. Rec.*, Sept. 22nd, 1883.)

In 1732 Arnaud excised from a rupture the cæcum, with some part of the colon and ileum. The patient, a man aged sixty, recovered ("Dissertation on Hernias," pt. 2, obs. xvii.).

Reybard in 1843 removed a carcinomatous growth of the sigmoid flexure, together with three inches of the gut. The patient survived the operation, and died of recurrence in twelve months (*Bull. Acad. de Méd.*, t. ix., page 1033).

Within the last twenty years resect
the large and the small intestine have
steadily-increasing frequency.

McArdle (*Dublin Journal of Mea*
1—123) has collected seventy-six ex
gangrenous hernia. Kendal Frank
vol. lxxii., page 224) has framed a tal
excision of the colon for cancer.

Billroth reports (*Brit. Med. Journ*
407) that he has himself performed 1
upon the stomach and the intestines.

Reichel as long ago as 1883 brou
of gut resection for various conditio
Chir., 1883, page 230).

Morton has collected sixteen exam
shot injury or penetrating wound ("
Traumatism," Chicago, 1890).

Mr. Croft's very admirable paper o
intestine (*Clin. Soc. Trans.*, vol. xxiii
of fourteen cases of abdominal secti
small intestine without wound. In fiv
performed.

Of individual cases, one of the mos
Koeberlé's. This surgeon removed ove
intestine from an adult suffering
stricture. The operation was succes
la Soc. de Chir. de Paris, 1881, page 9

I have dealt further with the subj
intestine elsewhere ("Intestinal Obst
page 476 *et seq.*).

The details of the operation will b
following headings :—

　　1. Enterectomy with circular
　　　　ends.
　　2. Enterectomy with the establi
　　　　anus.
　　3. Methods of uniting segments
　　　　size.
　　4. Colectomy.
　　5. Senn's operation.

1. ENTERECTOMY WITH CIRCULAR SUTURING OF THE DIVIDED ENDS.

1. The abdomen having been opened, the first step is to isolate the loop of intestine to be excised. This loop should be drawn well out of the parietal wound. Any adhesions which prevent it from being well exposed and isolated must be divided.

If any extravasation has taken place into the abdominal cavity, it should be dealt with before the resection is commenced.

The operator must, moreover, be prepared for the absolute necessity of abandoning the excision altogether.

The disease or gangrene may be found to be too extensive, or the bowel may be so bound down that it would be impossible to isolate it sufficiently to enable a resection to be performed, or the amount of extravasated matter found in the peritoneal cavity may be such that the thorough cleansing of the serous space and the rapid establishment of an artificial anus will be obviously the right course to adopt.

Not only must the loop to be dealt with be well exposed, but healthy bowel both above and below the seat of disease must be brought into view.

The mesentery of the part to be resected should be also examined.

In cases of malignant disease it is needless to say that no resection operation should be entertained in cases in which the disease is other than very clearly limited, or in instances in which the mesenteric glands are found to be involved.

The part to be resected is placed upon a thin Turkey sponge, and the whole wound through which the intestine has been drawn is well and carefully packed all round with fine sponges. It should be impossible for any intestinal matter to find its way into the peritoneal cavity.

If the parietal wound has been very large, it may be desirable that it should be closed in part by sutures before the resection is commenced.

2. The bowel must be occluded above and below the resection area. If sponges have been well packed all around

the coil, this precaution may sometimes, and in some special cases, be dispensed with.

Many clamps have been devised for the present purpose. No instrument, however, is so efficient as the fingers of an intelligent assistant. The holding of the gut by an assistant, however, is apt to involve two difficulties. In the first place, his hands may come very much in the surgeon's way; and in the second place, it is scarcely possible to retain a proper and equable hold of the gut during the long space of time involved by the operation.

Of the various clamps devised, the best is that introduced by Mr. Makins (*St. Thomas's Hosp. Reports*, 1884, page 81) (Fig. 342). The blades are covered with indiarubber tubing, and are long enough to compress the whole width of the

Fig. 342.—MAKINS'S INTESTINAL CLAMP.

bowel. They are simple, and are easily applied and removed. Other forms of clamps suitable for the intestine are figured in the chapter on Excision of the Pylorus (Fig. 366).

Some surgeons ligature the bowel lightly above and below, making use of a cord made of gauze, which is passed through a hole in the mesentery. Dr. Senn, in experiments upon animals, was most satisfied with ligatures made of indiarubber bands. The bands are about one-eighth of an inch wide, and are applied by perforating the mesentery at a point free from large visible vessels, and are then tied in a loop with sufficient firmness to obstruct the lumen of the bowel.

A simple clamp or the fingers of an assistant are, however, to be preferred to any form of ligature. The ligature not only exercises an undue amount of compression and involves an injury to the mesentery, but it throws the cut margin of the bowel out of line, and in the case of a dilated bowel is apt to throw it into folds.

Dr. Maunsell (Inter-colonial Medical Congress, 1889) adopts the following simple method:—A flat piece of sponge is placed over the bowel, and the two ends of the sponge, together with the intervening mesentery, are transfixed with the shaft of a large safety-pin. The body of the pin lies over the sponge. By closing the pin the bowel is clamped.

In adjusting clamps (should these instruments be used), the upper clamp will be applied first. The segment of bowel to be excised will then be gently emptied by passing the fingers along it, and the lower clamp will be fixed in position. Little matter should therefore escape from the isolated segment during the division of the coats of the bowel. Before applying the sutures, care must be taken that the bowel above the resection area is not greatly distended. If it be so, the distension must be relieved, as much gas and fæcal matter being allowed to escape as will find an exit. This is best effected by making an opening in the centre of the loop to be excised, and allowing the intestinal contents to escape into a gutter of thin indiarubber tissue which has been already prepared and put in position. This answers better than the method of loosening the upper clamp after the bowel has been excised.

3. The portion of diseased bowel is now excised. This is effected with blunt-pointed scissors. The cut must be made about three-fourths of an inch beyond the margin of the clamp. If it be much nearer, it will be found that the clamp interferes with the movement of the needles during the passage of Lembert's suture.

The bowel should be cut straight across, *i.e.*, at right angles to its long axis. After such a section it will be noticed that the divided coats retract a little more on the free than on the attached border of the bowel, and as a result the incision lines tend to diverge a little and to become oblique. It has been advised by some that the bowel be divided by two oblique and diverging incisions, in such a way that more of the intestine is cut away upon the free than upon the mesenteric side. Experiment will show that there is little to recommend this method, and that it involves a less complete restoration of the natural curve of the intestinal coil.

. The scissors cut their way from the free border towards the mesentery ; on approaching the mesentery, care must be

taken to save as much of that membrane as possible
(Fig. 343).

The segment of bowel to be removed may be almost—as
it were—enucleated. The mesentery may then be divided as
close to the wall of the bowel as is possible.

An account has already been given of the interspace which
extends along the whole length of the mesenteric attachment
(page 297). The scissors will open this interspace, and will
follow it, dividing the mesentery close to the bowel.

Another—and in most instances a better—method of treating the mesentery consists in excising a triangular portion of
the membrane together with the gut to be removed. The base
of the triangle will
be at the intestine,
but will be narrower
than the length of
bowel removed. By
allowing the mes-
entery to overlap
the divided ends
as it were, the vas-
cular supply of
those segments is
the less interfered
with. The margins
of the wound in the mesentery are then carefully brought
together by a continuous suture. This measure brings about
the neatest adjustment of the parts, and is most efficient in
preventing that kinking at the suture line which is so apt to
occur after resection operations. In cases of malignant disease it is an advantage to remove the mesentery which contains the lymphatics issuing from the growth. It is insisted
upon by some that it involves, however, a greater amount of
interference with the vascular supply of the divided ends of
the bowel than does the method of cutting the mesentery
close to the intestine; but it cannot be said that this point has
yet been proved.

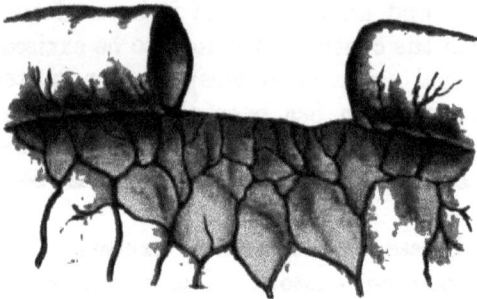

Fig. 343.—POSITION OF THE MESENTERY AFTER RESEC-
TION OF THE GUT. (*After MacCormac.*)

4. The divided ends of the bowel are now thoroughly well
cleansed, and all soiled sponges are removed and replaced by
fresh ones

The mucous membrane may be found to protrude considerably, and to appear to interfere with the proper adjustment of the sutures. On no account, however, should any portion of this membrane be pared away.

The sutures may now be applied. If it is intended to introduce a double row, then the surgeon proceeds at once to unite the margins of the divided mucous membrane.

In an operation like the present, where time is usually a matter of considerable importance, the inner row of sutures may be dispensed with, or may at least be replaced by a continuous suture, which can be rapidly introduced.

The surface sutures will be applied according to Lembert's method, and in the manner already described (page 306).

It may be once more pointed out that the weak part of the suture line will be at the mesenteric border. It is at the line of the attachment of this membrane that the first stitches are applied. Use must be made of any peritoneum which has been saved from the mesentery, and sufficient must be found to serve as a covering for the bare portion of the bowel. Not only must the muscular coats be well brought together at this part, but inturned flaps of peritoneum covering that coat must also be brought into direct and close contact.

After the mesenteric border has been dealt with, it is most convenient to turn next to the free or opposite border of the intestine, and to insert three or four sutures there.

The surgeon may then introduce a batch of three or four sutures upon the lateral parts of the bowel, at points on either side, midway between the first two sets of sutures. Finally, the gaps between the four isolated batches of sutures are filled up, and the union of the divided ends is completed.

The clamps are now removed.

The surgeon next turns to the mesentery. If a triangular portion have been removed, the margins of the gap are brought together by several points of suture—or, better still, by a continuous suture.

If the mesentery have been divided close to the bowels there will be a large redundant fold to be dealt with. The cut edges of this fold may be united by a continuous suture after the manner shown in the diagram (Fig. 344). This, however, must not be allowed to suffice. To prevent kinking, to prevent a pouch from being formed, and to give to the suture line the fullest degree of support, the base of this fold of mesentery—along the lines A, B (Fig. 344)—must be transfixed by a series of sutures, and the two layers of serous membrane in this situation be brought into close contact.

It will be obvious that in the majority of instances, and notably in cases of malignant disease, this large redundant fold should be removed; or, in other words, that a triangular piece should be cut out of the mesentery together with the bowel.

5. The bowel is well cleansed, the sponges that have held the coil in place are removed, and the sutured loop is allowed to drop back into the abdomen. The abdominal wound is then closed; and unless distinct reasons exist to the contrary, no drainage tube is introduced.

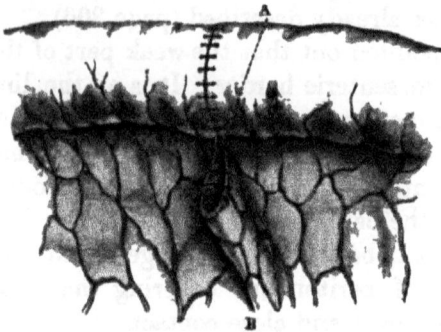

Fig. 344.—REDUNDANT FOLD OF MESENTERY LEFT AFTER THE INTESTINE HAS BEEN SUTURED. (*MacCormac.*)

There is nothing to recommend the plan advised by some of attaching the sutured coil to the parietal peritoneum, and of leaving the parietal wound partly open.

This is advised " if there is any doubt as to the perfection of the suturing." There should be no more doubt upon this point than upon the perfection of the ligaturing in hæmorrhage, or upon the perfection of the reduction in operating upon strangulated hernia. If there are irremediable weak points in the suture line, an artificial anus should be established at once.

2. ENTERECTOMY WITH THE ESTABLISHMENT OF AN ARTIFICIAL ANUS.

The early steps of the operation are precisely the same as in the procedure just described.

The removal of a triangular piece of the mesentery facilitates the subsequent operation for the closure of the artificial anus. The gap left in the mesentery should be united by suture, as already described.

After the excision has been carried out, the wound in the parietes is so far closed as to leave only a gap through which the divided ends of the gut project. The two sections of bowel—still clamped—should be brought together by their mesenteric borders, and are united by a few points of suture. If time and the condition of the patient allow, the union of the two ends may be carried a little to either side of the mesenteric border. The mucous membrane over the uniting isthmus should be brought together by a simple continuous suture.

The lower end of the divided bowel is now rapidly united to the parietes. The margin of the bowel is secured all round to the margin of the parietal wound. The serous covering of the intestine must be brought into contact with the serous lining of the abdominal wall. The sutures are most conveniently passed by means of a large curved Hagedorn's needle. The suture material which should be used in these cases is silkworm gut which is peculiarly well adapted for the purpose. The needle must first transfix the wall then the tissues of the parietes then the parietal peritoneum then the whole thickness of the wall of the intestine. If the needle is passed in the opposite direction—i.e. from mucous membrane to skin—the suture may carry intestinal matter into the depths of the wound. Each needle is previously armed in the usual and convenient manner and thread and it is not for more than one suture. It will suffice if these sutures are about half an inch apart. The mucous membrane is loosely attached to the skin at the margin of the wound.

The main sutures that are passed are the ones, and removed are the ones ... is withdrawn.

The upper end of the ... Every precaution must ... soon as the upper ... be in proper ... the lumen of the ... dry. The mucous ...

oiled lint, which is frequently changed. Beneath it the wound may be covered by a thick layer of iodoform.

This method of operating is commented upon in a subsequent section (page 320).

3. METHODS OF UNITING SEGMENTS OF INTESTINE OF UNEQUAL SIZE.

The bowel above the segment resected may be much dilated, while the tube below is much contracted. In such a case, the two parts to be united may be brought to more nearly the same size if the distension of the upper part of the bowel be relieved by allowing its contents to escape. Moreover, after the excision, and before the sutures are applied, the lower clamp may be loosened, and the contracted bowel gently stretched to the necessary size with the fingers, after which the clamp may be reapplied.

In actual practice, however, these measures are usually not called for. If the bowel above the part to be removed be greatly dilated, and the bowel below be greatly contracted, then there must have been a severe grade of intestinal obstruction, and in such a condition the enterectomy should be concluded by establishing an artificial anus.

When, however, the cæcum has been excised, and the ileum has to be united to the colon, one or other of the following measures may be adopted :—

A. **Wehr's Method.**—The end of the narrower part of the bowel is not divided transversely, but is cut obliquely. The obliquity must be such that the oblong opening which results shall correspond to the lumen of the other end of the bowel. This unequal division of the intestine must always be made at the expense of the convex or free margin of the gut.

B. **Billroth's Method.**—This is known as lateral implantation. Assuming that the cæcum has been excised, the end of the colon is closed by sutures. This is effected by invaginating the free margins of the divided gut, so that the serous coats are brought into close contact. The parts are united by sutures, preferably by a double row.

A slit is now made in the wall of the closed colon. This slit is vertical—i.e., in the long axis of the colon—is placed upon that margin of the gut which is opposite to the attachment of the meso-colon, and is situate about two inches from the closed end. The size of the slit will correspond to the size of the divided end of the ileum.

The end of the ileum is implanted into the slit, and is secured there by very careful suturing.

c. **Senn's Invagination Method.**—This is described on page 310. The rubber ring is introduced into the end of the ileum, and the walls of the colon are invaginated to receive it. The ileum may be thus inserted into the open end of the divided colon, or that end may be closed by sutures, and the ileum be implanted into a slit made in the colon above the closed end, as in Billroth's method. In such a case the margins of the colic slit must be properly invaginated.

d. **Senn's Method by Intestinal Anastomosis.**—This is fully described in the next chapter. (*See* also pages 310 and 334.) It is only necessary to state here how the two ends of the intestine are arranged with reference to one another. In one case of carcinoma of the cæcum Dr. Senn excised the whole cæcum, together with eighteen inches of the ileum. The patient recovered. After the diseased parts had been cut away, the operation was completed as follows:—

" After all hæmorrhage had been carefully arrested, both resected ends were closed by invagination and a few stitches of the continued suture (Fig. 345, a); the first stitch was made to transfix the mesentery at the point where it was invaginated into the bowel. Medium-sized perforated decalcified bone plates were used in making the ileo-colostomy by lateral approximation. An incision about two inches in length was made near the closed ends of both intestines at a point opposite the mesenteric attachment, and into each opening a bone plate was inserted, and the lateral sutures, armed with a needle, were passed about an eighth of an inch from the margin of the wound at a point half-way between the angles of the intestinal wound. The surfaces of the bowel corresponding to the parts covering the plates were freely scarified with an ordinary sewing-needle. The visceral wounds were now brought vis-à-vis in such a manner that both closed ends were directed downwards, bringing in this manner the free surface of the colon and ileum together. Before any of the plate sutures were tied, a number of Lembert sutures were applied posteriorly, sufficiently far back so that after the approximation they should be just beyond the borders of the plates, thus affording additional security in maintaining coaptation (Fig. 350). The posterior pair of transfixion sutures was now tied, after which both pairs of the sutures not armed with needles were tied. During the tying of these sutures, it is of the greatest importance that an assistant should keep the plates accurately and closely pressed together. The last sutures to be tied were the second pair of fixation sutures ; and as this was being done, the bowel on each side was carefully pushed in between the plates with a probe. The sutures were tied in a square knot, and only with sufficient firmness to bring the parts in apposition, as any undue pressure would have been detrimental, and might have resulted in gangrene of the tissues included between the plates. The sutures were cut short, and the ends brought as near the opening as possible, by pushing them in this direction with a probe. After all the approximation sutures were tied, it only remained to apply on the upper side a few Lembert sutures in the same manner as was done on the opposite side before any of the approximation sutures were tied" (Fig. 345, c).—(*Journ. of the Amer. Med. Assoc.*, June 14, 1890.)

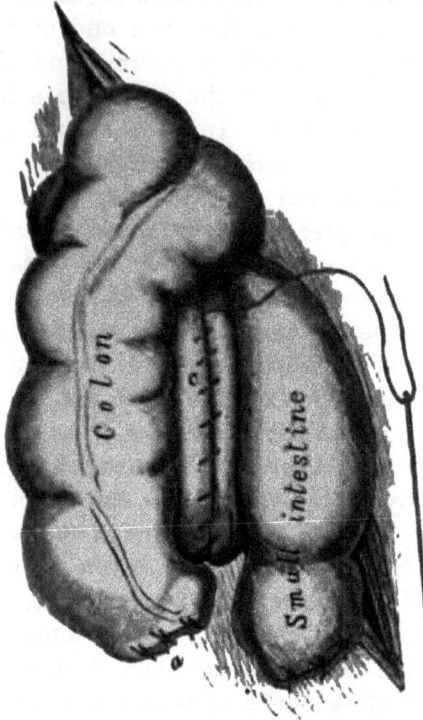

Fig. 345.—EXCISION OF THE CÆCUM; CLOSURE OF THE ENDS OF THE COLON AND ILEUM; INTESTINAL ANASTOMOSIS BY BONE PLATES. (*Senn.*)

4. COLECTOMY.

The operation for resecting portions of the colon differs in no essential particular from that applied to the small intestine.

After the diseased segment has been removed, the two divided ends of the intestine may be brought together and united by sutures, or any attempt at immediate union may be abandoned and an artificial anus be established. In colectomy, the latter procedure is more frequently carried out than is the case when the small intestine is dealt with.

An artificial anus may be established as a temporary measure, and may be followed by an attempt to close the opening at a later period by a second operation. In such a case the two ends of the divided colon are brought close together, and may even be united partially by a few sutures applied upon the deep or attached aspect of the gut.

If, on the other hand, it be intended that the artificial anus should be permanent, then it is well to close the opening in the distal segment of the bowel. This especially applies to resections carried out low down in the colon.

In closing the distal end it is well to turn in the edges a little, and to bring the serous coats of the bowel together so far as is possible.

The great majority of cases in which colectomy has been performed have been cases of malignant stricture of the bowel.

Mr. Kendal Franks, in a very valuable paper in *The Royal Medico-Chirurgical Transactions*, 1889, has collected fifty-one examples of this operation. The amount of intestine removed has varied from two to twelve or more inches. In one or two instances the whole cæcum has been excised, together with portions of the ascending colon and ileum.

The best position for the incision in the parietes offers some difficulties.

The most practical rule is that which would direct the incision to be made immediately over the tumour when a tumour exists.

In any case of doubt a small exploratory incision should be made in the median line, and this may be followed if necessary by a second incision directly over the seat of the disease.

Very little can be done through the median line. The transverse colon can be dealt with through an incision so placed; but with regard to other segments of the colon, much depends upon the mobility of the diseased part and upon anatomical conditions. The summit of the sigmoid or omega loop may be excised possibly through a median incision. It is conceivable also that under certain conditions the cæcum may be resected through a like incision. The circumstances, however, must be exceptional; while for the treatment of the ascending and descending portions of the colon the median wound is of no avail.

In every instance it is desirable that the diseased bowel should be reached by the shortest and most direct route.

Portions of the ascending and descending colon have been excised through the loin, through an incision identical with that used in lumbar colotomy. Sufficient room, however, is scarcely to be obtained through such a wound, the surgeon's movements are hampered by the restricted space in which he must manipulate, and the freeing of the bowel above and below the seat of the disease cannot be so efficiently carried out.

The details of the actual operation call for no especial remark, and the account above given of enterectomy will apply to the resection when performed upon the large intestine. The meso-colon, when it exists as a complete fold, is dealt with in the same manner as the mesentery.

Comment upon Resection Operations.—The operative measures above described are serious, and have been attended with a very high mortality. There is reason to believe that with improvement in the *technique* of the operation, and with an increased knowledge of the best means of managing the bowel, the death-rate will be considerably modified.

The main point which needs consideration is the question as to which is the better method of performing resection—the method which concludes by circular suture of the divided ends of the bowel, or that which leads to the establishment of an artificial anus.

It is obvious that the former of these two methods is the more complete, and is, from a theoretical point of view, the more perfect and satisfactory. The diseased portion of the bowel is removed, the continuity of the canal is restored by suturing, and the abdominal cavity is closed.

It will be obvious, however, that this method of performing resection involves a considerable expenditure of time, and that, to be surely successful, it requires all those conditions which contribute to the success of any extensive plastic operation. The general state of the patient should be favourable, and the local condition should be good.

Enterectomy, followed by circular suturing of the bowel, is a plastic operation in which perfect and immediate primary healing is essential; and such healing can scarcely be looked for when the patient is *in extremis* at the time of the operation, when the bowel is suffering from long-abiding distension or when the peritoneal cavity is the seat of fæcal extravasation.

In a large proportion of the cases the state of the patient is such that time is a matter of paramount importance, and every minute occupied by the operation adds to the danger, which is already great.

So far as resection of the small intestine is concerned, statistics and published cases have shown that the chief element of success in enterectomy depends upon the formation of a temporary fæcal fistula.

Enterectomy, followed by circular suturing of the divided ends of the bowel, may be advised under such conditions as the following:—

1. Cases of injury (*e.g.*, gunshot wound and stab) in which the whole of the damaged part can be readily excised, in which the injury is recent, and in which the condition of the patient is good.

2. Cases of growth involving the intestine, in which no degree of intestinal obstruction has been produced, and in which the general and local conditions are favourable.

3. Cases of resection involving the jejunum high up. The high mortality attending fistulæ in the upper part of the jejunum is well known.

In all these cases the state of the patient must be such as to enable him to withstand a long and tedious operation, and the local conditions must be such as would be required for the efficient performance of a plastic operation in other parts of the body.

In instances in which obstruction of the bowel exists, a temporary fæcal fistula should be established.

The lives of such patients are threatened by reason of the obstruction, and the artificial opening gives immediate and entire relief.

If the divided ends be united by suture directly after the resection, the distension to a great extent remains, the obstruction is but imperfectly relieved, since the gut at the suture line remains paralysed.

Such patients are, as a rule, already in a position of great danger when the operation is performed. They are not in a condition which would enable them to undergo a long and elaborate operation. The state of the intestinal wall is not such as would encourage sound and rapid healing, and the over-distended condition of the tube lends itself to the production of leakage at the suture line.

In resection for gangrene, also, it is obvious that the plastic part of the operation should be postponed, unless it be evident that the section is made through perfectly healthy intestine, and that the patient is in a condition to stand a long operation.

In colectomy, the objection to the formation of a temporary artificial anus is less obvious. At the same time the patient may be better able to submit to a procedure which involves so great an expenditure of time as does the suturing of divided bowel. The colic cases demanding operation are seldom so acute as the enteric.

One fact must not be forgotten, which is, that an artificial anus involving the large intestine is—other things being equal—less easy to close by a subsequent operation than is a like fistula in the lesser bowel.

The After-treatment. — The treatment of the patient after one of these operations is conducted upon the same general lines that are observed after all serious abdominal operations.

The patient must lie absolutely still upon the back, and must turn neither to the right side nor the left.

The knees may be bent over a large pillow.

The bandage around the abdomen should not be too tight.

The diet must at first be reduced to starvation limits. The food taken for the first week should be small in bulk, and of such a kind as to leave little *débris* in the alimentary canal. Milk in large amount is not to be advised. Ice, if indiscriminately administered, often appears to induce intestinal pain.

Nutrient enemata may be of value, and thirst may be quenched by rectal injections of warm water.

Morphia will probably have to be administered. The less given the better; but it must be sufficient to arrest intestinal movement. In some patients morphia appears to excite peristaltic movement, and after an injection of the drug a rumbling of the bowels takes place, and coils that were previously collapsed become distended.

Considerable relief usually attends the occasional introduction of the rectum tube.

The first action of the bowels should be spontaneous.

The Results of Resection Operations.—Dr. McCosh (*New York Medical Journal*, March 16th, 1889) has collected 115 cases of resection of gangrenous intestine in strangulated hernia. In every instance the bowel was united at once by sutures. Fifty-seven died and fifty-seven recovered (one was doubtful).

Reichel, in 1883, collected 121 examples of resection of the bowel for various causes. Out of this number fifty-eight died, fifty-eight are described as cured, and five recovered with a fæcal fistula (*Deutsche Zeitsch. f. Chir.*, 1883, page 230).

Resection of the small intestine for conditions giving rise to obstruction gave a mortality of 75 per cent.

Mr. Makins (*St. Thomas's Hosp. Reports*, 1884, page 81) has collected thirty-nine cases of resection for artificial anus. Of these fifteen died, three were left unrelieved, and the remaining twenty-one were cured.

In Dr. Morton's tables of 234 cases of "Abdominal Section for Traumatism" (Chicago, 1890) will be found sixteen examples of resection of the bowel for gunshot wound or stab. Of these twelve died and four recovered.

Mr. Kendal Franks has collected fifty-one examples of colectomy for malignant disease (*Med.-Chir. Trans.*, 1889). The mortality was about 57 per cent., and it is noteworthy that this mortality is not influenced by the method adopted —*i.e.,* it is the same when immediate suture was carried out, as when an artificial anus was established. So far as its influence upon the progress of malignant disease is concerned, resection of the intestine cannot claim to hold a satisfactory position. In those patients who survive the actual operation a speedy recurrence is the rule.

5. RESECTION OF INTESTINE BY SENN'S METHOD.

Two methods of dealing with the bowel after the diseased tissue is excised are carried out by Dr. Senn.

1. The ends of the divided bowel are entirely and permanently closed, and the continuity of the intestinal canal is then restored by means of "intestinal anastomosis by lateral approximation," bone plates being used.

This procedure has been already alluded to (pages 310 and 327), and the matter is further illustrated in the next chapter.

The closing of the divided ends of the intestine is carried out as follows, the case selected for illustration being one of excision of the cæcum and terminal part of the ileum :—

"After the peritoneal cavity is opened, the part to be operated on is brought into the wound, and prolapse of the small intestines is prevented by packing aseptic gauze, or a clean napkin wrung out in an antiseptic solution, around it. If a sufficient number of reliable assistants are not at hand, fæcal extravasation can be effectually prevented by elastic constriction of the intestine above and below where the communicating opening is to be made. The mesentery near the bowel at each of the places is perforated with a closed hæmostatic forceps, and with this a narrow aseptic rubber band is drawn through, which is then tied with sufficient firmness to prevent the escape of fæcal matter. If the cæcum is to be excised, two additional rubber bands are applied to the part to be removed, so as to prevent extravasation from this part after the bowel is divided. The spaces between the rubber ligatures must be carefully emptied by displacing the contents by passing the intestine between two fingers before the rubber bands are tied.

"The meso-cæcum must be tied in small sections with firm

Chinese silk before the cæcum is removed, as otherwise troublesome hæmorrhage is incurred from slipping of the ligatures. After excision of the cæcum and as much of the colon and ileum as may be necessary, both ends are permanently closed by invagination and a few stitches of the continued suture. The best way of effecting invagination is to grasp the margin of the bowel where the mesentery is attached with an ordinary catch forceps, and to carry this portion into the lumen of the bowel to the extent of an inch, when the remaining portion of the circumference of the cut end will follow, and by a little manipulation about an inch is evenly invaginated, when the first stitch is made on the mesenteric side in such a manner as to transfix the invaginated mesentery and the muscular and serous coats of the bowel. After this is tied, a few more superficial stitches are taken, and the first and last stitch are tied together, so as to pucker the end of the bowel somewhat in the manner done in tying a tobacco pouch.

"In making an anastomosis between the closed end of the ileum and colon after resection of the cæcum, both ends should be made to lie side by side, with the closed ends in a downward direction, and the surfaces to be united should correspond to the part of the intestine opposite the mesenteric attachment" (Fig. 345).—(*Journ. Amer. Med. Assoc.,* June 14, 1890.)

In the article from which this extract is taken two cases of excision of the cæcum are given. The method above described was carried out in both instances. One patient recovered from the operation, the other died from peritonitis in six days.

CHAPTER VII.

Intestinal Anastomosis.

By intestinal anastomosis is understood the establishment of a permanent fistulous communication between the intestine above and the intestine below the seat of some more or less permanent obstruction.

The general procedure may be illustrated by an imaginary case of malignant stricture at the junction of the jejunum and ileum (Fig. 346). Some obstruction has been produced. It is not considered advisable to excise the diseased segment. To overcome the occlusion, a loop of the lower part of the jejunum is brought to a loop of the upper ileum, and a permanent opening is established between the two.

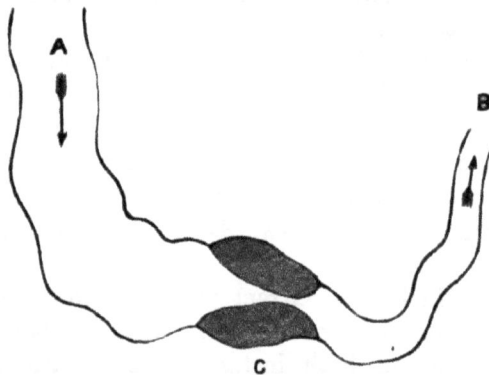

Fig. 346.—Intestinal Anastomosis.— Diagram of a Section of Intestine.

A, Upper end of bowel; B, Lower end of bowel; C, Malignant stricture.

The segment of bowel which is the seat of disease is thus excluded from the intestinal canal, and the intestinal stream is diverted into a new channel (Fig 347).

The idea of establishing such a communication between the bowel on either side of an obstruction originated with Maisonneuve, who performed the operation in two cases. Both patients died, and the proposed measure fell into contempt. The subject was revived in 1863 by Hacken, who carried out some experiments upon dogs. The operation, however, still remained in obscurity until it was revived by Dr. Senn, with whom must rest the credit of bringing intestinal anastomosis into the area of practical surgery.

Dr. Senn's chief communication was read at the Ninth International Medical Congress, held at Washington in 1887. A full account of his investigations will be found in a work on Intestinal Surgery, published in Chicago, 1889.

Dr. Senn brings about a communication between the two segments of the intestinal canal which are dealt with by means of perforated bone plates.

The suggestion of the use of such plates emanated from Dr. Connel, of Milwaukee.

Previous to the introduction of Senn's method, intestinal anastomosis was accomplished by *direct suturing*. The two loops to be united were brought together. An opening was made in each segment. This opening was in the long axis of the tube and upon its free border. Its length would be somewhat less than the natural diameter of the intestine. The margins of the two orifices were then united by a double line of sutures—one involving the mucous membrane, and the other the serous coat. The latter would be represented by very numerous points of Lembert's suture.

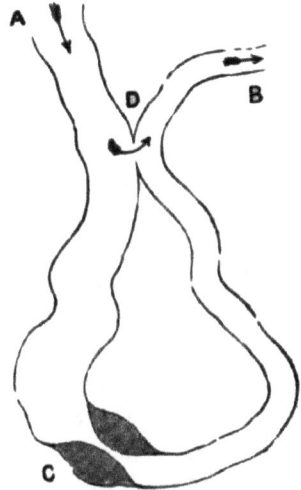

Fig. 347.—INTESTINAL ANASTOMOSIS.

A, Upper end of bowel ; B, Lower end of bowel : C, Malignant stricture ; D, Site of intestinal anastomosis.

This operation is very difficult and very tedious, and involves a considerable expenditure of time.

In practice it has yielded results which can only be described as eminently unsatisfactory.

Cases adapted for Senn's Operation.—The conditions in which intestinal anastomosis by means of perforated bone plates may be employed are very numerous. They may be classified in general terms under three categories.

w

1. When an obstruction exists which, for various reasons, cannot be removed.

2. As a better method than resection in certain cases of cancer of the intestinal canal.

3. As a better method than resection in certain examples of non-malignant disease producing obstruction, when the condition of the patient and the state of the parts would not favour the tedious and elaborate procedure involved by an excision of the affected tissues.

The advantages claimed for Senn's operation are these:—

The operation is readily performed, and is comparatively simple.

It is independent of any inequalities in the size of the tube above and below the seat of the disease.

It is efficient, and the junction at the seat of the anastomosis can be rendered so complete as to prevent much risk from the escape of the intestinal contents.

The operation is of very wide applicability.

The operation occupies but a short period of time, and a union can be effected n twenty minutes or less.

Dr. Senn maintains that the objection raised upon the grounds that an injurious accumulation of fæcal matter may take place in the excluded portion of the bowel is ill-founded.

Dr. Senn's conclusions as to the value of the operation are supported by very numerous experiments upon animals, and the few examples of the operation upon the human subject do not adversely affect his position.

The Bone Plates.—The compact layer of an ox's femur or tibia is cut with a fine saw into oval plates, a quarter of an inch in thickness, two and a half to three inches in length, and one inch in width.

The plates are decalcified in a ten per cent. solution of hydrochloric acid, which is changed every twenty-four hours until they are sufficiently soft to be bent in any direction without fracturing.

After decalcification they are washed and immersed for a short time in a weak solution of caustic potash, so as to remove the acid.

The plates are finally kept for use in a solution of equal parts of alcohol, glycerine, and water.

They then undergo no change in size when introduced into the alimentary canal. If inserted in a dry condition they swell, and tend to cause trouble by reason of their rapid increase in thickness.

After they have been inserted in the bowel, it is found by experiments that they are removed by absorption and dis-integration from the third to the tenth day.

The central open-ing in the plate is made as soon as they have been washed in the potash solution. It is oval in shape, and is readily made with a sharp penknife. The four perforations for the threads are made at the same time with a fine drill. They are placed close to the margin of the central aperture.

The relative size of the opening, and

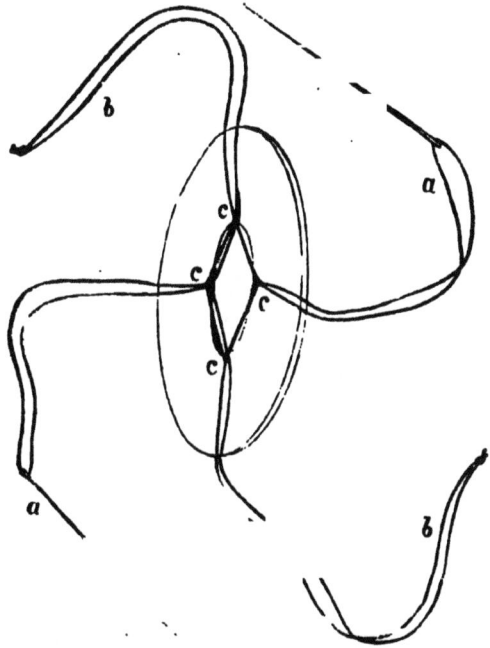

Fig. 348.—SENN'S BONE PLATE WITH THE SUTURES IN POSITION.

a a, Lateral or fixation sutures; *b b,* End or apposition sutures; *c c,* Perforations in the plate.

the position of the holes, are shown in Fig. 348. Before the plate is placed in the alcohol and glycerine solution, the threads are introduced, ready for use.

"The threads or sutures are attached by threading two fine sewing-needles, each with a piece of aseptic silk twenty-four inches in length, which are tied together; the knots become the ends of the *end* or *apposition sutures* (Fig. 348, *b b*), while the middle of such thread holds the needle, and becomes the terminal part of the *lateral* or *fixation sutures* (Fig. 348, *a a*) The fastening of the threads upon the plate is done by the lock-stitch by another thread passing through the perforations in the shape of a loop, and fastened at the back " (Fig. 348, *c c*).

Dr. Stamm (*Medical News*, Feb. 1, 1890) simplifies the method of introducing the sutures, and employs a plan which will be intelligible from an examination of Fig. 349. Two plates necessary for the operation are shown—one for the upper segment of the tube to be united, and the other for the lower. The method adopted causes the threads to correspond

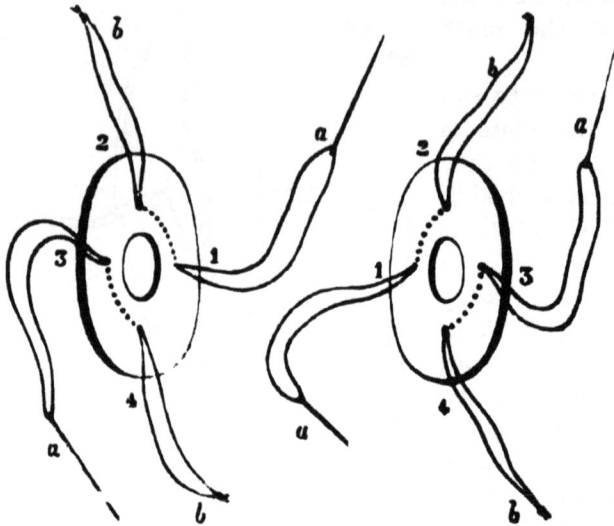

Fig. 349.—SENN'S BONE PLATES, THREADED AS ADVISED BY STAMM.
a a, Lateral or fixation sutures; *b b*, End or apposition sutures.

when the two plates are brought face to face. It will be seen that the needle introduced through hole 2 is brought out through hole 1; while that introduced through hole 4 is brought out at hole 3.

Dr. Stamm proposes to use black thread for 1 and 2, and white thread for 3 and 4.

Plates of three different sizes should be kept: the largest for gastro-enterostomy, the second for intestinal anastomosis, and the smallest for operations on children. The central opening in the plate should correspond to the lumen of the organ which is being dealt with. Thus, in gastro-enterostomy it would correspond to the lumen of the pylorus, and in ileo-colostomy to the lumen of the ileum.

When the plates are to be used, they are well washed in a two per cent. solution of carbolic acid.

1. **Incision of the Bowel.**—A loop of the bowel below the obstruction, and another loop above the obstruction, are brought into the wound. These coils should be as near to the seat of the disease as is convenient—that is to say, they should not be so far distant from one another as to exclude a large tract of intestine after the operation is complete, nor so near as to expose the actual area of disease or to render the manipulation of the parts difficult. It is probable that the upper coil will be distended and hypertrophied, and the lower empty and wasted.

The loops which are to be brought together by anastomosis must be emptied of their contents by drawing the fingers along them, and must be kept empty—either by digital compression, or by being constricted with indiarubber bands (page 334). Two of such bands are required for each loop. They are passed through the mesentery close to the bowel, are about four inches apart, are held in place by assistants, and are finally tied.

Before the bands on the proximal part of the intestine are secured, the incision into the gut may be made, and the contents be allowed to escape. After complete evacuation the rubber bands are tied and the parts well washed.

The incision is made in the long axis of the bowel, upon its convex or free side, and therefore along a line opposite to the attachment of the mesentery.

The cut must be large enough to readily admit a bone plate without using any force, and yet not too large, lest the plate escape through the incision after the sutures have been tied. Hæmorrhage from the wound is usually slight, and ceases spontaneously.

The best way to make the incision is to compress the bowel between the thumb and index finger of the left hand in the direction of the long axis, and then, with a sharp-pointed bistoury, to perforate the wall of the gut and cut from within outwards between the fingers in an upward direction.

2. **Insertion and Fixation of the Plates.**—The cavity of

the exposed bowel, isolated between the rubber bands, is cleared of mucus and any traces of fæcal matter by pledgets of cotton-wool.

The threaded plate is inserted while the bowel is held in the same position as when the incision is made. The plate is inserted edgewise, and when it is completely in the lumen of the bowel, traction is made on the sutures in such a manner that the disc makes half a turn, so that its upper surface faces the wound. It is now accurately adjusted, so that its ends are equidistant from the angles of the visceral wound.

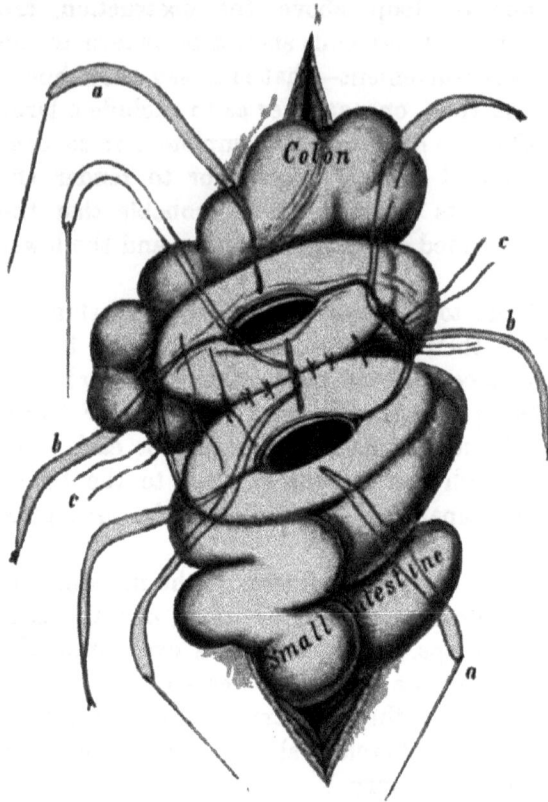

Fig. 350.—INTESTINAL ANASTOMOSIS WITH BONE PLATES.
a a, Lateral or fixation sutures; *b b*, End or apposition sutures; *c c*, Posterior sutures. (*Senn.*)

The plate is then fixed in this position by transfixing the entire thickness of the wall of the bowel, near the margin. of the wound, with each of the needles attached to the lateral or fixation sutures (Fig. 350, *a a*). One needle will, of course, pass through one margin of the wound, and the opposite needle through the other.

The apposition or end sutures hang out of the upper and lower angles of the wound (Fig. 350, *b b*).

The two coils of bowel which are to be united are each treated in precisely the same way.

The lateral sutures are intended to draw the margins of the wound asunder after tying, and prevent the slipping of the plates. They are hence called "fixation sutures." The end sutures serve to retract the angles of the wound, and to assist in holding the coapted parts in apposition after they are tied. Hence the name "apposition sutures." When all the sutures have been tied, and the operation is, in fact, completed, it will be found that the opening between the two intestinal tubes presents a diamond-shaped appearance (Fig. 350).

3. **Approximation of the Intestines.**—The serous coat of the bowel covering the plate is lightly scarified with the point of a needle. Both of the parts to be approximated are treated in the same manner, and the extent of the scarification will correspond to the area of the plate.

The scarification may be made in the form of crossed lines, and should not be so deep as to cause bleeding.

The intestines which it is intended to unite are brought together by an assistant in such a manner that the two wounds are exactly opposite each other.

"The approximation sutures are now properly arranged, so that when they are to be tied, the corresponding threads can be readily found. Before any of the sutures are tied, it is well to unite the serous surfaces along the posterior margins of the plates with a few superficial sutures (Fig. 350, c).

"After this has been done, the posterior pair of fixation sutures is tied with sufficient firmness to approximate, but not to compress, the parts between them. The sutures are to be tied always in a square knot, so as to prevent slipping of the knot. Next the pair of end or approximation sutures away from the operator is tied, and when this has been done the opposite pair is tied (Fig. 350). All the sutures are cut short as soon as they are tied. The last sutures to be tied are the remaining pair of fixation sutures; and while these are being tightened, the margins of the bowel are inverted between the plates with a director or probe. The cut ends of the last knot are pushed with a probe towards the opening.

"Approximation has now been completed, and all that is left is to reinforce the action of the plates by suturing the serous surfaces over the anterior margins of the plates by a few stitches of the continued suture " (Fig. 351).

The parts are well and carefully washed and cleansed, and the rubber bands or clamps are removed, and care is taken that the peritoneal cavity is free from blood clot or extravasated matter.

The loop is replaced in the abdomen.

In the case of ileo - colostomy, the colon may be fixed in place by a point of suture that involves the mesentery and the posterior parietal peritoneum.

4. **Treatment of the Parietal Wound.** —The use of a glass drainage-tube is advised in instances in which a considerable resection of intestine has preceded the establishment of the anastomosis. Under ordinary conditions the tube may be dispensed with on the third day.

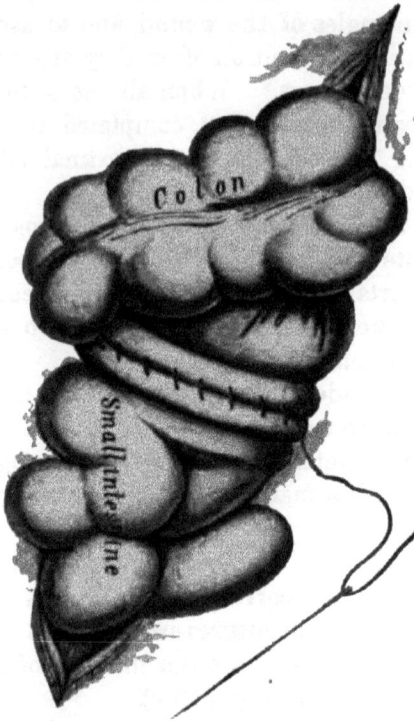

Fig. 351.—INTESTINAL ANASTOMOSIS BY BONE PLATES. (*Senn.*)

The wound in the abdomen is closed by sutures. Dr. Senn advises that the peritoneum be separately united with fine silk sutures, which are cut short and buried.

The main sutures are introduced in the usual way.

The mode of dressing the wound will depend upon the practice of the individual surgeon.

Dr. Sachs's Modification.—Dr. W. Sachs, Berne, describes (*Centralblatt für Chirurgie*, Oct. 4th) (*Brit. Med. Journ.*, Supp., Nov. 22nd, 1890) a modification of Senn's method of forming lateral anastomosis between two separated portions of intestine. Senn's procedure of applying two bone plates is held to be not free from danger. The sutures with which the plates are armed, after they have been passed through the intestinal walls and tied together, are enclosed within punctured walls, through which capillary communication may be established between the interior of the intestine and the peritoneal cavity. A small abscess may be set up around one of the threads cut very short and enclosed on every side by the opposed serous surfaces of the two portions of the gut. Another danger, pointed out by Helferich, is gangrene of the intestinal wall, due to pressure of the bone plates. Sachs proposes the use of an appliance resembling in form a sleeve stud perforated in the middle. This is made up of two bone plates fixed together, yet separated to a small extent from each other as far as the uniting portion immediately around the central perforation. A longitudinal incision having been made in each of the opposed portions of intestine, each disc is inserted into the intestinal canal on either side, and the intestinal anastomosis is thus readily and speedily established. Sutures are then applied through the serous membrane on each side wherever there is a tendency to protrusion of the mucosa. The following advantages are claimed for this method, which, however, has as yet been tested only in experiments on rabbits :— (1) The interior of the intestine is not exposed for so long a time as it is in Senn's operation. (2) The margins of the intestinal wound rest in the deep annular groove between the joined discs, and are thus protected against infection and the results of pressure. (3) There is no risk of the cut edges adhering together. (4) It is unnecessary to pass any suture through the whole thickness of the intestinal wall.

VARIETIES OF THE OPERATION.

1. **Gastro-enterostomy.**—(*See* Chapter XIII. upon the Operations on the Stomach.)

2. **Jejuno-ileostomy.**—The union is effected between the jejunum and ileum.

Dr. Senn found, in his experiments upon animals, that while the establishment of an opening between two coils of small intestine by means of incisions united by a double row of sutures occupied usually over an hour, the method by bone plates seldom took more than fifteen minutes.

3. **Ileo-colostomy.**—Union of the ileum with the colon. This is especially called for in obstructive conditions involving the ileo-cæcal region.

In cases where the obstruction is not amenable to removal, and where it is desired that no artificial anus should be formed, Dr. Senn advises one of two distinct methods:—

(a) The ileum is divided, the distal end is closed, and the proximal end is implanted into the colon after the manner already described (pages 310 and 327). This would be termed lateral implantation by the invagination method.

(b) The ileum is divided, both of the divided ends are closed, and the proximal end is brought into lateral apposition with the colon. An intestinal anastomosis is brought about by means of bone plates in the manner described above.

In instances in which the diseased segment of the bowel is resected, the continuity of the canal is established according to the plan detailed in Chapter VI., page 334.

4. **Ileo-rectostomy.**—Dr. Senn considers that in cases of intestinal obstruction situated low down in the colon, and due to conditions which cannot be relieved by simple operation, an intestinal anastomosis may be established between the ileum and the rectum, to avert the necessity of making an artificial anus.

The *modus operandi* is identical with that observed in ileo-colostomy.

This operation has been carried out in animals, but the conditions that would justify it in the human subject would have to be very extraordinary.

5. **Colo-rectostomy.**—" Among the many possibilities," writes Dr. Senn, " in the operative treatment of intestinal obstruction, a condition might be met with where the seat of obstruction is located low down in the colon, perhaps in the sigmoid flexure, and where it might be impossible or impracticable to remove the cause of obstruction, and where it becomes necessary to restore the continuity of the intestinal canal by establishing a communication between the permeable portion of the colon and the rectum."

The value of this operation must remain, like the last, a

ɔf theory. The case adapted for it must be most nal, and Dr. Senn takes no account of the anatomical es that would have to be surmounted in the human

Russell gives, in the *New York Medical Journal,* th, 1890, a case of complete recovery after jejuno- y by Senn's method, irf intestinal obstruction due to ception and sloughing of the intussusceptum in a boy een.

CHAPTER VIII.

ENTEROTOMY.

THE term enterotomy is applied to an operation carried out in cases of intestinal obstruction, a consists in opening the distended bowel above the occlusion and allowing its contents to escape. Th of course an abdominal section.

The procedure is sometimes known as "Nélato tion." It is assumed that the loop of bowel which will belong to the small intestine, and in the n instances this proves to be the case. It has al considered a feature of the operation that, after th has been opened, the most convenient distended presents should be incised and a fæcal fistula established. It will be obvious that the term er would more precisely represent this operation than enterotomy, which would imply the mere cuttin bowel, as in the removal of an impacted gall-stone.

The usage of many years has, however, estab position of the latter term, and the title enter employed by few.

Enterotomy for intestinal obstruction was first by Nélaton in 1840. He laid open the abdomen in inguinal region, and drew forth the first distend intestine which presented.

This mode of treatment was, however, first su Mannoury in 1819, but it was not carried into pract

The Operation.—The abdomen is opened in iliac region—if Nélaton's method be strictly follow incision parallel to and a little above the out Poupart's ligament.

The incision is placed to the outer side of th artery, and its length must depend upon the thick parietes. One inch and a half to three inches will represent the extremes. French surgeons advise a cut of 7 c.m. (2¾ inches).

As soon as the abdomen is opened, the first distended coil of intestine that presents is seized and drawn into the wound. It will probably belong to the lower ileum.

The convex part of the distended knuckle is drawn well into the parietal wound, but the convex or free border should alone project.

The gut should not be twisted from its natural position— that is to say, the spontaneous direction it has assumed should be preserved.

The wound in the abdominal parietes is now partly closed by means of silk-worm - gut sutures which are introduced at the two extremities of the wound (Fig. 352, B B).

The bowel will occupy the centre of the wound, and a sufficient number of sutures (two probably on either side) must be introduced to fix the gut in place by the mere narrowing of the parietal incision.

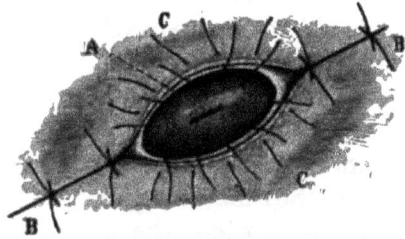

Fig. 352.—ENTEROTOMY.

A, Site of opening in bowel ; B, Sutures of parietal wound ; C, Sutures between the skin and the intestinal wall.

The sutures must include all the tissues forming the parietes, together with the peritoneum.

The latter membrane should be brought as near to the cut margin of the skin as is possible.

It will be found that a curved Hagedorn's needle of large size is the most convenient for introducing the sutures.

The wall of the bowel is now rapidly stitched to the margin of the skin, which tightly surrounds it on all sides. Very fine silk, passed by means of a small curved needle held in a holder, is best adapted for this purpose. The stitches should involve the skin and the serous and muscular coats of the bowel (Fig. 352, C C). Care should be taken not to open

the actual lumen of the g
great distension this is not
may be engaged simultane
cedure.

The gut is now opened I
be effected with a scalpel, a:

Before the incision is m
wound should be buried in
bowel should be allowed to
covered with vaseline.

The small sutures that
skin are for the purpose of
They would not suffice pre
in position.

To effect this latter obje
gut should be introduced
thickness of the intestinal
integuments.

These sutures should I
i.e., from the skin towards t
direction, they may carry fa

The opening into the b
should be upon the free or (

The smaller the knucl
wound, and the smaller tl
subsequent operation for the

The operation as above
remarkably short space of
amount of disturbance of in

After the gut has been i
ing of the abdomen, and no
of the bowel. The distended
in its own way, and the less
better.

A light dressing of abso
changed at first every few n

The skin around the op
and then covered with vasel

Modifications of the Op
conveniently made in the 1

The fingers are introduced, and an examination of the abdomen made. It is possible that a band or some equally simple cause of obstruction may be discovered and remedied, and the fæcal fistula be rendered unnecessary.

Such examination may enable the surgeon to select for his artificial opening a loop of intestine as near as is desirable to the seat of obstruction. The first loop which presents in the wound may be some distance from the place of occlusion.

Such a modification, although often advisable, is opposed to the chief principle of enterotomy, which is that relief be given to distended bowel in the simplest manner, with the least possible expenditure of time, and the least possible disturbance of parts. The opening has on many occasions been made in the left groin instead of in the right. In such a case it is probably the sigmoid flexure which is opened.

If time permit, it is well, before drawing a knuckle of gut into the parietal wound, to unite the peritoneum all round to the margin of the divided skin. When the bowel comes to be fixed in place, peritoneum is brought in contact with peritoneum, and a more speedy and certain sealing of the abdominal cavity is ensured.

Various methods of securing a loop of bowel in the parietal wound will be found described in the section on Iliac Colotomy, to which the reader is referred (page 371).

If the symptoms be not urgent, the operation may be performed *à deux temps*. The abdomen is opened and the bowel is fixed in place, but its lumen is in no way invaded. The part is dressed with iodoform. After an interval varying from a few hours to three days, the operation is completed by incising the gut and allowing its contents to escape.

In abdominal section for intestinal obstruction, in which the cavity has been widely opened up and determined attempts made to remove the cause of the obstruction, an enterotomy is often carried out as a last measure, all other attempts at relief having failed.

Dr. Curtis, of New York, in an excellent article on " Enterostomy for Acute Intestinal Obstruction " (*Medical Record*, Sept. 1st, 1888), gives the following particulars of the recorded cases he has collected :—

In all instances the symptoms were acute. The incision

was made in the right groin in twenty-eight cases, in the left
groin in twenty-one instances, and in the loin in seven cases
—total, fifty-six. In thirty-five cases in which full particulars
are given it was found that the small intestine had been
opened in thirteen cases, the cæcum in nine, the sigmoid
flexure in six, and the colon in seven.

The After-treatment.—This calls for no especial comment. The matter is considered in the chapters which deal
with " Resection of the Intestine " (page 332) and " Colotomy "
(page 368).

Value and Results of the Operation.

Enterotomy is of undoubted value in urgent cases of
intestinal obstruction when the patient is in immediate
danger of death from the actual obstruction. The operation
relieves the bowel rapidly and completely, and many lives
have thus been saved. It does not profess to touch the cause
of the disease, although there are not a few examples of acute
intestinal obstruction which are permanently relieved by
evacuating a distended bowel.

In many instances, enterotomy has been followed, in a
manner more or less mysterious, by complete cure. The
operation may, in many of its features, be compared to
the tapping of the bladder above the pubes in cases of extreme
distension of that viscus in which treatment has failed and
time presses.

It has been carried out in almost every form of intestinal obstruction, and is especially indicated in obscure and
extremely urgent cases, where not a moment has to be lost,
and where the patient can stand but a very brief operative
measure.

In the majority of cases it is true that the operation is
only palliative. In a few instances it has led to cure. It
has been urged against it—(1) That the fistula may be so
high up in the bowel as to lead to fatal marasmus. (2) That
a considerable length of the intestinal canal may be excluded.
(3) That the distended bowel between the opening and the
obstruction is left untouched. (4) That the original disease
is not dealt with.

A discussion of these objections would be out of place
in the present work.

Dr. Curtis's analysis of sixty-two cases of enterotomy for *xute* intestinal obstruction gives the following results :—

alieved by the operation	...		46 cases	=	72 per cent.	
xt relieved	...	...	...	6	„	
covered ...	...	...	...	32	„	= 61·7 per cent.
ssage of fæces per anum resumed in	19		„	= 60 per cent. of the recoveries,
ed	...	...	...	...	30	„ = 48·3 per cent.

In the fatal cases it is to be noted that the fistula has metimes failed to relieve the obstruction (in three instances ; was below the seat of it), and that gangrene of the gut mbsequent to the operation is a frequent cause of death.

CHAPTER IX.

COLOTOMY.

BY colotomy is understood the operation of establishing an artificial anus in the colon. This may be either temporary or permanent. But for the fact that the term colotomy has become firmly engrafted in the language of medicine, the more precise term colostomy might be advised.

Colotomy is carried out for the relief of obstruction in the colon of various kinds, and is most frequently employed cases of cancer of the rectum. It is performed also as a palliative measure in some examples of cancer of that part which no obstruction exists.

Under such conditions it is used to divert the course the fæces, and with a like object colotomy is performed in the treatment of recto-vesical fistula, and in intractable ulcers of the rectum and lower colon. It is performed also imperforate anus in infants after the local operations has failed.

Lumbar colotomy implies the opening of the ascending descending colon through the loin without wounding the peritoneum. This is known also as the extra-peritoneal operation, as posterior colotomy, or the operation of Amussat Callisen.

Iliac colotomy implies the opening of the sigmoid flexure or the cæcum, through an incision in the iliac region which involves the peritoneal cavity. This is known as the intra-peritoneal operation, as anterior colotomy, as Littre's operation, as laparo-colotomy, and as inguinal colotomy. The ridiculous terms, cæcostomy and sigmoidostomy, have acquired no position in surgical literature.

History of the Operation.

Colotomy was first proposed by Littre in 1710 (*M de l'Acad. des Sc.*, Paris, vol. x., page 36). He advised opening of the sigmoid flexure in the iliac region in certain cases of imperforate anus.

The method is said to have been first successfully practised by Dinet in 1793 (Sabatier's *Méd. Opér.*, vol. ii., page 336). In 1776 Pillore, of Rouen, opened the cæcum in the right iliac region through an incision which involved the peritoneum. The case was one of cancer of the rectum. (*See Brit. and For. Med. Review*, vol. xviii., page 452.)

The first iliac colotomies performed in England appear to have been carried out in 1821 by Freer and Pring (*Lond. Med. and Phys. Journ.*, 1821, page 9). The patients were adults, and the trouble was stricture of the rectum. Freer's patient died on the tenth day ; Pring's patient recovered.

Lumbar colotomy was first advocated by Callisen, of Copenhagen, in 1817 (*Systema Chir. Hodiernæ*, t. xi., page 842, Hafniæ, 1817). He proposed to open the descending colon through a vertical incision in the loin.

Jean Zalema Amussat carried out lumbar colotomy with success in 1839 (*Mémoires*—three in number—published in Paris, 1839-43). He employed a transverse incision, and extended the operation to the ascending colon. Out of six patients upon whom he operated, five recovered.

Among the earliest operators in England by the lumbar method were Curling, Hilton, and Bryant. Mr. Bryant's first lumbar colotomy was performed in 1859, and he believes that this was only the second operation of the kind performed in England—a colotomy by Hilton having been the first (Bryant, " Bradshaw Lecture," 1890, page 3).

In the last ten or fifteen years the operation has been very extensively performed.

Interest in the iliac operation was revived in England by Mr. Reeves, and the value of the method has been demonstrated, and the details of the operation improved, by Mr. Harrison Cripps, Mr. Allingham, Mr. Chavasse, and others.

The mortality attending colotomy has been in recent years very considerably improved, and the operation, once regarded as a desperate and uncertain procedure and a last resort, has come to be employed as a sure means of giving relief, and as a measure which may be carried out comparatively early in the progress of the diseases concerned.

x 2

Anatomical Points.—The chief details in the anatomy of the colon which are of importance in connection with the operation of colotomy have been already alluded to.

In lumbar colotomy, especial attention should be paid to the condition of the meso-colon upon the right and the left sides of the body (page 299).

The position of the ascending or descending colon in the loin may be approximately represented by a vertical line

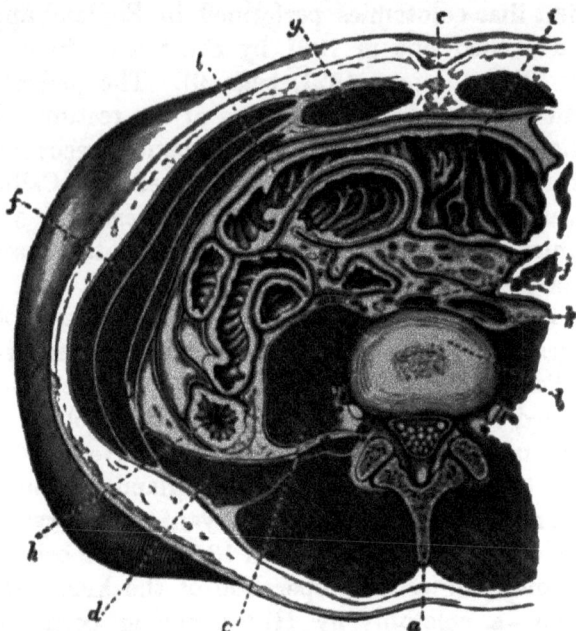

Fig. 356.—HORIZONTAL SECTION THROUGH THE BODY AT THE LEVEL OF THE UMBILICUS. (*After Braune.*)

a, Spine of the fourth lumbar vertebra; *b*, Disc between the third and fourth vertebræ; *c*, Umbilicus; *d*, Quadratus lumborum; *e*, Psoas; *f*, External oblique with internal oblique and transversalis muscles beyond; *g*, Rectus; *h*, Descending colon; *i*, Transverse colon; *j*, Aorta; *k*, Inferior vena cava; *l*, Ureter.

drawn upwards to the last rib from a point about half an inch posterior to the centre of the crest of the ilium. The centre of the crest will be indicated by a point midway between the anterior superior and posterior superior iliac spines.

LUMBAR COLOTOMY.

Instruments Required.—Scalpels; straight and curved scissors; dissecting, pressure, and artery forceps; tongue to hold the gut; broad rectangular retractors; curved needles in handles (right and left); Hagedorn's needles, of various sizes, and needle-holders; catgut; silkworm gut; blunt hooks; kidney-shaped receiver; sponges in holders; aniline pencil.

Position.—The patient should lie upon the sound side and close to the edge of the table. A small hard pillow or sand-bag is placed under the opposite loin, so that the region to be operated upon may be brought well into view, and the space between the crest of the ilium and the last rib be extended to the utmost (Fig. 354). In very corpulent subjects, and in cases in which there is considerable distension of the abdomen, this pillow may be dispensed with. The surgeon stands upon the side to be operated upon; the chief assistant is facing him, and upon the opposite side of the table. He attends to the sponging, and assists in holding the gut when it has been secured. An assistant may stand upon either side of the operator, and may attend to the retraction of the wound.

The patient's limbs and chest should be enveloped in small, neatly-folded blankets, completely covered with macintosh sheets. Three or four sponges may be wedged in between the hard pillow and the loin it supports. These sponges take up the blood which would otherwise find its way under the patient's body.

Before the operation, the bowel below the seat of disease should be cleared out by an enema.

When there is no distension of the abdomen, it is the practice of some surgeons to attempt to distend the colon with air introduced per rectum. The instrument best suited for this purpose is Lund's insufflator. I have never found any necessity to adopt this artificial distension, and in any case the use of the instrument may be dispensed with until the bowel is actually being sought for during the operation. The loin must be well scrubbed with an antiseptic solution. After the skin has been dried, the line of the bowel already alluded to may be marked out with an aniline pencil.

Incision.—Of the many incisions advised, the oblique incision of Bryant is the best. It affords more room, it follows the line of the vessels and nerves, and by lying in the line of a natural fold in the skin, it facilitates repair and tends to prevent prolapse of the bowel.

Operation.—*First Stage.*—The incision should be from three to three and a half inches in length. It is placed obliquely, midway between the last rib and the iliac crest. Its centre should correspond to the centre of the pencil line marking the site of the bowel (Fig. 354). It will be about parallel to the last rib, or will follow a line drawn from the anterior superior spine to the angle between the twelfth rib and the mass of the erector spinæ muscle.

The length of the incision will be mainly influenced by the thickness of the tissues, and this for the most part will

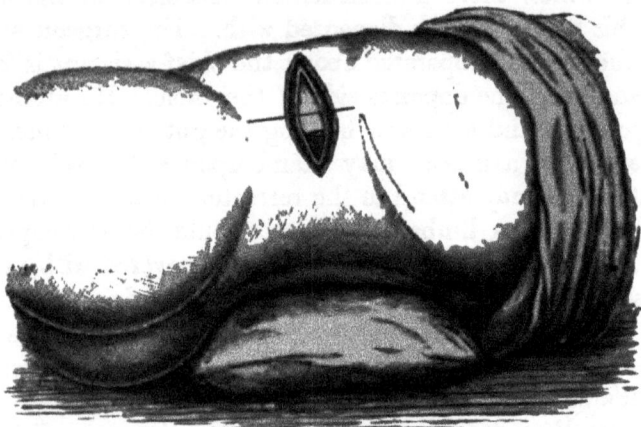

Fig. 354.—THE INCISION IN LUMBAR COLOTOMY. (The quadratus lumborum muscle is exposed.)

depend upon the degree of corpulency. The tendency is rather to make the incision too long.

After the skin and superficial structures have been divided, the external oblique and latissimus dorsi muscles will be exposed. The fibres of these muscles are in this situation vertical. They should be divided by a single clean cut through the whole length of the incision.

The layer of the internal oblique will next come into view. The fibres are found running somewhat obliquely upwards and forwards. This muscle is also cleanly divided through the whole length of the original wound. In the posterior part of the wound the fascia lumborum will probably come into view.

There are now exposed a few of the hindermost fibres of

the transversalis muscle, which are nearly transverse in direction, and the fascia lumborum. If the incision have been made as described, the actual amount of muscle tissue exposed in the depths of the wound will be slight.

The muscle and the fascia are now divided to the full length of the wound. Before this division is made it will probably be noted that the twelfth dorsal nerve, accompanied by the abdominal branch of a lumbar artery, are crossing the area of the operation. It is as well to avoid cutting the little artery.

In the posterior part of the incision the clear anterior border of the quadratus lumborum will be seen (Fig. 354). The fibres of that muscle seldom, if ever, need to be divided. Broad rectangular retractors will be found very useful at this stage of the operation.

A little fat may now come into view, and be mistaken for the subperitoneal tissue. It is the fat beneath the tranversalis fascia.

This fascia must be sought for and demonstrated, and cleanly divided to the full length of the wound. It is well to commence the division close to the anterior border of the quadratus lumborum.

The subperitoneal fat is now reached, and the first stage of the operation is completed.

The structures above named must be cut cleanly and deliberately. The experience gained by many dissections in the dissecting-room will enable the operator to perform this stage of the operation very quickly. A good anatomist can, from a general view of the body, judge of the thickness of the tissues through which he will have to pass.

The student will find that the muscular layers are comparatively thin, and totally unlike the thick plates of muscle which are depicted in anatomical text-books.

No director is needed, and in no operation is that dangerous weapon more out of place.

The parts should not be divided with scissors. All that is needed are a scalpel and a pair of dissecting forceps.

The operator will seldom be delayed by the need of applying pressure forceps to a bleeding point.

The chief error in this stage of the operation is due to the

ignoring of the transversalis fasc
pletely divide that structure.

Second·Stage.—The gut is no
distension of the abdomen exist;
bulges at once into the wound as
have been freed by the finger.

Failing such an appearance,
into the subperitoneal tissue ar
The finger follows the anterior
lumborum, and seeks for the angl
muscle and the psoas (Fig. 353).

It is towards this angle that the
colon faces in cases where no mesc
this part the lower end of the kidr
remembered that the bowel lies o
It is essential that the subpe
up with the examining finger or f
separated by means of two pairs
exposure of the non-distended bo
be done.

In corpulent subjects an imm
have to be ploughed through befo

The bowel may perhaps be rec
wound by the thickness of its co
scybalous mass. In such case it
drawn into the more superfici
examination.

The surgeon must be conv
behind the peritoneum—which h
the posterior parietes—and that
been fully opened up.

Assuming that the colon has
curved forefinger should be place
psoas and quadratus lumborum
should then be rolled over alm
upon. The bowel that falls int
other than the colon. (*See* Fig. 3.

Failing the rolling over of t
faces the surgeon may press up
parietes so as to force the intestin

The surest guide to the non-distended colon is the feeling which is communicated when its coats are picked up between the forefinger and the thumb.

The extent of the non-peritoneal surface of the colon will depend in part upon anatomical conditions, and in part upon the degree of distension of the gut. When the gut is not distended, this surface cannot be expected to exceed, and often not to equal, one inch.

The gut, when brought into view, may be identified by the thickness of its coats, by its non-peritoneal surface, and possibly by the existence of a longitudinal band.

The band which comes into view is that known as the posterior. The bands of the large intestine are well seen in the ascending colon, but are less clearly marked in the descending segment of gut, the longitudinal layer of muscle becoming more evenly spread over the colon as the rectum is approached. The colon can be recognised by many means, without wasting time over a search for the posterior longitudinal band.

The sacculi of the colon cannot be demonstrated, as a rule, through a lumbar colotomy wound. They are valueless as a means of identification.

The appendices epiploicæ can only be seen when the peritoneum has been opened, and when the colon has been drawn through the rent.

It is when great difficulty attends the identification of the bowel that Lund's insufflator may be used.

In the search for the bowel, great service is rendered by good broad rectangular retractors and a good light.

It is to be remembered that the colon may, on the right side, be absent from the loin, owing to a congenital deformity.

When a distinct meso-colon exists, and the colon is empty, the peritoneal cavity must almost of necessity be opened up and a loop of the intestine drawn through.

If, however, the meso-colon can be identified—and on the left side a branch of the inferior mesenteric artery may indicate it—the separation of its two layers is not as a rule difficult.

If the peritoneum have been opened, it is of little use to

waste time in attempting to sew up the rent as advised by some. In the deep wounds which are inevitable in corpulent subjects the closure of the gap in the membrane may be almost impossible. The rent made will most probably be large and irregular, and may be internal to the bowel.

I have never seen harm arise from neglecting to close an 'accidental or deliberate rent in the peritoneum in this situation, and it is remarkable how little such an opening of the serous cavity affects the results of the operation.

Should distended coils of small intestine protrude through the laceration in the serous membrane, and make their way into the superficial wound, the closure of the rent becomes still less possible. It is advised in one text-book that the distended loops should be reduced and the rent in the peritoneum closed by sutures. How this marvellous manœuvre is to be effected the writer does not state, nor is it explained how the inflated coils are induced to remain quietly in position while the surgeon is sewing up the peritoneum, nor how they escape injury from the surgeon's needle.

Such protruding coils reduce themselves when the distension of the abdomen is relieved.

Third Stage.—The bowel is fixed in position and opened. If the colon do not come readily into the wound, or if there be difficulty in retaining it, its walls should be seized in a vertical direction by self-holding tongue forceps. No more of the coat of the bowel should be picked up in the forceps than is required to give a hold for the instrument. It is in the part so held that the future opening may be made.

It is needless to observe that the opening must be made in the non-peritoneal segment of the bowel, and therefore upon its posterior surface.

Gentle pressure exercised upon the front of the abdomen will help to keep the gut in position. The more completely the subperitoneal tissue has been opened up, the more easily can the bowel be brought into view. The bowel should be merely drawn to the level of the skin. It should not be dragged out as a loop or even as a knuckle.

By means of a large curved Hagedorn's needle the two extremities of the parietal wound are now closed by sutures. Silkworm gut should be employed, and the needles should be passed very deeply, so as to include all the divided structures down to the fascia lumborum.

Probably two of such deep sutures on either side of the centre of the wound will be sufficient.

They should all be passed before any are tied. When they are tied, the skin should very closely embrace the small dome of protruding bowel which, still held by the tongue forceps, presents in the centre of the incision. The appearance presented will be nearly identical with that shown in Fig. 352, which illustrates the same stage in enterotomy.

As the edges of the wound, at its lateral extremities, are being brought together, the bowel should be drawn a little upon by means of the forceps, with the result that the skin and the bowel wall are brought into close contact.

By means of a small curved Hagedorn's needle, the skin is in the next place united all round to the intestine by many points of suture. The needle should only concern the skin on the one hand, and the muscular coat of the bowel on the other. The lumen of the gut should on no account be penetrated. Fine silk may be used for this purpose.

If this be well done, it is quite impossible for any fæcal matter to find its way into the depths of the wound; and should there be a rent in the peritoneum, it will at least be efficiently shut off from communication with the air.

The part is well dusted with iodoform, and, indeed, almost buried under that powder.

The hard pillow is removed, and the patient's body is a little inclined over to the affected side. A piece of lint well smeared with vaseline is at hand to form a surface over which the escaping fæcal matter may run.

Finally, the tongue forceps are removed from the gut, and an opening is made into the bowel by means of a small scalpel. The opening is quite large enough if it will admit the point of the little finger. The amount of flatus and fæces that escapes varies remarkably. If aperients have been administered, and the sickness has not been great, pints upon pints of fluid fæcal matter may gush from the opening. If, on the other hand, opium has been for some time employed, nothing but a little flatus may escape, and many hours, or even several days, may elapse before any solid matter escapes.

By means of a curved Hagedorn's needle of medium size, or a curved needle in a handle, the final sutures are introduced. They concern the whole thickness of the coats of the bowel on the one hand, and the skin on the other. Silkworm gut should be the material employed.

The needle is introduced through the skin, and its point is made to appear in the interior of the bowel. A fresh needle and a fresh thread are employed for each suture. If the suture be passed in the opposite direction—*i.e.*, from the mucous membrane to the skin—a fæcal seton is practically drawn through the tissues.

Silk should not be employed, as it favours the passage of intestinal fluid along its fibres by capillary attraction. Of all ligature materials, it is the one least well suited for the present purpose.

The method of passing a large curved needle armed with silk through the skin on one side, across the lumen of the gut and through the skin on the opposite side, is to be condemned. The silk becomes soaked with fæcal matter in its passage, and through the integuments upon one side of the wound at least this foul thread is drawn.

In securing the bowel, it is well to avoid too many stitches, too large needles, and too thick suture material. It is well also that the opening into the colon should be at first at least quite small. There is no object in opening the gut with the cautery.

On no account should any drainage-tube be employed. The wound should heal by first intention.

Comment.—The only difficult part of the operation consists in the search for the colon, when that part of the bowel does not readily present. In the great majority of the cases the colon at once makes itself evident.

It is remarkable that on the right side the duodenum has been opened in mistake for the colon, and on the left side the stomach. A hypertrophied and distended coil of small intestine has, with some better reason, been opened in the place of the large gut.

If the colon have been well freed from its connections in the depths of the wound, there is no need of any especial instrument for drawing the gut forward towards the skin.

The surgeon should aim at making the smallest possible opening in the colon. It can, if need be, be enlarged later.

The transversalis fascia may readily be mistaken for the peritoneum, especially where the bowel appears to glide beneath it. The recognition of this fascia is a matter of primary importance.

The bulging peritoneum may be mistaken for the bowel. This error will not happen to one who is familiar with the feel of the colon when picked up between the finger and thumb.

It must be remembered that the bowel may be empty when exposed, and this even when a cancerous stricture of the rectum is known to exist. This condition of empty colon is more usually met with on the left side, and in my experience I do not happen to have met with it except on that side.

A very fat loin introduces a difficulty in the operation. It must be met by a free incision, by a thorough division of each layer of tissue along the whole length of the original wound, and by the use of good retractors and a good light.

If, after every possible search has been made, and every expedient exhausted, no colon can be found, the best course is to open the abdomen in the middle line by a small incision, and to introduce two fingers to seek for the bowel. The segment needed may possibly be found, and be ultimately opened through the original lumbar wound. The median incision is then of course at once closed.

If, however, it be discovered that the part of the colon it is desired to reach from the loin is below the seat of the obstruction, or if a malignant growth is found to occupy the seat of the intended artificial opening, or if there be deformity of the colon, or any condition which may render the completion of the lumbar operation impossible or undesirable, then the surgeon should draw the cæcum to the median wound, and form an artificial opening in it there. Failing this, he should, through the median incision, open the lowest available coil of the ileum.

In these cases there is little to recommend the practice of opening the first coil of small intestine which presents through the loin after the colotomy has been abandoned.

Modifications of the Operation.

urgent, the operation may be carried out in two stages. The bowel is sought for, and is fixed to the skin by numerous superficial sutures precisely in the manner described. Care should be taken that no suture extends through the mucous lining of the bowel. The part is well dusted with iodoform, and after an interval of some hours, or some days, the operation is completed by opening the colon.

By this means the risk of suppuration in the wound, and in the connective tissue planes around it, is reduced to a minimum. Primary healing is more certainly secured: and if the peritoneum should have been opened in the operation, the prospect of any trouble following is greatly reduced.

In cases where the patient is stout and the loin deep, or where there has been difficulty in drawing the bowel to the surface, or where much restlessness is anticipated, the securing of the gut by numerous superficial sutures in the manner just described may not suffice. These fine stitches may be unduly dragged upon, and some of them may cut their way out. In such case the gut will be found to have retreated to the depths of the wound.

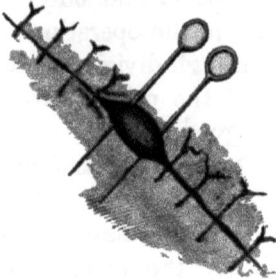

Fig. 355.—COLOTOMY IN TWO STAGES. The bowel secured by pins at the end of the first stage.

In these circumstances the bowel may be secured by means of hare-lip pins. Two pins are employed, and are passed through the bowel at the distance of about three-fourths of an inch from each other. They are at right angles to the line of the wound. There is no need to pass the pins through the edges of the wound; it will suffice if they simply lie across these (Fig. 355). A little gauze or a small length of drainage-tube is interposed between the ends of the pins and the skin. The pins must be exceedingly fine, and the punctures produced in the bowel should be at once buried by iodoform. Mr. Jacobson uses fine steel pins, which are "sufficiently tempered to be slightly flexile, thus yielding a little, a point of much importance when the knuckle of the colon has to be dragged up to the surface of a very fat loin, and thus exerts much tension on the pins."

Mr. Davies-Colley has shown that symptoms of strangulation may be induced by the forcible retention of a loop of bowel in the wound.

Mr. Howse adopts the following plan of fixing the colon:— Two pairs of pressure forceps are made to grasp small folds of the muscular coats of the colon. They should be applied with sufficient force to hold the bowel, but not to cause sloughing. They are placed about half an inch apart, and at right angles to the line of the incision. The forceps are laid flat on the skin, and kept in position by broad strips of plaster until the time comes for establishing the artificial anus.

(B) *The Closure of the Lower End of the Colon.*—In cases in which a permanent artificial anus has been established, fæces may collect between the fistula and the seat of the stricture, and severe symptoms, identical with those of intestinal obstruction, may be produced. Such symptoms may occur, as Mr. Bryant has pointed out, when a free outlet for fæcal matter exists at the new opening.

In cases of rectal cancer, also, much trouble may be occasioned by the continued passage of a little fæcal matter into the bowel below the artificial anus, by the trickling of the same over the ulcerated surface, and by the decomposition the retained matter induces.

To prevent the passage of fæces into the lower segment of the colon many means have been devised.

Mr. P. Jones (*Brit. Med. Journ.*, April 24th, 1886) detaches the mucous membrane from the upper segment of the bowel, and so adjusts it by sutures as to make it close over the opening into the lower portion of the colon. This operation can be best carried out when the artificial anus has been in existence for some time. The lower segment of the colon should be well flushed and emptied by a good irrigator before this measure is carried out.

Madelung (*Centralblatt für Chirurgie*, No. 23, 1884) advises that the colon be completely divided in a transverse direction, and that the distal end be closed by invagination and two rows of sutures, and be then dropped back into the abdomen. The proximal end is sutured to the wound.

There are many objections to this method. The operation involves time. The operation area is very limited. The peritoneal cavity is freely opened. Any fæcal matter which may be lodged in the lower segment of the bowel is permanently enclosed there.

In Jones's operation time may be allowed for the lower segment of the colon to empty itself, which it usually does. The closure may be postponed until all the urgent symptoms have passed away, and the distal end of the bowel may be well washed out before it is, as it were, sealed up.

The After-treatment.—The actual wound is dusted with iodoform, and all the skin around is well covered with vaseline. A large pad of absorbent wool is placed over the artificial opening, and retained by means of a many-tailed bandage.

So long as there is a copious escape of fæcal matter, no bandage should be applied.

The pad of wool must be changed as often as it is soiled, and the exclusive attention of one nurse may be occupied in keeping the patient always clean.

When the discharge is very free, a pad of loose " tenax," covered with a layer of wool, will be found to be more convenient.

The main feature in the nursing is that the part must be kept clean. The skin should not be *rubbed* clean, but should be cleansed by a stream of warm carbolised water, which is received in a kidney-shaped tray. This method involves no more trouble and no more time than the patting and rubbing process which is carried out with innumerable pledgets of cotton-wool.

After each washing, the skin is very gently dried, is once more covered with vaseline, and perhaps dusted with iodoform.

If the wound were to need to be washed every fifteen minutes during the first day or so, it would not be too often, and would certainly be better than to allow a freshly-united incision to remain for an hour or more poulticed with fæcal matter.

The use of a substantial flannel bandage will be found to be inconvenient.

During the first few days the patient should keep very quiet, should lie upon the back, or, if the position be altered at all should turn over towards the wounded side. The attachments of the gut will be dragged upon if the patient lie upon the sound side.

The discharge of fæcal matter from the bowel may be delayed for hours, or even for days.

The opening, as already stated, is at first very small; and if it suffice, well and good. If, however, hard scybalæ have to escape, then the opening must be in due course dilated, and this may be conveniently effected by sea-tangle tents. Two or more tents may be introduced at a time, and care must be taken that they do not slip into the bowel. The escape of large masses of fæcal matter is facilitated by means of enemata given through the artificial anus. Lund's forceps may in some special cases need to be used.

An aperient given on the fifth or sixth day after the operation has often an excellent effect.

Prolapse of the gut at the artificial opening is, so far as my experience goes, but rarely met with. A small opening in the gut, primary healing, and the maintenance of a healthy condition of the mucous membrane, appear to be the main factors which assist in preventing this complication.

The skin around the artificial anus may become very raw and inflamed. This is especially apt to be the case when the fistula is established near to a malignant growth, as when the cæcum is opened in the iliac region for cancer of the ileo-cæcal valve.

In these circumstances, a frequent washing-out of the bowel with an antiseptic lotion, and the most scrupulous attention to the cleanliness of the part, will effect much.

Properly-shaped pieces of lint soaked in oil may prevent some of the fæcal matter from running over the skin, but no contrivance that I have as yet seen has prevented it entirely.

An irritating condition of the intestinal contents may depend upon some grave digestive disturbances.

The matter that escapes from the bowel is sometimes almost as irritating as caustic potash. On the other hand, when the fistula has been made in the lesser bowel, I have observed the escaping fluid to be acid. It is well, in any case, that its reaction should be noted.

After a radical alteration of diet, I have noticed the matter escaping from the fistula to cease at once to be unduly irritating. Washing-out of the bowel has good effect, but more important is such good nursing that fæcal matter is never in contact with the inflamed skin for more than a moment.

In these cases of acutely-inflamed skin, ointments sometimes answer well, and an ointment made with balsam of Peru will be found as useful as any.

In some cases ointments appear to do harm ; and lotions, especially the lotion of rectified spirit and lead, may answer wonderfully.

In other instances the parts may be kept very dry, and may be dusted with bicarbonate of soda, or with boracic or benzoic acid.

The intense pain experienced when the skin is acutely inflamed may be in some degree relieved by cocaine.

The skin is apt to give more trouble when the fæcal fistula is in the median line, or in the iliac regions, than when it is in the loin.

I have seen the symptoms of iodoform-poisoning follow the liberal dusting of a colotomy wound with that powder ; and this danger is, I think, especially to be looked for when much mucous membrane is exposed. Iodoform may also produce an inflamed condition of the integument. In such case it may be discarded for creolin powder.

The disturbing symptoms produced by the presence of fæcal matter in the colon below the artificial opening may be relieved by the systematic washing-out of that part of the bowel, and by the subsequent closure, if need be, of its upper extremity.

The diet in these cases should be spare and nourishing, and of such a kind as to leave the least possible residue in the intestine. The consumption of milk in considerable quantity appears to encourage the formation of scybalæ. A liberal amount of vegetable matter should be a feature in the diet.

After the wound has healed, and the recovery from the operation is complete, the patient may be furnished with a simple belt which will permit a pad of wool or some folds of linen to be held in place when the patient is moving about. The simpler the belt the better, and it must be so constructed as to be readily unfastened. The various plugs, cups, bags, and pessaries which have been devised for the use of patients after colotomy are, so far as I have seen, more or less useless. After a short trial they are usually abandoned for some simple arrangement of cloths or pads which the patients have themselves devised.

ILIAC COLOTOMY.

Instruments required.—Scalpels; blunt-pointed bistoury; scissors; pressure, dissecting, and artery forceps; blunt hooks; rectangular retractors; straight and curved needles; needle-holder; sponge-holder; kidney-shaped receiver; sutures, etc.

Position and General Arrangements, as for abdominal section.

The Operation.—The following description of the operation is that given by Mr. Harrison Cripps ("Diseases of the Rectum," 2nd edition, page 452):— "As a guide, I take an imaginary line from the anterior superior spine to the umbilicus; the incision, two and a half inches long, crosses this at right angles, one inch and a half from the superior spine. Half the cut is above and half

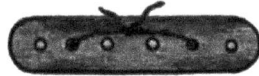

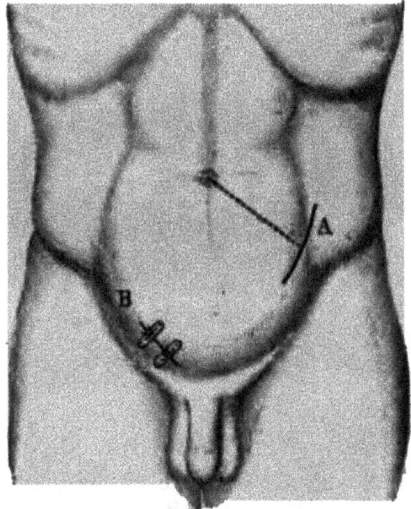

Fig. 356.—A, INCISION FOR ILIAC COLOTOMY; B, BALL'S OPERATION FOR THE RADICAL CURE OF HERNIA: THE WOUND IS CLOSED. (The suture plate is shown in the upper part of the figure.)

below the imaginary line, as shown in Fig. 356. In making the incision, the skin should be drawn a little inwards, so as to make the opening somewhat valvular. The peritoneum being reached, it is pinched up by fine forceps and an opening made sufficient to admit the finger. The intestines being protected by the finger, the peritoneum is divided by scissors to nearly the full length of the cutaneous incision. The colon may now at once show itself, and can easily be recognised by its longitudinal bands, its glandulæ epiploicæ. and by its regular convoluted surface. In about a third of my cases the large intestine presented at once; in the others, either the small intestine, omentum, or mesentery appeared first. If any of these latter present, they must be pushed back and the colon sought for by the finger. Sometimes it can be detected by the hard scybalous masses within it, or it can be traced up after passing the finger into the pelvis and feeling for it as it crosses the brim. Great care should be taken to prevent any of the small intestine from protruding, otherwise a considerable difficulty may be experienced in returning it into the abdominal cavity.

" The colon being found, a loop of it is drawn into the wound. In order to avoid the prolapse which is likely to occur if loose folds of the sigmoid flexure remain immediately above the opening, I gently draw out as much loose bowel as will readily come, passing it in again at the lower angle as it

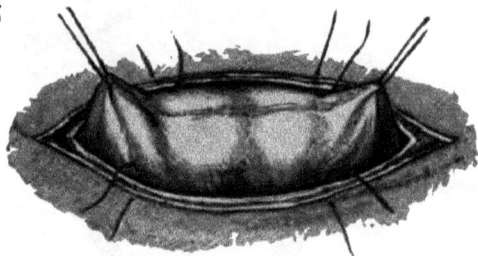

Fig. 357.—ILIAC COLOTOMY.
The four sutures securing the peritoneum to the skin are shown. (*Harrison Cripps.*)

is drawn out from above. In this way, after passing through one's fingers an amount varying from one to several inches, no more will come. Two provisional ligatures of stout silk are now passed through the longitudinal muscular band opposite the mesenteric attachment (Fig. 357). These provisional ligatures, the ends of which are left long, help to steady the bowel during its subsequent stitching to the skin, and moreover, are useful as guides when the bowel is ultimately opened. They should be about two inches apart.

" The bowel is now temporarily returned into the cavity. With a pair of fine forceps the parietal peritoneum is picked up and attached to the skin on each side of the incision, the muscular coats of the abdominal wall not being included. Four sutures of fine Chinese silk are sufficient, two on each side, an inch and a half apart (Fig. 357).

"The bowel is again drawn out, and fixed to the skin and parietal peritoneum by seven or eight fine ligatures on either side, the last suture at each angle going across from one side to the other. The bowel should be so attached as to have two-thirds of its circumference external to the sutures. By turning the bowel slightly over, the lower longitudinal band can be clearly seen, and it is best to pass the sutures for the lower side through this, since it is a strong portion of the gut (Fig. 358). The upper longitudinal band, through which the provisional ligatures have already been passed, is seen in the middle line of the wound. The bowel being now turned downwards, the opposite line of sutures are inserted close to its mesenteric attachment. No longitudinal band can, however, here be seen.

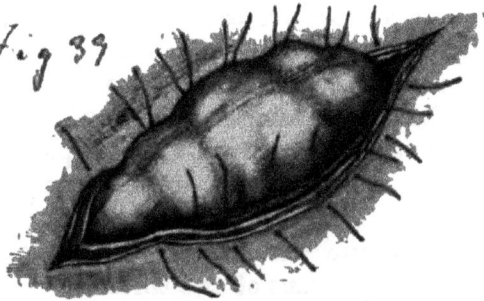

Fig. 358.—ILIAC COLOTOMY.
The sutures are in position, but not yet tied.
(*Harrison Cripps.*)

"The sutures, of the finest Chinese silk, are passed by small, partly-curved needles, the needle passing through the skin one-eighth of an inch from the margin, then through the parietal layer of the peritoneum, and lastly, partly through the muscular coat of the bowel, great care being taken to avoid perforating the mucous membrane. It is easier to pass all the threads before tying them up.

"The wound should be most carefully and gently cleaned; the threads can then be all tied with moderate tightness.

"If the case is urgent, the bowel may now be opened; if not, a piece of green protective is put over it—a necessary precaution, to prevent the granulations adhering to the gauze. The whole is covered with an antiseptic dressing, an additional thick pad being placed over the site of the wound. A broad flannel bandage is then wound firmly around the abdomen, so as to ensure considerable pressure."

The After-treatment.—Mr. Cripps then continues:—"The

wound is best dressed on the following day, to make sure that nothing has been unplaced.

"If all goes well, the dressings may be reapplied, and the bowel not opened till the fifth or sixth day. . . . All ligatures may be safely removed by the ninth day, or earlier if there is redness around them. Firm pressure with a pad and bandage will be required for some time later."

In many cases the wound heals by first intention; in the rest by granulation. In these latter cases much contraction of the orifice may take place.

Other points in the after-treatment of the patient and the artificial opening have been already considered (page 368).

Modifications of the Operation. — 1. Many surgeons advise an incision parallel with the outer third of Poupart's ligament, and only half an inch above it. Others place the incision an inch from the ligament.

Luke and Adams made use of a vertical incision external to the epigastric artery. Ball employs an incision about four inches in length in the left linea semilunaris.

2. In the older methods of operating, a loop of the sigmoid flexure was drawn well out into the wound, and was secured by means of two threads which transfixed the meso-colon close to its attachment to the bowel. This procedure has been revived by Mr. Allingham. The intestine, when fixed by the threads that transfix the meso-colon, is further secured by means of a number of interrupted sutures, which attach the intestinal wall to the skin.

Mr. Rose also secures the gut by means of a thread which is passed to and fro through the meso-colon, and also through the margins of the wound. By tightening this ligature, the parietal and the visceral peritoneum are brought into close contact (*Lancet*, Jan. 31st, 1891).

3. By drawing the knuckle of gut well forward into the wound, a good spur is formed at the point opened, and this spur serves to prevent fæcal matter from finding its way into the distal segment of the gut.

To obviate the tendency of the bowel to prolapse, Mr. Allingham recommends the excision of all the superfluous bowel with its meso-colon after it has been pulled out of the wound as far as is possible. As much as seven inches of gut have thus been removed. There is nothing to recommend this mutilation, and most surgeons will join with Mr. Bryant and others in their condemnation of this uncouth proceeding.

4. Maydl's operation (*Centralblatt für Chirurgie*, No. 24, 1888) is thus described by Dr. Senn :—

He opens the peritoneal cavity by Littre's incision, and draws a loop of intestine forwards until its mesenteric attachment is on a level with the external incision.

Through a slit in the mesentery close to the gut is inserted a hard rubber cylinder wrapped in iodoform gauze. A goosequill will answer the same purpose.

This device holds the intestine in the wound, and prevents its return into the abdominal cavity. By means of a row of sutures placed on each side of the prolapsed gut, and including the serous and muscular coats, the two limbs of the flexure, in so far as they lie in the abdominal wound, are stitched together beneath the rubber support.

If the intestine is to be opened immediately, it is stitched to the parietal peritoneum of the abdominal incision, and the latter protected by iodoform collodion. If the bowel is to be incised later, the latter is not stitched to the peritoneum, but surrounded by iodoform gauze packed in beneath the rubber support, the incision of the bowel being made four or six days later.

If the artificial anus is to be a permanent one, a transverse opening, including one-third of the periphery of the bowel, is made by the thermo-cautery, drainage-tubes are inserted into the two lumina, and the intestine is carefully washed out. If the progress of the case be satisfactory, the bowel is cut through completely in two or three weeks, the rubber support serving a useful purpose as a guide in making this incision. A few sutures will serve to secure the cut end to the skin.

If the direction of the muscular fibres has been respected in making the abdominal incision, the patient is provided with such an efficient sphincter that a large drainage-tube is required to keep the opening patulous.

Should the artificial anus be only a temporary one, the incision in the intestine is made in a longitudinal direction. When it has become desirable to close the artificial opening, the rubber support is removed, after which the bowel retracts.

and the opening often closes without any further treatment. If the adhesions are too firm for this, they are removed, and the bowel is sutured and returned into the peritoneal cavity.

5. Lauenstein first sutures the peritoneum to the skin, thus lining the external incision with that membrane. He then draws out a loop of intestine and closes the parietal wound by sutures passed through the meso-colon of the extruded portion of gut. Finally, the serous covering of each limb of the prolapsed loop is stitched through its entire circumference to the parietal peritoneum. The gut can now be opened (*Centralblatt für Chirurgie*, No. 24, 1888).

6. Verneuil employs a nearly vertical incision, and draws a knuckle of gut into the wound as large as a pigeon's egg. This is transfixed by two acupuncture needles, which lie on the parietes and keep the gut in place. The exposed bowel is united to the margins of the parietal wound by many sutures, and the protruding knuckle is then excised. The bowel wall bulging into the large opening thus made, effectually blocks the passage leading into the segment of the colon below the new anus (*La France Médicale*, 1887).

7. Ball secures the bowel above and below the future artificial opening by means of two special clamps. The gut is then fixed to the parietal wound by means of sutures which transfix the skin, parietal peritoneum, and whole thickness of the walls of the bowel. The intestine is opened, and the clamps are removed. The operation is described, and the instruments employed figured, in Mr. Ball's work upon "The Rectum and Anus" (London, 1887, page 366).

8. Mr. Paul divides the bowel, invaginates the distal end as in Senn's method, and returns it into the abdomen. Into the proximal end a glass tube one inch in diameter is tied. To the end of this tube a rubber pipe is fixed to carry the fæcal discharge away from the wound. This piece of the bowel is fixed to the parietal wound by sutures, and the margins of that wound are approximated around it.

After some three days the projecting piece of bowel is cut away (*Brit. Med. Journ.*, July 18, 1891).

The Opening of the Cæcum.—When the operation is carried out upon the right side, the cæcum is opened.

The steps of the procedure differ in no essential from the operation as above described.

The bowel has of course no meso-colon, and none of the measures which involve a dealing with that membrane can be carried out upon the right side.

The cæcum is always very readily to be found, and is easily drawn into the parietal wound, secured, and opened.

Under equal conditions, the operation is simpler upon the right side than upon the left.

When a doubt exists as to the position of the obstruction, it is well to remember that the cæcum can, in all ordinary anatomical circumstances, be opened through a median incision.

I have many times made an artificial anus in this situation. One of such cases is described in the·*Lancet* for Oct. 29th, 1887.

The Comparative Value of Lumbar and Iliac Colotomy.

A great deal has been written upon this subject, with the result that it is evident that extreme differences of opinion exist as to which of the two methods is the better.

It is urged that iliac colotomy is the easier and quicker operation, that the diagnosis can be verified, and that there is no risk of opening the small intestine, the duodenum, or the stomach.

On the other hand, it is pointed out that the lumbar operation involves, as a rule, no prolonged searching for the bowel, that the serous cavity is not usually opened up, that the opening is further away from the seat of the disease (in cancer of the rectum), and is more conveniently placed. Prolapse of the bowel appears to be decidedly more common in the iliac than in the lumbar operation, and the former operation is not well adapted for cases in which considerable distension of the abdomen exists.

Mr. Bryant has very fully considered the bearings of the subject in his Lecture on Colotomy, and with his final conclusion I, for one, am disposed to agree.

"The final conclusion," he writes, "is therefore clear that iliac colotomy is not yet proved to be superior to the lumbar operation. In doubtful cases, in which an exploratory incision is required for diagnostic purposes, it may be useful, but such cases are very few; in all others, lumbar colotomy has advantages which stamp it as the better measure. The single advantage that I can see in the adoption of the iliac method is that the question of operative interference will have to be taken into account at a far earlier period of the patient's trouble than it has been hitherto the custom to consider the propriety of the lumbar operation" ("Bradshaw Lecture," 1889, page 45).

Results.—The most elaborate statistics are those published by Dr. Batt (*Amer. Journ. of Med. Sciences*, Oct., 1884, page 423). Of his figures, the following is a general summary of a total of 351 operations:—

154	were for	malignant disease...	...	...	Mortality	31·6	per cent
20	„	fistula	...	„		10	„
52	„	imperforate anus ...	...	„		52·9	„
40	„	obstruction	...	...	„	50	„
72	„	stricture	...	„		43	„
4	„	ulceration	...	„		25	„
9	„	various other causes	...	„		44	„

Total... 351   General mortality ... 38   „

Form of operation.	Cases.	Result unknown.	Recovered.	Died.	Mortality per cent.
Amussat	244	2	165	77	31·8
Littre	82	1	38	43	53·1
Callisen	10	1	2	7	77·7
In umbilical region...	4	—	4	—	0·0
Not stated	11	—	6	5	45·4
Total	351	4	215	132	38·9

Of the patients who recovered from the operations for malignant disease—

13 died within six months.
15 „ between six months and twelve months.
10 „ between one and two years.
8 „ between two and three years.
1 „ four and a half years after the operation.

The statistics given by Batt extend back over many years, and do not therefore represent the value of the improvement which has been effected in modern surgery.

Mr. Cripps has performed colotomy for malignant disease of the rectum in forty-one cases, with the following admirable results :—

Lumbar method	14	...	Recovered 14	...	Died 0
Inguinal method	27	...	Recovered 26	...	Died 1
	41		40		1

The mortality of the operation being less than two and a half per cent.

CHAPTER X.

THE OPERATIVE TREATMENT OF INTESTINAL OBSTRUCTION.

IT would be beyond the purpose and limits of this book to enter into the question of the treatment of intestinal obstruction by operation with any attempt at precision or completeness.

The subject involves the indications for operation and the proper selection of a mode of procedure, rather than any definite or quite special surgical method.

In the account that follows, no more is attempted than an indication of the general lines upon which the operative treatment of intestinal obstruction is conducted.

The Purpose of the Operation.—It must be assumed that, in speaking of intestinal obstruction, reference is made principally to the acute or sub-acute forms of that affection. In chronic forms of obstruction a definite treatment can be carried out with greater precision: the diagnosis is usually more accurately made; there is less urgency; there is an absence of violent symptoms, and any proposed operation can be carried out with deliberation.

In the acute cases the progress of the trouble is often terribly rapid, the symptoms are violent, the need of immediate relief is very urgent, and symptoms which in a chronic case may assist the diagnosis are probably masked by narcotics in the acute form.

Many cases when seen by the surgeon are seen too late. Laparotomy for intestinal obstruction is regarded by some as literally a "last resource," and the patient is not considered to be ready for operation until he is *in articulo mortis*. In not a few instances the previous treatment has compromised the success of any interference by operation. The engorgement of the bowel has been increased by aperients, and the normal reflexes have been impaired or annihilated by excessive doses of opium and belladonna.

Operative treatment, to be successful, must be carried out early; and as soon as it is becoming evident that no relief is to be expected through natural means, then the sooner the assistance of the surgeon is called for the better.

It has been clearly enough shown that when once the symptoms of undoubted strangulation have appeared in connection with a hernia, nothing is to be gained by delaying the usual operation by even an hour.

The risks which attend delay, and the dangers which attend uncertainty, are greater than those which belong to the mere opening of the abdomen in the median line.

In the carrying out of an operation the surgeon will have two purposes in view—(1) the relief of the dangerously-engorged bowel above the occluded part, and (2) the removal of the cause of the obstruction.

It is true, in many cases, that the attainment of the second object will include the first, but it is not true in all.

The belly may be opened in an advanced and acute case, a simple band may be at once discovered and divided, and the abdomen closed. The case may appear very simple and very fortunate. It is true that the cause of the obstruction is removed, but the greatly distended and engorged bowel above the site of the divided band is not necessarily relieved.

It is filled up to the very stomach with a foul and fæculent fluid, by which the patient is being poisoned. The gut is paralysed, the normal reflexes are lost, toere is no peristaltic wave to free the many bends and twists which must be undone to secure a free passage, and the patient dies with some pints of the foulest and most putrid matter still lodged in a viscus possessed with an instinct to absorb its contents.

In such a case as this it is not the removal of the band which is the most urgent matter, it is the complete evacuation of the engorged bowel.

It is well in the acuter forms of intestinal obstruction to hold in mind that the patient is not dying because a band or an adhesion presses upon the bowel, and that it is not the cancerous stricture which has become suddenly blocked up, that is of itself bringing about death; but that the urgency depends rather upon the extreme engorgement of the bowel above the site of the obstruction.

It is obvious that the two conditions cannot be logically separated, but at the same time it is essential to recognise that the surgeon's first object should be rather to relieve the obstructed bowel than to remove the cause of the obstruction; and it must not be forgotten that the attainment of the latter purpose may not be followed by the attainment of the former.

There are cases, however, where another element may predominate, and these are represented by instances in which a vast peritoneal surface is implicated in the obstructive lesion. Such are volvulus of the sigmoid flexure and cases of obstruction by bands, where the constricted bowel is represented by many coils, and, indeed, by many feet of intestine. In such examples, death may follow apparently from the extensive peritoneal lesion before a period at which it becomes evident that the engorgement of the bowel above the obstruction is a predominating feature.

Still, in spite of what may be urged as exceptions, the facts remain that laparotomy in acute intestinal obstruction is attended by a terrible mortality, and that the best results so far have followed in those cases in which the contents of the distended bowel have been evacuated. Enterotomy may appear to be a somewhat unsurgical procedure, and not a very brilliant or complete operation, but still it can claim results which appear to indicate the direction in which surgical measures should tend.

In threatened suffocation attending the impaction of a foreign body in the larynx, experience has shown that it is better to perform tracheotomy first, and to search for the obstructing foreign body afterwards.

The Management of the Most Urgent Cases.

In these cases there is distinctly no time to be lost. The patient's condition is such as to forbid any but the slightest operation, and the surgeon's great object is to relieve the distended bowel with the least possible disturbance of the patient.

The patient is enveloped in warm blankets, and hot bottles are placed about the extremities. The operation, such as it is, is performed as the patient lies in bed. No anæsthetic can be administered. If one be attempted, it will be noticed that the patient becomes rapidly insensible, and very often, just as the surgeon takes the knife in his hand, there is a great rush of fæcal matter from the patient's mouth and nose, and the case is at an end. Some surgeons advise the use of cocaine, injected under the skin of the abdomen. The patients, however, in these cases are not in a condition to feel much pain. They stand the cutting part well, merely whining and moaning and wrinkling the brow as the surgeon proceeds.

A mask containing a drop or two of ether may distract their attention and cover their eyes while the actual skin incision is being made, but beyond this it is not well to go.

The *operation* consists in opening the abdomen in the median line below the umbilicus and performing an outer-otomy. The incision should be as small as possible—just large enough to allow one distended coil to be drawn forwards with the finger. There should be no searching for the cause of the obstruction. Every minute is of consequence in a case such as the present.

The bowel is rapidly fixed to the parietal wound by a few sutures, which do not penetrate beyond the sub-mucous coat, and the gut may be best evacuated by a large trocar and cannula, to the end of which a long indiarubber tube is fixed. The contents of the gut are thus carried away from the wound. A way for the trocar through the outer coats of the intestine must be made with a scalpel. As the bowel is emptying itself, it may be more accurately secured to the margins of the parietal wound by a few more sutures.

The wound is treated in the manner already described.

It is most important in these cases that the stomach should be washed out. This may be done either before or after the operation. The best apparatus is Leiter's irrigator, which acts upon the syphon principle. The washing-out should be effected by hot water, or hot water containing a little boracic or carbolic acid.

This measure usually gives great relief, and the introduction of a large amount of hot water into the stomach improves the pulse and tends greatly to revive the patient. In long-neglected cases of strangulated hernia with fæcal vomiting, I believe that a patient's life has been more than once saved by a thorough washing-out of the stomach with hot water at the time of the operation.

In cases of obstruction, which are a little less urgent, some search may be made for the cause of the obstruction prior to the establishment of the artificial anus. A band may be found, and a strangulated loop may be relieved, without adding perceptibly to the danger of the operation. But the search should be rapid; and if the site of the obstruction be not found almost at once, there should be no delay in opening the bowel.

The Management of the Less Urgent Cases.

In most of these cases the patient may safely be moved from the bed to an operating-table. The stomach should be washed out with hot water before the operation is commenced. An anæsthetic may be administered, but its use must be very cautious. Enough only is required to dull the patient's senses; and after the parietal wound has been made, enough only to restrain his movements.

The abdomen should be opened in the median line, between the umbilicus and the pubes.

The incision made should be large enough to admit the hand. Some surgeons advise a much larger incision. Kümmell recommends that the knife be carried from the xiphoid cartilage to the pubes. Such an excessive measure is obviously unnecessary; and it is difficult to conceive a case, unless it be one of extreme volvulus of a large sigmoid flexure, where such a wound would be other than embarrassing. Other surgeons have advised a very small median wound, one of not more than two inches, or one large enough to admit two fingers. If any search for the obstruction has to be made, a two-inch incision in a greatly-distended abdomen will be found of little use. If the belly were flat and shrunken, it might possibly be sufficient. A determined attempt to relieve a case of acute intestinal obstruction through an incision with a maximum length of two inches belongs to the performances of sensational surgery, and an urgent case of abdominal disease is hardly suited for the demonstration of surgical feats, or for showing, not so much what can be best done to relieve the patient, as what can be effected through a two-inch incision.

When the abdomen has been opened, search is made for the site of the obstruction.

Great difference of opinion exists as to the best method to adopt in carrying out this search. Among the multitude of counsellors there has as yet been little wisdom, and a plan that is vigorously advocated one year may be vigorously condemned the next.

In actual practice these cases present so many aspects, and are liable to such infinite variations, that it is, indeed, impossible to lay down hard-and-fast rules.

When the coils of intestine are greatly distended, they must be handled with infinite care. After a by no means rough manipulation, it may be found that the serous coat of the dilated coils has been split in twenty places. In the production of such lesions the operator's finger-nails often do no little harm.

The entire hand should not be introduced into the abdomen until every other means of examination has been exhausted; and an indiscriminate and purposeless pulling about of coils of intestine is to be avoided.

The method of making a very large incision, and of at once dragging out as much bowel as possible, has little to commend it.

As soon as the abdomen has been opened, three fingers may be introduced and the cæcum examined. If that viscus is found to be empty, the obstruction must be in the small intestine; if it be distinctly distended, then search must be made in the colon.

In the latter case the fingers may be passed into the left iliac region, and a stricture sought for in the sigmoid flexure or upper part of the rectum; or the empty colon below the obstruction may be detected and followed as far as is possible. In the case of colic obstruction, the operation will probably be at once completed by performing a colotomy in the median line. There can seldom be any object in closing the median incision, and then performing a lumbar colotomy.

If the obstruction be not in the colon, the surgeon should pass his fingers over the hernial orifices, should examine carefully the ileo-cæcal and umbilical regions, and explore so far as is possible all parts of the pelvis. The commoner forms of acute obstruction should reveal themselves after such an examination.

If the seat of the trouble be not yet discovered, search should be made in the pelvis for any collapsed coils of small intestine which may belong to the segment below the obstruction. Such coils are very often found hanging down in the pelvis, and, as Mr. Hulke has pointed out (*Med. Times and Gazette*, vol. ii., 1872, page 482), they often lead the surgeon to the occluded part, if they be carefully traced.

If so far no discovery of the trouble has been made, it may at least be urged that no injurious handling of the viscera has been carried out, and it will in many cases be desirable to desist, and to establish at once an artificial opening in the small intestine.

If, however, the patient's condition be such as to justify further search, the surgeon may, in the next place, allow some of the more distended coils of the bowel to protrude. They should be received in fine diaper towels which have been dipped in hot carbolised water. The escape of these coils may render an inspection and a further digital examination possible. Failing any clue to the site of the obstruction, he may, if the case admit, proceed to introduce his hand into the abdomen. Without this somewhat extreme method of examination, certain forms of obstruction, such as that due to hernia into the fossa duodeno-jejunalis, or hernia into the foramen of Winslow, could scarcely be made out. This fact I have illustrated by an example of the latter form of hernia, in which I performed laparotomy (*Lancet*, Oct. 13th, 1888). In cases of great distension, the introduction of the hand is almost impossible, or is likely to inflict considerable damage if persisted in. Such cases are not those in which the surgeon spends twenty minutes or more in searching for the obstruction, but are cases rather in which the gut is opened after a rapid and superficial examination.

Some surgeons (*e.g.*, Kümmell—*Deutsche med. Wochenschrift*, No. 12, 1886) conclude the examination by resorting to exventration. The abdomen is fully opened up, the distended bowels are allowed to gush forth, and the cause of the obstruction is sought for in the open and simple manner which is adopted at a post-mortem examination.

Madelung brings a prominent coil into the wound, and, having opened it, attempts to empty the distended part of the bowel. He considers that fifteen minutes might well be spent in efforts to effect a more or less complete intestinal drainage.

The escape of the contents is aided by turning the patient upon the side, by pressing upon the dilated loops, and by passing a Nélaton's catheter.

Another plan is to expose the whole of the free part of the small intestine inch by inch until the loop occluded is reached. As the bowel is drawn out at the upper angle of the wound, it is passed back into the abdomen again at the lower. This plan is almost impossible when there is great distension; it involves considerable handling of the gut, and much expenditure of time.

The surgeon may, moreover, proceed with his investigation in the wrong direction, and may find himself, at the end of a tedious examination, at the duodenum.

Mr. Rand (*Brit. Med. Journ.*, Dec. 22nd, 1883) has advised an examination of the root of the mesentery as a means of avoiding the last-mentioned error. The attached border of the mesentery is only about six inches in length, and it is so obliquely placed that the right layer is directed a little upwards, and the left layer a little downwards. If a loop of the bowel be drawn forwards, and its mesentery be followed backwards to the spine, it may be often possible to tell which is the upper and which the lower segment of the loop, and also to form some idea as to whether it belongs to the higher or to the terminal parts of the lesser bowel. This is usually spoken of as the method by straightening the mesentery.

In acute cases, these, and other very extended and time-consuming methods of searching for the obstruction which are described, can be but rarely justifiable. In chronic cases they may be appropriate enough.

After the cause of the obstruction has been found and relieved, it will in very many instances still be wise to evacuate the distended bowel.

The opening made may be closed as soon as the gut is considered to have sufficiently emptied itself; but it may with greater safety be left open for the time being, and be closed by a subsequent operation.

t 2

As Mr. Greig Smith ha
intestinal obstruction is
leaves the operating-table

In reducing such loop
assistant should draw forw
wound with large blunt
into a slit, just as a man w
into which something is t
back one by one by the kn
manipulate the bowel thro
the coils are few, or a diap

If the protrusion be c
prolapsed intestine may be
the edges of which are tu
abdominal incision.

This reduction of prot
siderable time. If, howeve
relieved, the process shonl
lation which is called for in

The sponges employed
hot, and any cleansing solu
Special means must be t
from exposure to cold.

The surgeon should no
the parietes. It must be
for the seat of the trouble
depths of the abdomen
examination the nearest c
spatulæ, and the margins
retractors.

The Removal of the

Strangulation by Ban
bands and adhesions may
The same may be said of s
adhesions, and large cord
need to be divided in secti
be cut short whenever po
period.

When either the Fallo
obstructing band, an attem

by traction, or by breaking down or dividing the adhesions which hold the organs in place. Failing this, the parts must be severed. It may be noted that after a strangulation under the appendix has been relieved by simple reduction, death has occurred from gangrene of the little tube itself. In such a case it would have been better if the process had been excised.

The Fallopian tube may be treated as a simple band, and divided between two ligatures.

The appendix, after it has been cut across, should have its proximal end closed by a double row of sutures—a continuous suture involving the mucous membrane, and a series of interrupted sutures involving the outer coats.

Meckel's diverticulum, when met with in the condition of a band, should be divided and treated as such ; when it exists as a patent tube, its severed end should be closed with as much care as would be observed in closing divided intestine.

It is not wise to leave a long diverticulum attached to the bowel. If time permit, it should be cut short. Gangrene and perforation of this process have followed in cases where the obstruction has been relieved, but the diverticulum left undisturbed. When very large, the removal of the diverticulum involves an operation of some gravity and duration, and this it may be undesirable to attempt. The larger diverticula may be divided, and the proximal end clamped and brought into the parietal wound, where it plays the part of an artificial anus. Such an opening is more easily closed than one in the bowel itself. In such a case the distal end would be excised entirely.

In cases of strangulation through slits and apertures, it is well, when possible, to close the abnormal aperture with a few points of suture after the gut has been reduced.

Much difficulty may be experienced in dealing with retro-peritoneal herniæ. In a case of strangulated hernia at the foramen of Winslow, I not only could not reduce the gut through a laparotomy wound during life, but after death reduction was not effected until I had severed the hepatic artery, the portal vein, and the bile duct.

Volvulus.—In only the very simplest cases can volvulus be unfolded by mere manipulation.

No persistent attempts should be made to effect such a reduction. The huge coil formed by the distended sigmoid flexure cannot be dealt with through the comparatively small wound made in abdominal section. The involved bowel should be tapped and emptied. Its contents are mainly gaseous. The hole made can be clamped temporarily and the volvulus reduced. If the reduction be perfect, and if it show no disposition to return, the opening may be closed. Failing such evidence, an artificial anus must be established in it. I have found it impossible to reduce a volvulus of the sigmoid flexure on the post-mortem table until the bowel had been emptied.

It must be remembered that the reduction of a volvulus does not usually remove the anatomical condition that led to it.

Intussusception.—Many cases of intussusception may be successfully treated by insufflation and injections of water per rectum. Some undergo spontaneous reduction, aided possibly by medical measures; a few cures have been ascribed to manipulation and galvanism, and still fewer to a process of natural recovery after gangrene.

Assuming that it is decided to open the abdomen, an attempt is at first made to reduce the invagination. The surgeon draws upon the intussuscipiens with one hand, while he squeezes and kneads the intussusceptum with the other. The latter part of the invagination should be straightened out as much as possible, and reduction should be attempted rather by gentle pressure applied to the intussusceptum than to persistent traction upon the entering tube. It is of little use to break down any adhesions which may exist between the two tubes of the intussusception. Reduction is only possible in comparatively early cases in which little structural alteration has taken place.

If, after many patient attempts, reduction cannot be accomplished, one or other of the following plans may be carried out:—

1. An intestinal anastomosis may be effected by Senn's method. A successful example of this operation has already been alluded to (page 347).

2. The involved segment of the gut may be resected and

an artificial anus established. This measure is of limited application, and could hardly be advised in a case where the invagination is extensive.

3. The establishment of an artificial anus without resection. This measure would appear to be recommended in irreducible cases where resection is contra-indicated and where time is pressing. It cannot claim to possess, on *à priori* grounds, any advantages over the first method named.

4. The resection of the intussusceptum, and the immediate restoration of the canal by suture of the divided ends of the bowel. This procedure, which must of necessity be very limited in application, and occupy a considerable period of time, has little to recommend it, and is not in accord with the principles that influence the general treatment of intestinal obstruction by operation at the present time.

Mr. Barker, in a very valuable paper (*Lancet*, August 11th, 1888), has collected seventy-three examples of intussusception treated by operation. The following is a summary of his tables :—

Laparotomy—Bowel reduced, 34 cases ; 22 died, 12 recovered.
      „   Intussusception irreducible, 29 cases—
              (*a*) Abdomen closed, 5 cases ; 5 died.
              (*b*) Intussusceptum resected, 14 cases ; 13 died, 1 recovered.
              (*c*) Artificial anus formed, 10 cases ; 10 died.
Artificial anus with laparotomy—10 cases ; 10 died.
            Total—73 cases ; 60 died, 13 recovered.

In chronic colic invagination into the rectum the invaginated part has been resected with success. Failing this attempts at reduction having already proved abortive, colotomy may be carried out.

Foreign Bodies.—In the case of some foreign bodies, *e.g.* gall-stones and the softer form of enterolith, it may be possible to break up the substance or to crush it without opening the intestine.

The bowel at the site of impaction will most probably be inflamed, the mucous membrane may be deeply ulcerated, or the coats of the intestine may be passing into a condition of gangrene. No attempt should therefore be made to disintegrate the calculus at the seat of impaction. The surgeon should endeavour to displace it upwards into the distended but healthier bowel above the obstruction, and deal with it there. Failing this measure, the foreign body may be removed by an incision made on the free border of the bowel and in its long axis. This incision also should be made through healthy intestine, and not directly through the gut at the seat of impaction. It is usually more convenient to make the incision in the dilated bowel above the obstruction.

The question of closing the incision in the gut at once by sutures, or of establishing an artificial anus, must depend upon the state of the intestinal wall at the seat of the impaction, and upon the degree of engorgement of the canal above that point.

If the gut be gangrenous at the seat of the obstruction, the part involved should be resected and an artificial anus established.

Other Forms of Obstruction.—Under this heading may be included in a general way varieties of obstruction due to causes which are less easily dealt with than is the case in the instances above given. In this category may be placed stricture, matting of adjacent coils of bowel together by many adhesions, direct compression of the gut by contracting adhesions, some complex forms of volvulus, and other allied conditions.

In these cases (1) an artificial anus may be established, and nothing more attempted. Such a procedure would be adopted for the more urgent and the more complex cases. (2) The involved part of the bowel may be resected and an artificial anus established. This measure may be advisable in cases of stricture, and in other instances where the resection can be carried out with ease and completeness. (3) Resection may be followed by immediate suture of the divided bowel. There is very little to be said in favour of this method in cases where any degree of obstruction exists. (4) The involved parts may be left undisturbed, and an intestinal anastomosis established by Senn's method. This procedure appears to have before it a fair prospect of success.

When the involved bowel is gangrenous, resection cannot be avoided; and such excision should be followed by establishing an artificial opening.

The Results of Operative Interference in Acute Intestinal Obstruction.—Statistics dealing with this subject are apt to be somewhat misleading. The general mortality which is to be adduced from the various published tables is without doubt lower than that met with in actual practice, and does not represent the actual death-rate. It may be inferred that the majority of the successful cases are published, but that a very large proportion of the fatal cases are left unrecorded.

Among the examples which would be reckoned as ending favourably are not a few which were—to judge from the published accounts—not instances of acute intestinal obstruction at all, but were examples rather of peritonitis. In such cases "much effusion into the peritoneal cavity" is reported, adhesions are encountered, and the cause of the imagined obstruction is not uncommonly ascribed either to adhesions or to volvulus of the small intestines.

One of the best collections of cases is that published by Dr. Curtis in the *Annals of Surgery* for May, 1888. He deals with the results of laparotomy in intestinal obstruction since 1873.

In a total of 328 cases there are 226 deaths and 102 recoveries—a mortality of 68·9 per cent.

It is made evident that the failure of the operation was due directly to the unfavourable condition of the patient; some were in a dying condition, others were exhausted, in many gangrene of the bowel was advanced. Dr. Curtis's tables afford a strong argument in favour of early operation.

In 247 cases where the cause of the obstruction was removed the mortality was 62·7 per cent.; while in seventy-four instances in which this was not done, the mortality was 86·4 per cent.

The highest death-rate was associated with cases where from any cause suturing of the bowel was carried out. The total number of such cases was forty-five, with a mortality of 86·6 per cent.

CHAPTER XI.

OPERATIONS FOR FÆCAL FISTULA AND ARTIFICIAL ANUS.

THE nature of the operation carried out in these cases will obviously depend upon the character, situation, and degree of the artificial opening.

For the purposes of classification, with a view to treatment, fæcal fistulæ may in the first place be divided into (A) those which involve the jejunum and ileum, and such parts of the colon as are normally provided with a free meso-colon, viz., the transverse colon and sigmoid fiexure; and (B) those which implicate the more fixed segments of the large intestine—that is to say, the ascending colon, the descending colon and the cæcum.

A. **Fæcal Fistula involving the Small Intestine and the Free Parts of the Colon.**

These unnatural openings may be roughly placed in three categories.

1. In the first the loss of substance in the wall of the bowel is small; the gut is not acutely bent upon itself; the orifice is small, and the opening in the skin is connected with the opening in the bowel by a sinus-like tract (Fig. 359, 1).

Such a form may be illustrated by the following case :—A surgeon made an exploratory incision in the median line of the abdomen in a young woman. The cut was small, and was below the umbilicus. It was probable, from her account, that the mass which was the subject of speculation was a fæcal accumulation. It would appear also that a loop of the lower ileum was accidentally wounded and the wound at once closed—the injured intestine lying close to the parietal wound, which was also sutured. Some days after the operation the wound broke down. Fæcal matter then began to escape, and a permanent fistula resulted, which when I saw the patient, had been discharging for nearly

twelve months. Through this opening practically the whole
of the intestinal contents ·were evacuated, since a small
motion was only passed per anum about once a fortnight.
I closed this artificial anus at one sitting by the method
described as *Method No.* 1, and the patient made an uninter-
rupted recovery.

It is to this form of the trouble that this method is
especially applicable.

2. In the second class of case the loss of intestinal
substance has been greater, the opening is larger, and the
mucous membrane of the bowel is more directly in contact
with the skin, and is more extensively exposed. There is no

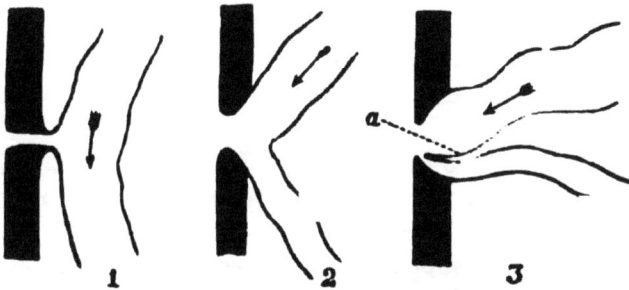

Fig. 359.—THREE FORMS OF FÆCAL FISTULA.

very considerable "spur," if any, separating the upper segment
of the gut from the lower (Fig. 359, 2).

This form of artificial anus may be illustrated by that
which is left after enterotomy, especially when followed by
some sloughing of the bowel. It may result, also, after a resection, when the bowel has been partly united, and a fæcal
fistula has been carefully established, with a view to a subsequent operation for closure. For this variety the procedure
described as *Method No.* 2 is applicable.

3. In the third form there has been a little or a great loss
of substance. The opening is probably extensive, the two ends
of the gut meet at the orifice at a very acute angle, and the
lumen of the proximal segment is separated from that of the
distal segment by a fold formed of the coats of the bowel at
its mesenteric border. This fold is known as the spur, or
éperon (Fig. 359, 3, *a*). It forms a real septum, and prevents
the contents of the gut from following their natural course,

while it is a potent factor in the maintenance of the artificial orifice.

The treatment of this variety is especially considered in the section headed *Method No. 3.*

The best instance I have seen of this form was in a man who had suffered from strangulated inguinal hernia. He declined treatment. The gut sloughed, the coverings of the sac gave way, and the parts of the intestine which were concerned in the fistula were those which had formed the pedicle of the loop of strangulated bowel. This case was remarkable from the fact that, although the patient continued to prefer the nostrums of a herbalist to the uncertainty of what was termed "a necessary operation," the fistula, at the end of many months, closed spontaneously, to the gratification of the patient and the discomfiture of scientific surgery. It is probable that this case may be an example of cure by the use of powerful caustics.

B. **Fæcal Fistulæ involving the Fixed Parts of the Colon.**
The most frequent of these are such as result from intentional or accidental wounding of the colon through the loin, and such as follow suppurative typhlitis. The abnormal opening will, therefore, be usually found either in the right iliac region or in the left loin.

So far as its characters are concerned, it will most commonly accord with the first of the three types mentioned above. There is a sinus, of varying dimensions, leading down to the bowel, which is comparatively deeply placed. In the right iliac region this is, perhaps, the form which the lesion will take without exception, the segment of gut involved being the cæcum.

The fæcal sinuses in the right inguinal district which result from typhlitis have a distinct tendency to undergo spontaneous cure, and of this termination I have seen many examples.

The fistulæ which are placed in the loin exhibit little of this disposition.

These colic sinuses are very difficult to close by operation. The great thing needed for success in any such operation is a ready supply of peritoneum. Two serous surfaces must be brought together.

In the sinuses which result from typhlitis the bowel is commonly buried in a mass of adhesions. The true peritoneum has been lost, and little material is available to meet the requirement that, in closing the opening in the gut, two surfaces of serous membrane should be brought into contact.

The procedure adopted for the majority of these cases is that described as *Method No. 3.*

An artificial anus in the loin is also, as a rule, very difficult to close. There may be no opportunity of making a complete union by means of united serous surfaces, and the obstacles in the surgeon's way when there has been much destruction of the bowel are almost insurmountable. In one case, that of a woman, an incision had been made in the left loin, with the intention, it was reported, of exposing the left kidney. By some surgical misfortune the descending colon was cut across by the operator. It was probably empty and cord-like, and may have been mistaken for other tissue. The kidney had not been disturbed. I made the most persistent attempts to close the resulting fistula; but although the sinus was diminished in size, the object of two tedious operations was never realised.

Methods of Operating.

Method No. 1.—For some time before the operation every means is taken to put the skin around the abnormal opening in as healthy a condition as possible. The eczema, which is often present, may be much relieved by constant attention to cleanliness, by keeping the part dry, and by dressing it with dry boracic acid powder, with boracic ointment, or such other application as may seem indicated. The diet must be so regulated as to allow of the formation of the least possible amount of intestinal *débris.* By careful dieting, moreover, much can often be done to diminish the irritating properties of the escaping matter. (*See* page 369.)

The lower bowel may be well cleared by enemata. Mr. Makins advises that no food be given by mouth for a couple of days before the operation, and that the strength meanwhile be maintained by rectal feeding. This precaution, however, can seldom be necessary. The diet must be very spare for twenty-four hours before the operation, but the patient is likely to suffer in strength and in resolution if all food be denied.

The bowel above and below the opening should be washed out as well as is possible, both before the operation and during the administration of the anæsthetic. For this purpose a weak carbolic solution may be used.

The opening in the bowel is now plugged with non-absorbent cotton-wool. An elliptical incision is made in the skin. This incision will circumscribe the abnormal orifice, and will include the skin immediately around it (Fig. 360). This skin is seldom healthy, and the surgeon can well afford to sacrifice it. The long axis of the ellipse will be placed as is most convenient. It will, when in the median line, be vertical; when in the iliac region, it will probably be oblique. The sacrifice of skin should be liberal. The lateral parts of the cut (*d* and *c*, Fig. 360) are cautiously deepened till the peritoneum is reached, and the peritoneal cavity well opened.

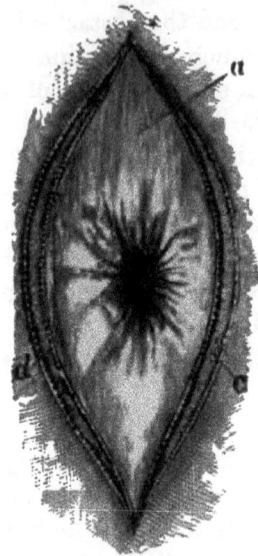

Fig. 360.—METHOD OF CLOS-
ING AN ARTIFICIAL ANUS.

a, Eczematous skin around
fæcal fistula : *d, c.* skin
wound.

A portion of a gum-elastic bougie is introduced into the artificial anus, and made to serve as a guide.

There is often difficulty in clearly opening the peritoneum on both sides. It is desirable, however, that the lateral incisions (*d* and *c*) should be sufficiently wide apart to render it probable that the surgeon is clear of the adhesions which surround the sinus.

The utmost caution must be observed in opening the abdomen, as a coil of adherent bowel may easily be cut into.

The tip of the finger is introduced through one of the lateral cuts, and the part explored. The position of the gut can be made out, and, if it be not closely adherent to the abdominal wall, the tract of the sinus can be traced.

The skin wound is now deepened all round, and, guided by the finger which is introduced into the abdominal cavity, is carried throughout through the peritoneum. There is thus isolated a little oval island, made up of the tissues of the abdominal parietes. Owing to the retraction of the skin, the actual sacrifice of muscular and aponeurotic tissues is small, and the parts concerned are usually found to be so modified by inflammation and atrophy that little normal-looking muscle tissue comes into the isolated patch. The tissues of the parietes about the abnormal opening are, as a rule, much altered, and such as are sacrificed can probably well be spared.

The bowel is now liberated as far as is possible, and is drawn into the wound with the island of skin attached to it. Sponges are wedged in around the bowel, to prevent the entrance of any fæcal matter into the peritoneal cavity. The surgeon now isolates, as well as he can, the mass of adhesive tissue which binds the gut to the parietes. This he does without opening the sinus, the position of which is indicated by the bougie.

The gut is clamped above and below by the fingers of an assistant. A small elliptical piece is excised from the intestinal wall. In the centre

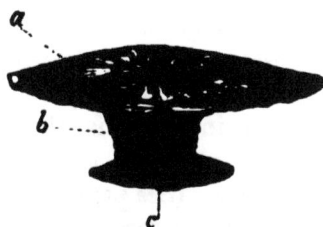

Fig. 361.—METHOD OF CLOSING AN ARTIFICIAL ANUS.

a, Skin with fæcal fistula ; b, tissues around the sinus ; c, bowel with internal orifice of the sinus.

of this ellipse will be the orifice into the gut. The long axis of the ellipse will coincide with that of the bowel. The parts are cleaned, the plug of wool is removed, and the gap made in the bowel is closed by a double row of sutures. The edges of the parietal wound are also united by sutures.

In the case of a deep sinus—such an one, for example, as may be met with in the iliac region leading to the cæcum—it is often possible to so cleanly divide the tissues around the sinus as to remove the diseased parts in a single piece, which will have the outline and arrangement shown in Fig. 361.

When a sinus burrows or follows a devious course, or is double, then this operation cannot be carried out without an accidental opening of the fistulous passage.

It is well, however, that the ill-conditioned inflammatory tissue in which the sinus is, as it were, buried, should be

Various plastic operations have been proposed for closing, the simpler forms of fæcal fistula, but I am not aware that much success has attended the practice. Attempts at closure, brought about by means of simple or reversed skin flaps, are not, on common surgical grounds, likely to be attended with satisfactory results.

Method No. 2.—The patient is prepared in the manner already described, and the skin around the opening is placed in as healthy a condition as is possible. The bowel is lightly plugged. The integument is excised by means of an elliptical incision, and the isolated part of the parietes thus defined is entirely removed before the conclusion of the operation. The abdomen is opened as in the previous operation. The involved loop of bowel is freed from adhesions as far as is necessary, and is drawn forwards, together with the oval isolated piece of the parietes which still adheres to it.

The intestine is clamped above and below, the plug of wool is removed, and as much of the gut is excised as is necessary. (*See* page 321.)

After the resection the divided ends of the intestine are united by suture in the manner described in a previous section (page 323).

The most convenient clamps are those introduced by Mr. Makins (Fig. 342).

After the bowel has been united, the wound in the abdominal parietes is closed by sutures in the usual way. It is to be remembered that the lower segment of intestine will be much narrower than the upper.

The resection is carried out upon the lines already laid down.

Mr. Makins, in a valuable paper in the *St. Thomas's Hospital Reports* for 1888, has collected thirty-nine examples of resection of intestine for the cure of artificial anus. The mortality was 38·4 per cent. Of the twenty-four patients who recovered, three were still left with a fæcal fistula.

Method No. 3.—The procedures described in this section are concerned with the removal of the obstructing spur or *éperon.* After the removal or obliteration of that fold, spontaneous closure of the artificial anus has many times followed.

The simplest method consists of introducing a substantial

piece of thick indiarubber tubing into the two orifices of the bowel. The tube tends to straighten itself, and, as a consequence, the bowel also ; it presses at the same time upon the *éperon*, and encourages its removal by displacement and absorption. A piece of silk is attached to the tubing, to prevent its slipping out of reach. Mr. Mitchell Banks has obtained some excellent results from the use of this simple measure.

Various methods of disposing of the spur by means of caustics, the ligature, and incision with a bistoury, need only be mentioned to be condemned.

The use of the enterotome is strongly advocated by some. Few illustrations of the use of this uncouth instrument have, however, been provided in Great Britain. Nevertheless no account of the treatment of artificial anus would be complete unless it revive this old-world mode of treatment. The following account is from Mr. Greig Smith's work on "Abdominal Surgery":—"Since the introduction of this instrument [the enterotome] by Dupuytren, and the great success that followed its use, the mode of destroying the spur by slow crushing has enjoyed a considerable amount of favour. Dupuytren's well-known instrument has been modified and improved by Blasius, Delpech, Reybard, Gross, and others. Probably the best of these is Gross's enterotome, which not only divides the spur, but removes it. Its structure is simply that of a large torsion forceps, the points of which are transformed into two circular opposing rings. These are made to include the spur, and are left till the compression of the blades cuts their way through, removing the greater part of the spur between them. As the compressed portion sloughs away, protective inflammation is set up in the neighbouring peritoneum. In a few cases, however, perforation has been caused by the enterotome, and death has resulted."

CHAPTER XII.

THE REMOVAL OF THE VERMIFORM APPENDIX.

DISEASED conditions of the appendix are of very common occurrence, and the important part played by this little process in the production of typhlitis has been fully recognised.

It would be out of place here to detail the conditions under which an excision of the appendix may be carried out.

The treatment of cases of relapsing typhlitis by removing the appendix during the period of quiescence offers, probably, more admirable results than are to be obtained in the treatment of any other form of the disease. I first advised this operation in 1887, and have elsewhere very fully dealt with the circumstances and details of the procedure (*Med.-Chir. Trans.*, vol. lxxi., page 165; *Lancet*, Feb. 9th, 1889; *Brit. Med. Journ.*, Nov. 9th, 1889; "The Surgical Treatment of Typhlitis," London, 1890).

In deciding upon this operation it must be borne in mind that the measure is only justifiable in properly-selected cases.

The Operation.—The chief points in connection with the operation itself are the following :—

1. Before the operation the position of the diseased appendix should be made out, if possible. Its position might have been indicated during one of the attacks.

2. The operation should not be performed until all inflammatory and other symptoms have quite subsided.

3. The incision should be made obliquely from above downwards and inwards over the cæcal region, its lower extremity ending just external to the epigastric artery. The incision should not be always made directly over the appendix or over the dullest region. If it be so placed, a number of adhesions will probably be encountered, and the demonstration of the peritoneal cavity might be difficult. The cæcum

or the appendix might be actually adherent to the anterior abdominal wall. The incising of the peritoneum should, therefore, be conducted with the very greatest care. It is well that the parietal cut should open the abdomen at a point just beyond the diseased area, and where no adhesions exist.

4. When the appendix and cæcum are exposed, the area of the operation should be cut off from the general abdominal cavity by sponges. If this plugging with sponges be well carried out, no blood should enter the peritoneal space.

5. All adhesions should be divided by cutting; none should be "broken down." The latter measure is apt to tear the bowel—or at least, to bare it of peritoneum.

6. The appendix should be lightly clamped close to the cæcum, and should be divided about half an inch from that intestine; it should not be secured by a simple ligature. The mucous membrane should be united by many fine sutures, or by a continuous suture; then the divided outer walls of the process should be brought together by a second row of sutures. When the wall of the little tube is greatly thickened by inflammatory exudation, it is practically impossible to bring the serous coats together. To still further secure the orifice, the stump of the appendix might be lightly attached to any adjacent surface of peritoneum, or it may be covered by an omental graft.

7. The abdominal wound should be closed; no drain is required.

During the progress of the operation any adhesions likely to give rise to future trouble might be dealt with; this more especially applies to adherent omentum, or to adhesions binding down coils of small intestine. If the appendix be closely adherent to the ureter, or to a coil of the ileum, or be found deeply attached in the pelvis, its removal may be attended with very considerable difficulties. The management of such a case must be left to the judgment of the individual surgeon.

Before commencing the operation the surgeon must be prepared for such difficulties. Some cases are remarkably simple, and the removal of the diseased process can be effected in a few minutes. In other instances the surgeon's movements are seriously hampered by adhesions. Parts are

a a 2

densely matted together in such a way that their recognition is very difficult. The confusion may be almost inextricable, and the risk of wounding the bowel or the ureter, or important vessels, is considerable.

In two cases in which I was attempting to remove the appendix for the relief of relapsing typhlitis I was compelled to abandon the project.

I have excised the appendix in a large number of cases, and up to the present time have to record no death as resulting from the operation.

CHAPTER XIII.

Operations on the Stomach.

Anatomical Points.—The position of the stomach, and its relations to surrounding parts, are much influenced by the degree of distension which it exhibits, and are further apt to be modified by the effects of disease, either in its own walls or in the structures which surround it.

When empty, the stomach lies at the back of the abdomen, beneath the liver, and some little way from the surface. When distended, the greater curvature is elevated and carried forwards, the anterior surface is turned upwards, and the posterior downwards. The direction of the rotation depends mainly upon the fixity of the smaller curvature.

Normally, the lesser curvature looks upwards, backwards, and to the right. When distended, the anterior surface is brought well against the anterior belly wall, and the viscus may occupy the whole of the median line as far as the navel. In obstruction of the pylorus the dilated stomach may nearly fill the abdomen, and its greater curvature may reach to the groin. (*See* Fig. 378.)

Under normal conditions, the *cardiac orifice* is situate behind the seventh left costal cartilage, about one inch from the sternum. The *pylorus*, when the viscus is empty, lies just to the right of the middle line, from two to three inches below the sterno-xiphoid articulation, and on a level with a line drawn between the bony ends of the seventh ribs (Fig. 362). When distended, the pylorus may be moved nearly three inches to the right of this point (Braune).

The *fundus* of the stomach reaches on the left side to a point as high as the level of the sixth chondro-sternal articulation.

The *uncovered area of the stomach* is normally represented by a triangle, the right side of which is formed by the edge of

the liver, the left a
ninth costal cartila₃
drawn between th₄
(Fig. 362).

The tip of *the α*
landmark, and it is
points out that it ha₄
ninth cartilage by ₄
width, that it plays
under the finger a s₄

The position of
subcostal angle is 1
conditions it may be
ninth right cartilage

The *pyloric* open₄
of 16 m.m. This a₄
sixpenny-piece.

Operations.—Th₄
will be described :—

    1. Gastrosto₄
    2. Gastrotom
    3. Loreta's o
    4. Resection
    5. Gastro-en₄

This operation co
ing (*stoma*) in the s
purpose that the p
' mouth."

Gastrostomy is c
gullet, especially in ₄

History of the
abbreviated from t₄
' Abdominal Surgery.
advocated this meas₄
which were beyond l₄
of the operation with

A little later, Blo₄
forming gastric fistul

In 1849 Sédillot performed the first operation upon the human subject. The patient died. The same result followed in a second and a third case. Fenger carried out the operation in 1853. This patient also died.

In 1858 Mr. Cooper Forster, of Guy's Hospital, performed the first gastrostomy in England, but with a fatal result. The operation was attempted by Günther, Gross, Curling, Bryant, and others, but in each case death ensued. The first satisfactory result was obtained in 1874 by Mr. Sydney Jones.

The operation has since this date advanced, and the establishment of the procedure as a justifiable surgical measure is largely due to Mr. Howse, who advocated the performance of the operation in two stages.

The practice of delaying the opening of the stomach had been previously advised by both Egebert and Nélaton.

Preparation of the Patient.—If the patient is no longer able to swallow, the strength should be supported by nutrient enemata. One such injection, containing an ounce of brandy, may be given just before the operation. There is no need to adopt any especial means for distending the stomach. The less the patient is disturbed the better. He should not be placed upon cold macintosh sheets spread upon an exposed operating-table; the operation can be well enough done as the subject lies in bed. The dragging of the patient from the bed to the table and back again can do no other than harm. The body should be well covered up with blankets, and the limbs surrounded by hot-water bottles.

Deep anæsthesia is not required, and ether is to be preferred to chloroform. I have performed the operation when so small an amount of ether has been given that the patient, while complaining of no great pain, has yet been dimly conscious of all the steps of the operation.

The quicker the operation can be carried out, within reason, the better.

The skin of the abdomen must be thoroughly cleansed before the operation, and a pad of lint, soaked in some warm antiseptic solution, may be placed over the region of the stomach some hours before the anæsthetic is given.

The patient lies in the recumbent position, close to the left

side of the couch.   The left arm may be placed behind the
back.   The surgeon stands to the left of the patient, and the
chief assistant to the right.

The Instruments Required.—Scalpels ; blunt-pointed
bistoury; dissecting forceps ; toothed or "nibbed" forceps ;
pressure and artery forceps ; scissors ; metal retractors; blunt
hooks ; curved needles and needle-holder ; straight needles for
the parietal wound ; sponges in holders ; sutures; ligatures,
etc.; sharp tenotome to open the stomach.

The Operation.—The operation is described as it is carried
out when performed in two stages.

1. **The Parietal Incision.**—The surgeon should endeavour
to mark out the lower
edge of the liver by per-
cussion and palpation.
The normal position of
this edge has already
been given (page 400)
The liver, however, in
the operation area may
be found, as high up as
the level of the xiphoid
cartilage, or as low down
as the level of the
ninth costal cartilage.
In cases of stricture of
the gullet, the organ is usually a little lower than normal
owing to the empty condition of the stomach and intestines.

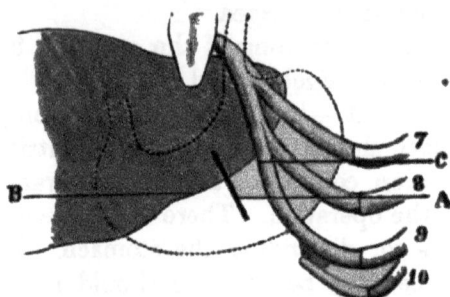

Fig. 362.—A, The incision for gastrostomy ; B,
The margin of the liver ; c, The margin of the
costal cartilages ; 7, 8, 9, and 10, The seventh to
the tenth costal cartilages.

The incision is oblique, is parallel to the margin of the low
costal cartilages, and is about one inch from that margin. Its
length is about two and a half inches, and may be modified
according to the thickness of the parietes.

The centre of the incision should correspond to a point
from three-fourths of an inch to one inch below the margin of
the liver (Fig. 362).

If the cut be too near to the ribs, the wound is apt to be
needlessly disturbed by the movements of the thorax, and too
little tissue is left on the outer margin of the wound to give
hold to the sutures. The edge of the cartilages comes also
in the surgeon's way.

If the cut be too low down, the stomach is missed, or undue traction is made upon its walls. If it be too high up, the liver comes in the way; and although the stomach may be dragged up from beneath the liver, yet the sharp margin of that organ is apt to bear with injurious pressure upon the line of sutures which unite the stomach to the parietes.

The incision is carried through the tissues of the abdominal wall. The fibres of the external oblique muscle will be found to run almost at right angles to the line of the wound, and the fibres of the internal oblique to be nearly parallel with that line. The transversalis muscle will be cut transversely. The incision will probably cross the left semilunar line, in which case some fibres of the rectus are exposed.

The peritoneum is reached, and is divided to the full length of the original wound.

Modifications of the incision are described in the Comment upon the operation.

2. **The Exposure of the Stomach.**—Retractors are introduced into the wound, and search made for the stomach. The liver will come into view, and below the margin of that organ the stomach may at once be detected. It is recognised by the smoothness and absolute opacity of its surface, by its faint pink colour, and by the thickness and stiffness of its wall, as demonstrated by pinching up a fold between the thumb and finger. To make the identification more certain, the relations of the viscus to adjacent structures, and especially to the liver, should be made out.

The colon has been mistaken for the stomach, and has been opened under the influence of that error. The stomach is usually contracted, and lies high up, under cover of the left lobe of the liver. In such case, the omentum or the transverse colon commonly presents. By means of a piece of fine Turkey sponge in a holder, the colon may be thrust downwards into the abdomen, and the stomach thus brought into view; or the surgeon may draw the colon downwards with his fingers. The omentum is more conveniently pushed away by means of the sponge, to the rough surface of which it readily attaches itself.

In any case of doubt the surgeon should follow the under-surface of the liver with his finger as far as the portal fissure.

Thence he is conducted to the stomach by the gastro-hepatic omentum. Farabeuf advises the following method:—The forefinger is passed back along the under-surface of the left lobe of the liver to the vertebral column, where, through the thin gastro-hepatic omentum, the aorta may be felt. It is then carried a little to the left, still keeping to the depths of the abdomen and high up under the diaphragm, when a fold (*une cravate*) more or less thick is met with. This is the lesser curvature of the stomach.

The stomach should be drawn to the wound, and the spot at which to open it must be determined upon.

This spot should be as near the greater curvature as possible, and at a part free from large veins. It is most important, however, that the new opening should be so placed as to avoid any traction upon the stomach.

As soon as the situation of the "stoma" has been determined upon, the stomach wall may be lightly seized at the centre of the selected area by means of pressure forceps. By means of these forceps the organ can be drawn forwards and held in excellent position while the sutures are being introduced.

3. The Fixing of the Stomach.—This is best effected by means of silkworm-gut sutures and Hagedorn's needles. The needles should be of moderate size (about No. 5), and fully curved. They are conveniently introduced by means of Hagedorn's needle-holder.

The stomach is drawn well forwards into the wound, and each needle is made to take a good hold of the gastric wall. It should penetrate all the coats except the mucous. The needle is then carried through the peritoneum, and ultimately through the muscular layers of the parietes and the skin. In order to make the inclusion of the peritoneum simple and certain, it is as well to fix it on either side with pressure forceps, by means of which the membrane can be brought well into view while the needles are being passed.

The sutures should be so inserted as to circumscribe an area on the stomach about equal to a shilling-piece. From six to ten sutures will suffice. It is as well to introduce several of the main sutures before any are tied. The sutures should take up enough of the stomach wall to secure a good hold. The mucous coat must not be punctured, and each stitch must be very securely tied. There should be no dragging upon any part of the stomach. The centre of the area circumscribed by the sutures will be represented by that part of the stomach wall to which the pressure forceps are attached. In the place of these forceps a long silkworm-gut suture is passed through the serous and muscular coats. It is left in the form of a long loop, and serves as a sure guide to the spot to be opened when the second stage of the operation is reached.

Before the stitches are introduced into the stomach, the upper and lower extremities of the parietal wound will have been transfixed by silkworm-gut sutures, introduced by means of straight needles passed through the whole thickness of the abdominal wall.

After the stomach has been secured, these sutures are drawn tight and are tied.

The wound and the exposed surface of the stomach are now dusted with iodoform, and the part is covered by a substantial pad of wool supported by a flannel roller.

This completes the first stage of the operation.

4. The Opening of the Stomach.—This constitutes the second stage of the gastrostomy.

The time that is allowed to elapse before the stomach is opened must depend upon the circumstances of the case. There can be no particular object to be gained by delaying the opening beyond the fifth day.

In a large number of cases the second stage of the gastrostomy may be carried out on the third day.

No very valid arguments have been advanced in favour of effecting the opening at the time of the first operation, and of completing the procedure at one sitting.

If the case be in any way suited for gastrostomy, the patient will be well able to postpone direct feeding through the stomach for eight or twelve hours. Even this period of time will suffice to form such a barrier of lymph about the suture line as will prevent the entrance of fluid into the peritoneal cavity during the act of feeding. Moreover, such a space of time will allow the patient to recover from the effects of the anæsthetic and the disposition to vomit, which is often noticed.

If care be observed there is practically no risk of any extravasation taking place during the feeding; and even if it be assumed that the peritoneal cavity is not securely sealed there is still no difficulty in preventing such an accident.

If it be determined to effect an opening into the stomach within a few hours of the first operation, the mode of suturing above described will be found to suffice. The attachment of the viscus to the parietes may in such case be rendered doubly secure by a series of fine silk sutures which are interposed between the main stitches and which connect... the parietal peritoneum and the outer coats of the stomach.

Should the surgeon be doubtful as to the security afforded by the method of suturing detailed he may make use of the more elaborate measure advised by Mr. Greig Smith. This measure is a modification of that introduced by Mr. Howse and is described as follows:—

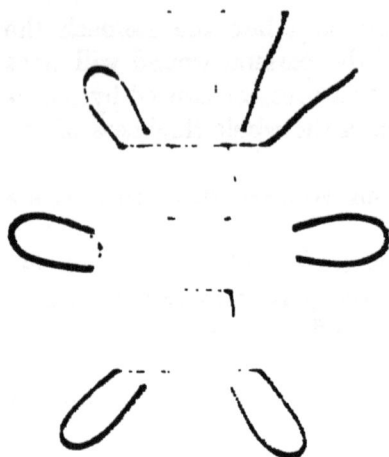

Fig. —— A DIAGRAM TO SHOW THE ... OF STOMACH TO PARIETES ...

"First, having devised a suitable ... insert ... loops of suture very near the spot where the opening is to be made. By these the stomach is manipulated during the process ... suturing and they serve to ... when the opening is made. Then with a round needle threaded with ... silk ... pass a continuous suture ... about two inches in diameter under the peritoneum ... At every third ... the needle is taken out and re-inserted so that ... loops, each about half an inch ... length are ... in the serous surface. This ... corresponding ... in the ... with a ... round-bodied needle ... an eye is passed through ... each of the loops ... and when the ... is ... through a piece of ...

rubber tubing is slipped under it. The loops are pulled with moderate tightness over the rubber tubing from each end of the incision. Finally, the ends of the silver sutures are hooked under the tubing, and serve to keep the exposed part of the stomach well up to the gaping wound " (Fig. 364).

In cases in which it appears to be necessary to feed the patient at once, some surgeons introduce, every few hours, a small amount of food through a large hypodermic syringe capable of holding two drachms. The puncture must be repeated at each occasion of feeding.

If it be intended to postpone the opening of the stomach for a week or so, the viscus may be secured in a very simple way by means of two hare-lip pins. These pins must be stout, and are inserted under the serous and muscular coats of the stomach in lines transverse to the direction of the wound, and they enclose a square area of the gastric wall whose sides measure about three-quarters of an inch.

The ends of the pins are protected by short lengths of india-rubber tubing.

During the time that elapses between the first and second stages of the operation the patient may be fed through the mouth if he can

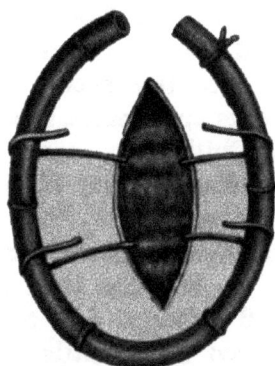

Fig. 364.—METHOD OF FIXING THE STOMACH TO THE PARIETES IN GASTROSTOMY. (*Greig Smith.*)

still swallow, and in any case nutrient enemata must be regularly given.

Feeding through an œsophageal tube is to be avoided, as it usually causes retching and coughing.

No morphia is required. Every means must be taken to support the heat of the body.

The actual opening of the stomach is a very simple matter. It is painless, and no anæsthetic is required. Assuming that four or five days have elapsed, the wound will be found to be somewhat contracted and puckered in. The depths of the wound will be occupied by a dry crust of iodoform mingled with a considerable quantity of lymph. The

parts are well and carefully washed, and then as carefully
dried. For this purpose nothing answers better than pledgets
of Tillmann's dressing.

The guiding suture is drawn upon, and the gastric wall is
pierced close to it by means of a sharp tenotome. Care must
be taken that the instrument penetrates all the coats of the
stomach, and does not force the undivided and loose mucous
coat before it. The knife is withdrawn, and a director introduced; and, guided by the latter instrument, an indiarubber
tube, the size of a No. 8 catheter, is passed into the stomach.
The hole made should be as small as possible, and the tube
should be gripped firmly by the walls of the stomach. Before
effecting the opening, the bottom of the wound may be
packed with Tillmann's dressing, which will absorb any blood,
and, later, any fluid which may escape from the tube.

The tube should be about eighteen inches in length, and
to its upper end a small glass funnel is affixed, covered at the
top with thin gauze.

The Feeding of the Patient and the After-treatment.—
The amount of food introduced on the occasion when the
stomach is opened must depend upon the patient's condition.
If no food has been swallowed for a considerable period, it
will suffice at first to introduce only a few drachms of milk
mixed with a little brandy. The quantity can be gradually
increased. If, however, the patient has been able to take
some food through the gullet up to the time of the operation,
his first meal may consist of from four to eight ounces of a
mixture of milk, egg, and brandy. This is slowly poured in
through the funnel, the gauze covering of which prevents any
semi-solid particles from entering and blocking the tube. A
pad of Tillmann's dressing packed around the aperture in the
stomach will absorb any fluid which may escape. As a
matter of fact, however, such escape is very seldom to be
anticipated.

After the feeding the tube is left in place. It is secured
to the ribs in the form of a coil by means of strips of plaster.
Its end is left open, and serves to afford escape to any fluid
which the stomach might attempt to reject. This open end
is received by a pad of absorbent wool.

The skin around the margin of the "stoma" is smeared.

with vaseline, is kept very clean, and well dusted with bi-carbonate of soda. A plug of Tillmann's dressing occupies the depths of the wound.

The feeding should be repeated frequently, but the quantity administered each time should be small.

The diet will consist of milk, eggs, beef-tea, soups, tea, cocoa, and a proper allowance of water.

The tube must be removed every day and a new one substituted. When the fistula is established, the tube may be left out—if it causes irritation—and be introduced when required. When the tube is removed, a pad of *non*-absorbent wool dressing should be placed over the orifice, and be kept in place by a large pad of some absorbent material in cases of regurgitation.

All food administered should be of the temperature of the body. As time advances, more food may be given, but at less frequent intervals. The fistula will in process of time become enlarged, and then very finely-minced meat and pulped vegetables may be introduced into the stomach by means of a suitable syringe.

The patient's own feelings afford the best guide to the value of certain foods and the amount and mode of their administration.

Leakage of gastric juice and regurgitation of food are often due to the stomach having been opened too near to the pylorus. The patient who is the subject of such trouble should be fed in the recumbent position, and lying upon the left side.

The irritation produced by the escape of gastric juice is best met by constant attention to cleanliness, to the very frequent changing of dry absorbent pads, and to the liberal powdering of the part with bicarbonate of soda.

Comment.—Many forms of incision have been advised and carried out. Some have employed an incision in the median line, others a vertical incision in the left linea semilunaris. Sédillot used a cross cut below the xiphoid cartilage. Howse prefers a vertical incision in the sheath of the rectus, a little to the inner side of its outer border. The vertical fibres of the rectus are exposed and are separated (not cut) with the handle of the scalpel. The posterior part of the sheath is thus reached. It is divided vertically, and the abdominal cavity opened. By this method it is hoped that a kind of sphincter action may be obtained for the fistulous opening.

The incision has the disadvantage of bringing the wound area somewhat closer to the pyloric region.

In carrying out the incision advised in the text, it should be remembered that, owing to the emaciation of the patient and the sunken condition of the abdomen, the part of the belly wall attached is—as the patient lies upon the back almost vertical. The integument, after passing over the margin of the ribs, turns suddenly backwards towards the spine, following the sunken abdominal wall.

There does not appear to be any especial advantage attending the practice of stitching the divided edges of the peritoneum to the margins of the skin wound before the wall of the stomach is secured in place. It may be claimed, however, for the method, that it brings the largest possible amount of peritoneum in contact at the suture line.

By many surgeons the area of the stomach circumscribed by the sutures is larger than that described in the text, and may equal in extent the surface of a penny.

The many different methods adopted of feeding the patient only serve to emphasise the fact that no rigid rule can be adhered to, and that this factor in the after-treatment must be modified according to the particular circumstances of each case.

Results of the Operation.—Gastrostomy cannot be said to occupy a very exalted or favoured position among surgical measures. It belongs to the forlorn category of last resource. It is for the most part carried out in patients who are dying of cancer, and whose death is being hastened by starvation.

One thing is certain, and that is—the operation is usually carried out too late. The condition of mal-nutrition into which the patient is allowed to sink is eminently favourable for the growth and progress of a cancerous mass. The stomach is allowed to pass into a state of atony before an attempt is made to introduce food into it.

The operation often gives great comfort to the patient, and relieves him of the distress attendant upon feeding by an œsophageal tube.

The troubles arising from the establishment of the fistula, the acute gastritis, the prolapse of the stomach wall, the inflammation of the skin caused by the escape of gastric juice, are all to a great extent preventable, and these after-evils have been considerably reduced as the *technique* of the operation and the management of the case have been improved.

The most elaborate statistics of the operation are those collected by Gross (207 cases) and by Zesas (162 cases). Gross gives a mortality of 29·47 per cent., and reckons that life is prolonged for an average period of eighty-two days in the cases of malignant disease.

The mortality of the operation in cases of cicatricial stricture was about the same, and the average duration of life after the stomach was opened was 295 days.

Zesas finds that the mortality of the operation (since the introduction of antiseptics) is as high as 70 per cent. It is evident that he adopts a different method of distinguishing death from the operation from death from the disease to that adopted by Gross. The periods of dying are divided as follows:—under 24 hours, 17 cases; under 30 hours, 69; between 1 and 12 months, 19; between 12 and 18 months, 1. The majority of the deaths are due to exhaustion, pneumonia, or peritonitis.

In one case of cancerous stricture of the gullet, the patient lived for 403 days after the stomach had been opened. The obstruction was complete at the time of the operation, which was performed by Dr. James Murphy (*Brit. Med. Journ.*, Oct. 28th, 1888).

2. GASTROTOMY.

This term is applied to the operation of opening the stomach for the purpose of removing a foreign body, or for exploration.

The cutting into the stomach for the removal of a foreign body is an operation of some antiquity.

"A surgeon and lithotomist named Shoval" removed a knife-handle measuring six and a half inches in length from the stomach of a young peasant on July 9th, 1635. No sutures were applied to the stomach, and five only to the external or parietal wound. The part was dressed with tepid

b b

balsam, bolar earth, white of egg, and alum. T
completely recovered (South's edition of Cheliu
page 391).

Many successful cases have been reported fre
time since that date.

The foreign bodies removed have included fo
handles, spoons, plates of false teeth, and masses of

The anatomical relations of the parts concerned
already dealt with.

The preparation of the patient, and the ii
required, are considered in the section on Gastrosto

There is no need to attempt to bring about a
distension of the stomach before the operation.
been effected by introducing ether into the visci
an œsophageal tube, or by causing the patient
measured quantities of tartaric acid and bicarbonat

The Operation.—The parietal incision may be n
same position as is advised in gastrostomy, with tl
cation—that it may be conveniently placed a little l
the margins of the ribs.

If the foreign body can be distinctly felt th
parietes, then the incision may be made directly ov
cut has been made in the left semilunar line. I
unusually large foreign bodies, such as are repr
masses of hair, the incision may be conveniently n
median line.

The incision should be at first about two and a
in length. It may be enlarged subsequently as req

The peritoneum is divided and the stomach
If the contained foreign body be sharp-pointed, the
tion of the stomach must be conducted with great

When the surgeon has determined upon the sp
the opening into the stomach is to be made, two sil
sutures may be passed through the serous and mus
of the viscus, one on either side of the area select
incision. These sutures are allowed to form lon
means of which the stomach can be drawn forward
in place.

The stomach wall should be gently drawn we
parietal wound, and before the opening is made

between the viscus and the margins of the parietal incision must be plugged with small Turkey sponges. The number of sponges introduced must be noted. In a case reported by Mr. Thornton, a sponge was left behind in the abdomen. It was removed on the next day, and the patient made a good recovery.

The incision into the stomach should be transverse to the long axis of the viscus, *i.e.*, in the line of the blood-vessels.

As soon as the organ has been opened, the forefinger is introduced and the position of the foreign body made out.

It should be so manipulated as to place it in the position best suited for ready removal.

Forceps will probably be required to effect the extraction. Care must be taken not to damage the wall of the stomach by careless manipulation, or by attempts to drag the foreign body through too small an incision.

If necessary, the stomach may be washed out after the foreign body has been extracted.

The next step is the closure of the wound by suture. Fine silk may be used for the purpose. The divided mucous membrane is first of all brought together by means of a continuous suture. This is best introduced by a small, fully-curved needle, held in a needle-holder. Hagedorn's needles and holder answer the purpose very well. The sutures must be well secured at each end, and must be tightly drawn throughout. The laxity of the gastric mucous membrane renders the application of this suture an easy matter.

The outer part of the gastric wound is closed by many points of Lembert's suture. These are of fine silk, are introduced by means of an ordinary milliner's needle, and include both the serous and the muscular coats. The details of the suture have been dealt with in the section on Enteroraphy (page 306).

Any of the methods employed for suturing the intestine may be adapted to the stomach. It is desirable, however, in any case that a special suture should be employed to unite the edges of the mucous membrane.

The parts having been well cleansed, the sponges are removed from the abdomen, and the guiding loops of silkworm gut from the stomach wall.

h h 2

The parietal incision is closed in the usual way.

After-treatment.—This should be carried out upon the lines indicated in other abdominal operations. (*See page 242*) Little or no food should be given by the mouth for three days. The patient should not be allowed to suck ice incessantly; on the other hand, there is no object to be gained by practically starving the patient; the stomach becomes irritable under such treatment. The diet for some two to three weeks should be of the very simplest and most easily-digested character, and the food should be given in small quantities and at frequent intervals.

Comment.—The incision in the stomach may need to be of considerable size. In Mr. Thornton's case the foreign body consisted of a ball of hair, and the gastric wound, after it had been closed by sutures, measured three inches.

Some thirteen or fourteen examples of gastrotomy have been recorded, and out of this number two died from the operation. The procedure cannot rank as a specially dangerous one.

SPECIAL APPLICATIONS OF GASTROTOMY.

1. For the Removal of Foreign Bodies impacted in the Cardiac Opening of the Œsophagus.

Dr. Richardson, of Harvard, succeeded in 1886 in removing a plate of teeth which were impacted in the lower end of the gullet, and which were reached through an opening made in the stomach. The whole hand was introduced into the stomach before the removal could be effected. Dr. Richardson advises a long oblique incision close to the margin of the left costal cartilages.

Dr. Bull, of New York, performed a very similar operation in 1887.

2. For the Treatment of Gastric Cancer by means of the Curette.

Dr. Bernays (*Annals of Surgery*, Dec., 1887) has attempted to treat cancer of the stomach as other malignant growths affecting mucous membranes in more accessible positions have been treated, viz., by curetting.

The stomach is exposed in the usual way, and its serous coat is then united by many sutures to the parietal peritoneum and muscles. An opening, about one inch and a half in length, is then made in the stomach wall, and the margins of the visceral wound and.of the parietal incision are united by many points of suture. The stomach is well washed out and its interior examined. The growth is removed partly by the finger-nails, partly by the sharp spoon. The stomach is finally irrigated with cold carbolised water. The fistula may be left open, in order that the process of curetting may be repeated; or it may, on the other hand, be closed.

In one case Dr. Bernays removed fourteen ounces of growth, and in another case fourteen drachms. Both patients were considerably relieved.

It appears likely that the operation may prove of value in selected cases, and may be placed in comparison with gastro-enterostomy and pylorectomy.

3. LORETA'S OPERATION.

By this term is understood an operation by means of which digital or instrumental dilatation of the orifices of the stomach can be carried out.

The operation was first performed by Professor Loreta, of Bologna, on Sept. 14th, 1882. The matter was brought to the notice of English surgeons by Mr. Holmes, who published a summary of Loreta's monograph in the *British Medical Journal* for Feb. 21st, 1885.

It is reported that Loreta himself has carried out the operation in more than thirty cases. It has been successfully adopted by many surgeons. Up to the present time the operation appears to have been performed twice only in England. The first case was by Mr. Hagyard, of Hull (*Brit. Med. Journ.*, Feb. 19th, 1887), and the second was by myself (*Brit. Med. Journ.*, May 18th, 1889). Both these cases were entirely successful.

An interesting case of digital exploration of the pylorus is reported by Mr. John Taylor (*Lancet*, May 3rd, 1891).

Dr. McBurney, of New York, has also operated twice, and his paper (*Annals of Surgery*, May, 1886) must be referred to. Dr. Barton, of Philadelphia, has operated twice, and his article upon the operation, published in the *New York Medical Record*, May 25th, 1889, is a valuable contribution to the literature of the subject.

The operation is carried out in cases of non-malignant stricture of the pylorus or of the cardiac orifice of the stomach. The measure may claim to have been attended with a considerable degree of success.

For matters relating to the preparation of the patient and the instruments required, the reader is referred to the section on Gastrostomy.

The Operation.—1. **The Dilatation of the Pylorus.**

The chief features of the procedure may be illustrated by the operation as it was carried out in the case of my own patient :—

I made a vertical incision, four inches in length, in the median line. The lower end of the cut reached as far as the umbilicus. The greatly-dilated stomach was at once exposed. The pylorus was at first difficult to define. It appeared to be embedded in a mass, of almost cartilaginous hardness, which was firmly adherent to the under-surface of the liver. Not only was the actual pyloric extremity of the stomach adherent to the liver, but a portion of the viscus itself, to the extent of some three square inches, was in like manner attached.

I divided the adhesions as freely as was possible. The segment of the liver to which they were attached was pale, and had the appearance of being atrophied. It was found impossible to quite free the pylorus, and to separate entirely the stomach from its attachment to the liver.

I then made a vertical opening into the stomach, midway between the two curvatures and about two inches from the pyloric orifice. Before this opening was made, the stomach was drawn as far forwards into the wound as possible, and was gently held by a small pair of dressing forceps, the blades of which were protected by indiarubber. The interval between the viscus and the parietes was plugged with sponges, so that any fluid escaping from the stomach would have been prevented from reaching the peritoneal cavity. To avoid bleeding, in opening the stomach I think that the incision should be vertical, and should not be too near the pylorus. It should be scarcely large enough to admit the index finger, with which it is at once plugged. In Mr. Hagyard's case, the bleeding at this stage of the operation is described as " terrific." A rush of escaping gas followed the opening of the stomach ; but as the wound was at once plugged with the right forefinger no fuid escaped, and there was no bleeding. Within the stomach, the portion of the gastric wall still adherent to the liver could be well made out. It was perfectly smooth.

The pylorus was surrounded by a ring of very dense tissue, and appeared as if set in cartilage. It would not take the point of the forefinger. I steadied the pylorus with the left hand while I gradually bored the right forefinger into the constricted orifice. The process of dilatation was slow, but in time the finger was introduced into the duodenum. Without withdrawing the finger from the stomach I enlarged the wound in the viscus with a bistoury, held in the left hand, and passed the middle finger into the stomach. The wound even now was small, and the fingers were closely embraced by the gastric wall. Under such conditions hæmorrhage was scarcely possible. The middle finger was passed through the pylorus and the forefinger inserted slowly after it. In a little while the orifice was sufficiently dilated to take the two fingers. During the process the pylorus was steadied by the left hand. This dilatation appeared to me to be quite sufficient, because an orifice admitting the two fingers together would have a circumference of about four inches. Loreta is reported to dilate the pylorus with the two forefingers until they are more than three inches apart. This would represent an opening with a circumference of not less than seven inches. Had dilatation to this extent been attempted in the present instance, the walls of the viscus would certainly have been ruptured. The normal pylorus has a diameter equal only to that of a sixpenny-piece.

The wound in the stomach was closed in the manner already described (page 419). The sponges were removed, the operation area cleansed, and the wound in the parietes closed by sutures in the usual way.

Morphia was administered for some days, and the patient was fed by nutrient enemata. Thirst was relieved by sucking a little ice. The stitches were removed on the seventh day. Milk and soda-water were given by the mouth on the ninth day. Solid food was taken on the eleventh day. The nutrient enemata were continued until the fourteenth day.

Loreta commences to feed his patients by the mouth on the fourth day.

Mr. Hagyard's patient took nothing but ice b
until the seventeenth day.

My patient made a good recovery, and when l
years after the operation, had had no return of b
and had an excellent appetite.

Comment.—It may be possible to effect t
manipulations through a parietal wound small
made in the present case.   Loreta at first made hi
inches in length, and placed it on the right of
line, the upper and inner end being about four c.
xiphoid cartilage, and the lower and outer end th
the ninth costal cartilage.

He subsequently abandoned this incision for
the linea alba.

Dr. William Gardner, of Adelaide (*Brit.*
Dec. 14th, 1889), made a transverse incision abou
in length "in the epigastric region."

It has been advised that the stomach shou
out before the operation.

The operation requires much patience, and it
that the utmost gentleness be exercised throughc

Some difficulty has been experienced in
adherent omentum.

If the finger cannot be at once introduc
pylorus, a catheter may be passed, and after
dressing forceps may be inserted in order t
necessary dilatation.   A urethral dilator was us
the opening in Mr. Hagyard's case.

The stomach has been opened in a case
stenosis, and the pylorus found to be norn
Dr. Marten, *Lancet*, August 2nd, 1890).

The pyloric orifice may be found to be exce
and may only be discovered with great difficulty.

In a case reported by Dr. Hale White a
(*Clin. Soc. Trans.*, 1891) the pylorus was
so small that it would only admit a No. 4 cat
was considered to be impossible to dilate th
tracted orifice at the time, the margins of the g
were united to those of the parietal incision. It
to dilate the pylorus gradually through the ｐ

thus established. The patient, however, died seventy-six hours after the operation.

In a case of fibrous stricture of the pylorus under my care, I opened the stomach, but could not find the orifice leading into the duodenum. A most careful search, in which every possible means of investigation was exhausted, failed to demonstrate any pyloric opening. The search extended over half an hour. The stomach was enormously dilated, and reached nearly to the groin. The viscus was emptied and well washed out. The wounds in both the stomach and the parietes were closed. The patient was relieved by the operation to a surprising extent, and remained for some months free of her distressing symptoms. In due course, however, all the troubles returned. I then proposed to make an attempt to find the pylorus through the duodenum, but the patient would not entertain the idea of another operation. In cases of recent stricture of the pylorus due to the swallowing of caustics, I would urge that the operation should be postponed until the symptoms of ulcer of the stomach have passed away, and that the stomach should then be opened and a temporary gastric fistula established, through which the stricture might be *gradually* dilated.

In a recent case of this character the tissues around the constricted part were so soft that the wall of the stomach gave way while I was endeavouring to force my forefinger through the narrow strait.

2. **Dilatation of the Cardiac Orifice.**—This operation has been successfully performed by Loreta in at least four cases. Two cases under other Italian surgeons also recovered. From Mr. Holmes's paper the following account is derived :—

The patient, aged twenty-four, had swallowed a caustic alkali. A stricture at the gastric end of the œsophagus followed, and failed to yield to treatment by means of bougies.

The operation was performed eleven months after the accident. An oblique incision, five inches in length, was made downwards and to the left, from the xiphoid cartilage.

The stomach was much contracted, and was found with difficulty. It was drawn out of the wound, and opened by means of a longitudinal incision, midway between the two curvatures, and as near the cardia as possible. The cardiac orifice was only discovered after a prolonged search. A dilator was then introduced into the opening. The instrument was like that used by Dupuytren in lithotomy, only longer. It measured eight inches from the joint to the ends of the blades, and was so constructed that the blades could not be separated more than five c.m. (A figure of "Dupuytren's lithotome" is given in Weiss's "Catalogue," Feb., 1888, page 148.) When the stricture had been dilated, the wound in the stomach was closed, and the operation completed in the usual way. Recovery was complete in eighteen days.

In two cases, on about the fourth day the patient was seized with dyspnœa, attended by abundant mucous expectoration from the trachea and bronchi, with serious disturbances of the circulation. These symptoms lasted some days.

4. RESECTION OF THE PYLORUS.

This operation consists in removing the pylorus, together with the adjacent parts of the stomach and of the commencement of the duodenum. After the excision the divided walls of the stomach and the bowel are brought together, and united by sutures.

The operation has been performed on account of non-malignant disease in a few isolated cases, the condition being that of pyloric ulcer or of pyloric stenosis. Apart from these unimportant exceptions, the operation has been limited to cases of cancer involving the pyloric orifice of the stomach.

The possibility of excising the diseased pylorus was suggested by more than one surgeon about the beginning of the present century. Experiments upon animals made by Günther, Gussenbauer, Winiwater, Wehr, and others, at a later period, demonstrated the possibility of the operation.

The first operation upon the human subject was performed by Péan in 1879, and the second by Rydygier in 1880. Both patients died. The first successful operation was carried out by Billroth in January, 1881.

Pylorectomy has been somewhat extensively performed in Germany, but the operation has not been received with much favour in Great Britain.

The operation, as it is described in the following sections

represents the method which has been practised and elaborated by Billroth.

Preparation of the Patient.—The stomach at the time of the operation should be empty. For a week or more previous to the operation, the diet should be very carefully regulated; and if sufficient food cannot be taken by the mouth, such feeding must be supplemented by nutrient enemata. Peptonised milk appears to be the most suitable food to be given by the mouth, and it may be supplemented by meat extracts, beef-tea, custard, and such other simple articles of diet as are readily taken by the patient, and are well borne.

For one week previous to the performance of the excision the stomach should be washed out daily, either with warm water or with some very weak warm antiseptic solution.

This washing is best effected by means of a syphon irrigator, or "syphon stomach-tube." Reversible stomach-pumps—or, indeed, all forms of stomach-pumps—are to be avoided.

The stomach should be washed out for the last time one or two hours before the anæsthetic is given.

The bowels must be thoroughly evacuated.

The abdominal wall will need to be carefully cleansed, and well washed and rubbed with a 1 in 30 solution of carbolic acid.

Every arrangement must be made to prevent undue loss of heat from the patient's body. The extremities should be enveloped in warm flannels, and a good supply of hot bottles should be at hand, to be employed directly after the operation.

It must be remembered that the operation involves a considerable time, and is attended with no small degree of shock.

The general arrangement of the table, the accessories of the operation, and the position of the surgeon and his assistants, are the same as in other abdominal operations. (*See* page 225.)

The Instruments Required.—Scalpel; blunt-pointed bistoury; dissecting and artery forceps; twelve pairs of pressure forceps; large pressure forceps; volsella; blunt-pointed scissors, straight and curved; sharp-pointed scissors;

broad spatulæ; rectangular retractors; intestinal clamp; fine-toothed forceps; three dozen rounded intestinal needles; needle - holder; aneurysm needle; blunt hooks; sponge-holders; fine silk; catgut; straight needles and suture material for the parietal wound; sponges, etc.

The Operation.—The operation may be divided into the following stages :—

    1st. The opening of the abdomen.

    2nd. The isolation of the pylorus.

    3rd. The excision of the diseased parts, and the uniting of the stomach and duodenum.

    4th. The closure of the parietal wound.

First Stage.—**The Opening of the Abdomen.**—The pyloric tumour having been defined, an incision is made in the skin over it. This incision should follow the long axis of the pyloric end of the stomach, and its centre should correspond to the most conspicuous part of the growth. This parietal wound will, therefore, be more or less transverse. The full incision will be about four or five inches in length, will be above the umbilicus, and will incline from above and from the left downwards, and to the right. The upper third of it will be to the left of the median line (Fig. 365, *a b*).

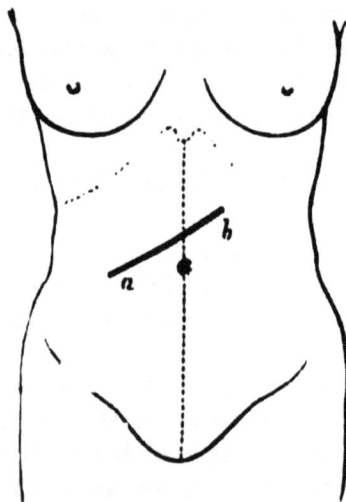

Fig. 365.—PARIETAL INCISION FOR PYLORECTOMY. (*Billroth.*)

If the pyloric tumour be very low, an attempt should be made to raise it before the skin is incised.

The incision should at first be only about two inches in length, in order that the fingers may be introduced for exploration. Such examination may reveal a condition which would induce the surgeon to abandon the operation.

The cut given is that known as Billroth's. Some surgeons employ a less transverse incision, others a vertical one in the median line, above the navel, or one just to the right of the median line, through the fibres of the rectus.

The right semilunar line has been employed, and by some operators a cruciform incision has been adopted.

The transverse incision, when compared with the vertical one, gives the surgeon more room, and permits of a readier exposure of the parts. It is, however, more difficult to close; it involves a greater division of muscle fibre, a more free bleeding, and it leaves a greater disposition to ventral hernia.

As soon as the abdomen has been opened, the diseased district is carefully explored, and its relations are noted.

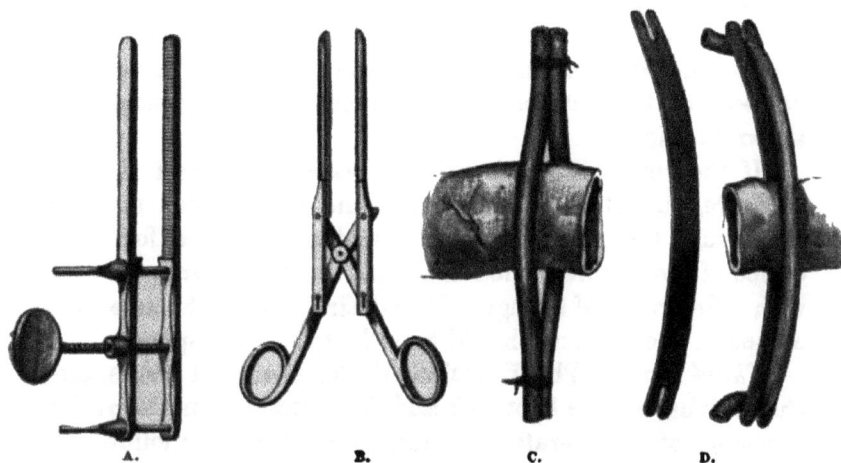

Fig. 366.—CLAMPS USED FOR THE DUODENUM AND PYLORUS IN PYLORECTOMY, ETC.
A, Billroth's; B, Gussenbauer's; C, Rydygier's; D, Heinecke's.

Second Stage.—**The Isolation of the Pylorus.**—This is the most difficult and the most tedious part of the procedure.

The growth is drawn as far as possible into the wound, and a number of sponges are carefully packed around the stomach and pylorus, in order to prevent extravasation into the peritoneal cavity. The number employed must be noted.

Slight adhesions to adjacent parts are divided, and the pylorus freed as far as is possible.

The great omentum is now divided close to the greater curvature, and over as small an area as is consistent with the efficient removal of the growth. It should be clamped in segments by means of two pairs of pressure forceps. The

omentum is divided between the forceps, and is then ligatured
upon the distal side of either pair.   In the place of this the
epiploon may be dealt with in sections, which are isolated by
means of double ligatures passed on an aneurysm needle.
The segments thus secured are divided between the ligatures,
which must be carefully tied.

The lesser omentum is treated in the same manner.

Any enlarged gland observed must be removed.

When the pyloric mass is free, a large flat sponge is
passed beneath it, and the other sponges, packed around the
part, must be rearranged.

Some surgeons now clamp both the stomach and the duodenum upon either side of the part to be removed.   Others
clamp the duodenum only.   Various clamps have been
devised for this purpose.   Those most usually employed are
shown in Fig. 366.

If the stomach has been well washed out, and if, as is
probable, but little food has for some time passed into the
duodenum, the use of clamps can seldom be called for.   The
orifice of the divided duodenum can be temporarily blocked
with a fine piece of sponge.   It is desirable that the area concerned in the excision should be well isolated by sponges.

Third Stage.—**The Excision of the Diseased Parts, and
the Uniting of the Stomach and Duodenum.**—In describing
this stage of the operation, I cannot do better than follow the
very lucid plan adopted by Mr. Barker in his " Manual of
Surgical Operations," and divide the procedure at this stage
into four steps.   It must be noted that the cut surfaces, to be
united after the excision, are of very unequal extent, and that
the normal disproportion between the stomach and duodenum is increased by the distension of the former and the
contraction of the latter.   It is desirable, whenever possible,
that the duodenum should be attached to the greater curvature of the stomach.

1st Step.—The stomach is divided about three-quarters of
an inch from the border of the growth—or, at all events, in
sound tissue.   This is effected by means of strong, straight,
blunt-pointed scissors.   The cut is made obliquely from above
downwards, and from left to right; it divides only about
two-thirds of the depth of the organ, and leaves a wide gaping

opening in the lesser curvature (Fig. 367). Bleeding vessels are secured with pressure forceps, and are subsequently ligatured if necessary. If the stomach be not empty, it may now be freed of its contents, and be very gently swabbed out with cotton-wool.

2nd Step.—The wound made is at once closed by means of a double row of sutures introduced in the manner already described, *i.e.*, a

Fig. 367.—PYLORECTOMY: THIRD STAGE, FIRST STEP.
(*Barker.*)

continuous suture for the mucous membrane, and interrupted sutures for the serous coat (page 419).

When all the sutures are in place, the end of the stomach is reduced to about the size of the lumen of the duodenum. The sutures are not cut short at once, but are collected together and held in a bundle by a pair of pressure forceps. They serve to secure and steady the stomach during and after the division of its remaining third (Fig. 368). The best material for the sutures is very fine silk. The continuous suture should be introduced by means of a straight milliner's needle, and the outer row of Lembert's sutures by means of curved intestinal needles held in a handle.

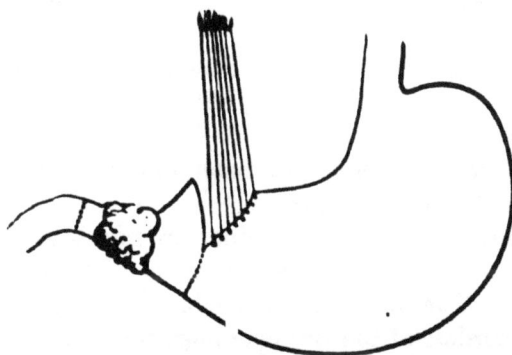

Fig. 368.—PYLORECTOMY: THIRD STAGE, SECOND STEP.
(*Barker.*)

3rd Step.—The remaining part of the stomach is now divided with the scissors, the cut following the oblique line of the incision already made in the viscus.

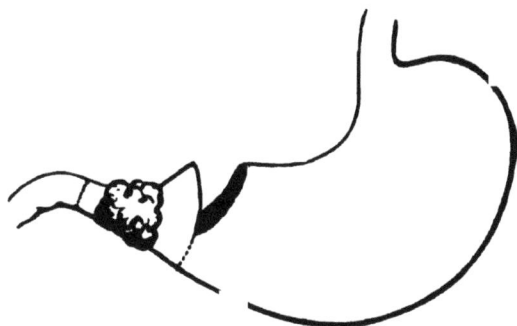

The stomach is now free, and its inner surface may be further cleansed if necessary. The growth is grasped by means of the volsella.

The duodenum is now severed by an oblique incision which runs from above downwards and to the right. It corresponds to the incision in the stomach, and must be entirely clear of the growth. The division at this stage concerns only the upper half of the intestine.

The lower half remains unsevered, and it is by means of it, or rather of the growth which is still attached to it, and which is grasped in the volsella, that the duodenum is held in place while the first sutures are being introduced (Fig. 369).

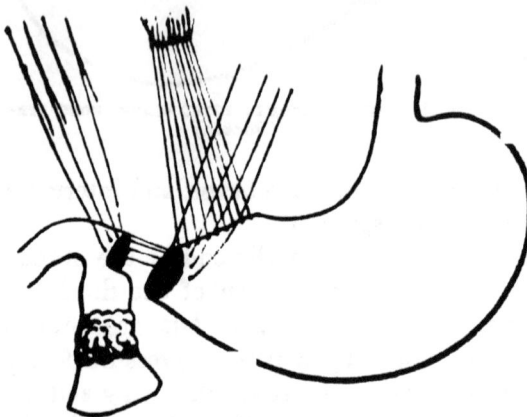

Fig. 369.—PYLORECTOMY : THIRD STAGE, THIRD STEP. (*Barker.*)

The margin of the orifice in the stomach is now adapted to that of the freshly-divided duodenum.

Where their upper borders come together, a series of close-set sutures are passed across from the one to the other, but are not yet tied. They are introduced after the manner of Lembert's suture, and involve all the coats of both the stomach and duodenum, with the exception of the mucous coat.

The posterior borders of the two openings are now brought into contact, and here the union is effected at once by means of Woelfler's sutures. The united sutures, which already pass between the upper borders of the two openings, serve to hold the two viscera together. Woelfler's sutures are applied from the inner side by means of curved needles armed with fine silk and carried in a needle-holder (Fig. 370).

The needle should pierce each layer about a centimètre from the cut edge. By this means a considerable breadth of the serous coats is brought into apposition. The needle is inserted between the mucous and muscular coats of the stomach, is carried through the muscular and serous coats of the viscus, then transfixes the same coats in the duodenum, and is brought out between the muscular and mucous layers of that bowel close to the cut edge (Fig. 371, a).

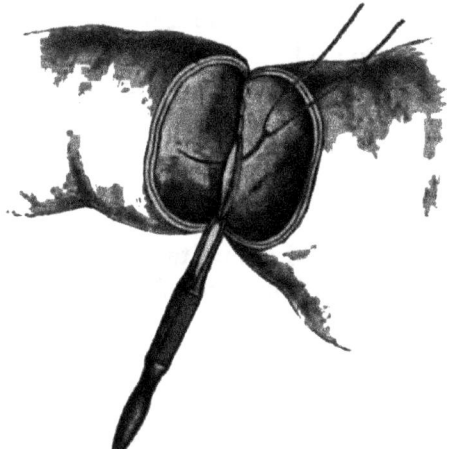

Fig. 370.—PYLORECTOMY: MANNER OF INTRODUCING WOELFLER'S SUTURES. (Billroth.)

The edges of the mucous membrane fall naturally into apposition; for, owing to the strong retraction of the muscular coat, the mucous lining always projects a little.

If at any point this be not the case, a very fine suture can be carried through the mucous membrane and the ends cut short (Fig. 371, b).

These sutures, both deep and superficial, are all tied tightly as soon as they have been inserted.

The sutures which already pass between the upper margins of the two openings may now be tied, and the superior and posterior margins of the orifices of the two viscera will thus be united.

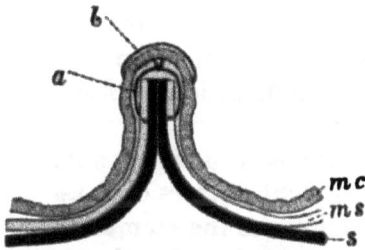

Fig. 371.—WOELFLER'S SUTURES.

a, Deep suture; b, Superficial suture: mc, Mucous coat; ms, Muscular coat; s, Serous coat.

4th Step.—The remaining half of the bowel is cut through in the same line as the first half. The parts are brought into close contact, and the remaining portions of the cut edges (i.e., the anterior and inferior parts) are united by means of a double row of sutures applied in the manner just described.

c c

All the sutures are now firmly tied, and all ends are short. Extra sutures may be introduced at any spot wh the union appears weak. A few additional sutures may conveniently be introduced at the spot where the transv row of sutures in the duodenum meet the longitudinal in the stomach.

Fourth Stage.—**The Union of the Parietal Wound**— edges of the omenta are united to the edges of the alt stomach by a few points of suture.

The whole field of the operation is most carefully clean the stomach is replaced, and finally the margins of parietal wound are united in the usual way.

Modifications of the Method—The appearance of the p after the u operation is ab in Fig. 372 may not be al possible to u the duodenum the greater cu ture in the ma described. The tent and the position of growth may n it more conven

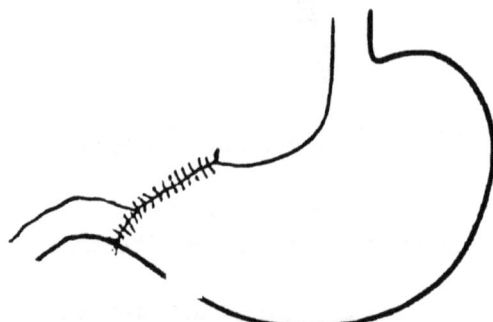

Fig. 372.—PYLORECTOMY. (*After Billroth.*)

to attach the bowel to the lesser curvature, as shown in 373, or to suture it to the divided margin of the stou midway between the two curvatures, as shown in Fig. The methods involved in these modifications differ i essential from that already described.

The After-treatment.—This will be conducted upon general lines laid down in the treatment of cases of abdou section, and especially such as implicate the stomach. pages 242, 414, and 420.) Every measure must be taken to vent the effects of shock. The operation is of long dur lasting two and even three hours.

The feeding of the patient is a matter of great import The strength cannot be maintained by nutrient ene and upon ice taken by the mouth. The best results followed in cases where food was early administered, and was well borne. In one of Billroth's earlier cases a tablespoonful of cold sour milk was given every hour the day after the

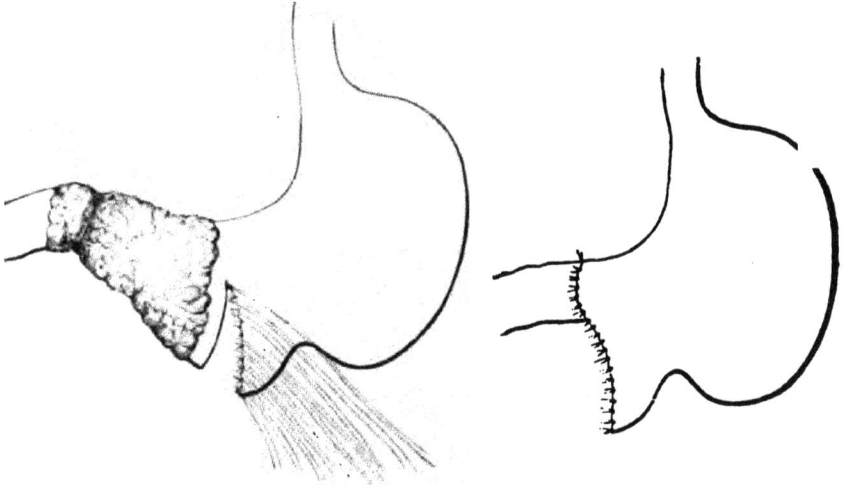

Fig. 373.—PYLORECTOMY. (*After Billroth.*)

operation. The quantity was gradually and cautiously increased. In fourteen days the patient was taking meat.

As Mr. Butlin observes: "No definite rules can be laid down with regard to the kind or amount of food which should be administered; but, in all probability, the food which the

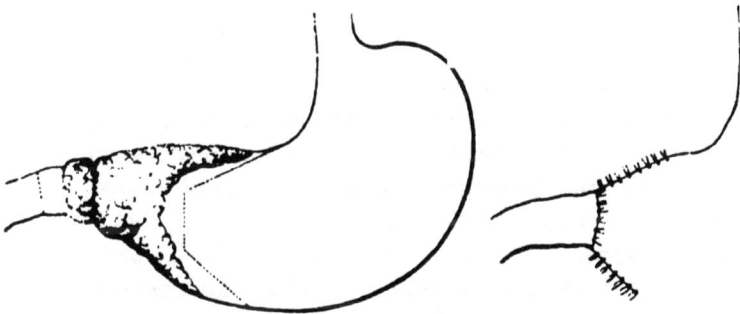

Fig. 374.—PYLORECTOMY. (*After Billroth.*)

patient could best tolerate before the operation will be the most useful during the first few days after it; and it is for this reason that the recommendation has been made that great

c c 2

care should be taken in the stages of preparation to discov
the variety and form of food which suits best each individu
patient."

Results.—Dr. Winslow (*Amer. Journ. Med. Sci.*, 18
lxxxix., page 345) has collected fifty-five cases of pylorecto
for cancer. Of these, forty-one died from the effects of
operation, a mortality of about 76 per cent.

Saltzmann (*Centralblatt für Chirurgie*, No. 33, 1885) de
with a larger number of cases, and states that the death-r
of the operation has fallen from 100 per cent. in 1880 to
per cent. in 1884, and 20 per cent. in 1885. Of the fatal ca
the greater number have died within the first twenty-f
hours. The chief causes of death have been collapse, in
tion, and peritonitis.

The influence which extensive adhesions have upon
result of the operation is well shown by Saltzmann.

In fourteen cases without adhesions the mortality
35·7 per cent., in seventeen with slight adhesions the morta
was 64·7 per cent., and in twenty-six cases with exten
adhesions it was 91·5 per cent.

The final results in the cases of those who have survi
the actual operation have not been good.

No case of cure has been reported. In all a more or
rapid recurrence has been the rule. So far, one patient o
appears to have survived the operation for a longer pe
than eighteen months.

Mr. Butlin, after an exhaustive examination of the
tistics of this operation, comes to the following conclus
which I would venture to endorse :—

" The excessive mortality due to the operation, the rapi
of recurrence in what have appeared to be most favour
cases for operation, the return of the symptoms of obstruct
in some, if not many, of the cases, and the fact that th
does not yet appear to be one case which can be claimed
genuine cure, lead me to doubt whether the operation
resection of the pylorus for cancer is ever a justifi
operation."

5. GASTRO-ENTEROSTOMY.

This operation consists in establishing a perma

fistulous opening between the stomach and some part of the small intestine.

The operation is advised in cases of cancer of the pylorus, and was first proposed, and for some time considered, as a substitute for excision of that part of the stomach.

The procedure was first devised and carried out by Woelfler in 1881 (*Centralblatt für Chirurgie,* Nov. 12th, 1881). It was found that the obstruction was overcome by diverting the course of the food matters, that the patient was greatly relieved, that life was prolonged, and that no grave gastric symptoms supervened. In course of time it became evident that gastro-enterostomy was not so much a mere substitute for pylorectomy, or a *dernier ressort* when excision could not be practised, but an operation that in its results could be fairly compared with the older operation, and that could be considered to be in many respects superior to it. Latterly the conviction has arisen that the majority of the cases of pyloric cancer can be better and more successfully treated by gastro-enterostomy than by excision of the diseased parts.

The published results of this operation, which are given on a subsequent page, tend distinctly to support this view.

· The procedure has now been carried out in a large number of cases, and it has been especially favoured by German surgeons.

A very admirable collection of the reported cases has been made by Mr. Herbert Page (*Med.-Chir. Trans.,* vol. lxxii., 1889), who also adds a successful case of his own to the list.

Two methods of performing the operation will be described, viz., the method of Woelfler, and that of Senn.

1. **Woelfler's Operation.**—The *preparation of the patient* is conducted upon the lines already laid down in the account of excision of the pylorus.

The *instruments* required are the same.

The Operation.—One of the most successful cases of Woelfler's operation as yet recorded was reported by Mr. Barker, and it may be safely said that his particular modification of the original measure represents the best method of performing the operation. The following is an account given by that surgeon (*Brit. Med. Journ.,* Feb. 13th, 1886).

The incision made in the
employed in excision of the
already made as to the compa
a vertical wound apply equally
Barker himself employed a med
of the cases collected by Mr. Pa
has been somewhat extensively

The stomach is exposed. the
relations of the parts to one and

" After pushing the omentu
to the left," writes Mr. Barker,
was caught in the fingers, a
incision. The middle of the an
was also drawn out and su
carbolised sponges. I now p
tubing through the mesentery
having emptied the portion o
the ends of the tubing tight ei
contents of the bowel into the
fixed each piece of tubing wi
loop of gut was now laid upon
opened, and a longitudinal fold
and a half from the great curv
the finger and thumb of the
collapsed gut. These incisions
serous and muscular tunics, and
viscera intact for the present
before, between finger and thi
sponding posterior edges of
suture, the needle entering
between mucous and muscular
the cut edges of the muscular
the serous surfaces were closely
either viscus was opened. Th
about one-eighth of an inch ape
of an inch beyond each end of
bowel.

" The moment had now com
intestine completely, and this
scissors through the mucous co

being ready to receive any fluid which might escape. A few drachms of succus entericus flowed from the bowel, little or nothing from the stomach opening. After careful cleansing, the anterior borders of both openings were now united by a row of interrupted fine silk sutures, introduced according to Czerny's method. When this was completed, the two openings were securely closed; but, as an extra precaution, the intestine was turned over, and the posterior suture was reinforced by a second row of interrupted sutures, placed about a quarter of an inch away from the first. The anterior was then similarly reinforced by a row of continuous sutures, taking up, as before, only the serous and muscular tunics. Lest there should be any 'kinking' of the latter, as in one of Billroth's cases, I stitched the efferent portion to the stomach wall, about three-quarters of an inch from the right extremity of the opening between the stomach and jejunum."

The operation is completed as in the procedure for excising the pylorus.

The After-treatment is much the same as that observed after pylorectomy. Food is given by the mouth as soon as the vomiting has passed off, and as soon as it is well borne. Solid food has been given as early as the sixth or eighth day. The recovery of some of the patients has been remarkably rapid.

Comment.—Considerable care should be exercised in selecting the loop of intestine which is to be attached to the stomach wall. It should be as near to the pylorus as is possible and convenient. It is quite impossible to make any use of the duodenum, and the first twelve inches or more of the jejunum can hardly be pressed into the service of the operator. It is best to bring the selected loop of bowel round the edge of the omentum, this structure having been pushed to the left. There is nothing to recommend the suggestion that the loop of bowel should be brought through a rent artificially made in the great omentum.

The loop of small intestine has been brought through a rent made in the transverse meso-colon (*Brit. Med. Journ.,* April 11th, 1891—Mr. Clarke's case).

The surgeon should not be satisfied with drawing out the very first loop of bowel which presents. In one case the

post-mortem revealed that tl
the stomach was only nine i
In another instance the point
above the valve.

Before incisions are made
bowel, it should be ascertain
brought readily and perfectly
without undue traction upon
Mr. Clarke, of Huddersfield, ir
used, it was found that the
and jejunum could not be ap
the stomach had to be closed,
convenient spot.

In the place of the india
text, Makins's clamp, or one
rectomy, may be convenientl
(*See* pages 320 and 429.)

The bleeding from the di
be copious and very troubleso:

In a case reported by
hæmorrhage from the ston
ligatures had been employed i

In two of the cases collect
the transverse colon was f
compressed by the loop of bo
been drawn across it.

In a patient operated o
revealed a stinking gaseous
In this case the loop of bow
opening made in the transven
that gangrene of the parts co

In one of the reported cas
the gut, the patient dying on

A considerable expenditi
operation. In Mr. Page's c
operation occupied three hou

Results.—Mr. Page has c
Woelfler's operation. Of thes
the operation, and twenty-tl
death ascribed to the immedi

ollapse, exhaustion, peritonitis, and kinking of the bowel.
n twelve cases of recovery, in which a full history is given,
t is to be noted that the average duration of life after the
operation was twenty-two weeks.

In Lücke's case the patient lived for fifty-six weeks in
comparative comfort, and was enabled to resume her house-
hold duties. In Barker's case an equally good result followed.
The patient survived the operation fifty-three weeks, and for
eight months may be said to have been perfectly comfortable.

The relief given in the majority of the cases has been very
noteworthy. One patient gained 21 lbs. in four weeks, and
another 19 lbs. in three weeks. A third patient was allowed
to get up on the twelfth day.

In some of the fatal cases the operation had certainly
been postponed until too late.

2. **Senn's Operation.**—The method of effecting an anastomosis between two more or less distant parts of the alimentary canal by means of perforated bone plates has been
already described (page 336).

The following is Dr. Senn's description of the operation as
applied to gastro-enterostomy :—

"The evening before the operation the stomach was
washed out by the syphon-tube, and again just before the
anæsthetic was administered. For the last irrigation, a five
per cent. solution of salicylate of soda was used.

"In all of the cases the incision was made through the
median line, and extended from near the ensiform cartilage
to the umbilicus. The opening in the stomach was made
parallel to the long axis of the organ, and at least an inch
and a half distant from the margin of the tumour. A continued suture of fine silk was applied around the whole
circumference of the opening, both for the purpose of arresting
hæmorrhage, and preventing bulging of the mucous membrane. In the intestine the opening was made between two
rubber ligatures, so as to prevent any extravasation of intestinal contents, and the margins of the wound were sutured in
a similar manner. The opening in the intestine was made
first, and the plate introduced and sutures adjusted, and the
loop retained in the lower angle of the wound, covered by a

warm compress. The large curvature of the st
pyloric orifice was then drawn sufficiently fo
wound to make the incision and introduce th
everything was ready for adjustment, the pa
visceral wound were carefully disinfected, dried
surface lightly scarified with an ordinary needl
corresponding to the size of the plate; the
(wounds) were then brought opposite each o
silk suture, embracing only the serous and
was applied behind the lower middle plate s
the middle lower suture was now tied, wh
approximated the two openings; the lateral su
tied, and lastly the anterior middle. The sutu
short and the ends buried. During the tying
it is necessary to exercise caution, that the
visceral wound are well embraced by the plate

" As in these cases the weight of the intest
siderable tension, I have taken the precaution
cases to apply a superficial continuous suture
tying the four sutures, so as to approximate
faces over the anterior margins of the plates.

"The necessary preparations being ███
assistance the operation can be finished in
thirty minutes. Neither shock nor peritoni██
any of the cases. Usually on the third day
of peptonised milk and beef-tea were given a
and solid diet during the second week."

Comment and *Results.*—This method
advantage of being completed in a compara█
and when the *technique* of the operation has
it seems probable that it will present the be█
forming gastro-enterostomy. It is quite ██
details of the operation are susceptible of im
the number of cases at present published is
would be scarcely fair to attempt a decided ██
general value of the procedure.

In one case (Senn, "Intestinal Surgery," p
fistula formed, and through the opening wh█
plate ligatures were expelled. In another ██
the plates were vomited up on the ninth day.

reported by the same surgeon fragments of the plates were passed per anum on the thirteenth day.

In more than one of the recorded cases severe and continued vomiting followed the operation. In two of these instances (cases by Mr. Clarke, of Huddersfield, *Lancet*, Dec. 9th, 1890; and *Brit. Med. Journ.*, April 11th, 1891) the vomiting was incessant from about the twelfth day until the patient's death, on the thirtieth day. Mr. Clarke concludes that in these cases the artificial opening must have closed. He adds that "in two, at least, of the failures of this operation, closure of the opening has occurred."

In one of Mr. Clarke's cases, after the plates had been introduced, it was found that the two openings could not be brought together. The gastric plate was removed, and the wound closed. A second opening was made in the stomach at a more convenient place, and the plate introduced afresh. The patient lived thirty days (*Brit. Med. Journ.*, April 11th, 1891).

I have collected nineteen examples of this operation. Three patients died from the immediate effects of the operation. The others are reported to have recovered.

In ten of these the accounts of the termination of the case are complete; and from these it would appear that the average duration of life after the gastro-enterostomy was less than ten weeks.

In one instance the patient's death did not take place until forty weeks after the operation.

CHAPTER XIV.

DUODENOSTOMY AND JEJUNOSTOMY.

THESE operations consist, as the names imply, in the establishing in the duodenum or jejunum ot an artificial opening or stoma, through which food can be introduced. The measures have been carried out in cases of stenosis of the pylorus of various kinds.

Duodenostomy was first performed by Langenbüch in 1879. The operation has been carried out in two stages. In one the bowel is attached to the wound in the parietes; in the other it is opened.

The operation has been performed several times, but in no instance does the patient appear to have survived.

In jejunostomy the artificial opening is made lower down in the intestine. This operation has not been performed many times, but it has been attended by some degree of success. It is claimed for this measure—when compared with gastro-enterostomy or pyloric resection—that the operation is very simple, that it is readily carried out, and, above all, that it may be very quickly performed. There is no risk of extravasation from the stomach, or of kinking of the bowel; the colon cannot be compressed, as has been the case in some of the examples of gastro-enterostomy; and more complete rest is given to the malignant growth.

The stomach is, however, excluded from the digestive process, and unless the artificial opening be made quite high up in the jejunum, the probability of gradual starvation is considerable. The stomach is not relieved, and no food can be taken by the mouth.

One of the most fully reported cases of this operation by Mr. Golding Bird was published in 1885 (*Clin. Soc. Trans.*, vol. xix.).

An oblique incision was made, in the same position as in pylorectomy. The malignant growth was examined, the transverse colon was drawn upwards, and the omentum was pushed to the left. The jejunum was sought for, and the gut was followed until its commencement was reached. The post-mortem in this case showed that the opening had been made two inches from the termination of the duodenum.

The bowel was attached to the margins of the parietal wound in the usual way, but the opening of the gut was deferred until the third day.

Mr. Golding Bird gives a very interesting account of the feeding of the patient, and of the indigestion which at first followed. The man improved, but died on the ninth day, through an accidental opening of the peritoneal cavity.

Anatomical Points.—The
of the diaphragm. Its c
right side by the ribs, fr
inclusive, and in front b
costal cartilages, from the
diaphragm being interpose

The liver extends to
two inches beyond the lef
middle line the gland lies
the stomach, and reaches a
cartilage and the navel.

The lower edge, as i
represented by a line dra
eighth left costal cartilag
the lower edge on the righ
inch below the margins
recumbent position the liv
entirely covered by the cos
It descends also on expirati
this disposition for mover
becomes necessary to stit
parietes.

" The extent of the live
of the body, is indicated b
close to its lower end, and
of the fifth chondro-stern
that of the sixth " (Quain).

The right lung lies in fr
upper border of the sixth r
as far down as the fifth int

Behind, the liver comes

at a part corresponding, both in position and width, to the tenth and eleventh dorsal vertebræ. On the extreme right the liver descends to the level of the second lumbar spine (Fig. 378).

It is needless to say that the relations of the viscus may be greatly altered by diseased conditions, especially by such as are attended by enlargement of the organ, or the development of abscesses or tumours within its substance.

The gall-bladder, when moderately distended, is pear-shaped, and measures about 10 c.m. in length and 3 c.m. in width at its fundus. It is capable of holding about 20 c.c.m. of bile.

The fundus touches the abdominal wall below the free end of the cartilage of the tenth right rib, and near the outer border of the right rectus muscle.

The fibrous coat of the gall-bladder is thin, but is remarkably firm and tough.

The cystic duct is about one inch in length, and turns a little towards the left. It joins the hepatic duct at an acute angle. The common bile duct measures about three inches. It descends in the lesser omentum in front of the portal vein, and to the right of the hepatic artery and its gastro-duodenal branch. It enters the right pancreatico-gastric fold behind the first part of the duodenum, and is crossed by the pancreatico-duodenal artery as it approaches and pierces the second part of the duodenum about its middle.

Operations upon the Liver.—The following operations will be described :—

1. Operations on hydatids of the liver.
2. Operations on hepatic abscess.
3. Hepatotomy.
4. Cholecystotomy.
5. Cholecystectomy.
6. Cholecystenterostomy.

1. OPERATIONS ON HYDATIDS OF THE LIVER.

The surgical measures adopted in the treatment of this affection may be considered under two headings :—(A) Measures intended to bring about the destruction of the parasite *in situ ;* and (B) The treatment by incision and the evacuation of the contents of the cyst.

A. **The Destruction of the Parasite** *in situ.*

The procedures carried out to effect this end may be spoken of as being of a comparatively mild nature. Many remarkable examples of cure have been reported in connection with these modes of treatment, but, on the whole, they must be regarded as somewhat speculative, as distinctly uncertain, and therefore as unsatisfactory. The two principal measures will be described:—

1. *Simple Puncture.*—The skin having been cleansed, a convenient spot is selected over the most prominent part of the tumour. An aspirator needle is driven in, and a certain quantity of the fluid contents of the cyst withdrawn. The amount removed has varied from a few ounces to three pints, and must obviously be influenced by the size of the cyst. Pain, faintness, cough, or the escape of blood or bile affords an indication to desist.

After the removal of the needle the puncture is covered with collodion, or with a pledget of wool dusted with iodoform.

The puncture is of no avail when suppuration is established. This simple tapping has been repeated many times in the same case.

The operation is not free from danger. Leakage into the peritoneal cavity has followed, and has led to a fatal peritonitis; the portal vein has been punctured (*Clin. Soc. Trans.*, vol. xi., page 230); and in more than one case sudden and fatal syncope has occurred.

After the evacuation of the fluid of the cyst some iodine solution has been injected, but the results have not been especially favourable.

2. *Electrolysis.*—This method of treatment has been fully investigated by Dr. Fagge and Mr. Durham (*Med.-Chir. Trans.*, vol. liv., page 1). The same may be said of the results as has been said of treatment by puncture.

In one case Mr. Jacobson made use of this method after a previous tapping had failed. Two electrolytic needles were passed into the most prominent part of the swelling, about two inches apart, and were then attached to wires, both connected with the negative pole of a galvanic battery of ten cells. A moistened sponge connected with the positive pole was placed on the skin at a little distance. The current was passed for half an hour. There was no constitutional disturbance, the tumour steadily diminished in size, and a good recovery took place.

B. **The Treatment by Incision.**

The operation may be performed in one or in two stages.

The first deliberate operation upon hydatids of the liver was performed by Mr. Tait in 1882.

He demonstrated the possibility and also the safety of the method of operation in one stage.

The subject has been very fully dealt with by Dr. W. Gardner, of Adelaide, and others, in the *Transactions of the Second Inter-Colonial Medical Congress* (1889).

1. *The Operation by One Stage.*—This measure is termed by some hepatotomy. It involves the opening of the abdominal cavity, the incision and evacuation of the hydatid cyst, and the suturing together of the margins of the hepatic and parietal wounds.

The skin having been well cleansed, an incision, about four inches in length, is made over the most prominent part of the tumour. The wound will probably be longitudinal, *i.e.*, in the long axis of the body. It should fall upon the abdominal part of the swelling—that is to say, should the most prominent portion of the tumour present in an intercostal space, it should not be incised there, owing to the difficulty of ensuring adequate drainage when the fluid is evacuated between two ribs.

The knife is carried through the parietes, and an examining finger is cautiously introduced into the abdominal cavity. The incision should at first be only about one inch and a half in length. It is extended in whatever direction appears most advantageous after the preliminary digital examination has been made.

The incision may fall upon a spot where the liver is already adherent to the parietes. If so, it is well. Should the digital exploration show that the viscus is adherent to an adjacent part of the abdominal wall, then the incision may be carried in that direction; or another and entirely distinct incision may be made over the adherent area.

In the majority of the uncomplicated cases of hydatids there are no adhesions.

d d

The liver is exposed, and the most convenient spot for evacuating the cyst determined upon. This area is circumscribed by many Turkey sponges, which are carefully wedged in all round, so as to prevent the escape of any fluid into the peritoneal cavity.

It will now be convenient to introduce the largest needle of an aspirator, and to withdraw enough of the contents of the cyst to remove all tension. The more fluid removed by the cannula the better, so long as too much time be not expended in the process.

The cyst is drawn as far forwards as possible, the needle puncture is enlarged with a scalpel, and the left forefinger is at once introduced into the opening. This digit serves to act as a plug, and at the same time it is a means of hooking or dragging the cyst forwards, so as to bring its opening well into the parietal wound.

The margins of the cyst wound should now be seized by two or more pressure forceps, and by means of these the lips of the cyst wound are drawn forwards, and are kept well approximated to the parietes while the main bulk of the contents of the cyst is escaping. By this means the whole cyst may often be evacuated without any fluid entering the peritoneal cavity.

Hæmorrhage from the hepatic incision may be arrested by sponge pressure, or by pressure forceps; or, failing these, by a continuous suture of catgut.

The cyst is now so far empty that no more fluid spontaneously escapes. The opening in the cyst is enlarged as far as is required, and its margins are held by means of additional pressure forceps, as one would hold the mouth of a bag. The finger is introduced, and the interior of the cyst is examined. Additional cysts may be discovered, and broken down and evacuated. The whole of the interior of the cyst should be well but gently cleared out. Dr. Gardiner advises douching the interior of the cyst with warm water, and the cautious use of forceps applied to the mother cyst, and guided by the operator's left forefinger.

The time is now come for uniting the margins of the hepatic wound to the margins of the parietal incision.

The edges of the cyst wound are still held with forceps,

and into the mouth of this wound a sponge is wedged. The sponges which have been packed around the operation area are now removed, and are carefully counted, as one or more may readily slip out of sight. The peritoneal cavity is cleansed. by means of sponges in holders in the usual way (page 231), and to this part of the operation special attention must be paid.

The margins of the opening in the cyst are now sutured to the edges of the parietal wound. The stitches may be interrupted, and of silkworm gut closely applied; or they may be continuous and of silk. Care must be taken that peritoneum is brought in contact with peritoneum. A curved Hagedorn's needle will be found useful in this part of the operation. If the cyst wall have been firmly secured, the cavity may be further evacuated and cleared out by means of Turkey sponges in holders; but all such manipulations must be conducted with the utmost gentleness.

A large drainage-tube is introduced and is fixed in position. For large cysts I use a tube with a diameter of one inch. It is useless to attempt to drain a cavity which has contained some pints or quarts with a tube with a lumen of one quarter of an inch.

The wound is dusted with iodoform, and covered with a large absorbent dressing of wool or of Tillmann's linen. It is secured in place by means of a many-tailed bandage.

The After-treatment consists of the frequent washing-out of the cyst cavity with some antiseptic solution, and the maintenance of the most absolute cleanliness and the most perfect drainage. An irrigator which provides a large stream is essential; and the cleansing solution may be composed of carbolic acid, creolin, corrosive sublimate, or weak iodine.

2. *The Operation by Two Stages.*—This operation aims at securing adhesion between the parietal peritoneum and the hepatic peritoneum over the seat of puncture.

The procedure to effect this end constitutes the first stage of the operation. The second stage is undertaken after an interval of some days, and is simply represented by the incising of the now adherent cyst.

It is claimed for the measure that it does away with the

risks attending the escape of blood or c
peritoneal cavity.

The operation in two stages has been
Volkmann, and is often known by his name

The parietal incision is made, and the p
opened. The cut edges of this part of the
may then be attached by a few points of sut
of the parietal wound. A dressing of gau
so firmly as to keep the abdominal wall a
contact with the liver.

Some surgeons prefer to secure the p
of the liver to the parietal peritoneum by
fine catgut. These are passed by mean:
Hagedorn's needle. Mr. Godlee advises th
pretty deeply into the substance of the li
stitches be in a double row.

The cyst is incised at the end of three, fo
no anæsthetic being, as a rule, required.

The exact method adopted by Mr. Gc
by the following account of the procedure
case of abscess of the liver (*Brit. Med.*
1890, page 123):—" I made a vertical in
and a half below the margin of the ribs.
most prominent part of the swelling, *i.e.,*
(from side to side) of the rectus, and
abdominal wall, found no adhesions at the
exposed. I therefore separated the rectus
layer of its sheath, so as to expose a portion
in Fig. 375. Then with Hagedorn's needles υ
were applied—the outer being interrupted
inner continuous and of catgut (*f*). The
into the liver substance, and the closure
be ascertained, complete." In this particul
was opened at once.

For the purpose of producing adhesions,
of the tumour through the parietes has
Bardeleben and others are in favour of prodi
means of Vienna paste or caustic potash.

The former method is uncertain, and
the latter is slow and painful, and in many

Should it be found, on examination, that stitches will not hold, two courses are, according to the practice of Dr. Gardner, open to the surgeon. In the first place, to pass a stitch on each side through the peritoneum and muscle only, and keep the sides of the incision apart by a tampon of sublimate gauze, sprinkled with iodoform.

If successful in securing adhesions, the cyst is opened later; but if no adhesions form, then the following method must be adopted:—The cyst having been exposed, and the abdominal walls pressed against it by means of a circle of sponges, the operator—who must be rapid in his movements—plunges in his knife, and cuts downwards sufficiently to enable two fingers of his left hand to be introduced. He then, by the side of his fingers, inserts four cardinal stitches, and ties them. The remaining steps of the operation are similar to those already described.

Observations and Comment upon the Two Methods.

Hydatid cysts of the liver have been successfully evacuated through the pleural cavity. This is illustrated by a case of Mr. Edmund Owen's. The incision was made in the right intercostal space; the pleura was sound and free from adhesions. The diaphragm was incised, the cyst exposed, and the tension upon its walls relieved by aspiration. The face of the sac was then "drawn through the diaphragm, and across the shallow pleural cavity to the skin wound, to which it was secured by four hare-lip pins. Thus the pleural wounds were placed in mutual contact."

On the fourth day the pleural surfaces were found to be firmly adherent; the cyst was then incised, and twenty-eight ounces of fluid were evacuated. No part of a rib was

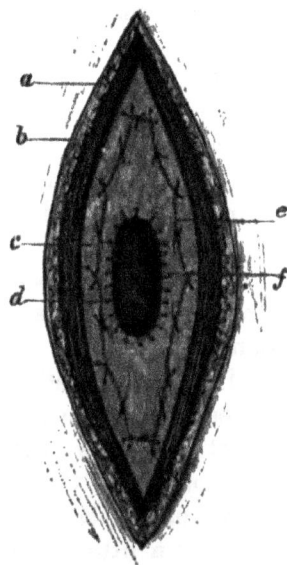

Fig. 375.—METHOD OF ATTACH-ING THE LIVER TO THE PARIETES. (*Godlee.*)

a, Subcutaneous fat; *b*, Rectus; *e*, Sheath of rectus; *d*, Liver; *e*, Interrupted suture; *f*, Continuous suture.

removed. The patient mac
Trans., vol. xxi., page 78).

Mr. Thornton has report(
of the pelvis was successfully
liver which had been opened
his cases a large hydatid cy:
cated with a large hydatid
through the abdominal sac (/
page 5).

In exposing the cyst by t|
tum has more than once beei
tumour, and to have hamper(

(For an account of the re:
see page 457.)

Of the two methods abo
by one stage would appear
to carry with it no particula
words, it has not been sho\
characteristic of the method
founded.

This latter method som
surgeon's movements; whe
extent and the stability (
variation, and those whic|
to completely shut off the
is acting a little in the dar
wall to the parietes is not
is secured by sutures, and
the contents of the cyst
Above all, much time is
of little moment in the (
may be of paramount impo
abscess.

If care be taken during t|
the escape of fluid into the |
minimum; and it must be di
is not done away with enti
mann's operation, especially '
out at so early a period as t
sutures are employed.

The direct operation by one stage may claim to be the more thorough and the more satisfactory, and to effect with more completeness the object the surgeon has in view.

It does not appear that these advantages are discounted by any unusual or special risks.

Mr. Godlee's method undoubtedly represents the best plan of carrying out the operation by two stages.

2. OPERATIONS ON HEPATIC ABSCESS.

What has been said about the treatment of hydatids of the liver may be said of hepatic abscess.

The abscess may be opened in three ways:—

1. **By Direct Incision,** when the abscess is "pointing," and when from the local tenderness, redness, and œdema, it is evident that adhesions exist, and that the pus is close under the skin. This measure needs no further comment.

2. **By Incision and Drainage carried out at One Sitting.**

The method observed is precisely similar in all points to that already described in connection with hydatid cysts (page 449). If care be taken, and if the operation be conducted upon the lines laid down, there is little danger of any pus finding its way into the peritoneal cavity.

After the abscess has been evacuated, a gentle examination of its interior may be made, to ascertain if another abscess or cyst exists. The abscess cavity should be well cleared out by means of a soft sponge in a holder. The manipulation must be gentle, as the abscess wall is readily damaged, and bleeding ensues.

The after-treatment of the case is the same, the main points being free drainage, frequent and free flushings-out with the irrigator, and the use of antiseptic measures throughout.

3. **By Incision and Drainage carried out in Two Stages.**

The proceeding employed is precisely identical with that already described in the account of hydatids of the liver (page 451). The best method is that employed by Mr. Godlee.

It has been pointed out that in dealing with the parasitic cyst, this method in two stages has no very great advantages. The same observations may apply to the case of hepatic abscess.

In addition to such objections as have been al
lated, the following may be noted :—

The adhesions which form, when no sutures a
may be insignificant, and may cover but a ver}
When the incision is made, that area may be
gressed.

Such adhesions cannot be firm until many
elapsed, and this delay may prove a serious matt
of an abscess which is rapidly approaching the su
over, after adhesions have been secured, the absce
signs of pointing at another spot distant from 1
site of the incision. If Mr. Godlee's method be a
objections cease for the most part to hold good.
has shown that if the sutures are introduced in
described, the abscess may be at once opened, a
thus avoided.

Observations and Comment.—The method by
at one sitting offers undoubtedly the best mear
with hepatic abscess. Attempts to open the abse
of the actual cautery or by caustic potash ar
demned. The aspirator is only of use as an aid
and as a palliative means. Its employment h;
compromised the success of a subsequent opei
incision. There is nothing to recommend the c
of tapping the abscess with a trocar, and of
through the cannula, or through a drainage-tub
in the place of the cannula.

The drainage thus secured is very inefficie
leak out into the peritoneal cavity, the surgeoi
thrust with the trocar in the dark, and importa
may be punctured; the cannula may slip, and
would not meet a case where multiple abscesses
apparently slight operationis—like most timid, sp
meddlesome half-measures—probably more dai
the complete operation.

A valuable series of lectures on hepatic absee
by Mr. Godlee in the *Brit. Med. Journ.* for J
should be consulted by those who are intere
branch of surgery. To the following points in t
especial attention may be directed :—

Mr. Godlee demonstrates by means of an illustrative case that even when an abscess is actually "almost pointing," it is impossible to be certain that the liver will be found to be adherent. In the case quoted there were no adhesions.

Several of Mr. Godlee's cases illustrate the evacuation of the abscess through the chest wall. It is urged that in these cases the incision should be made below the normal limit of the pleura; but that if by chance either pleura or peritoneum be opened, the opening must be closed with a double row of stitches before the liver is incised.

In one illustrative case an exploring-needle had revealed the presence of deep-seated pus in the chest. An incision was made over the ninth interspace, and a portion of the ninth rib was removed. The diaphragm was then stitched with some difficulty to the costal pleura, and the abscess was opened by cutting through the attached diaphragm. The patient made a good recovery.

In another case, in which the abscess was opened through the seventh intercostal space, profuse hæmorrhage occurred.

In a third case, in which an incision was made into the abscess through the seventh or eighth space at the lower part of the axilla, "terrific hæmorrhage" attended the enlargement of the opening into the abscess.

3. HEPATOTOMY.

Although the term hepatotomy is usually applied to cases in which an incision is made into a hepatic abscess or a hydatid cyst, it may be conveniently adopted for such *unclassified cases* as are cited below. In not a few of the so-called examples of hepatotomy for abscess and hydatid, no actual liver tissue is incised.

Excision of Hydatid Cysts *en masse.*—Dr. Tansini (*Gazetta degli Ospitali,* January 21st, 1891) exposed in a woman, aged twenty-five, an epigastric tumour the size of a fœtal head. It was found to be firmly adherent to the great omentum; and when the attachments to this membrane had been divided and ligatured, the tumour was demonstrated to be a hydatid cyst of the liver. The cyst was then deliberately dissected out, the liver substance being freely incised. The bleeding, which was considerable, was checked by ligature and

temporary pressure. The great wound in tl
closed by a double series of catgut and silk
sutures in all were employed. The abdoi
closed, and the patient made a good recover}

M. Terillon (*Brit. Med. Journ.*, Suppl.
removed, by means of an elastic ligature, a p
containing numerous small hydatid cysts.
wound was six inches in length. The portio
was about the size of two fists. It was eucii
ture, and was fixed outside the wound in the

It sloughed off in due course, and the
perfectly.

Excision of Protruding Portions of
Duplay, in commenting upon the above case
ten instances in which protruded portions o
site of penetrating wounds of the abdomen h
by the knife. All the patients recovered.

He mentions also three cases in which th
growth of the liver had been attempted. In
was attended by alarming, and in one by fat

Excision of Cancer of the Liver.—Pr
cised in November, 1890, a considerable po
for malignant disease in a woman, aged thirty
für Chirurgie, No. 6, 1891). The liver was
otomy, and a cancerous growth was disco
lobe. The mentum was adherent to the
membrane some enlarged glands were found
lobe was without difficulty brought throu
wound, and was fixed *in situ* by sutures, ar
base by iodoform gauze, in order to shut
cavity. An elastic tube was then fastened
or pedicle of the affected lobe. On the four
elastic tube was applied, and on the eighth
ligature was substituted. On the twelfth d
ration of the mass was effected by means of t
The wound healed up in four weeks, at whicl
left the hospital.

4. CHOLECYSTOTOMY.

This operation implies the making of ar

gall-bladder through a wound in the parietes. It is carried out for the removal of gall-stones, and for the relief of dropsy and empyema of the gall-bladder. By its means various forms of obstruction in the common bile duct have been relieved. The operation has been successfully carried out in certain cases of wound or perforation of the gall-bladder, and in one instance at least the gall-bladder was opened, and a temporary biliary fistula established, in order to relieve extreme congestion and enlargement of the liver (*Bull. de l'Acad. de Méd.*, Nov. 4th, 1890). The terms cholelithotomy and cholelithotrity have been employed in instances in which gall-stones have been removed by cutting, or have been crushed *in situ.*

History of the Operation.—So long ago as 1733 Petit suggested the possibility of dealing with certain disorders of the liver by surgical means ; and in a memoir published in 1743 he suggests that the distended gall-bladder should be relieved by puncture, and that stones lodged in that viscus should be removed by lithotomy (*Mém. de l'Acad. Roy. de Chir.*, 1743, page 163). Operations upon the gall-bladder were discussed in a casual and flighty manner during the early part of the present century, but it was not until 1867 that the modern operation of cholecystotomy was first performed. The operator was Dr. Bobbs, of Indianapolis. The patient recovered (*Trans. Indiana State Med. Soc.*, 1868, page 68). Dr. Marion Sims appears to have performed the second recorded operation (*Brit. Med. Journ.*, 1878, vol. i., page 811). The patient died, but Dr. Sims's paper may be said to have laid the foundation for the performance of the operation in Europe, since he detailed with great clearness and precision the various steps of the procedure. The first successful operation in England was performed by Mr. Tait on August 23rd, 1879 (*Med.-Chir. Trans.*, vol. lxiii., page 17). Mr. Tait adopted Dr. Sims's plan, and in subsequent cases he further elaborated the operation and extended its possibilities. The operation as now practised may be said to be a most successful one, and the mortality is probably not higher than five or six per cent.

Condition of the Gall-Bladder.—Mr. Tait (*Lancet*, vol. ii., 1885, page 239) divides gall-stones into two classes:—(1) The

solitary, and (2) the numerous. The former
than two or three in number, and may b·
size. They are liable to block the cystic ·
great distension of the gall-bladder, but not ·
bile still finds its way along the commo·
duodenum. The latter are small, and m·
hundreds. As they allow some bile to
jaundice may be absent, and the distension o·
is usually intermittent.

The distended gall-bladder may attain ·
tions, may contain some pints of fluid, and
occupy the abdominal cavity as to be mistak·
cyst. Mr. Taylor has pointed out that the ·
enlarges, tends to follow a line extending fr·
right tenth cartilage across the median line
below the umbilicus.

The distended viscus may be pyriform, g·
form in outline. It may be hard and firm,
elastic. The tumour, if of no great size,
liver on respiration.

On the other hand, the gall-bladder ma·
as to be scarcely recognisable. It may be c·
by adhesions, and these adhesions may be ·
extending to entirely confuse the anatomy of
small gall-bladder has been found to be encl·
omentum and intestine, and is not infrequen·
enlarged liver. The walls of the bladder m·
case, and very hard and thick in another.

Stones may be discovered to be impact·
cystic or the common duct, or in both at the·

Some surgeons have advised a prelimin·
gall-stones by means of a needle; the practi·
be condemned as uncertain, unsatisfactory·
unsafe. An extensive examination of the r·
bladder by means of a needle is a more dang·
than an exploratory incision.

Instruments Required.—Scalpels; bisto·
artery, and pressure forceps; long-bladed di·
large pressure forceps for extensive adhesio·
tum; rectangular retractors; spatulæ; blunt·

intestinal and other curved needles; needle-holder; needles in handles; sponge-holders; small lithotomy scoops and lithotomy forceps; nasal polypus forceps covered with india-rubber; Lister's sinus forceps; grooved directors; strong needles for breaking up gall-stones; aspirator.

The polypus forceps are used for crushing stones; other forms of forceps may answer equally well.

The Operation.—The general management of the opera-tion, the preparation of the patient, the position of the surgeon and his assistants, conform to the lines already laid down in dealing with abdominal section.

The parietal incision is about three inches in length, and can be enlarged as required. It is best made vertically over the most prominent part of the tumour, when one exists, or over the fundus of the gall-bladder when no swelling is evident.

Various incisions have been recommended—notably an oblique one parallel with the ribs—but the great majority of operators have adopted a vertical wound.

The peritoneum is opened, and the area of the operation is explored with the forefinger. The wound is enlarged as required. Intestine may protrude and hamper the surgeon's movements, or the omentum may be found in the way, or an enlarged liver may overshadow the operation region.

If the gall-bladder be found to be of great size, or very tense from over-distension, it should be carefully aspirated. The site of the needle puncture is protected by sponges, which are wedged in position. As the cyst is emptied, its wall is gradually and gently brought into the parietal wound. This is not always an easy matter, or even a possible matter; and as the cyst wall is often very thin, it must needs be handled with great gentleness.

Care must be taken that no fluid escapes into the peri-toneal cavity.

If the bladder be but slightly distended, its wall may be brought to the surface without previous aspiration.

The wall of the gall-bladder is best held and drawn for-wards by means of pressure forceps. The amount of traction exercised must be very judiciously regulated.

The wall of the gall-bladder is then opened by an

incision made between
points are dealt with, and
the cyst may be drawn
between the lips of the
perly-applied sponges the
cavity is prevented.

The finger introduced
stones, notes their positio

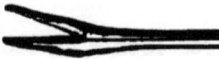

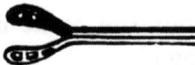

Fig. 376.—TAI

removing them.   Loose
finger, or by means of sc
pattern.   If a stone be dis
gall-bladder, it is well, befc
the margins of the wound
wound in the parietes.

Inasmuch as the walls
weak, the greatest care n
difficult part of the operat

It is often well to sut
wound to the skin margi
the unsutured interval, so
of forceps and scoops in
viscus.   Before the sutur
must be removed and cou

In dislodging stones, Tait's special forceps (Fig. 376) are of great service, and their movements within the bladder may be guided by the finger introduced into the abdomen, and placed against the outer wall of the cyst at the site of the impacted stone.

Sometimes the stone may be prised upwards by means of the finger so introduced.

If the calculus cannot be dislodged, then it may be very slowly and cautiously chipped into fragments by means of forceps, the action of which is controlled by the finger without the gall bladder; or the disintegration of the stone may be effected by the needle, controlled in like manner by the finger.

In some cases the impacted stone has been broken up by means of padded forceps applied to the stone outside, and therefore through the walls of the neck of the gall-bladder.

The detritus which results from these procedures is got rid of by repeated washings.

Attempts to push the stone onwards through the duct by means of a probe or director have not met with much success. The proceeding also is not entirely free from risk.

Mr. J. W. Taylor succeeded in dislodging an impacted calculus in the cystic duct by means of frequent syringing through the fistulous opening after the operation had been completed.

Mr. Thornton has dilated the cystic duct, and has then succeeded in removing the impacted stone through the wound in the gall-bladder.

The treatment of such stones as are impacted so low down in the duct as not to be reached from the gall-bladder is dealt with in the succeeding section.

The operation is concluded by completing the suturing of the gall-bladder to the edges of the skin wound. The gall-bladder is held in position while the sutures are being introduced.

The best suture in a straightforward case is a continuous suture of fine silk, which includes the cyst wall, the parietal peritoneum, and the skin. A drainage-tube is introduced into the gall-bladder, the parts are cleared, and a simple absorbent dressing capable of being frequently and readily changed is applied.

Modifications and Complications of the Operation.

1. *When the Stone is impacted in the Duct, and cannot* *reached through the Gall-Bladder.*

Small stones so placed have been gradually worked bac into the gall-bladder by manipulation.

When this cannot be done, the calculus may be broken with a needle introduced through the duct wall. Incision the duct may in this way be avoided, but the method coul only be adopted, in the case of small stones. In one ca Mr. Thornton found two stones lodged in the common du He broke them to pieces by needling, and then crushed th fragments with protected forceps. The fragments were n moved through the gall-bladder, and the duct was not incise (*Lancet*, April 4th, 1891, page 763). The gall-bladder wa however, so much damaged that it had to be removed.

In many instances the duct has been opened, the ston removed, and the wound in the duct closed by sutures. Th following cases by Mr. Thornton (*loc. cit.*) serve to illustra this practice :—

A stone was found impacted in the common duct, ju below the entrance of the cystic duct. Failing either t reach it through the cystic duct, or to break it up, M Thornton incised the duct and needled the stone into fra ments. It was found impossible to extract all the fragmen through any reasonable opening in the duct; the majorit were therefore left in the duct, the wound in which was close by sutures. The gall-bladder had been already opened. Th patient did well .

The second case is reported as follows. The patient wa woman aged forty-three, and a good recovery followed :—

" I found the liver so large that the gall-bladder and duc were quite covered ; there was much adhesion of omentu and intestines, a large oval stone impacted in the commo duct, and, failing to define the gall-bladder accurately, and fee ing sure that it would be impossible to get at the ston through a contracted cystic duct, I decided to incise th common duct at once, and so remove it. I was much hamper by the large liver, and had to work entirely by touch, deep the abdomen, guiding the knife on the left index finger. T first incision was followed by such a rush of dark ven blood that I feared for the vena cava, but, having introduced a small Fergusson's glass speculum, I saw that it proceeded from a vein in the adherent omentum, and this I easily secured. I had great difficulty in loosening the stone, which was firmly adherent to the lining membrane of the duct over a great part of its surface. After removing it I could see the termination of the duct in the duodenum quite distinctly through the speculum. I closed the opening in the duct by six fine interrupted points of silk suture, and a continuous one over all, using the omentum to strengthen the closure, as I had done in the previous case of duct incision. I drained the peritoneum by a glass tube " (*loc. cit.*, page 764).

The third case is of a similar character. The patient, a woman aged thirty-six, made a perfect recovery.

"I found two stones impacted one above the other in the common duct. The gall-bladder was so shrunken that it was difficult to recognise it, and I at once decided to open the common duct, remove the stones, and suture the opening. This procedure I carried out with much difficulty, owing to the matting of parts by adhesions; and not being very well satisfied with the security of the suturing of the duct, I passed a rubber tube into the pouch, at the bottom of which it lay, and brought it out through the upper part of the abdominal incision, and I also passed a glass tube into the pouch of Douglas through a counter-opening above the pubes. The latter was hardly required, but a very heavy discharge of bile-stained serum flowed from the rubber tube for many days after the operation, showing that my fears as to the security of the duct sutures were well founded."

2. *When the Gall-Bladder cannot be Dealt with.*—The following case, also reported by Mr. Thornton (*loc. cit.*, page 821), illustrates this difficult complication. The patient was a lady aged thirty-four. She made an excellent recovery :—

"On opening the abdomen, I found everything so matted together that I at first mistook the head of the pancreas for a thickened gall-bladder. Finding my mistake, I proceeded to carefully make my way through some fresh adhesions between the stomach, the omentum, and the right lobe of the liver, and at last found the gall-bladder, deeply placed and packed with gall-stones. In searching for it I opened a small abscess

e e

under the edge of the liv
thick pus, and cleared
clearing-out of the stones
the aid of various scoops
and washed it out, I foun
remove it, suture it, or sut
and I therefore merely pas
the gall-bladder, and brou
wound; this of course lef
the general peritoneum,
opening above the pubes,
also with a glass tube. 1
bladder open seems at first
and one other prove that v
the tube, and with the aux
when necessary, be safel
wound in the gall-bladder
expect from its being so m
to the incision; but there
age from the open gall-bl
the discharge of bile-stain
was very free from the firs

3. *When it may be P*
Bladder.

In several instances, aft
and the stones removed,
at once closed by sutur
turned within the abdomei
closed.

This method has bee
and has been practised
Winkelmann, and others.

Roux employs three r
membrane, one for the fibr
covering. He has report
Méd. de la Suisse Romand

An interesting article b
also be referred to (*Deuts*
xxi., page 383).

Although the operatio

described, may be considered to be, from a certain standpoint, an ideal one, it is not a procedure to be indiscriminately recommended. Many fatal cases have been reported. The sutures may give way, and death result from the escape of bile into the peritoneum, as occurred in one of Mr. Thornton's cases (case 8, *loc. cit.*, page 764).

If any small stone which occludes the duct should be overlooked, or if the ducts be not left perfectly clear, the measure may be disastrous.

The general results of the ordinary operation, in which a temporary biliary fistula is established, have been so good that the measure must be very nearly perfect which can compare favourably with it.

The " ideal cholecystotomy " may be entertained in simple cases in which the walls of the gall-bladder are sound and have not been much handled, and in which it is perfectly evident that the ducts are quite clear. Whenever it is carried out, it would be wiser to have a drainage-tube in the parietal wound, rather than to close it entirely.

In connection with this procedure may be mentioned that of Zielewicz, who, having performed cholecystotomy, applies a ligature to the cystic duct, to prevent any regurgitation of bile into the wound (*Centralblatt für Chirurgie*, No. 13, 1888).

Comment.—Few operations present wider possibilities or a greater degree of uncertainty than does cholecystotomy. The surgeon who embarks upon this operation will proceed with a speculative spirit. The operation may prove to be quite simple, and to be readily carried out and completed; on the other band, it may present difficulties of an almost insuperable character, and may even have to be abandoned.

Everything depends upon the anatomical condition of the parts, upon the thickness of the abdominal parietes, the size of the liver, and the presence and extent of adhesions.

In one case (Dr. Parkes's, *Trans. Amer. Surg. Assoc.*, vol. iv., page 299) "the most careful and diligent search failed to find the gall-bladder."

In other instances the gall-bladder has been opened, but no stones have been found.

In some cases the cause of the obstruction in the duct could not be relieved.

It is not uncommon to f
the gall-bladder into the ape

In certain of the reported
been occupied by the operati

A stricture of the duct h
tion by means of instruments
tract (Dr. Parkes's, *Amer. J*
page 100).

The After-treatment ca
sutures are removed in due
dispensed with as soon as t
sound. The sinus is frequen
kept scrupulously clean.

The fistula usually close
fourteen to twenty-one day
patent for months or years.

5. CHOLE

The operation of the rem
posed by Langenbüch in 18
him in at least twelve cases.
by many other surgeons, alt
given by Langenbüch have n

So far as collections of pu
it would appear that the mo
ten per cent.

Cholecystectomy is of lin
posed that it should take the
a more tedious and more ser
teoted stones still be lodging
one way of escape. It does r
every nidus for future calculi

The operation has been
found to be impossible to uni
to that in the parietes, and ir
gall-bladder have been too
the manipulations of the
possible.

The Operation.—Two pa
the peritoneum covering the

The viscus is thus bared, and is rapidly enucleated. The separation begins at the fundus and ends at the cystic duct. The two peritoneal flaps are then united by a continuous suture of fine silk, the cystic duct is secured between two ligatures and divided, and the gall-bladder is removed.

The operation may be almost bloodless (as in Mr. Thornton's first case, *Brit. Med. Journ.*, Jan 5th, 1889), or, on the other hand, the hæmorrhage from the liver substance may be free, and may need to be controlled by pressure or by the actual cautery (as in a case by Roux, *Revue Méd. de la Suisse Romande*, Oct. 10th, 1890).

It is well to carry a glass drainage-tube down to the site of the gall-bladder, and to leave it in position for two or three days.

6. CHOLECYSTENTEROSTOMY.

By this term is understood the establishment of a fistula between the gall-bladder and the intestine. The not less uncouth, but less precise, term of entero-cholecystotomy has also been applied to this operation.

The procedure has been carried out in cases in which there is an insuperable obstruction in the common bile duct, such as may have been brought about by destructive inflammatory changes, or be due to the pressure upon the duct of a malignant tumour. In Tillaux's case, for example, the duct was entirely occluded by a cancerous growth, springing from the head of the pancreas. The same condition existed in Kappeler's case, and in others. Mr. Mayo Robson has carried out the operation with success in the treatment of a biliary fistula, through which, apparently, the whole of the bile was discharged.

The operation of cholecystenterostomy appears to have been first suggested by Nussbaum. The first actual operation was, however, performed by Winiwarter (*Prag. Mediz. Wochens.*, No. 21, 1882). The procedure has since been carried out by Tillaux, Terrier, Socin, Kappeler, Bardenheuer, Robson, and others.

The Operation.—The operation has been performed in many ways, and no settled practice can be said to be established. Cholecystenterostomy has been carried out in

one, two, and three stages. The mode (
cases of biliary fistula requires also some
tion.

1. **The Method in One Stage.**—This m
by Kappeler's operation (*Centralblatt für*
page 18; and 1889, page 591). The case wa
of the common duct by a growth from th
abdomen is opened by a vertical incision alo
of the right rectus muscle. The parts c
operation are carefully examined. The diste
is drawn out of the wound, is punctured w
emptied.

A loop of the highest part of the jejunu
and is isolated by means of two loops of catg
the mesentery at some distance from one am
the bowel. The catgut is introduced by mear
needle, and the loops enable the surgeon to d
segment of gut forwards to fix it, and to o
after it has been emptied by pressure.

The trocar wound in the gall-bladder i
suitable incision is made in the bowel. Tl
two wounds are then united by means of
sutures. The parts are cleansed and replace
wound is closed by sutures.

2. **The Method in Two Stages.**—This n
by the operation advised by Winiwarter
abdomen having been opened, the gall-bladd
convenient loop of the upper jejunum, over
2 square c.m. The sutures are so introduced
the mucous membrane of either viscus, and a
form of a circle.

The parts thus united are fixed to the pa
by several points of Lembert's suture.

The parietal wound is left open. This co
stage.

The second stage is carried out at the
days, when the bowel is incised, and a free
into the gall-bladder, at the spot at which tl
to it. If possible, the mucous membrane of
is united to the mucous membrane of the bo

in the free part of the intestine is closed by sutures, and the parietal incision is encouraged to heal.

3. **The Method in Three Stages.**—This is the method carried out by Tillaux in a case in which the common bile duct was entirely obliterated by a malignant growth springing from the head of the pancreas.

1st Stage.—Laparotomy is performed, and an examination and exploration of the parts concerned are made. The nearest convenient loop of the jejunum is fixed to the gall-bladder by sutures, in such a way as to unite a fairly wide surface of the one to the other. The gall-bladder is now opened and emptied. The margins of the incision in the bladder are united to the parietal wound, and a biliary fistula is established.

2nd Stage.—Some nine days later the bowel is opened into the gall-bladder through the fistula. The knife, of course, must not transgress the area of adhesion between the two viscera. Means are taken to ensure that the opening between the bladder and the bowel will remain patent.

3rd Stage.—Some eighteen days later the biliary fistula is closed by a plastic operation.

4. **The Method in Dealing with Persistent Biliary Fistulæ.**—This is illustrated by Mr. Robson's case (*Med.-Chir. Trans.*, vol. lxxiii., page 64).

In this instance cholecystotomy had been performed for empyema of the gall-bladder. There was a stricture of the common duct, and apparently the whole of the bile was discharged through the fistula. Cholecystenterostomy was performed fifteen months after the first operation. Mr. Robson's account is as follows:—" On March 2nd, 1889, I opened the abdomen in the right linea semilunaris, through the old scar, in the centre of which was the fistula, prolonging the opening two inches beyond the lower end of the cicatrix. The gall-bladder was detached from the parietes, and found to be much contracted and thickened. There was so much matting of the viscera that it was found impracticable to bring up and fix the duodenum or jejunum to the gall-bladder; hence the hepatic flexure of the colon, lying near, was raised and encircled by an elastic ligature, after its contents had been squeezed upwards and downwards. Convenient spots having been selected on the gall-bladder and colon, a circle the size of a florin was marked by a scalpel on each viscus. Along these lines, sutures of fine chromicised catgut were passed, about one-eighth of an inch apart, but they were not tightened until openings, one-third of an inch in diameter, had been made in the centre of the circles, quite through all the coats of the two viscera concerned, and the cut edges of the mucous membrane of the colon had been sutured by a number of interrupted stitches of fine catgut to the edge of the mucous membrane of the gall-bladder. . . . The outer row of ligatures, only involving the serous and muscular coats, was tied and cut off short." The freshened edges of the old fistula were not brought together by sutures; a glass drainage-tube was introduced, and the parietal wound was closed around it.

Bile and fæcal matter were discharged from the wound for some time, but it ultimately closed after a period of two months.

CHAPTER XVI.

SPLENECTOMY.

SPLENECTOMY, or extirpation of the spleen, has been carried out in cases of injury or prolapse of the spleen, in certain instances of movable spleen, in simple hypertrophy of the organ, and in some cases of tumour of the spleen. Experience has shown that the extirpation of the leucocythæmic spleen is an unjustifiable operation.

The history of the operation is thus given by Sir Spencer Wells in his "Surgical Treatment of Abdominal Tumours," page 182 :—" I think we may look upon the case of extirpation of the spleen attributed to Zaccarelli in 1549 as apocryphal. We do not find anything authentic till 1826, in which year Quittenbaum, of Rostock, removed a diseased spleen from a woman, who died of shock in six hours. Then, in 1855, Kückler, of Darmstadt, reported that he had done the operation on a man who had enlarged spleen from ague. He encountered no special difficulty in his undertaking, but lost the patient from hæmorrhage two hours after operation." The first operation in England was performed by Sir Spencer Wells in 1865. The patient lived six days. Péan, who operated in 1867, had what may be termed the first successful result in modern times. Since then the operation has been extensively practised, and with a considerable degree of success.

Anatomical Points.—The spleen most closely approaches the surface in the parts covered by the tenth and eleventh ribs. Above this it is entirely overlapped by the edge of the lung. It is in all parts—when of normal size—separated from the parietes by the diaphragm.

Its long axis coincides very nearly with the line of the tenth rib. "Its highest and lowest points are on a level, respectively, with the ninth dorsal and first lumbar spines; its inner end is distant about one and a half inch from the median plane of the body, and its outer end about reaches the mid-axillary line " (Quain).

The three surfaces of the spleen—gastric, renal, and phrenic—are well shown in Fig. 377.

The peritoneum which invests the spleen is reflected at the hilum, and, passing on to the stomach, forms the gastro-splenic omentum. This omentum contains the splenic and other vessels, and forms the pedicle, which has to be dealt with when the organ is excised. The splenic artery breaks up into branches—which vary from five to seven in number—just before it reaches

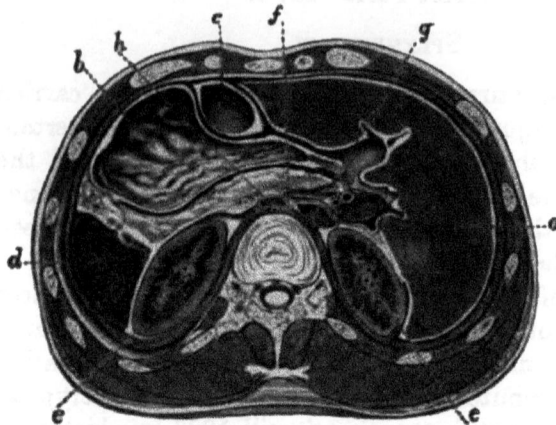

Fig. 377.—HORIZONTAL SECTION THROUGH THE UPPER PART OF THE ABDOMEN. (*Rüdinger*.)

a, Liver; b, stomach; c, transverse colon; d, spleen; e, kidneys; f, pancreas; g, inferior vena cava; h, aorta with thoracic duct behind it.

the gland. These branches vary in length and size, and will probably have to be dealt with individually in cases of great enlargement.

The vasa brevia, from four to six in number, are directed forwards and to the right, and lie also in the gastro-splenic omentum. Some issue from the trunk of the splenic artery, some from its terminal branches. They all reach the left extremity of the stomach. Some or all of these branches may be divided in the pedicle.

The gastro-epiploica sinistra artery also occupies the gastro-splenic omentum for a small part of its course.

The splenic vein is placed below the artery. Its tributaries correspond to the branches of the artery, and the trunk of the vessel is of considerable size.

The comparative thinness of the spleen capsule, and the peculiar friability of the splenic tissue, must be borne in mind.

The Instruments Required.—Those required for ovariotomy, with the exception of such special instruments as the ovarian trocar.

The Operation.—The parietal incision is conveniently made along the outer edge of the left rectus muscle. It is vertical, and may need to be of considerable length. Its upper extremity should lie near to the ribs. In many of the reported cases a median incision has been made use of.

The peritoneum having been opened, the tumour is examined. If any adhesions exist, they must be at once dealt with. If very extensive adhesions are discovered, which serve to connect the spleen with adjacent viscera, and to obscure the anatomical details of the part, the operation had probably better be abandoned. The omentum is not infrequently found to be adherent to the tumour, and some trouble has arisen from the accidental division of the large vessels which may be found in that structure.

The enlarged spleen is now gently drawn through the wound. The organ must be handled with the greatest care, and any attempts to force it through a comparatively small incision must be avoided. The spleen has been ruptured during removal as the result of too severe pressure brought to bear upon it. This occurred in one of Sir Spencer Wells's cases.

The tumour must be allowed to escape slowly, and as it protrudes the pedicle must be from time to time inspected, lest undue traction be made upon the vessels therein, and especially upon the thin-walled veins.

Dragging upon the pedicle has produced alarming symptoms of collapse, due, no doubt, to injury to the splenic nerve plexus, which is derived from the solar plexus.

The most important feature of the whole operation is concerned with the treatment of the pedicle.

In general terms, the practice advised by Sir Spencer Wells may be followed. He recommends "temporarily securing all the blood-vessels by pressure forceps as near to the spleen as possible, then removing the enlarged organ, afterwards applying silk ligatures by transfixion behind the forceps, and tightening them as the forceps are removed. All the ends of the silk should be cut off near the knots." He condemns the practice of Langenbeck, who advises that the splenic artery be tied as close to the cœliac axis as possible, and before it divides into its many branches. He points out that this could not be often done without much disturbance of the pancreas, and a ligature applied close to so large a trunk as the cœliac axis is likely to be followed by secondary hæmorrhage (*Med.-Chir. Trans.*, vol. lxxi, page 262).

In more than one case a small artery has slipped out from its ligature, and severe bleeding, difficult to check, has followed.

Some surgeons tie the pedicle in two intertwined ligatures and then add a separate ligature around the whole stump.

No especial advantage has been shown to attend the practice of ligaturing the artery and the vein separately.

Care must be taken that the structures of the pedicle are relaxed at the moment that each ligature is tied. It is better to err in the direction of applying too many ligatures than to attempt to include the whole pedicle in one or even two knots.

In dealing with the pedicle, the pancreas has been wounded, and the tip or tail of that organ has even been included in the ligature.

The ligatures having been all cut short, the peritoneal cavity is well cleansed, and the abdominal wound is closed.

Comment.—The great risk of the operation is hæmorrhage from the pedicle. In twenty-nine cases collected by Collier, no less than fourteen died directly from bleeding.

The treatment of the pedicle constitutes the main feature of the operation, and next to it must rank the treatment of such adhesions as may exist.

Results.—Mr. Wright, of Manchester, has collected sixty-two cases of splenectomy. In twenty-two cases the operation was for leukæmia, and all the patients died. In twenty-three cases the spleen was the seat of simple hypertrophy, and fifteen patients died. Of seven who were operated on for malarial disease, five recovered; and of three on whom splenectomy was performed for cystic disease, all recovered (*Med. Chron.*, Dec., 1888).

The operation in cases of wounded or prolapsed spleen has been very successful. Ashhurst has collected twenty-one cases of splenectomy performed for traumatism, and in all recovery followed.

CHAPTER XVII.

OPERATIONS ON THE KIDNEY.

Anatomical Points.—The kidneys are deeply placed, and are most accessible to pressure at the outer edge of the erector spinæ just below the last rib. They rest about equally upon the diaphragm and the anterior layer of the transversalis aponeurosis, which latter structure separates them from the quadratus lumborum. They rest to a slight extent also upon the psoas.

The upper edge of the kidney corresponds with the space between the eleventh and the twelfth ribs, and with the eleventh or twelfth dorsal spine. The right kidney is a little lower than the left. The lower end of the kidney is about on a level with the middle of the third lumbar spine (Fig. 378). The hilum is about opposite to the gap between the first and second lumbar spines.

The inner border of the gland at its upper part is about one inch from the middle line; the outer border at its lower part is three and three-quarter inches from that line.

A horizontal line passing through the umbilicus will probably correspond to the lower end of the right kidney, but will be entirely below the left.

A vertical line carried upwards from the middle of Poupart's ligament has one-third of the kidney to its outer side, and two-thirds to its inner side.

The area corresponding to the kidney on the posterior surface of the body is indicated in Fig. 378.

In relation with the anterior surface of the right kidney are the under-surface of the liver, the second part of the duodenum, the commencement of the transverse colon, and the ascending colon.

In the same relation on the left side are the fundus of the stomach, the pancreas, and the descending colon.

Crossing the posterior surface of the kidney obliquely from above, downwards and outwards, are branches of the last

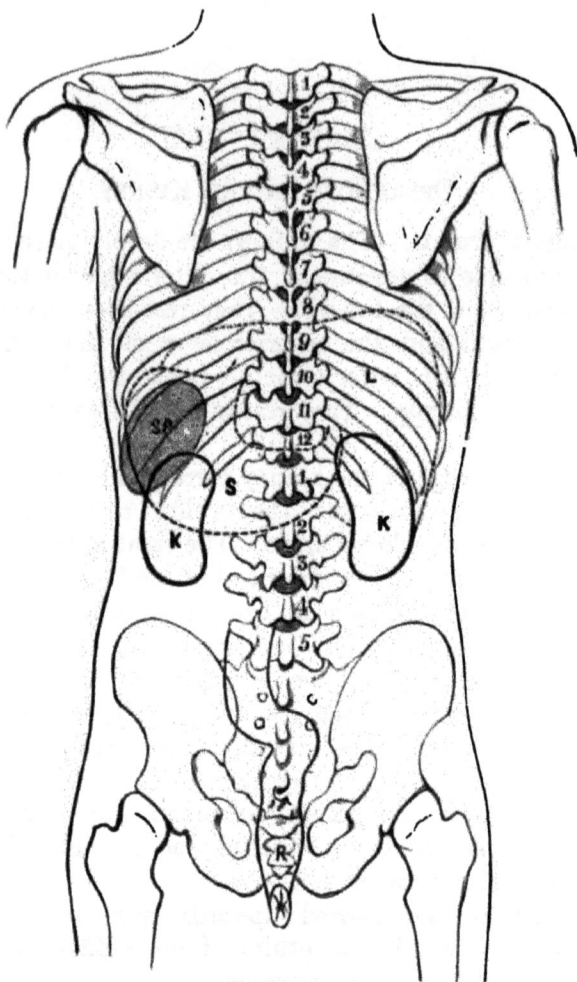

Fig. 378. —DIAGRAM TO SHOW THE RELATIONS OF THE VISCERA TO THE PARIETES.
(Posterior view.)

s, Stomach; L, Liver; K, Kidney; sp, Spleen; R, Rectum.

dorsal nerve, and of the first lumbar artery, together with the ilio-hypogastric and ilio-inguinal nerves.

The fatty tissue in which the kidney is embedded is of much surgical importance. It is more abundant behind than in front, and the laxity of its substance permits of the ready enucleation of the organ. In certain diseased conditions this fatty area may be occupied by inflammatory tissue, which is found to be intimately and inconveniently adherent to the kidney.

The structures which enter the hilum of the kidney form also the surgical pedicle of the kidney. They consist of the renal vessels, the pelvis of the ureter, lymphatics, nerves, and connective tissue.

The renal artery is the size of the brachial, and divides just before reaching the hilum into four or five branches. These branches lie behind the corresponding branches of the vein and in front of the pelvis of the ureter. They give small branches to the capsule and the ureter.

The renal vein corresponds closely to the artery, and is a vessel of considerable width.

The renal artery may be replaced by two, three, four, or even five branches. These usually arise from the aorta, but may take origin from the lumbar, iliac, or inferior mesenteric arteries.

The branches of the renal artery may enter the upper end or the anterior surface of the kidney instead of the hilum, and may give off supernumerary branches to adjacent parts.

The ureter loses its cylindrical form on a level with the lower end of the kidney, where it begins to expand into the funnel-shaped cavity called the pelvis (Fig. 379). After entering the hilum the pelvis divides into two, or even three, primary tubular branches, which in turn end in several truncated short and wide pouches, the calyces. In the pelvis of the ureter, or in the calyces, calculi are frequently lodged. The calyces are too narrow to admit of the introduction of the finger for exploration.

The abnormalities of the kidney are of considerable surgical importance. They are very fully dealt with in Mr. Henry Morris's work on "The Surgical Diseases of the Kidney."

One, or less frequently both, kidneys may be misplaced. The left is more often out of place than the right, and the organ may be found over the sacro-iliac synchondrosis, or the promontory of the sacrum, or be discovered in the iliac fossa or pelvis. The misplaced kidney is often mis-shapen.

The kidney may exhibit a more or less extreme degree of lobulation. The ureter may be double.

The two kidneys may be fused. "The lowest degree of fusion is seen in the horseshoe kidney. The two kidneys are united at their inferior portions by a flat, riband-like, or rounded bridge of tissue, which crosses the vertebral column. In the higher degrees the two lateral portions approach one another more and more, until they reach the highest degree, in which a single disc-like kidney, lying in the median line, and provided with a double or a single calyx, represents complete fusion" (Rokitansky).

When the two kidneys are united by a web of connective tissue, the condition is no bar to operation.

There may be an entire absence of one kidney. The single kidney may be lateral or median in position.

Mr. Henry Morris gives the following estimate of the frequency of these abnormal conditions.

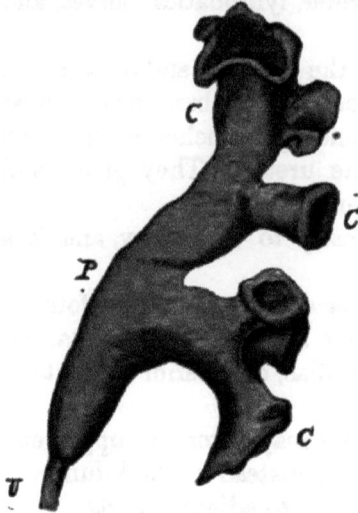

Fig. 379.—CAST OF THE INTERIOR OF THE UPPER END OF THE URETER. (*Henle.*)
u, Ureter; p, Pelvis; c, Calyces.

Congenital absence or extreme atrophy of one kidney may be expected to be present in 1 in about 4,000 cases.

The horseshoe kidney may be looked for in the proportion of 1 to every 1,600 cases, and the single fused kidney in 1 in about 8,000 cases. Examples of wasted, small, and shrunken kidneys are a little more common.

The Operations Performed.—The following operations will be described :—

1. Nephro-lithotomy, or incision of the kidney for stone.
2. Nephrotomy, or incision of the kidney, including puncture of the kidney.
3. Nephrectomy, or removal of the kidney.
4. Nephrorrhaphy, or fixation of a movable kidney.

History of Operations upon the Kidney.

It would appear that during the earlier days of surgery

incisions had been made from time to time into fluctuating swellings in the loin, and through such wounds abscesses and cysts were evacuated, which were subsequently shown to have had origin in the kidney.

In like manner ancient records contain accounts of cases in which renal calculi were removed through the loin, their discharge having followed the evacuation of an abscess in that region. Those early operations were all more or less casual.

The possibility of removing stones from the kidney is discussed by more than one ancient writer, and such a measure of treatment was now and then advised in the vague, haphazard, and irresponsible language that marks many of the earlier surgical records.

A case is recorded in the *Philosophical Transactions* for 1696 by a Dr. Bernard, which would seem to have been one of nephro-lithotomy. Some discredit has been cast upon the case, and the details of it are not sufficiently complete to make it of scientific value. The case certainly had no influence upon surgical practice.

The first operation of nephro-lithotomy was performed by Mr. Henry Morris in 1880. The operation was deliberately undertaken and carefully planned, and it forms the basis and starting-point of the modern procedure.

Nephrectomy had been performed unintentionally several times before it was deliberately carried out as a precise operation by Gustav Simon, of Heidelberg, in April, 1869. The operation was performed for an intractable fistula of the ureter, and the patient made an excellent recovery. In Mr. Barker's article in the *Med.-Chir. Trans.*, vol. lxiii., will be found an account of the first twenty-eight reported cases of nephrectomy.

Nephrorrhaphy was first performed by Dr. Hahn, of Berlin, in April, 1881.

Since the various operations were introduced, the development and application of each measure have been very rapidly extended.

1. NEPHRO-LITHOTOMY.

The operation of incising the kidney for the purpose of

f f

removing renal calculi has been carried out with remarkable
success in a large series of cases.

Discrimination must be exercised in selecting subjects for
operation, and the diagnosis should be as clear as possible. In
not less than twenty-five instances a nephro-lithotomy has
been performed and no stone discovered.

The circumstances in which the operation may be
carried out are admirably discussed by Mr. Jacobson in a
paper published in the *British Medical Journal* for January
13th, 1890.

It will be convenient to take this operation as the type of
the series about to be described.

The Instruments Required.—Scalpels; bistouries; dissecting, artery, and pressure forceps; toothed forceps; two rectangular metal retractors; metal or ivory spatulæ; syringe.
The following special instruments are used in dealing with the
stone:—A stout slender needle in a handle, or a hare-lip pin
for sounding for the calculus; long-bladed tenotome; suitable
probes and scoops; steel director; the smallest-sized bladder-
sound (*see* page 486); small lithotomy forceps; Lister's sinus
forceps; dressing forceps; nasal polypus forceps. A small
periosteal elevator may be useful in detaching some stones,
and a No. 3 Duncan's uterine dilator has been recommended
as a convenient sound.

The Preparation of the Patient.—The preparation of the
patient should be upon the lines already laid down in dealing
with Abdominal Section (page 221).

It is desirable that the bowels, and especially the colon,
should be as well emptied as possible.

The skin over the site of the intended incision should be
well cleansed and washed with an antiseptic solution.

Two methods of operating will be described, viz., the
lumbar method, and the abdomino-lumbar method.

A.—THE LUMBAR OPERATION.

1. The Exposure of the Kidney.—The patient lies upon
the sound side, as near to the edge of the table as possible.
The loin of the affected side is well exposed, and to widen the
interval between the last rib and the crest of the ilium a
narrow hard cushion may be placed under the loin of the

und side. This pillow may be a little in the way in the
ter stages of the operation, in which case it may be
moved.

The surgeon stands by the patient's back, leaning over the
unk. An assistant stands on each side of him, to sponge
d assist in retracting the wound. A third assistant is
aced on the other side of the table, opposite to and facing

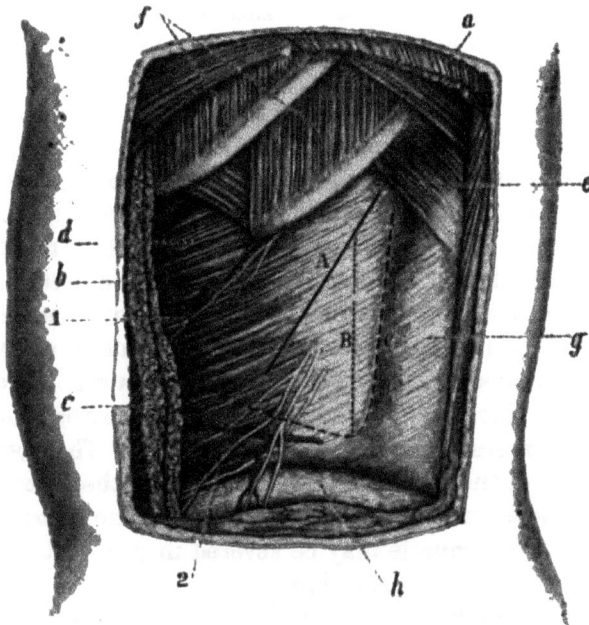

Fig. 380.—OPERATIONS UPON THE KIDNEY.

Incision for exploration, for nephrotomy and nephro-lithotomy; B, Additional incision for nephrectomy; c, König's lumbo-abdominal incision for nephrectomy.

Latissimus dorsi; b, External oblique; c, Internal oblique; d, Transversalis; e, Serratus posticus inferior; f, Intercostals; g, Fascia lumborum over erector spinæ; h, Crest of ilium; 1, Intercostal nerve and artery; 2, Twelfth dorsal nerve and lumbar artery.

he surgeon. His chief duty is to press the kidney towards
he loin when the organ has been exposed.

The twelfth rib should be definitely recognised and well
defined.

An oblique incision is made across the costo-iliac space.
The cut commences above, about half an inch below the
st rib and close to the outer border of the erector spinæ. It

f f 2

is continued downwards and forwards towards the crest of t
ilium (Fig. 380, A). Its length must depend upon the sp
available, and upon the depth of the tissues of the loin
will suffice if it be at first three inches in length, and it m
be subsequently enlarged to four or five inches as required.

Other forms of incision are alluded to in the Comme
upon the operation (page 489).

After dividing the skin, superficial fascia, and fat, the ou
border of the latissimus dorsi and the hinder border of t
external oblique muscles are exposed. The fibres of both
vertical, and they are divided to the full length of the d
incision. The sheath of the erector spinæ muscle should
be opened. The internal oblique muscle and the poster
aponeurosis of the transversalis muscle (fascia lumborum)
now laid bare. The fibres of the former muscle run up
and inwards. Piercing the fascia near the rib there may pos
be seen branches of the last dorsal nerve and last interc
artery, and nearer the iliac crest, the first lumbar nerve an
branch of the last lumbar artery. Both muscle and apo
rosis are divided to the full length of the wound. No dire
need be employed, and any bleeding points may be ligatured
pressure forceps are apt to be in the way. The anterior
outer edge of the quadratus lumborum, and the anterior l
of the fascia lumborum, are exposed. The latter is fr
divided. The muscle may be severed in part if it encroad
upon the field of the operation.

As each layer of tissue is divided, the severed parts
retracted by means of broad, rectangular metal retractors.

The fascia transversalis is now reached and divided, wl
the peri-renal fatty tissue is exposed.

The retractors are made to take up the whole of
severed structures down to the exposed fatty capsule, and
depths of the wound are laid open to the utmost.

The peri-renal adipose tissue is now opened up with
forceps and finger, and the kidney is reached and laid b
In order to bring it well into the field of the operation
assistant should press the anterior wall of the abdomen
the palms of both hands towards the exposed loin,
endeavour, as it were, to force the kidney into the incision

Through the free opening made in the peri-renal fat

finger is introduced and the whole kidney systematically examined.

As the surgeon approaches the back of the kidney, there will be sometimes noticed, writes Mr. Morris, a difference in the character of the fat, that immediately in contact with the kidney being finer in texture and of a delicate primrose colour.

If long-standing inflammation have been present, the surrounding tissues will be confused, will be matted together, and will offer a more or less firm resistance to the exploring finger.

2. **The Detection of the Stone.**—The posterior surface of the kidney is first examined with the finger, whilst the organ is well supported in front by the hand of the surgeon or his assistant. The finger-tip is then passed over the anterior surface of the gland while the kidney is supported by the psoas muscle and the spinal column. "To do this satisfactorily, it is best to turn the patient on his back, so that the kidney may fall into its natural place. The examining finger is thus left free to test the degree of resistance of the renal structure without having to use any force in keeping the kidney against its counter-resistance, viz., the vertebræ and muscle " (Morris).

If no indication of the stone be afforded upon either of these surfaces, the whole organ is tilted forward, and the pelvis is examined from behind. Each part of the kidney is squeezed and rubbed between the fingers, and any unduly hard or unduly soft spot noted.

A small stone may be readily overlooked, and, indeed, the presence of such a calculus may not be apparent to the finger even when the kidney has been removed and is examined upon a table.

If any hard or raised area be made out, the exploring-needle may be at once thrust into it to establish the presence of the stone.

Should no result follow the examination so far, the exploring-needle may be used. It is driven systematically into the substance of the kidney from many points. Twelve or more of such exploratory punctures may be made. While the needle is being used, the kidney must be fixed firmly in the wound. The instrument, which should not be more than

two and a half inches in length, is best introduced from one
end to the other of the posterior border, and each thrust
should be towards the hilum. The length of the needle will
scarcely allow of the renal vessels being reached.

As a next step, the plan advised by Mr. Jordan Lloyd may
be adopted. "The procedure is analogous to the method of
detecting stone in the bladder, differing from it only in one
particular, that we reach the kidney's interior through an
opening artificially made. When the kidney is exposed
through a lumbar wound, I puncture its lower end with a
long-bladed tenotome in a direction upwards and inwards,
making for the lowest of the calyces. If the surgeon is
observant and his knife is keen, he will readily appreciate the
moment when a cavity is struck by the altered resistance
offered to the puncturing instrument. . . . Into this opening
I pass a child's bladder-sound, and systematically explore the
whole interior of the pelvis. This sound should be of special
construction, having a beak not more than one-third of an
inch in length, a stem about seven inches, and the size of a
No. 3 English catheter. It should be passed at once to the
top of the kidney cavity, a distance of nearly four inches, and
the exploration should be carried out systematically
above downwards, the point being rotated in all directions so
as to investigate both tubes and calyces as the instrument is
withdrawn."

Supposing that still no stone is discovered, an incision
may be made into the posterior border of the kidney, sufficiently deep to reach the calyces. These cavities may then
be explored by the finger, aided by a sound or bougie.

This plan is advised by Mr. Morris, who urges that a
wound so made may be expected to heal well, and that it
involves a less risk of a urinary fistula than when the pelvis
is incised, although it undoubtedly involves more haemorrhage.
Mr. Jacobson prefers in such cases to open the pelvis or the
thinner kidney tissue close by, on the grounds that an incision through the substance of the organ may lead to bleeding, which directly or indirectly may prove to be serious.
Mr. Thornton also prefers an incision through the pelvis, and
maintains that wounds so placed heal well enough.

If an incision has already been made through the

tissue, in order to carry out the method of examination advised by Mr. Lloyd, then it is needless to say that that wound should be made use of in order to carry out a more complete investigation.

3. **The Removal of the Stone.**—Having detected the stone by one or other of the methods described, "the overlying part of the kidney should be cut into with a narrow straight bistoury; then with a scooping movement of the finger, introduced through the incision, the stone, unless a branched or very large one, can be raised to the surface of the parietal wound on the point of the finger; or a pair of forceps might be passed into the kidney by the side of the finger, and the stone seized and withdrawn. The finger is, however, much to be preferred; and if the incision is small, as it ought to be, the finger serves the purpose of plugging the renal wound, while it lacerates the renal tissue to the necessary extent. By this plan the hæmorrhage is minimised, and the rent made with the finger heals as readily as the cut" (Morris).

In the place of the forceps a small scoop may be used, and may be made to supplement the action of the finger. Whenever possible, it is most desirable that the calculus be removed entire.

If the stone be felt in the pelvis of the kidney, the steps taken to effect its removal must depend upon the surgical bias of the individual operation. Some surgeons, as already stated (page 486), advise that the pelvis should be reached by cutting through the renal tissue; others recommend an incision direct into the pelvis itself. This incision must always be very cautiously made. Whenever possible, the opening should be from behind, and the instrument used should not be sharp. It often happens that the pelvic wall overlying the stone can be opened by means of the finger-nail, or at least by means of a steel director or a sharp spoon or scoop.

If the stone be irregularly branched, it is better to break it up into two or more fragments, and to remove them separately, so as to avoid undue laceration of the kidney. Such removal should be followed by a free irrigation of the part with a warm and weak antiseptic solution. In this way Mr. Kendal Franks removed a stone weighing, when complete, 171 grains (*Lancet*, vol. ii., 1880, page 1223).

Some of the largest stones met with have
entire. The great calculus, weighing no less tl
removed by Mr. Jacobson in 1886, was extracte
Soc. Trans., 1889, page 203).

The number of stones removed may b
In one of Mr. Jacobson's cases no less than fc
most of them of large or fair size, were rein
kidney of a boy aged fifteen.

When the calculus is found to block up th
ureter, its removal is often a matter of the
culty, involving infinite patience and no littl
skill.

The bleeding which follows upon the remov
will usually yield to the well-applied pressure o
sponge. If, however, the oozing cannot be cl
means, the wound in the kidney may be plug
of iodoform or simple gauze, which can b
twenty-four hours.

In any case in which the wound has beei
renal pelvis, no attempt should be made to clos
This measure has been carried out, and has
with disastrous results (*Westminster Hospital*
page 161).

4. The Closure of the Wound.—After the w
well washed out, a full-sized drainage-tube sh
duced to the very bottom of the incision. It
contact with the wound in the kidney; and
opening has been made in the pelvis of the org
abscess in the gland has been opened, it ma
actually to introduce the deep end of the tube i
Much pain is, however, apt to follow the int
tube into the kidney substance.

The wound in the parietes is then closed in
and the drainage-tube secured in place by a
worm gut forms the best suture material.

The wound may be dressed with large spong
iodoform, or with pads of absorbent wool or
linen of considerable thickness.

The dressing in any case is best secured l
many-tailed bandage.

Complications and Modifications of the Operation.

1. *The Exposure of the Kidney.*—It is important that the incision made in the parietes should be sufficient to meet the needs of the particular case. When the patient is stout and the loin deep, a considerable incision may be called for.

Additional room may be gained by converting the usual lumbar incision into a T-shaped one by cutting downwards towards the crest of the ilium (*see* Nephrectomy, page 497); or the quadratus lumborum muscle, when exposed, may be freely incised in a line at right angles to its fibres.

Occasionally the lower end of the kidney barely reaches below the twelfth rib. In such case Mr. Morris advises that an upward incision be made over the last rib, a little posterior to the front extremity of the oblique wound.

It is important that the twelfth rib be clearly defined and identified by counting the ribs from above downwards. The last rib is not infrequently rudimentary, and when the pleura descends in such a case below the lower edge of the eleventh rib, it may readily be wounded if the incision be carried upwards. This happened in a case reported by Dr. Dumreicher. Dr. Holl has shown that the last rib is often so short as not to reach as far as the outer margin of the sacro-lumbalis muscle, and such a structure may readily be mistaken for the transverse process of a vertebra. Even when the last rib is of normal size, the pleura may descend below it; and this would appear to have been the condition of things in a case of Mr. Thornton's, in which he wounded the pleura, but in which no costal abnormality is noted ("Surgery of the Kidneys," page 83).

The operation may be somewhat complicated by an excessive amount of subcutaneous fat. "If this fat is very abundant," writes Mr. Jacobson, "some of it should be ligatured with chromic gut and removed; poorly vitalised, it is prone to suppurate tediously and to delay healing."

Rigidity and possible thickening of the muscles in some cases of long-standing disease may raise a difficulty in the way of the operation, and a still more serious obstacle may be due to the matting of the tissues together around the kidney. These inflammatory adhesions and organised deposits of plastic lymph may greatly complicate the operation.

Some difficulty has been experienced in finding the kidney through the lumbar incision. Mr. Bruce Clarke mentions a case in which "an hour elapsed before even the kidney could be found."

The organ when found may be difficult to deal with. It may be unduly covered by the ribs, or may be firmly fixed by inflammatory tissue to the surrounding structures

The kidney, on the other hand, may be unusually motile. it may be difficult to fix, and, when counter-pressure is applied, the organ may repeatedly slip up under the ribs.

2. *The Detection of the Stone.*—The calculus may be very difficult to detect, especially if it be of small size, or if it be lodged in a calyx, or if it be fixed in a very indurated kidney. The kidney often becomes hard and tough under the continued irritation of a stone, and this very hardness of the renal substance should raise suspicion. The kidney may be sacculated, and in one of the sacculi a small stone may fall, and be difficult to find.

The stone may be lost in the rush of fluid which escapes when the pelvis of a much-distended kidney is opened.

Mr. Morris draws attention (*Brit. Med. Journ.*, Nov. 16th. 1889) to the following difficulties that may stand in the way of a ready detection of the stone:—

Deposits of tubercle, or even small abscesses, just beneath the renal surface may, from their hardness or outline, give the same tactile sensation as a calculus.

In sacculated kidneys the renal cavity may be wholly or partially filled by a soft mortary phosphatic calculus, which gives no sound nor resistance to the scalpel or trocar.

"There is a condition of impaction which absolutely baffles detection," writes Mr. Morris, " unless by chance the stone is struck on probing the kidney. This is when the calculus is fixed in a recess of the kidney of normal size and consistence with a thick layer of renal tissue all around it."

3. *The Removal of the Stone.*—The hæmorrhage from the wound in the kidney may be very severe.

When the kidney tissue has suppurated, and the calculus lies in the abscess sac, the operation is usually easy and the situation of the abscess more or less readily indicated. Difficulty in removing the stone may depend upon a very mobile kidney which is hard to fix, upon the stone being very small or very large, and especially upon the calculus being branched. Very special difficulties will nearly always attend the attempt to remove a large branched calculus embedded in the calyces or near the outlet of the pelvis.

Multiple calculi may give rise to difficulty, as may also a stone situated in the anterior part of the kidney near the entrance of the blood-vessels.

Soft calculi, which break up readily, and which exist rather in the form of a calculous deposit than of a distinct stone, are also very difficult to deal with efficiently.

B.—THE ABDOMINO-LUMBAR OPERATION.

This method, as the name to some extent implies, involves the exposure of the kidney through an incision in the anterior abdominal parietes, and the subsequent removal of the calculus through the ordinary lumbar wound.

The kidney is most conveniently exposed through Langenbüch's incision. The details of this operation are given in the section on abdominal nephrectomy (page 502).

The present procedure is conducted upon the following lines:—The abdomen is opened by Langenbüch's incision over the suspected kidney. The hand is introduced into the peritoneal cavity, and both kidneys and both ureters are carefully examined. The calculus is sought for by the fingers of the hand so introduced, and by means of this hand the kidney is fixed, and the colon guarded during the second step of the operation. This step consists in cutting down upon the stone from the loin.

The lumbar incision does not implicate the peritoneum, and may be made of much smaller dimensions than the wound usually required. The opening in the abdominal cavity is primarily for the purposes of exploration and diagnosis, and secondarily it allows of the stone being extracted from the loin with greater readiness and certainty.

This method of nephro-lithotomy is advocated by Mr. Thornton, who has performed the combined operation in ten cases. Of this number, eight recovered, one died, and one was left with a permanent fistula, for which nephrectomy was subsequently performed.

The following advantages have been claimed for this method :—The condition of both kidneys can be ascertained; the stone is detected with greater ease and certainty; there is no fear of an accidental wound of the colon or peritoneum. The lumbar incision is smaller, and there is consequently less risk of extravasation of urine, and of a subsequent lumbar hernia.

The objections urged against the operation are that two incisions are made instead of one, that the peritoneal cavity is opened up, and that the extent and severity of the operation are increased. The advantages of a smaller lumbar incision would be negatived when much manipulation is required to extract the stone, and when severe bleeding followed the wounding of the kidney. If the surgeon has one hand in the abdomen, he has only one free for the necessary manipulation in the loin; and in a complex case the single hand would scarcely suffice. It is, moreover, a matter of question whether the stone could be detected more readily through an abdominal than through a lumbar incision.

The After-treatment.—This concerns mainly the lumbar wound. If an incision has been made into the abdomen, it is closed by sutures and treated in the usual way.

For the first few days the whole or the greater part of the urine secreted by the wounded kidney will escape through the loin. It soon, however, diminishes, and after a period varying from a few days to a few weeks it usually ceases altogether. The wound must be kept very clean. The dressings should be large and absorbent, and must, so long as urine is escaping, be changed very frequently. To protect the skin, lint spread with boracic ointment or vaseline may be applied over the wound, a hole being provided for the tube to pass through. As soon as the escape of urine has very distinctly diminished, the tube may be gradually shortened, and then finally removed. The wound, as a rule, heals quickly and without complication.

The Results of nephro-lithotomy have been remarkably good in cases in which the kidney has been otherwise healthy. Newman has collected forty-two examples of such operations without a death. Where suppuration was present, sixty operations were followed by twenty-six deaths, a mortality of over forty-three per cent.

Mr. Tait records fourteen operations for stone, with one death (*Brit. Med. Journ.*, Nov. 16th, 1889).

The chief dangers of the operation would appear to be due to hæmorrhage, cellulitis, uræmia, septicæmia, and renal fistula.

2. NEPHROTOMY.

This term is conveniently applied as well to the mere exposure of the kidney through the loin for the purposes of examination, as to the making of an incision into the organ so exposed for certain therapeutic reasons.

Nephrotomy in the latter sense is applied to the treatment of cases of calculous suppression, of simple or hydatid cysts, of hydro-nephrosis, and certain examples of pyo-nephrosis. The operation of puncture of the kidney is dealt with at the end of this section.

The Operation is carried out in the manner already indicated (page 482). The general circumstances of the operation, the position of the patient on the table, and the instruments required, are all considered in the section referred to.

1. *In Cases of Suppuration.*—In some cases of suppuration the presence of redness and swelling may indicate a deviation from the usual incision.

In such instances the tissues between the skin and the kidney will be more or less matted together, and may, indeed, form little more than the wall of an abscess.

When the presence of pus is less distinctly indicated, the kidney is exposed in due course and is examined for evidence of abscess. At any suspicious spot a fine grooved needle may be introduced into the kidney, and be followed, if pus escape, by an incision, and then by dilating forceps.

Thick or caseous pus may be evacuated by the scoop or finger-nail. In any case the interior of the abscess should be explored by the finger. This examination may reveal other abscess cavities or pockets of pus, or may demonstrate the presence of an encysted calculus.

After the evacuation of the pus and the exploration of the cyst, the kidney should be well flushed out with a warm and weak antiseptic solution; a drainage-tube is then introduced up to the kidney, and the parietal wound is closed around the tube.

In some cases it may appear d
into the renal cavity, but the pi
can be but seldom necessary.

In cases in which the kidne
the organ must be steadied whi
dealt with ; and before the tube
to secure the too movable gland
two deep sutures introduced in
mended by Mr. Pearce Gould.

The after-treatment of these
from that indicated in nephro-li

The tube should be short
must be frequently changed, a
quently and freely irrigated.

2. *In Cases of Cyst.*—The k
steadied and examined. A porti
of the fatty tissue which covers
wall so exposed may be brougl
there after having been opene
the scalpel or tenotome, and
enlarged with Lister's sinus for
As the contents escape, the cyst
forceps and is drawn towards
sutured directly to the skin, it r
points of thin catgut suture to t
depths of the wound.   This
kidney is unduly mobile.   Whe
by adhesions, it will suffice mere

In any case, the interior of t:
the forefinger.

A large drainage-tube is
wound is closed around it.

The after-treatment of the
already indicated.

In cases of simple cyst the c
and closes, and the wound heal
hydatid cyst a like result may 1
suppuration.

When done for hydro-nephr
some permanent obstruction in

of urine and pus must ensue. Unless this fistula is treated by
nephrectomy, it is well that some receptacle for the discharge
from the loin should be employed. Mr. Morris's apparatus made
for this purpose answers well.

In cases of nephrotomy carried out for tubercular disease
of the kidney, it is scarcely to be expected that the resulting
sinus will close. The abscess cavity should be not only well
evacuated, but its walls well scraped. The healing of the sinus
may possibly be hastened by a few injections of tuberculin.

Puncturing the Kidney.—The following account of this
measure—which, although slight as an operation, may prove
serious as a means of treatment—is derived from Mr. Morris's
work on the kidney:—

" Puncturing the kidney with a trocar or the aspirator is
performed for the relief or cure of hydro- and pyo-nephrosis,
large isolated serous or blood cysts of the substance of the
kidney, and hydatid cysts. When, from their degree of distension, such swellings are causing serious consequences by
pressure, or there is risk of the cyst wall rupturing, the contents ought to be evacuated.

" The point selected for puncturing will depend on circumstances. If there be any spot over the swelling which is thin,
soft, prominent, or fluctuating, the trocar should be there
inserted. A point which is not seldom indicated is midway
between the umbilicus and the anterior superior spine of the
ilium; or half an inch below, and an inch and a half to the
side of, the navel. When no particular spot is suggested by
discoloration or prominence, no better place can be selected on
the left side than an inch in front of the last intercostal space;
but if the tumour be of the right side, this is too high, as the
liver would probably be traversed. If there is no indication
for operating elsewhere, the best spot to select when the
kidney is of the right side is half-way between the last rib and
the crest of the ilium, between two and two and a half inches
behind the anterior superior spine of the ilium.

" In performing the operation the aspirating trocar should
be inserted without any previous incision of the skin; if a
larger trocar be used, an incision through the integument
and muscles is sometimes made before introducing the instrument.

" The dangers of the operation are very slight. If, however, the puncture be made too far forwards, and through non-adherent peritoneum, some of the contents of the cyst might be extravasated into the peritoneal cavity on withdrawing the cannula, an accident which has proved fatal in more than one case. There is also the danger of wounding the intestine, which, as a rule, is in front of and adherent to the tumour; and if the trocar be long, and be thrust too far inwards, it might penetrate some important blood-vessel, and cause dangerous, if not fatal, hæmorrhage. The penetration of the thin edge of the liver with an aspirating needle, though to be avoided, is not an accident likely to be followed by any ill consequence. The instrument should not be introduced too near the ribs, for fear of wounding the pleura."

3. NEPHRECTOMY.

The operation of removing or excising the kidney has been performed for tumour of the kidney, for renal or ureteral fistula, and for disorganisation of the organ by injury, suppuration, or urinary infiltration. Nephrectomy has also been carried out in cases where nephrotomy or nephro-lithotomy has failed, and in certain examples of movable kidney.

Nephrectomy may be performed in two ways:—

    1. By incision through the loin—lumbar nephrectomy.
    2. By incision through the anterior abdominal parietes —abdominal nephrectomy.

1. LUMBAR NEPHRECTOMY.

The Instruments Required.—Scalpels; bistouries; dissecting, artery, and pressure forceps; toothed forceps; large pressure or clamp forceps, straight and angular; broad metal rectangular retractors; metal or ivory spatulæ; blunt hooks; stout aneurysm needle in a long handle; pedicle needle; stout silk ligatures; flat director or periosteal elevator. Sharp spoons and Paquelin's cautery may be of service.

The position of the patient, and of the operator and his assistants, is the same as has been already described. The hard pillow under the loin should be used, in order to extend the space between the last rib and the iliac crest to its utmost

The Operation.—1. **The Exposure and Isolation of the kidney.** — The incision made is the same as has been already described in the account of nephro-lithotomy (page 482). Through this incision the kidney is exposed, and through it an organ of normal size may be removed.

When the organ is reached and has been superficially examined, it will usually be found necessary to enlarge the original incision. This may be done in many ways.

The oblique incision may be extended to the full length admitted by the conformation of the individual.

Morris advises that to the original cut be conjoined a second incision, running vertically downwards from the first, and starting from it about one inch in front of its posterior extremity (Fig. 380, B). This second incision is left until the kidney has been reached and explored, and is made by cutting from within outwards with a blunt-pointed bistoury, guided by the index finger of the left hand. This vertical incision affords increased facility for dealing with the pedicle (page 499).

The position of the vertical incision with reference to the original oblique cut may be modified according to circumstances. It may be more convenient that it should start from the centre of the oblique cut, or from its actual posterior extremity.

Other incisions, more or less closely resembling the above have been advised or carried out.

Some surgeons carry a short transverse incision forwards from the lower end of the oblique one. The actual form of incision is a matter of little moment, provided that sufficient room is obtained and that the peritoneum is not opened.

König divides the soft parts vertically along the border of the erector spinæ down to a point just above the iliac crest. He then curves the incision forwards towards the umbilicus, and ends it at the outer border of the rectus muscle (Fig. 380, c). All the muscles are divided down to the peritoneum. The vertical part of the wound is completed first, and the fingers being introduced, the peritoneum is detached and is pushed forwards, so as to be free of the anterior part of the incision when that comes to be made.

This incision—known as the retro-peritoneal lumbo-abdominal incision—gives plenty of room, but it is needlessly extensive. It involves a very considerable division of muscular fibre, and is very likely to be followed by a ventral hernia. When such an extensive exposure of the renal region is called for, it is better that Langenbüch's incision should be employed.

The kidney is exposed in the manner already described (page 482).

It is now necessary to examine it and to separate it from its connections. Good broad rectangular retractors should be used, so as to expose the parts well, and an assistant should at the same time press the kidney into the wound by the hands applied over the front of the abdomen. If there have been no inflammation in the peri-nephritic tissue, the separation of the kidney is easy.

The fatty tissue around the kidney can readily be detached by means of the index finger of one hand introduced into the depths of the wound, and swept round the organ in close contact with its capsule. In this manner the gland is readily enucleated and isolated.

Even when no inflammation has occurred, it is possible—as Mr. Morris points out—that some of the renal capsule may be torn off and left behind when this manœuvre is carried out. When there has been much inflammation, as in cases of calculous or scrofulous pyo-nephrosis, the tissue surrounding the kidney will be found condensed and adherent, and the enucleation of the organ will then be difficult or impossible. In such case the kidney should be enucleated from its thickened and firmly-adherent capsule, and the latter left behind with the pedicle. In effecting this enucleation, a flat hernia director, or a round-pointed periosteal elevator, will be found to be of service. The only guide in such enucleation is the exposed kidney tissue itself.

It may be possible, in some of these cases, to isolate the kidney, together with its capsule, entire, by means of cutting-scissors curved on the flat being employed for the purpose; but the satisfaction of removing every trace of the disease is hardly sufficient to justify the risk incurred by such proceeding.

In any instance, the enucleation must be conducted with caution; the capsule may be stripped off in one place, and the adherent tissue cut through in another. The kidney must not be violently torn out; and, indeed, in such cases, but little traction can be brought to bear upon the organ.

When the kidney has been already exposed by a previous operation, it will probably be easier to enucleate the organ from its own capsule than from the peri-nephritic fatty tissue.

2. **The Treatment of the Pedicle.**—The kidney, having been freed, is drawn as far into the wound as possible, and the pedicle is isolated with the fingers, and examined carefully. To obtain more room, the lower ribs may be drawn forcibly upwards with a strong retractor.

When convenient, an assistant may draw the kidney forwards while the surgeon manipulates the pedicle. A suitable aneurysm needle, in a long handle, is passed cautiously between the ureter and the vessels. It is passed naked, and when its point is exposed upon the other side of the pedicle, the eye is threaded with carbolised silk, which is carried through the pedicle in the form of a double loop as the needle is withdrawn. The loop is divided and the needle removed. One ligature should enclose the vessels, and the other the ureter. The ligature on the vessels is tied first. It should be carried as deeply as possible, in order that sufficient room may be provided between the kidney and the ligature for safe division of the pedicle.

As the ligature is being drawn tight, all traction upon the pedicle must be taken off.

The more completely the ureter is isolated, the better. The ligature which surrounds it may be at once drawn tight, or the ureter may be clamped in the line of the ligature.

The pedicle is now divided with blunt-pointed scissors close to the hilum of the kidney.

Before severing the pedicle, some surgeons apply a separate single ligature around the whole of the already ligatured parts.

The kidney is now removed. Its delivery may be assisted by pressure exercised upon the anterior wall of the abdomen, and by drawing up the lower ribs.

The pedicle is examined. Any bleeding point detected should be at once seized with pressure forceps, and secured later. Such hæmorrhage may depend upon the existence of aberrant or abnormal branches that have escaped the ligature on the pedicle.

If the ureter has been clamped, it may be left to be dealt with at this stage of the operation. If it appears healthy, the ligature which surrounds it may be drawn tight, and the clamp removed. If it be dilated and occupied with foul or tubercular pus, the stump should be carefully cleansed, and then scraped with a sharp spoon. It may, after this treatment, either be ligatured and dropped back into the wound in the usual way, or it may be brought into the parietal incision, and retained there by a few points of suture.

Silk is the most convenient material for the ligature of the pedicle, but other substances have been used with success, and notably, among them, kangaroo tendon.

No attempt should be made to ligature the artery and the vein separately, and in most instances such a practice would be impossible.

The possible existence of abnormal veins and arteries must always be borne in mind. These vessels may escape the clamp or the ligature, and yet be severed when the kidney is removed. In more than one recorded case, fatal hæmorrhage has resulted from this cause.

In the event of bleeding persisting after the kidney has been removed and the pedicle tied, the wound must be well exposed, dried, and illumined. In nearly every instance it will be possible to pick up the bleeding vessel with pressure forceps, and subsequently to tie it. If the hæmorrhage persists, and it is impossible to secure the bleeding point so, the wound must be well plugged from the bottom with gauze, which is kept in place by firm bandaging.

The wound in the parietes is now closed by sutures. These should be of silkworm gut, and should be passed deeply, so as to embrace the various layers of tissue divided. A few superficial sutures will in addition be required. A drainage-tube is introduced into the depths of the wound, and the part is dressed in the usual way, and is supported by a firm flannel bandage.

Complications of the Operation.—It may be found to be impossible to remove the kidney after it has been exposed. This complication is illustrated by a case of Mr. Howard Marsh's. The case was one of pyelitis. When the kidney was incised, much fœtid pus escaped, and the gland was found to be so extensively diseased that its removal was necessary.

Owing to the size of the kidney and the firmness with which it was embedded, this was found to be impossible. That part of the kidney which had been exposed was transfixed with a double ligature and cut away. A fatal suppression of urine followed. At the post-mortem the remainder of the kidney was dissected out only with the greatest difficulty.

If, when the kidney is exposed through the loin, it is found to be of so great size as to render removal through the lumbar incision doubtful, it is better to perform the abdominal operation than persist at all hazards in the attempt to extract the organ from the loin.

There is little to recommend the advice that in these cases, after the vessels have been secured by a temporary ligature, the kidney should be cut away in separate portions.

When the pedicle is very short and thick, and perhaps overlapped by the kidney, a preliminary ligature should be applied, and then the kidney itself be cut away well in front of it. After the removal of the diseased organ the stump can be brought into view, the vessels can be secured by fresh ligatures more conveniently applied, and the stump trimmed by removing as much tissue as the position of the ligatures will allow. No evil appears to have followed when small portions of the kidney have been of necessity left behind when dealing with a very short pedicle.

Mr. Greig Smith mentions a case in which the aorta and vena cava were adherent to the capsule of a much-enlarged suppurating kidney, and in which it was found to be impossible at the autopsy to dissect apart the vascular walls and the renal capsule. In such a case a provisional pedicle must be made out of the kidney tissues, and Mr. Smith advises that the base of the organ be surrounded by a temporary ligature attached to an écraseur while the diseased tissues are cut away close to it.

A serious complication arises in cases in which tl
has become adherent to the peritoneum or to sor
abdominal viscera. In excising such an organ, the pt
must of necessity be opened up, and must needs be
fine catgut sutures.

In one instance (*Amer. Journ. Med. Sc.*, 1882,
the removal of a kidney was found to be impossible
autopsy revealed that it was not only adherent to t
around it, but also to the colon and pancreas.

After-treatment.—The patient must be kept i
cumbent position until healing is complete. The
tube may be removed on the second or third da
cases. The wound usually heals well, although som
'four weeks may elapse before the drainage-track is
closed. The recumbent position should be insisted t
the healing is firm.

2. ABDOMINAL NEPHRECTOMY.

The list of instruments required has already b
(page 496). The operation is conducted upon the ge
observed in other abdominal operations. The prep
the patient, and the general disposition of the p
surgeon, and his assistants, have been considered in t
section (page 221).

The operation here described is that known a
buch's operation.

The Operation.—The incision—known as Lan
incision—is vertical, is made in the semilunar line
four inches in length, and is commenced just l
margin of the ribs. The centre of the incision will
be about the level of the umbilicus. The abdomen
and when all bleeding has been checked the hand
duced.

As a first measure the hand may be passed aci
opposite side of the body, and the opposite kidne
examined. If this organ be found to be extensive
or if it be discovered that the patient has but o
then the nephrectomy must needs be at once aband

The kidney on the affected side is now exa
size is estimated, its general characters as regard

consistence, etc., are ascertained, and the condition of its pedicle is demonstrated.

The small intestines are kept aside by means of a large flat sponge, which is introduced into the abdomen.

The colon is made out, and is pushed towards the median line. The surgeon then incises the outer layer of the meso-colon vertically over the renal region. Into the rent thus made the fingers are introduced, and the kidney is laid bare.

If the parts around the gland are in a fairly healthy condition, it is well at once to clear the pedicle and to ligature the vessels. When this has been done, the enucleation of the kidney becomes an almost bloodless procedure. The vessels are reached by stripping off the peritoneum in the direction of the aorta. They may be tied in two segments, the ligatures being passed on an aneurysm needle through the centre of the vascular part of the pedicle. No advantage appears to attend the attempt to secure the artery and the vein separately. The enucleation of the kidney can now be pro-ceeded with, and the organ can be cleared up to the pedicle. The vessels on the renal side of the ligatures are secured by pressure forceps applied close to the kidney, and between the forceps and the ligatures the vessels are divided with blunt-pointed scissors. A sponge placed beneath the site of the section will absorb any blood that may escape.

Nothing now attaches the kidney but the ureter. When it is found to be in a fairly healthy condition, it is well isolated, and is ligatured at the most convenient spot. Pressure forceps are now applied on the renal side of the ligature, and between the ligature and the forceps the duct is divided. A sponge placed beneath the scissors will absorb any fluid that may escape from the ureter. The ligatured stump is then dropped back into the abdomen, and the kidney is removed.

Should the ureter be found to be diseased or be filled with putrid pus, or be in any condition that would probably give rise to further trouble, it may be turned out through an opening in the loin, as advised by Mr. Henry Morris, and fixed there. The lumbar opening, in such a case, should be placed just at the outer edge of the quadratus lumborum muscle, and it can be conveniently made by cutting down externally upon forceps that have been thrust towards the skin in that position.

Mr. Thornton's proposal to bring the end of the diseased ureter into the parietal wound, and to fix it there, has been properly condemned—on the grounds that the ureter so fixed would form a rigid and possibly troublesome intra-abdominal band, and that the septic discharge from the tube might interfere with the healing of the abdominal wound.

When the kidney is found to be very adherent, and to be embedded in a mass of inflammatory tissue, it should be enucleated before the pedicle is dealt with, or before any attempt is made to secure the pedicle. The vessels in such a case may be very difficult to demonstrate, and may only be discovered when they are cut across.

In any case, the cavity left by the removal of the kidney is at once plugged with one or more sponges. Should any bleeding points be detected, they are at once secured with pressure forceps. The sponge will have been some little time in position by the time the ureter has been secured. The sponge is removed, the sac is well cleaned out, and if any septic matter is likely to have found its way into it, the whole cavity is well washed out with a weak and warm antiseptic solution. When the operator has convinced himself that all oozing has ceased, and that the operation area is absolutely clean, the wound in the parietes may be closed in the usual way, and a suitable dressing applied.

If, however, the parts involved have been much disturbed, if there has been much oozing, or if some little oozing still persists, or, above all, if any septic material from the kidney has escaped into the cavity left by the removal of the kidney, then drainage should be employed. The drainage-tube is best carried through the loin at a convenient spot close to the anterior or outer edge of the quadratus lumborum muscle.

There is nothing to recommend a drainage-tube introduced through the abdominal wound.

There is no need to close by sutures the rent made in the peritoneum, nor to attempt thereby to shut off the wound cavity in the loin from the general peritoneal cavity. It is better that the sac should be left open.

Mr. Barker states that " it is well to unite the anterior lip of the wound in the meso-colon with the anterior lip of the peritoneal layer of the abdominal wound, so as to shut off the peri-nephral space from the general cavity of the abdomen."

This plan appears to have been carried out by Mr. Thornton in one case, with the result that acute intestinal obstruction followed, of which the patient died, although enterotomy was performed.

Comment.—In dealing with cysts of the kidney, with cases of pyo-nephrosis, and with such tumours as are represented by soft sarcomata, it is very important that the capsule of the gland be not opened. If a rent be accidentally made, the cystic fluid or the pus escapes into the abdomen, and in the case of a sarcoma a far greater calamity may happen.

Thus, in a case operated on by Czerny, the capsule was broken through, and the soft sarcoma growing within was laid bare. A profuse hæmorrhage ensued, which could only be arrested by temporary compression of the aorta, and which returned as soon as this was taken off. The aorta was finally ligatured. The bleeding ceased, and the patient lived ten hours.

In this operation the close proximity of the vena cava must be borne in mind. In one case Mr. Thornton accidentally included a small piece of the vena cava in the pressure forceps, which had been applied about the renal vessels. When the vessels were divided, a small V-shaped piece was cut out of the wall of the vena cava, and the patient bled to death.

The After-treatment resembles that observed after other abdominal operations. It is well, however, to avoid opium in any form, even in small doses, and to keep the bowels at rest, if possible, for the first five to seven days.

OTHER METHODS.

1. **By Median Incision.**—This operation is very fully dealt with in Mr. Barker's paper in the *Med.-Chir. Trans.*, vol. lxiii. The abdomen is opened in the median line, the intestines are pushed well over to the opposite side by means of sponges, and the kidney is exposed. The colon is displaced to the outer side, and the meso-colon is opened through its inner layer. The rest of the operation does not differ materially from that just described.

When compared with Langenbüch's operation, that procedure may claim the following advantages over the method of the median incision :—

In Langenbüch's operation the kidney is more directly exposed, and the pedicle is more easily reached; the peritoneal cavity is less extensively exposed; the kidney is reached through the outer layer of the meso-colon, and therefore the main colic vessels are not met with, and consequently not exposed to damage.

The median operation has one small advantage—the opposite kidney can be more readily examined.

2. **By Lateral Extra-Peritoneal Incision.**—This operation is performed as follows :—A vertical incision is made from the anterior superior iliac spine up to the eighth rib. The various layers of the parietes are cut through until the peritoneum is reached. This membrane is not incised, but is stripped up from the iliac fossa, and from the anterior surface of the kidney, and is displaced inwards.

The kidney is thus exposed, and the pedicle is dealt with in the usual way.

No especial advantage can be claimed for this method. The wound is deep, and the risk of ventral hernia is increased. The fact that the peritoneum is not opened is the only point that can be urged in favour of the procedure.

COMPARATIVE VALUE OF LUMBAR AND ABDOMINAL NEPHRECTOMY.

The advantages and disadvantages of these two methods of operating may be expressed as follows :—

Lumbar Nephrectomy.—*Advantages.*—The peritoneum is not opened. Excellent drainage can be provided. If putrid pus escape, the area infected is small. If nephrectomy be abandoned, the possibly-diseased organ is left in a convenient position. The operation is of special service when dense posterior adhesions exist. The wound is large enough for all ordinary purposes.

Disadvantages.—The operation is difficult in the corpulent. There is some danger of wounding the pleura. The kidney is not always very easily found. The peritoneum and the colon are in danger when extensive anterior adhesions exist. The pedicle is less easily reached and less safely secured. The kidney is more likely to be torn in the act of removal. The operation is not adapted for large tumours. Above all, the opposite kidney cannot be examined.

Abdominal Nephrectomy.—*Advantages.*—Ample room is provided, and the kidney is readily found. The pedicle is easily reached and easily dealt with. If the incision be in the semilunar line, a series of muscular planes are not divided. The opposite kidney can be examined. Tumours of any size can be removed.

Disadvantages.—The peritoneum is opened, and may be contaminated should putrid pus escape during the operation. Unless a second incision is made in the loin, efficient drainage is not provided. When dense posterior adhesions exist, the operation may be difficult. The disposition to a ventral hernia is probably greater than is the case in lumbar nephrectomy.

Results of the Operation.—The most complete statistics have been provided by Dr. Newman ("Surgical Diseases of the Kidney," 1888). They show the following results:—

	Cases.		Deaths.
For hydro-nephrosis and cystic disease ...	46	...	18
For suppurative disease without calculus	54	...	18
For „ „ with „	61	...	22
For tubercular disease	33	...	12
For tumours	74	...	24
	268		94

In general terms, the mortality attending the operation of nephrectomy may be placed at about 40 per cent.

Dr. Newman gives the mortality after lumbar nephrectomy as 30·5 per cent., and after the abdominal method as 47·1 per cent. It must be remembered, however, that the abdominal operation will probably represent the more serious class of case.

Death has been due to shock, to hæmorrhage, to uræmia and anuria, to peritonitis, and to the results of septic inflammation.

4. NEPHRORRHAPHY.

This operation is practised in cases of floating, movable. or wandering kidney, in which the organ is the seat of frequent, severe, and spasmodic attacks of pain, or of more or less continuous discomfort, and in which all other measures—such as the use of pads and belts—have failed.

A full consideration of the whole subject will be found in a paper by Dr. Keen, published in the *Annals of Surgery*, Aug., 1890, and in a monograph by Max Sulzer, *Deutsch. Zeit. f. Chir.*, 1891, page 506.

The latter author refers to eighty cases of nephrorrhaphy, and to thirty-seven instances of nephrectomy for movable kidney.

The mortality of the operation has been very low. The results are dealt with on page 510.

Mr. Morris claims that the measure "has proved very successful in its ultimate results, as well as in the readiness of recovery from the operation."

The Operation.—The kidney is exposed through the loin in the manner already described (page 482). When reached, it is well forced into the wound by an assistant, who presses upon it with both hands applied over the anterior abdominal wall. The fatty capsule is well opened up. Often very considerable difficulty will be experienced in fixing an unusually mobile organ. In one instance I found it necessary to fix the kidney with a tenaculum while the suture was being applied.

Among the many methods that have been employed to fix the gland, that advocated and practised by Mr. Morris appears to be the most certain. The following is this surgeon's description :—

"In the first three operations I contented myself with drawing the adipose capsule well up into the wound, and cutting some of it away, so as to diminish the size of the space in which the kidney had wandered, then stitching the shortened capsule to the cut edges of muscles and skin by three or four sutures, leaving a considerable part of the loin wound to heal by granulation, with the view to thereby secure a firmer hold on the kidney by the new-formed tissue of the wound. Finding this was not a sufficient holdfast, in my subsequent operations I inserted sutures into the kidney substance in the following way :—Three kangaroo tendons are passed through the posterior surface of the kidney—one nearer the upper, the other nearer the lower end, and the third midway between the other two, but nearer the hilum. Each suture is buried for a length of three-quarters of an inch within the renal substance, and penetrates about half an inch into the thickness of the organ. The upper suture passes through the upper edge of the shortened adipose capsule, the transversalis fascia, and the muscles, and is tied to them; the lower suture is similarly passed through and tied to the lower edges of the cut structures; and the intermediate suture is passed through both edges of the divided capsule, fascia, and muscles, and laces all up together. The ligatures are then cut short and buried in the wound; one or two catgut sutures bring the rest of the cut edges of the muscles together, and the skin is closed by silk sutures, one or two of which are made to fix the adipose capsule well up between the edges of the skin. The wound is covered by iodoform cotton-wool, and a large elastic pad of cotton-wool is fastened over the front of the kidney, so as to steady and support it in its new position. The wound heals without suppuration, except that a track is sometimes left for a few weeks along the course of the drain-tube."

The plan of using kangaroo tendon sutures, which were inserted permanently, originated with Mr. Pearce Gould. In performing this operation, I have used silkworm gut in the place of kangaroo tendon; and I have found it most convenient to pass the sutures by means of a large, curved Hagedorn's needle. I have not made use of a drainage-tube.

Dr. Newman employs a method that has been attended with excellent results, which he describes in the following words:—" In addition to stitching the kidney to the abdominal parietes, I split the fibrous capsule, and separate it from the surface of the kidney, as I find it is of little use to stitch the adipose capsule, on account of its being so loose. I have no doubt that the failures in fixing the kidney have arisen from neglect of this precaution. When the fibrous capsule is not divided, the granulations of the wound in the parietes fail to form a firm attachment to the surface of the dense fibrous capsule; but when the raw surface of the kidney is exposed, a most intimate band of adhesions is formed. The amount of granulation tissue occupying the lower portion of the wound should be increased by keeping a large drainage-tube between the deeper parts of the wound and the surface of the kidney. By so doing, a wedge-shaped mass ot granulation tissue forms, the apex corresponding to the cutaneous surface, while the base lies against the raw surface of the kidney. In all the cases in which I have operated, the result has been most satisfactory."

Some of the other methods employed require a brief notice. Mr. Thornton has found ordinary silk sutures, deeply passed into the substance of the kidney and left in for a fortnight, to answer admirably. He advises that the areolar tissue in the vicinity should be "stirred up," and that several thick drainage-tubes should be inserted, "so as to obtain the maximum of aseptic irritation."

Silk sutures, when introduced with the idea of being permanently retained, have excited suppuration, and have led to troublesome sinuses.

Catgut sutures have proved a little untrustworthy, having been too quickly absorbed.

The plan of fixing the kidney by means of catgut sutures which merely included the capsule, and of then stuffing the wound from the bottom with gauze to induce granulation, has not proved trustworthy.

The After-treatment.—The treatment of the wound is conducted upon the usual lines. When drainage-tubes are employed, these are not removed until evidences of inflammation appear. It is essential that the patient should rest in the recumbent position for a period of not less than four to six weeks after the operation. During convalescence the colon should be kept empty, and after the patient gets up, a supporting belt should be worn for some few months.

Results.—Dr. Keen has collected 134 cases of nephrorrhaphy. Of this number, four died, representing a mortality of 2·9 per cent. Of 116 cases reported in detail, and reviewed after a period of at least three months, 57·8 per cent. were cured, 12·9 per cent. were improved, and 19·8 per cent. failed.

The cases treated by suture of the fatty capsule only, present 26·6 per cent. of failures; those treated by suture of the fibrous capsule yield 25·9 per cent. of failures; while in those treated by suture involving the kidney substance, the failures are represented by 13·5 per cent.

Part XL
OPERATIONS ON HERNIA.

CHAPTER I.

OPERATIONS FOR STRANGULATED HERNIA.

THE operation for strangulated hernia is not only very frequently performed, but it ranks also as one of the urgent measures of surgery which often need to be carried out at a moment's notice, and possibly under unfavourable conditions. The operation itself is comparatively simple, and needs for its performance but few and simple instruments.

The mortality of the procedure, however, is higher than would at first sight appear probable. In the practice of large hospitals the death-rate will stand at between thirty and forty per cent.

This fact depends not upon the gravity of the operation itself, but upon the condition of the patient at the time of treatment. In numerous cases the hernia has not been discovered; in many the early management of the case has been unwise, taxis has been persevered with unreasonably, and the question of operation has been too long postponed.

The operation itself can carry with it very little danger; it is the delay that is fatal.

The mortality will unquestionably become lower in proportion as the operation is carried out early, and a purposeless expectant treatment is abandoned.

The death-rate is higher after operations upon inguinal than upon femoral hernia, and it reaches its maximum in connection with the umbilical rupture.

In the early part of the present century the great question in connection with the operative treatment of strangulated hernia was whether the sac should be opened or not.

The introduction of improved methods of treating wounds

has rendered this matter one
rule the sac should be opened
strangulation is recent and th
which but slight attempts at
may be left unopened, and
inspecting the gut. In any
should be exposed; and the s
which, after the relief of the
carry out a measure for radic

The Instruments Requir
dissecting forceps; fine-tooth
forceps; blunt-pointed bist

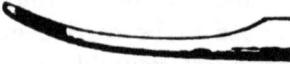

Fig. 381.—coo

hooks; needles; needle in ha
event of its being necessary
lapsed intestine, clamps, inte
suitable sutures should be at

The hernia knife should b
and should have a short cu
"herniotomes," and other co
the stricture should be avoide

The two most convenient
those known as Cooper's and

Preparation and Position
The skin over the area of
cleansed and washed with an

When the region of the g
pubes and on the scrotum or
far as is necessary.

It is well that the bladd
standing cases, in which the
very desirable that the st
washed out. This is the mo
the natural reflexes has bee
cases the stomach may cont

with this poisonous compound still in the viscus, the patient may be sent back to bed after the operation.

In the worse class of case the foul contents of the stomach gush forth by the mouth and nose as soon as anæsthesia is established, and death often follows thereon. The washing-out of the stomach may be accomplished either before or after the operation, and when the patient is wholly or partially anæsthetised.

In the severest cases it is perhaps safest to do it before the herniotomy. Considerable relief follows this measure, and the shock present is often distinctly modified by flushing the stomach with warm or hot water.

The best apparatus to employ is a syphon irrigator, and after the organ has been emptied some pints of water at a temperature of 100° F. can be passed through the stomach. I have found no difficulty to attend this measure, nor is much time occupied in its execution. With the beneficial results I have been distinctly satisfied. If the washing is carried out after the operation, *e.g.*, while the dressings are being applied, it is often to be noted that the after-vomiting due to the anæsthetic is greatly lessened, or even absent.

The patient's limbs and chest should be protected by blankets covered with macintosh sheets. Every care must be taken to avoid exposure to cold, and it may even be well to have a few hot bottles in contact with the body during the operation in cases attended by much collapse.

The patient lies upon the back, close to the right-hand edge of the table. The surgeon stands to the patient's right, and this position he should assume in dealing with all the usual forms of hernia, with those of the left side as well as those of the right.

To take up a position between the patient's legs in operating upon a left hernia is very inconvenient; to stand on the left side is still more awkward. If the pelvis be brought close to the edge of the table, a left hernia is dealt with with the greatest ease from the right-hand side. The assistant stands, opposite to the operator, upon the other side of the table. One assistant alone is required.

Before the operation is commenced, it is well to wedge three or four large sponges between the patient's buttock and

л л

perineum and the table. These sponges will absorb any fluid
which may find its way towards the perineum, and will save
much of the time usually devoted to the cleaning of the
patient after the operation has been completed.

THE OPERATION.

The general details of an operation for strangulated hernia
will now be described. The special features that belong to
the herniæ of particular regions will afterwards be dealt
with. The operation may be conveniently considered under
these headings :—

1. The exposure and opening of the sac.
2. The division of the stricture, and the treatment of
   the contents of the sac.
3. The treatment of the sac and the closure of the
   wound.
4. The treatment of complications.

1. **The Exposure and Opening of the Sac.**—An incision is
made over the neck of the sac, and as a rule in the long axis
of the tumour. The various layers between the integument
and the sac are divided by clean and precise cuts that
involve the whole length of the incision. Any vessels that
are liable to be divided are secured with pressure forceps.

There is no need to use a director in dividing the tissues
which cover the sac, and that dangerous instrument can very
well be dispensed with.

It is needless to say that the various precise anatomical
coverings of the sac cannot be identified as they are divided.
The subcutaneous tissue can of course be recognised, and
in the inguinal region the intercolumnar fascia and the
cremasteric fascia can often be made out; but beyond this
the surgeon will be but little reminded of the coverings which
are so elaborately displayed in the dissecting-room.

"The great mistake in one's first operations," writes Mr.
Banks, in dealing with the exposure of the sac, " is in thinking
that the sac has been reached long before it has. In this way
two or three extensive strippings are often made, and then,
after all, another layer or two are found. By these strippings
the cellular tissue is torn up, as a result of which troublesome
sloughing and suppuration are apt to occur."

The incision should be sufficient in size, and may be enlarged with a probe-pointed bistoury as occasion demands.

Many means of recognising the sac, when it is exposed, have been given. Not a few of these are fallacious and uncertain. The " shining surface " and the " arborescent vessels " of the older text-books will be found to be false guides. The *inner* surface of the sac is smooth and shining, and when such a surface is demonstrated and fluid escapes, it is more than probable that the sac has been opened. There may, however, be no fluid in the sac, as is often the case in umbilical herniæ ; and on the other hand, bursal or lymphatic accumulations of fluid may be found outside a hernial sac, especially in the femoral region, when an ill-fitting truss has been long worn. There are vessels ramifying in the wall of the sac, but they are not always distinct ; and, misled by the appearance of vessels ramifying on a smooth surface, the bowel has been cut into, under the impression that its wall was the wall of the sac. When a plastic form of peritonitis has invaded the hernial sac, the smoothness of the lining membrane may be entirely lost.

The sac, when well exposed, has usually a distinct capsule-like outline, its walls are tense, and when they are thin, the blood-stained fluid contained therein, or the purple gut, may give to the structure a bluish aspect. In a thick-walled sac, that somewhat characteristic bluish tint may be entirely absent.

The sac is best identified by the fingers, rather than by the eyes. As the hernia is laid bare, the surgeon should from time to time pinch up the coverings yet left undivided between the finger and thumb, and estimate their thickness.

Even when adhesions exist, he will be able to find a spot where no such attachments have been formed, to feel the contents of the sac slipping from his grasp, and to appreciate the thickness of the tissue still covering the hernia. When, after repeated examination, he finds that this layer has been reduced to very slender limits he should open it. It may represent not only the sac, but the layer of tissue outside it ; or it may represent an unduly thick sac reduced by dissection. Before actually incising the

A A 2

supposed sac, he may follow up its neck and note its
nections with the surrounding parts; he may endeavo
insinuate a narrow director by the side of the neck of th
and thus ascertain the exact relations of the tissue in qu
with the interior or exterior of the abdomen. If this
precaution be taken, it is scarcely possible to open the
in mistake for the sac.

The more frequent error, however, is to mistake a
mobile bluish sac for the bowel, and to make attemp
reduce it.

Any attempt to demonstrate the sac by counting
supposed anatomical layers that are divided in exposi
is almost sure to be fallacious.

The identification of the sac is usually not difficult, i
corpulent, when allowance has been made for the depth
incision, since the sac tissue often stands out in di
contrast with the mass of loose and fatty tissue
surrounds it. Greater difficulties in the way of identifi
may exist in the emaciated, and in those that have
worn an ill-fitting or unduly tight truss. In
herniæ the sac wall may be expected to be very thin,
it is not infrequently opened prematurely.

The sac, having been identified, is well exposed, an
neck is well cleared. In most herniæ this is a very ea
step; and in cases in which it is intended to divide the
ture without opening the sac, it must of necessity
important step in the operation.

Before opening the sac, the operator pinches up a
portion of the wall between his finger and thumb, in
estimate its thickness and to demonstrate that it is clear
attachments to the contents of the sac. A like fold in th
wall is then picked up by dissecting forceps and open
means of a scalpel, the blade of which is held nearly
operator pulls the little fold of sac away from the bowel
makes the division. When once an opening is made
readily enlarged by means of a blunt-pointed bistou
blunt-pointed scissors. The sac should be cleanly opene
not torn open. The operation up to this point shoul
carried out by careful incisions, and not by tearing.

The method of exposing a hernial sac by tearing

tissues asunder with the forefingers or with a pair of forceps and a director does not belong to operative surgery.

2. The Division of the Stricture, and the Treatment of the Contents of the Sac.—When the contents of the hernia are adherent to the sac wall, some difficulty may attend the full display of the protruded parts. (*See* page 521.)

The exposed bowel is carefully examined and its treatment determined upon. The less it is handled the better. If it be in a condition suitable for reduction, the next step will be to divide the stricture. The neck of the sac is examined with the point of the left forefinger, and the density of the stricture and the best point for introducing the hernia knife is determined upon. The finger must be used gently. There must be no attempt made to dilate the stricture with the finger, or to force the finger through the constricted aperture. The part of the bowel that usually suffers most in strangulated hernia is the part directly embraced by the stricture, and this is the part that will be crushed and bruised if persistent attempts be made to force the finger into the stricture.

The forefinger lies with the nail towards the bowel, and the most the surgeon does is to make clear a point at which the hernia knife can be inserted. The finger is the best director: the hernia knife is passed along it with the blade flat against the finger. The point of the knife at last reaches the pulp of the finger that is pressed against the stricture, while the nail lies against the bowel. The point of the knife is passed, still on the flat, past the finger and into the ring. It is then turned with its edge towards the stricture, and by a slight movement of the blade the stricture is divided. The position of the knife and the left forefinger during this manœuvre is shown in Fig. 382.

The left forefinger acts throughout as a guide. It is retained in position after the knife has been withdrawn, and is then employed to ascertain that the division of the stricture has been sufficiently complete.

upon, and a director must be used. This especially applies to cases where the neck is deeply placed, where the stricture is narrow and tight, and where a place for the introduction of the hernia knife cannot be made out by the forefinger.

The choice of the director employed must depend upon the habit of the operator and the nature of the case in hand. It is introduced with the right hand, guided by the left fore-finger, and must be most carefully manipulated. The left fore-finger and the director are employed in exactly the same manner and relation as the forefinger and the knife.

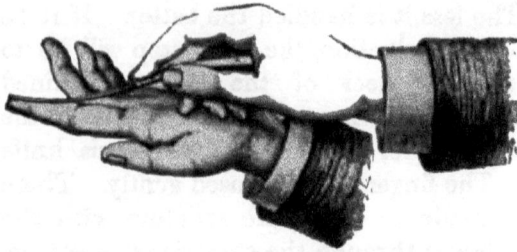

Fig. 382.—METHOD OF HOLDING THE HERNIA KNIFE.
(*Fergusson.*)
The knife is represented too long in the blade.

When once the director has been passed through the stricture, and is in place, it is held in position with the left hand, while the hernia knife is used in the right.

The knife must be cautiously introduced. It is possible for the bowel to overlap the director and the knife, and to be cut by the movement of the blade. It is well to have but a very limited cutting edge, and to see that the whole of the cutting edge is well within the stricture before the division is attempted.

After the knife has been withdrawn, the stricture may be further dilated with the director, which is forced against the divided fibres and therefore away from the bowel.

It should be a rule to endeavour to make as slight a division of the stricture as possible, such a division as will allow of the gut being reduced, and no more.

The loop of bowel should now be gently drawn down and the constricted part examined, since it is here that the injurious effects of the strangulation may be most manifest.

The next step is to reduce the gut, the fibrous and muscular structures around the hernial orifice being relaxed as far as possible. In inguinal and femoral ruptures this is effected by flexing the thigh upon the pelvis. An attempt is then made to squeeze the bowel by a kind of kneading movement with the thumb and fingers through the opening.

The manipulation must be of the gentlest, and the surgeon must be prepared to exercise considerable patience. If the coil will not return by pressure applied at one extremity, it may yield by pressure applied at the other end of the loop.

In some cases of difficulty, the reduction is rendered easier if the margin of the hernial orifice is held up by means of a small blunt hook introduced into it. This especially applies to large inguinal herniæ.

In other cases more bowel may be drawn down from the abdomen, and the reduction may then be directed in the line in which the withdrawal of the intestine appears to be the more easily effected.

Sometimes the reduction is simplified by returning the mesentery first and then the actual loop. In other cases it is desirable that the cut edges of the sac be held asunder with forceps, to prevent the walls from being folded in.

If the bowel be much distended, that part nearest to the ring can often be emptied of some portion of its contents by judicious manipulation.

Any flakes of lymph that may be disturbed in handling the gut should be washed away with a weak carbolic solution.

After the reduction the finger should be passed through the ring into the abdomen, to make sure that all is clear. The sac is now washed out.

If any omentum exist in the hernia, it must be dealt with as its condition demands.

If it appear healthy, is small in amount, and is quite free from adhesions, it may be reduced. Nothing better can be done for it. In the majority of cases, however, it will need to be removed. It will be found to be altered in structure, to be inflamed, or to be matted into a granular kind of mass, or to be adherent.

Small portions may be ligatured *en masse* with one catgut ligature, and then cut off. Larger portions are most conveniently dealt with if split up into many strands, often six or more in number, each segment being separately

ligatured with ca
ligatures should
omentum shoul
lest they slip.

It is well to 1
mass may be, it

The number
" In splitting th
of several ligatur
exercised not to
excessively thin,
empty one can l
as one side goes
open ; and when
off, it bleeds furi

The neck of
clamp, be excisec
multiple ligature
individual vesse
them separately.

The reduction
every case comp
the abdomen. 1
its neck. All ad
sac must be caut
must be free. T
plug to close th
which has nothi
fruitful source of
to a hernial orifi

3. **The Treat
Wound.**

In very sever
exhausted, and ii
tion with as litt
is, and the woun

In cases of a
tion exists that
with according to

In the majo

The "breaking-down" of such adhesions must be a matter of infinite care, as the bowel is, as a rule, more readily torn than is the wall of the sac.

Many of the adhesions can be divided with scissors or a scalpel, and some may be torn through after partial division. In the case of a very large and neglected labial hernia, which had been many years irreducible and had become strangulated, I found that a loop of colon contained in the sac had become firmly adherent to the coverings of the hernia, which were so very greatly thinned that the gut was practically attached to the skin.

As separation would have been dangerous, I divided the skin all round the attached area. I then reduced it to the smallest possible dimensions by trimming with the scissors, scraped off its epithelial surface to ensure its being clean, and returned the bowel into the abdomen with the disc of skin still adherent to it.

In another case I returned a loop of bowel with a considerable portion of the sac still adhering to it—it having been found to be easier to separate the sac from the tissues outside it than to detach it from the bowel. The adherent tissue was reduced to the smallest possible dimensions by dissection before the gut was replaced.

In any case in which long-adherent gut is reduced, it must be remembered that it is reduced with a raw surface, and that it will probably acquire a fresh attachment within the abdomen.

No loop of intestine should be returned the limbs of which are united by adhesions; and the same observation applies to reducible bowel which is adherent to reducible omentum.

"A few cases remain," writes Mr. Jacobson, "in which adhesions should be left alone. When gangrene is threatening, their presence, especially about the neck of the sac, is the chief safeguard against extravasation into the peritoneal cavity. In some cases of large hernia, if the patient is much collapsed, as long as any recently-distended loop is returned, any long-adherent intestine may be left. And in other cases of collapse from delay of the operation, where there is much difficulty in returning a loop of intestine, especially if this is not in good condition, it may be left after the stricture has been sufficiently divided."

B. *When the Gut is Gangrenous.*—Much has been written upon the subject of the treatment of gangrenous intestine in hernia, and very remarkable differences of opinion have been expressed upon the question. It would be out of place to enter into a discussion of this subject, or to consider minutely the physical signs that may distinguish intestine which is gangrenous from that which may still recover.

If the bowel, when exposed, be in what may be termed a doubtful condition, it had better be reduced into the abdomen. It is in a more favourable position for recovery within the peritoneal cavity than within the inflamed sac. Before replacement, the parts concerned should be well washed with an antiseptic solution. Such a coil of bowel seldom travels far from the hernial ring. The sac should be left open, and a drainage-tube of large size be introduced. If the gut at a later period gives way, it will do so gradually; and as adhesions are rapidly formed, the intestinal contents will escape along the course of the open sac. Whatever theoretical objections may exist to this procedure, practice has shown that it may be safely carried out, assuming that it applies to bowel which is not actually gangrenous, but in a condition which may be termed doubtful. It is remarkable to what an extent these loops of "doubtful" intestine recover. Some cases reported by Mr. Bennett (*Lancet*, October 18th, 1890) illustrate very forcibly the points just dealt with.

If the bowel, when exposed, be found to be gangrenous, two courses are open to the operator:—

(1) The stricture may be divided, and the gangrenous bowel be resected.

In carrying out the resection, either an artificial anus may be established, which can be closed by a subsequent operation, or the divided ends of the gut may be at once united and returned into the abdomen. The union may be effected by means of sutures, or by means of Senn's decalcified bone plates. (*See* pages 319 and 327.)

(2) The sac having been well opened up and well washed out with an antiseptic solution, the bowel is left *in situ* after having been incised. The parts are well dusted with iodoform,

and means are taken to pro
Several surgeons of eminence
stricture should be divided, ar
situ, having been first secured
stitches passed through the
then fastened to the skin.
the abdominal cavity is open
from the putrid contents of tl
have already shut off the gan
tective barrier is broken dov
doubtful condition, the plan ls
but when it is actually gangre
much to recommend it. It l
stricture be not divided, th
relieved. This argument in fs
however, not supported by ex
when gangrene has set in, nea
the parts, especially when tb
which attend the process are
is usual to observe fæcal m:
putrid bowel is incised.

If there be no immediate
tents, such discharge will tak
of the parts has subsided, as
gut.

As to which method is t
bowel or the leaving of the
must depend upon the precise
patient with so advanced and
hernia that the bowel has bec
in a condition to undergo s
operation. If the gut be re
young and in good conditio
tion, and the local conditior
method adopted will probab
resection, with the establishm
employment, after the excisio
necessary union. The union c
of sutures involves a considera
hardly applicable to this clas

occupied as long as three hours, and McCosh states that the average duration is not less than an hour and a half.

A consideration of this question will be found in the following papers, among others :—Mr. Banks, "Clinical Notes," page 86, and *Med. Soc. Proc.*, vol. viii., 1885 ; Mr. Lockwood, *Med.-Chir. Trans.*, 1891 ; Dr. McCosh, *New York Med. Journ.*, March 10th. 1889, with a table of 115 cases of resection of

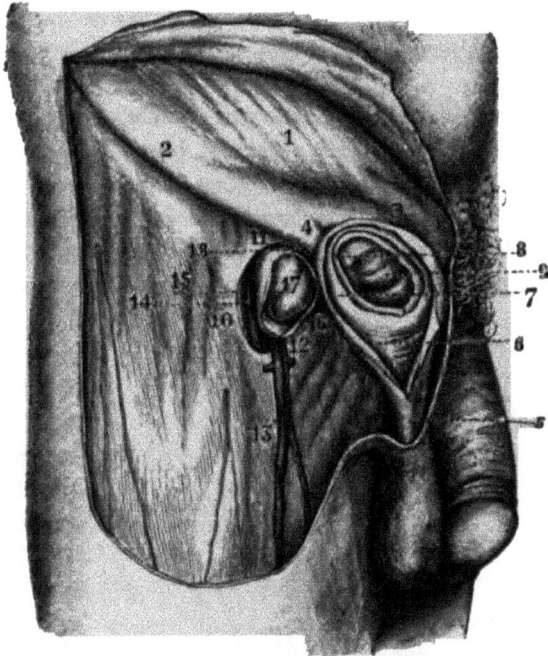

Fig. 383.—INGUINAL AND FEMORAL HERNIA.

1, External oblique muscle ; 2, Poupart's ligament ; 3, Inner pillar of outer abdominal ring ; 4, Outer pillar of the same ; 5, Spermatic cord ; 6 and 7, Coverings of the sac ; 8, Sac ; 9, Intestine ; 10, Falciform process ; 11 and 12, Boundaries of saphenous opening ; 13, Saphenous vein ; 14, Femoral vein ; 15, Femoral artery ; 16, Sac ; 17, Intestine ; 18, Abnormal obturator artery. (*Rüdinger.*)

gangrenous intestine in hernia; Mr. Bennett, *Lancet*, Oct. 18th, 1889.

c. *When the Intestine is Wounded.*—The bowel may be accidentally wounded when too rash a division of the superficial parts is made, when adhesions exist between the gut and the sac, when the altered gut is mistaken for the sac, and when the loop of bowel comes into accidental contact with the edge of the hernia knife as it is being passed through the stricture.

The opening made should in each case be closed by means of Lembert's suture, the loop of gut should be returned into the abdomen, and if the wound has been extensive, it will be as well to leave the sac open, and to introduce a large drainage-tube, in case the intestine might give way at a later period (*See* cases reported by Mr. Bennett, *Lancet*, Oct. 18th, 1890.)

THE OPERATION AS APPLIED TO PARTICULAR HERNIÆ

1. **Inguinal Hernia.**—The anatomy of the hernia is shown in Fig. 383. The patient having been prepared in the manner already described, an incision is made over the centre of the tumour, and in the long axis of the tumour, and is so arranged that the centre of the wound will about correspond to the external ring (Fig. 384). The cut may at first be some inch and a half in length, and may be enlarged subsequently if required.

The sac is exposed; the only layers of tissue which will probably be recognised are the intercolumnar and

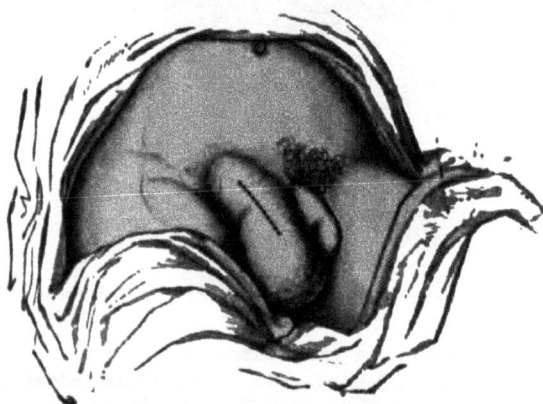

Fig. 384.—INCISION FOR INGUINAL HERNIA. (*After Ferguson.*)

the cremasteric. The superficial external pudic artery will probably be severed in dividing the subcutaneous tissues.

The sac is opened and the contents are dealt with in the manner already described (page 514). In dividing the stricture, the knife should be made to cut in a direction upwards, *i.e.*, parallel with the median line.

To relax the parts about the inguinal ring as the bowel is being reduced, the thigh should be a little flexed upon the abdomen, and should be at the same time a little adducted and rotated in.

In the case of a large scrotal hernia, any redundant skin may be excised.

After the wound has been closed, the dressing is applied, and is fixed in place by means of a spica bandage, which should be applied while the thigh is in the position of flexion.

When the limb is brought again into the extended posture the bandage is drawn tight.

Comment.—There is nothing to commend the practice of dividing the skin by picking up a fold of integument and transfixing it, nor in exposing the sac is it wise that the over-lying tissues should be "torn through with the nails of the forefinger."

The various anatomical forms of inguinal hernia must be borne in mind. In the congenital varieties the sac has nearly always a long neck, which corresponds to the length of the inguinal canal. The internal and external abdominal rings are separated by a normal distance, and the canal has a distinct existence. In these herniæ strangulation is often acute and urgent, and the protrusion has to be followed up to the end of the inguinal canal before the stricture can be properly dealt with.

In the acquired hernia, on the other hand, the two abdominal rings become soon approximated. The inguinal canal can scarcely be said to exist, and when the rupture is reduced, the breach in the abdominal wall presents the features of a more or less simple hole. In such cases the neck of the sac is short and easily reached, since it is practically within the grip of the external ring. The acquired hernia is, other things being equal, more easily treated by operation than the congenital form, and the thinness of the sac in the latter variety adds to the difficulties of manipulation.

In a form of what is known as the encysted hernia, more than one layer of peritoneum may be met with in exposing the gut.

In inguinal hernia the stricture is very often situated in the neck of the sac itself, and in such cases no reduction can be effected until the sac has been opened up.

The exact site of the stricture, and the precise anatomical

structure which produces it,
moment. The operator will s
tain its position and density, a
of dividing it.

In dividing the stricture, th
damaged is the deep epigastri
within proper limits, this dange

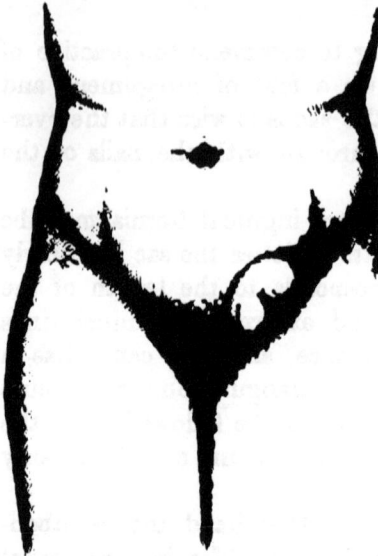

Fig. 385.—INCISION FOR FEMORAL HERN

placed that the centre of the
the upper border of the s
The wound will be at first
length, and may be enlarged a

As a rule, no vessels of an
the sac.

The operation is complet
scribed (page 514).

The stricture is usually for
nat's ligament, and should be d
inwards, *i.e.*, towards the medie

In reducing the bowel the
adducted, and rotated in.

A similar spica is applied to that employed in inguinal hernia.

Comment.—The operator may be reminded that the femoral vein lies to the outer side of the femoral ring, that the spermatic cord (in the male) lies just about its anterior border, and that the epigastric artery skirts its upper and outer part. The little pubic branch of this artery passes round the ring to ramify over Gimbernat's ligament. In one case out of three and a half the obturator artery arises from the epigastric. Out of 101 cases where the vessel so arose, it reached its destination in fifty-four instances by passing along the outer side of the crural ring, a position quite free from danger in herniotomy. In thirty-seven cases it passed backwards across the ring, and in ten instances around its inner border (R. Quain) (Fig. 383, 18). When in the last-named position, the vessel could hardly escape being wounded in the operation upon a femoral hernia, and such wounds have led to fatal hæmorrhage. In one case the pulsations of the abnormal artery were felt before the parts were divided.

The bleeding may best be dealt with by enlarging the wound and ligaturing the bleeding point, or by making a special incision parallel to Poupart's ligament and exposing the vessel through it. The hæmorrhage has also been checked by the application of pressure, and in a less satisfactory manner by means of acupressure.

The subject of the wound of this artery has been fully dealt with by Mr. Barker in a paper in the *Transactions of the Clinical Society* (vol. xi., page 180).

The After-treatment of Cases of Herniæ of the Groin submitted to Operation.

The patient should observe the recumbent position, and must avoid all exertion and straining during the period of convalescence. He should not be allowed to lift himself in bed. It often happens that the comfort of the patient may be increased by allowing the thighs to be kept a little flexed by introducing a pillow beneath the knees. In male patients retention of urine is occasionally complained of.

The dieting of the patient should be upon the lines observed in the after-treatment of cases of Abdominal Section (page 243). Opium should not be administered unless distinctly indicated. The bowels should be opened on the fifth day by an enema, unless previously relieved. Flatulent distension of the belly may be relieved by the use of the rectal tube, or, if severe and persistent, by means of a saline aperient. In some rare cases a severe diarrhœa sets in within a day or so of the operation, and is not only very difficult to cope with, but may soon lead to death from exhaustion.

The drainage-tube should be removed within forty-eight hours in ordinary cases that are doing well. The sutures may be taken out on the eighth day, or even later. The wound should be dressed whenever the bandage becomes loose, and the parts around must be frequently washed and kept scrupulously clean.

The patient should not be allowed to get up until three weeks have elapsed after the operation, and then only if the wound is sound.

The question of a supporting bandage or a truss will then have to be considered.

3. **Umbilical Hernia.**—To appreciate properly the operation carried out for the relief of strangulated umbilical hernia, it is desirable to draw attention to the three forms of rupture met with in this situation.

1. *The Infantile Hernia.*—This, the common hernia in infants, appears some time after the separation of the umbilical cord, and is due to a yielding of the umbilical cicatrix. The rupture is generally small and simple. It exhibits a decided tendency towards spontaneous cure, is very efficiently treated by means of strapping so applied as to approximate the margins of the opening in the abdomen, and appears to have demanded operative interference of any kind very seldom indeed.

2. *The Congenital Form* is observed at birth, and depends upon a defect in the anterior abdominal parietes. The hernia, which commonly contains the cæcum, is forced between the structures of the cord, and with those structures the sac is more or less imperfectly covered. These herniæ, when dealt with by operation, need to be treated by means of the method of radical cure described below. The gut is reduced, the sac is cut away, the edges of the opening in the abdominal wall are freshened, and the gap is closed by many deep sutures.

to call for immediate treatment. The strangulation will usually be found to be at the lower part of the neck of the sac, i.e., to be brought about by the lower margin of the rigid hernial orifice.

In such case it may suffice to displace the hernia upwards, to make a vertical incision over the lower part of the tumour to expose the sac, to open it or not as occasion suggests, and to divide the stricture by cutting from above (i.e., from the hernia) directly downwards. These ruptures are, however, exceptional, and the great majority of the umbilical herniæ that come under the surgeon's notice belong to the next category.

The hernia is large, and possibly of enormous size; the patients are most frequently women past middle life. They are usually corpulent, and often excessively so; their tissues are flabby; their muscular development is feeble; their digestive organs are deranged; and they are not infrequently the subjects of embarrassed breathing. They make bad subjects for operation, and the unwieldy character of the huge and pendulous abdomen, which is shaken terribly by every cough, adds a difficulty to the after-treatment. The contents of these herniæ are usually in whole or in part irreducible. They generally contain omentum as well as bowel, and often present a loop of the transverse colon. Adhesions of an extensive and complex character may be anticipated, and the symptoms of strangulation are generally of a sub-acute character. The symptoms, indeed, are more allied to those that are associated with the so-called incarcerated or obstructed herniæ than with distinct strangulation. The coverings of the hernia are usually thinned, unhealthy, and discoloured; the mass is pendulous, and its general outline is lobulated.

is most desirable, wher
should be carried out.
enormous sac behind, is
healing, and to perpetua

My results in dealir
uncommon among the
London Hospital—have
every instance not only 1
the operation for radical

The Operation.—In
enumerated, the surger
spatulæ, curved needles
dorn's needles.

The patient is prepar
general disposition of th
be the same as is obse
will always stand to the

The parts must be
class of patients, the 1
unpleasantly evident.

After the whole herr
soap and water, the skir
of lint soaked in a warn
be in place for an hot
the better.

Nearly the whole of
now marked off by me
axis of which will corres
will extend, indeed, on
the swelling; and as it
wall on either side, but
is such as would be mad
dimensions situated in 1

The first incision is
be moved from one sic
occasion requires.

The surgeon now de
base of the mass, and 1
tissue, aims at exposir
little way beyond, *i.e.*, tr

To effect this, such skin as covers the base of the protrusion is turned back. When once the aponeurosis is reached, it is followed all round the stalk of the tumour by deepening the incision. When this has been done, the hernia, covered by perfectly-undisturbed skin, will be entirely isolated from all the tissues outside the abdomen, and will be attached only by its neck. The neck must be well cleared, and the aponeurosis which bounds it, and which, therefore, forms the margin of the hernial orifice, must be laid quite bare.

The sac may now be opened at any convenient spot where it can be proved to be free from adhesion to its contents. The contents are exposed, and are dealt with in the manner already described. Adhesions are divided, the bowel is freed, and, if in sound condition, is reduced into the abdomen. Before this can be done, the hernial orifice will need to be divided; and this can be effected by enlarging the opening above and below the neck of the sac in the median line with a probe-pointed bistoury. This division may be extra-peritoneal. After the gut has been replaced, the omentum is excised, or is dealt with in a manner suited to its condition (page 519).

The sac is at last emptied, and the hole leading into the abdomen is then plugged with a large Turkey sponge secured in a holder.

The next step is to excise the whole of the sac and its coverings, including the elliptical portion of the skin, down to the level of the aponeurosis. This may be effected with the scalpel at one sweep.

The margins of the ring are now freshened, as in plastic operations involving the skin, and the opening in the aponeurotic part of the abdominal parietes is closed by sutures. These sutures should be of silkworm gut. They may be introduced on a curved needle in a handle, or by means of a large curved Hagedorn's needle. Before they are inserted, the sponge should be removed and be replaced by the end of an ivory spatula, which will serve to protect the intestines from injury. As many sutures as possible should be introduced before any are tied. They must be closely placed—four to six to the inch—and must include the whole thickness of the aponeurosis and the peritoneum.

The operation is concluded by suturing the skin and

subcutaneous tissues. The wound is entirel
drainage-tube is required. The dressing of tl
subsequent treatment are conducted upon th
in other abdominal operations.

It is well that the patient should wear a
for some months ; but in the majority of the
number—in which I have operated this has
time dispensed with.

4. Obturator Hernia.—In this form t
through the obturator canal, between the hor
the os pubis and the uppermost fibres o!
externus muscle. The obturator vessels ma}
on the outer or inner side of the sac, or abo
Among the cases collected by Dr. Charles :
Journ., April 19th, 1890) the vessels were to
six cases, to the outer side in six cases, and b
three cases. The proximity of the nerve
liable to be pressed upon, and pain along the
marked symptom of the rupture.

The hernia presents beneath the pectine!
inner side of the capsule of the hip, behind
side of the femoral vessels, and to the o!
adductor longus tendon. This hernia is n
females, and it is worthy of note that the obt
be examined to some extent through the vagi

The *operation* for exposing the hernia *in*
gulated, is carried out as follows :—

The parts having been duly cleansed, a
from three to four inches in length, is made o
midway between the line of the femoral arter
of the pubes. The subcutaneous tissues and !
been divided, the upper edge of the adductor
reached. The deep external pudic artery we
severed. The upper border of the long ad
downwards and inwards with a wound retract

The fibres of the pectineus muscle are eit!
using the handle of the scalpel, or are divided

The obturator muscle is then defined, and
by a little careful dissection. The hernia ma
that muscle or through its uppermost fibres.

The thyroid membrane is then nicked in a downward direction, and the gut reduced. The sac may or may not be opened. Care must be taken not to wound the femoral or saphenous veins. In dividing the constriction, a lateral incision should be avoided. The sac may be dissected out, and its neck ligatured, as was done in Dr. Firth's case. Before the wound is closed, a drainage-tube should be inserted.

Dr. Firth states (*loc. cit.*) that out of twenty-five cases recognised during life, seventeen were subjected to operation, eight were relieved by taxis, but only five altogether were saved by the two methods of treatment.

The bowel may be reduced through an incision made in the median line of the abdomen, traction being made upon the gut while pressure is brought to bear upon the tumour in the thigh. This method would appear to possess distinct advantages if carried out in suitable cases and at an early period. The operation has been performed by Mr. Hilton and by Mr. Godlee. In both cases, however, death resulted.

5. **Other Forms of Hernia.**—It is unnecessary to allude to other forms of hernia, which, although exceedingly rare, may be, or have been, treated by operation.

It may suffice if reference be made to recent papers dealing with these herniæ.

Lumbar Hernia.—Mr. Macready (*Lancet*, Nov. 8th, 1890) has collected twenty-five examples of this hernia. In six, strangulation occurred ; of these, two were operated upon: one recovered and one died. One case appeared to have been untreated, and the remaining three were successfully dealt with by taxis.

Sciatic Hernia.—M. Wassilieff (*Revue de Chirurgie*, March, 1891) describes a case in which strangulation occurred. The rupture was successfully reduced. He enters fully into the anatomical relations of this uncommon hernia, and the operation which should be carried out, should such treatment be demanded.

Perineal Hernia.—M. Winckel (*Annales de Gynécologie*, Aug., 1890) deals very fully with the subject of this hernia, with its varieties and anatomical relations. He advises the treatment of this form of rupture by a radical operation.

CHAPTER II.

The Operations for the Radical Cure of Hernia.

From the earliest days of medicine surgeons have concerned themselves with attempts to cure hernia by means of operation. The methods either advised or actually employed are legion, and no chapter in the literature of surgery contains more remarkable measures, or more extravagant and varied efforts of invention.

Chelius, in his "System of Surgery," has given a very interesting history of this strange development of surgical practice, and has endeavoured to classify the innumerable operations which the restless activity of one generation after another has brought before the medical world.

The majority of the methods of treatment are no longer of any but historical interest.

The treatment by increasing pressure, which was maintained by means of a conical linen pad until the skin ulcerated, has been entirely abandoned. The same may be said of the terrible and barbarous methods by caustics and the actual cautery.

The method of "healing-in" a detached portion of skin, or of a portion of infolded skin, into the abdominal ring, was very extensively practised. One of the last of these operations, that designed by Wützer, was attended by a slight success, and the account of the method has but recently disappeared from surgical text-books.

The treatment by injection is of old date. The fluid originally employed was red wine. Injection methods have been revived of late years, and have been advocated by several surgeons. But the procedure has not met with any general support, and does not compare favourably with other methods now in vogue. It is founded upon principles which are not quite in accord with the instincts and inclinations of modern surgery.

The treatment by ligature of the sac is of some antiquity, and, in view of the operations now carried out, the early modes of effecting this object are of interest.

Berard laid bare the hernial sac by an incision, and surrounded the neck of the sac and the spermatic cord with a golden thread. This was drawn sufficiently tight to close the ring, but not to compress the cord. This was the method by "the golden puncture." Paré separated the hernial sac from the surrounding parts, and after tying it with a leaden thread closed it with the glover's suture. This was the method by "the royal stitch."

Sir Astley Cooper dissected out the entire sac in a case of femoral hernia, and "passed stitches through its mouth so as to bring the edge into perfect contact." The wound healed, but the hernia returned. Petit carried out the same operation. Neither surgeon formed a favourable view of the measure, and it was condemned by Lawrence and others of his time.

Within recent years the development of the operation for the radical cure of hernia is closely associated with the name of Professor Wood, of King's College. He adopted a method of closing the hernial aperture by means of a wire suture passed subcutaneously. The procedures devised by Mr. Wood were ingenious although complicated, and represented for some years the best known means of attempting to cure ruptures by operation.

Wood's operation, and such like measures as are founded upon the principles underlying his operation, were never very extensively adopted, and it may be said that they have now given place to simpler and surer modes of treatment.

With the advent of antiseptic surgery and of improved methods of treating wounds, there soon arose a series of operative measures, from which those procedures which are now in extensive use have been rapidly developed. The work of Sir Joseph Lister rendered these operations possible, and conspicuous among the pioneers of the modern operation is Mr. Mitchell Banks. Mr. Banks was one of the earliest and foremost operators, and to him is largely due the credit of demonstrating the possibility of what may be termed the open method of operating.

Within the last ten years the "radical cure" of hernia has

been developed with
operations which ar
among the most succ

It is acknowledge
little too ambitious, a
operator that the me
every year that passe
to a title with whic
beginning.

Without enterin
operations are perfe
that they are restr
not adapted for indis

It would be out c
very many operatio
title of radical cures

A large number
and more or less wel
few operating surgeo
nor is it to be ex
operation at all tim
the originator.   T
methods employed r
operandi must of ne
gical habits of each c

Methods of Oper
ing will be described

      1. Mitchell l
      2. Barker's c
      3. Ball's ope
      4. Macewen'
      5. Modified
         lation.

A brief prelimina
operations may be gl

1. *Mitchell Ban*
from the surroundir
neck high up.   The
inguinal ring is closed

2. *Barker's*—Thi

neck of the sac is ligatured, and the sac below the ligature is divided, but it is not dissected out. The hernial orifice is closed by means of the suture used to ligature the neck of the sac, the stump of the sac acting as a plug.

3. *Ball's.*—The sac is well separated up to the abdominal part of the neck. It is then twisted around its own axis, and the fundus having been cut away, the twisted stump is secured *in situ* by sutures which pass through the margins of the hernial ring.

4. *Macewen's.*—The sac is dissected out and separated from its connections. It is then puckered up by means of a suture, and is so drawn upwards as to form a pad upon the abdominal aspect of the hernial opening. The ring and canal are then closed by means of sutures.

The methods dealt with will be described as they apply to

THE RADICAL CURE OF INGUINAL HERNIA.

1. **Mitchell Banks's Operation.**—The parts having been shaved and well cleaned, the sac is exposed through the usual incision, and all bleeding is controlled before the sac is opened. The sac, when reached, is carefully separated from the surrounding tissues. "At its lowest part the sac is always more or less adherent to the tunica vaginalis, and at that point requires very careful separation, otherwise the tunica and its contained testicle are apt to be pulled bodily out of the scrotum. As regards the structures of the cord, the only one about which there need be any anxiety is the vas deferens. Very early in the process of clearing the sac it ought to be found, and kept carefully in view during the whole operation. As for injury to the vessels or other constituents of the cord, this does not seem to affect the testicle at all. In the case of congenital inguinal herniæ, there is always much more difficulty in separating the cord than in any other form ; and in young children, in whom the peritoneal tube is very thin, it is most difficult.

" In congenital herniæ it is necessary to divide the tube a little way above the testicle, so as to make a tunica vaginalis, which ought to be stitched up with fine catgut. The rest of the tube is then stripped up to the ring, and tied and cut off in the usual manner. When the sac has been dissected out and the contained bowel pushed up into the abdomen, there is often a strong temptation to ligature at once without opening it. I think the sac should always be opened and examined, because, although one may feel absolutely certain that no bowel remains, there is often a very thin slip or tag-end of flattened omentum lying just outside the ring and adherent around the neck of the sac. Now if this be cut across with the sac, its inner end still remains attached to the abdominal wall opposite the internal inguinal aperture, and acts as a pioneer for more omentum and for bowel to come down. Concerning the removal of omentum, whether adherent or not, not the slightest dread need be entertained of cutting away any amount of it. . . . (*See* page 519.)

"The sac having been thoroughly separated and opened, and its contents having been disposed of, it should be well pulled down and tied as high up as possible, whether at the femoral or the inguinal apertures. The great object of the whole proceeding is to restore a uniform surface to the peritoneal wall; and hence the higher up the sac is tied, the better is the chance of this being permanent.

"Turning next to the pillars of the ring, I employ two, three, or four silver-wire sutures to pull them together. These are inserted with a curved needle in a handle. Room must, of course, be left at the lower part of the ring for the spermatic cord to pass through. The wire should be thick— so thick that a single knot on it will suffice to make it hold without any second knot or without twisting. Then it should be cut very close to the knot, so as to leave no sharp projecting ends."

These deep sutures are left in position. They are intended to hold the pillars of the ring together, and are not introduced with the idea that they will lead to a union of one pillar with the other.

In cases of large inguinal hernia, care must be taken that the epigastric artery is well pushed aside before the needle carrying the deep sutures is thrust through the tissues. The operation is completed by uniting the skin wound with superficial sutures.

When an undescended testicle exists in connection with an inguinal hernia, it is better always that the testicle should be removed at the time that the operation for radical cure is carried out.

The wound is dressed in the usual way. A drainage-tube is not required, or, if introduced, may be removed at the end of twenty-four hours.

Good pressure should be kept up by means of a spica bandage. The after-treatment is conducted upon the same lines as are observed after the operation for strangulation. Mr. Banks advises that all patients should wear a light support after the operation.

2. **Barker's Operation.**—This procedure closely resembles that just described. The details of the operation are thus given by the author (*Brit. Med. Journ.*, Dec. 3rd, 1887). The silk used is of the hard twisted variety:—

"The first step is the exposnre of the sac close to the inguinal opening. This is done through the usual herniotomy incision in the direction of the cord. The neck of the sac is cleared by careful peeling with the thumb-nail, special care being taken to disturb the vas deferens and the nervous and vascular structures of the cord as little as possible. A stout silk thread is now passed under the neck of the sac close to the external ring, great care being taken that the vas deferens is not included. Before this thread is tied round the neck of the sac, the latter is opened longitudinally below the thread, sufficiently to see clearly that the neck is free from gut or omentum, which, if present, is reduced completely, or the omentum may be cut away When the neck is quite clear, the thread is tied firmly round it *en masse*, the threads being left uncut for the present.

"The sac is now cut across half an inch below the point of ligature, and the lower scrotal portion is left to take care of itself. I have never been able to see any possible gain from dissecting it out, and I have, I believe, seen injurious effects follow from the laceration of the scrotal tissues consequent on dissecting it out. One of the threads hanging from the stump of the neck of the sac is now threaded in a Liston's needle, and the latter is passed up the inguinal canal in front of the vas, guided by the left index finger, which pushes the stump of the sac before it, and feels for the inner aspect of the abdominal opening—that is, the internal ring.

Here the needle is forced through one borde
and out through the external oblique musc
unthreaded and withdrawn, and is again filled
thread hanging from the stump of the sac
carried, in the same way as the first, up the
through the border of the opening opposite to
its fellow already lies, and through the exter
before. Both threads being now pulled upon
the sac is drawn well within the abdomen;

threads are kno
the first step—e
closing the int
complete (Fig. ■

" The needle
with another pice
carried up the e
guided by the ■
which keeps ■
the way. It is
transfix the wal
to the operato
appear on the es
about a quarte
below the first i
the thread is se
needle is withdi
canal, and then :
the outer wall o
the operator's le
unthreaded and

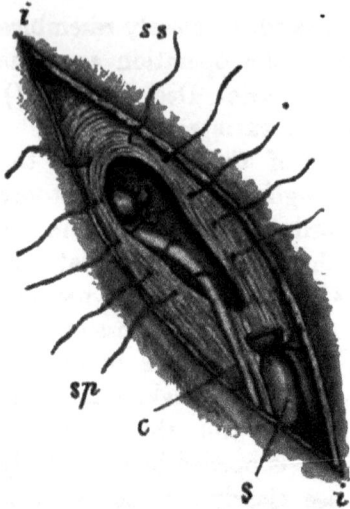

Fig. 386.—BARKER'S OPERATION FOR
THE RADICAL CURE OF HERNIA.

i, Skin incision; *c*, Spermatic cord;
s, Sac of hernia; *s s*, Suture for the
sac; *s p*, Sutures for closing the canal.
(*After Barker.*)

be used with a fresh piece of silk in the sai
third stitch a quarter of an inch from the
way from four to seven stitches are passed
opposed walls of the inguinal canal, until
room is left for the structures of the cord
(Fig. 386). The threads (all still untied, excep
now examined, to see that they are all in front o
then are tied from above downwards one a
Before this is done, of course, all blood or seru
sponged away from every part of the wound.

are then cut short, and stitches are passed through the lips of the skin wound. A sponge is left in the latter until all these are *in situ*, and is only removed as they are tied.

" All drainage is unnecessary in almost all these cases if the wound is completely dried up to the moment of closure, and is well padded with antiseptic wool from the first. But a strand of gut or silk may be left in the lower angle if there is any doubt upon this point. A carefully-adjusted salicylic wool dressing, and firm bandaging complete the operation. This dressing is usually left for a week or ten days untouched, and on its removal the wound is found almost invariably perfectly healed, and the stitches through the skin may be removed. The patient should remain recumbent for three weeks or a month from the time of the operation, so that the parts may have no strain."

The skin sutures are removed between the tenth and the fourteenth day. Primary healing is the rule. In a few instances the deep silk sutures have suppurated out.

No truss or support is used after the parts have healed soundly.

3. **Ball's Operation.**—The following description of the method carried out by Dr. C. B. Ball is derived from the author's account published in the *British Medical Journal* for Dec. 10th, 1887 :—

" 1. The sac must be completely isolated from the structures comprising the spermatic cord ; this, which is frequently a matter of considerable difficulty, must be done very thoroughly ; for this dissection I have found a narrow-bladed, blunt-pointed scissors the most convenient instrument ; by means of the finger the separation can be carried up right to the internal abdominal ring, and the peritoneum loosened from its attachments for a little distance from that opening.

" 2. Having ascertained that the sac is empty (by opening it if necessary), grasp its neck with a broad catch-forceps, and gradually twist it up ; while this is being done, the left forefinger should be used to free the upper portion of the neck. In ordinary cases four to five complete revolutions are sufficient, but this in great measure depends upon the thickness of the sac, and the portion of it to which the torsion forceps is applied ; the twisting should be continued until it is felt to be quite tight, and that any further torsion would produce rupture.

"3. The torsion forceps is now transferred to an assistant, who is to maintain the twist; a stout catgut ligature is placed round the twisted sac as high up as possible, tied tightly, and the ends cut off short.

"4. Two sutures of strong aseptic silk are now passed through the skin at a distance of about an inch from the outer margin of the wound, through the outer pillar of the ring, through the twisted sac in front of the catgut suture, and then through the inner pillar of the ring and skin upon the inside. As these sutures effectually prevent the sac from untwisting, it may now be cut off in front of them; and a catgut drain is brought out through a separate opening at the back of the scrotum, and the two sutures closed over lead plates (Fig. 356), which lie at right angles to the wound. If necessary, a point or two of superficial suture may be put in to close the wound completely (Fig. 356, B). Dry dressings are employed, retained by a double spica bandage, which is painted over with a solution of silicate of potash; this keeps the dressings in place, and the parts effectually at rest. The after-pain is not very severe.

"As a usual result the dressings are allowed to remain on for ten days or a fortnight, after which time the wound is commonly found healed, and the sutures can be removed; of course, should the temperature go up, or discharge appear, the dressing must be taken down earlier.

"The immediate effect of this procedure is best studied upon the dead subject, and I have had four opportunities of thus investigating it. The operation was performed as above described, and the abdomen was then laid open, and the hernial orifice inspected from above; in each case it was found that the peritoneum was thrown into a number of spiral folds radiating from the internal abdominal ring in all directions. These extended for a distance of over four inches, and in two instances were observed to pass over the internal abdominal ring of the opposite side. The entire length of the inguinal canal was occupied by the twisted sac, which completely filled it, and the sides of the inguinal canal were closely approximated. There was no depression at the internal abdominal ring; indeed, this portion was more prominent than the rest of the peritoneum in the neighbourhood. This can readily be understood from the way in which the final sutures are passed, which have the effect of pressing back the twisted cord towards the abdominal cavity.

" Some surgeons have expressed a fear that in twisting up the sac there would be danger of including a portion of the intestine, and so strangulating it; this, however, I am convinced is quite impossible if the sac is first thoroughly emptied, and the twisting carefully followed and guarded by the left forefinger.

" In the treatment of bubonocele, a difficulty may be found from the fact that sufficient of the fundus of the sac does not protrude from the external abdominal ring to permit of efficient torsion; or when the sac is very small, and returns with the hernia, it may be quite impossible to twist it. Upon two occasions this difficulty has occurred to me, but it must be remembered that in this class of case it is only in exceptional circumstances that the operation for radical cure is called for; a truss usually perfectly controls the rupture. It is the very large and bulky herniæ that are the real test of any operation of the kind; and in these cases torsion of the sac answers admirably, and I believe that the only contraindication to operation on account of size is that very-rarely-met-with condition in which the abdominal cavity has become so contracted that the hernia is incapable of being replaced within it.

" A modification of the above procedure is obviously necessary in the case of congenital hernia, and upon four occasions I have treated this form successfully. The sac is divided circumferentially close to the testicle, and the serous lining of the upper portion is stripped off from the inside, separated well up to the internal ring, and twisted as before.

" In my first case I sutured up the lower portion to form a tunica vaginalis; but, as it was followed by acute hydrocele and suppuration, I have discontinued the practice, and now only take care that the drain communicates with it. In the first case upon which I operated there was, in addition to a very large right inguinal hernia, a bubonocele upon the left side, and I was very much surprised to find that the twisting

j j

of the large hernia effe
side ; this I consider t
far-reaching effect of to

"When both the he
of course, too much t
sufficient. I have only
first operation decreas
opposite side ; at a sul
also twisted. I do not

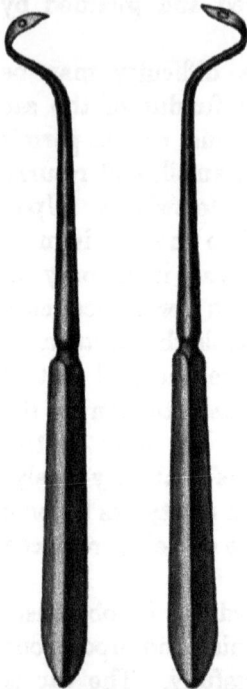

Fig. 387. -- MACEWEN'S
HERNIA NEEDLES, RIGHT
AND LEFT.

duced through the cana

The operation may
one relating to the esta
aspect of the internal
inguinal canal.

The steps of the
Macewen (*Brit. Med. J*

"A. *The Formation of a Pad on the Abdominal Surface of the Circumference of the Internal Ring.*—(1) Free and elevate the distal extremity of the sac, preserving along with it any adipose tissue that may be adherent to it; when this is done, pull down the sac, and, while maintaining tension upon it, introduce the index finger into the inguinal canal, separating the sac from the cord and from the parietes of the canal.

"(2) Insert the index finger outside the sac till it reaches the internal ring; there separate with its tip the peritoneum for about half an inch round the whole abdominal aspect of the circumference of the ring.

"(3) A stitch is secured firmly to the distal extremity of the sac. The end of the thread is then passed in a proximal

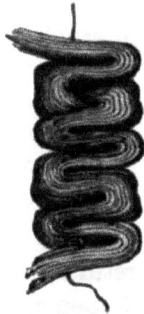

Fig. 388.—MACEWEN'S OPERATION. (The sac transfixed and drawn into folds.)

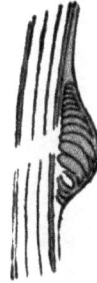

Fig. 389.—MACEWEN'S OPERATION. (The pad covering the abdominal aspect of the internal ring.)

direction several times through the sac, so that, when pulled upon, the sac becomes folded upon itself, like a curtain (Fig. 388).

" The free end of this stitch, threaded on a hernia needle, is introduced through the canal to the abdominal aspect of the fascia transversalis, and there penetrates the anterior abdominal wall, about an inch above the upper border of the internal ring. The wound in the skin is pulled upwards, so as to allow the point of the needle to project through the abdominal muscles without penetrating the skin.

" The thread is relieved from the extremity of the needle when the latter is withdrawn. The thread is pulled through

j j 2

the abdominal wall; and when traction is made upon it, the sac, wrinkling upon itself, is thrown into a series of folds, its distal extremity being drawn furthest backwards and upwards. An assistant maintains traction upon the stitch until the introduction of the sutures into the inguinal canal; and when this is completed, the end of the stitch is secured by introducing its free extremity several times through the superficial layers of the external oblique muscles. A pad of peritoneum is then placed upon the abdominal side of the internal opening, where, owing to the abdominal aspect of the circumference of the internal ring having been refreshed, new adhesions may form (Fig. 389).

"B. *The Closure of the Inguinal Canal.*—The sac having been returned into the abdomen and secured to the abdominal circumference of the ring, this aperture is closed in front of it in the following manner :—The finger is introduced into the canal, and lies between the inner and lower borders of the internal ring, in front of and above the cord. It makes out the position of the epigastric artery, so as to avoid it. The threaded hernia needle is then introduced, and, guided by the index finger, is made to penetrate the conjoint tendon in two places; first, from without inwards, near the lower border of the conjoint tendon; secondly, from within outwards, as high

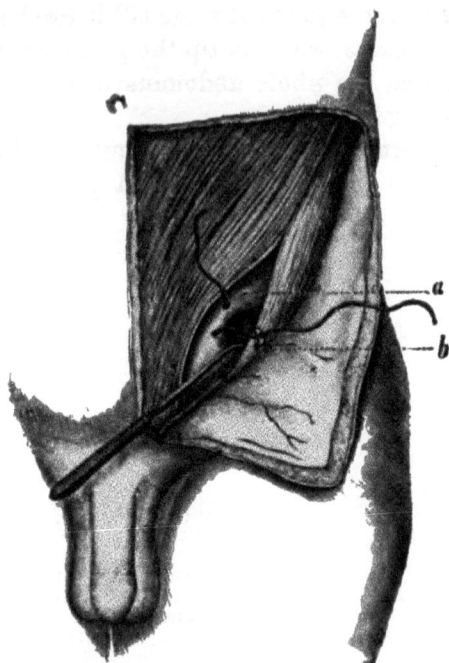

Fig. 390.—MACEWEN'S OPERATION FOR THE RADICAL CURE OF HERNIA.

a, Point at which double penetration of the conjoined tendon is made, and site of the loop on the abdominal aspect of that tendon; *b*, Thread from lower border of conjoined tendon being carried through the outer pillar of the ring.

up as possible on the inner aspects of the canal (Fig. 390, *a*). This double penetration of the conjoint tendon is accomplished by a single screw-like turn of the instrument. One single thread is then withdrawn from the point of the needle by the index finger; and when this is accomplished, the needle, along with the other extremity of the thread, is removed. The conjoint tendon is therefore penetrated twice by this thread, and a loop left on its abdominal aspect (Fig. 390, *a*).

"Secondly, the other hernia needle, threaded with that portion of the stitch which comes from the lower border of the conjoint tendon, guided by the index finger in the inguinal canal, is introduced from within outwards, through Poupart's ligament, which it penetrates at a point on a level with the lower stitch in the conjoint tendon (Fig. 390, *b*). The needle is then completely freed from the thread and withdrawn.

"Thirdly, the needle is now threaded with that portion of the catgut which protrudes from the upper border of the conjoint tendon, and is introduced from within outwards through the transversalis and internal oblique muscles, and the aponeurosis of the

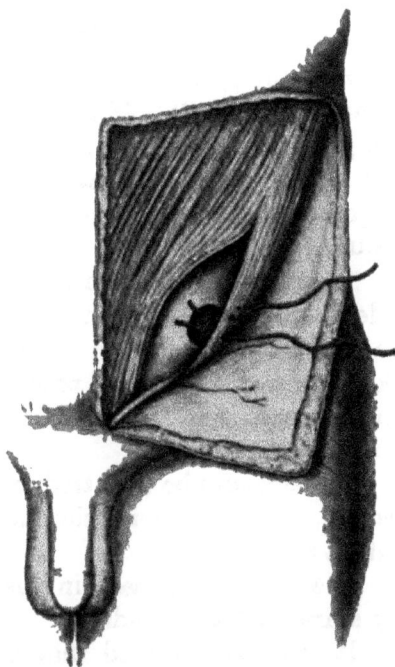

Fig. 391.—MACEWEN'S OPERATION FOR THE RADICAL CURE OF HERNIA. (The threads ready for tying.)

external oblique at a level corresponding with that of the upper stitch in the conjoint tendon. It is then quite freed from the thread and withdrawn (Fig. 391).

"There are now two free ends of the suture on the outer surface of the external oblique, and these are continuous with the loop on the abdominal aspect of the conjoint tendon

(Fig. 391). To complete the suture, the two free ends are drawn tightly together and tied in a reef knot. This unites firmly the internal ring.

" The same stitch may be repeated lower down the canal if thought desirable. In adults it may be well to do so when the gap in the abdominal parietes is wide. The pillars of the external ring may likewise be brought together.

" In order to avoid compression of the cord, it ought to be examined before tightening each stitch. The cord ought to lie behind and below the sutures, and be freely movable in the canal. It is advisable to introduce all the necessary sutures before tightening any of them. When this is done, they might be all experimentally drawn tight, and maintained so, while the operator's finger is introduced into the canal to ascertain the result. If satisfactory, they are then tied, beginning with the one at the internal ring, and taking up in order any others which may have been introduced. In the great majority of cases the stitch in the internal ring is all that is required.

" During the operation the skin is retracted from side to side, to bring the parts into view, and to enable the stitches to be fixed subcutaneously. When the retraction is relieved, the skin falls into its normal position, the wound being opposite the external ring. The operation is therefore partly sub- :utaneous."

A drainage-tube is introduced into the lower part of the wound, and the skin incision is closed by a few chromicised catgut sutures.

The wound is dressed in the usual way, and is supported by a firm pad and bandage.

It will be observed that the external wound is small. It is described as " sufficient to expose the external abdominal ring."

After-treatment.—When no contrary indication exists, the dressings are left undisturbed for fourteen to twenty-one days. From four to six weeks after the operation the patient is allowed to rise from bed, but he is not permitted to work until the end of the eighth week.

Adults engaged in laborious occupations are advised to wear a bandage and pad as a precautionary measure. Those who are not so engaged are not required to wear a belt except when of very lax habit. All are recommended not to overstrain themselves. In the majority of children (six to fourteen years) the closure is so complete and firm that further treatment by pad or belt is quite unnecessary.

In congenital inguinal hernia the sac is first isolated from the cord. As this structure is generally intimately connected with the posterior surface of the sac, often by close organic adhesion, the sac should be divided longitudinally by two parallel incisions, one on each side of the cord, and the latter permitted to lie behind clear of the sac. The isolated sac should then be divided transversely about an inch above the testicle. The lower part is formed into a tunica vaginalis. The upper is pulled down as far as possible, and dealt with quite as the sac of an acquired hernia, additional precautions being necessary to clear the cord at the internal abdominal ring. It is freed of its connections, and placed as a pad on the abdominal aspect of the circumference of the internal ring.

5. **Modified Procedures adapted to Cases of Strangulation.**—Any one of the above described operations may be, and has been, carried out in cases where the hernia is exposed for the purpose of relieving acute strangulation.

It will be obvious, however, that in many cases of strangulation the time spent over the operation is of considerable importance, and that in a patient who is greatly exhausted by a long continuance of urgent symptoms, it would not be wise to attempt to carry out so elaborate an operation, for example, as that last described.

In certain of the most severe cases the gut is found to be gangrenous, and the question of an operation for radical cure does not arise. To render it possible, the gut would have to be resected, and the divided ends united: the parts would be restored to the abdomen, and then the treatment of the sac, which had contained the putrid bowel, could be commenced. Upon such a long and hazardous procedure few surgeons would probably care to embark, especially as the patient would be already much exhausted.

In cases which are less urgent, but are still in such a position that the operation needs to be completed in as short

a time as possible, it will usually suffice merely to l
neck of the sac, and then to close the wound, or a
to dissect away the sac after the ligature has been

Cases so treated often do as well, so far as
of the rupture is concerned, as cases dealt with
elaborate method.

In instances in which the operation for the
strangulation is carried out, in what may be termed
circumstances, one or other of the operations already
may be performed.

As the operation for strangulated hernia has us
carried out at a moment's notice, that measure wl
least complex has much to recommend it. A surg
gency is not the best time in which to recall the va
of a complicated operation.

THE RADICAL CURE OF FEMORAL HERNIA.

1. Mitchell Banks's operation is carried out in
manner as in inguinal hernia. The sac is separate
away, and a ligature is placed round the neck of the
attempt is made to close the femoral ring. This v
measure answers well enough in a large proportio
and is especially well adapted for cases attended by
tion.

2. Barker's operation for femoral hernia is thus
("Manual of Surgical Operations," 1887, page 342):-

"When the sac is opened and quite clear of l
omentum, it may either be separated completely fr
roundings, and removed after its neck has been c
stout silk ligature, or this may be passed round tl
the sac and the latter be left in its bed, being simp
below the ligature at the ring. But whether take
not, the stump of the ligatured sac is thrust under t
arch, while the latter is being sutured. This is no
as follows :—A long Liston's handled needle, thr
carbolised silk, is passed through the posterior la
femoral sheath and pubic portion of the fascia lata
about an inch below Poupart's ligament, and a little
the femoral vein, which is protected by the index fi
then thrust upwards nearly as far as the peritoneal r

there made to emerge across the crural opening, and pass through the lower border of Poupart's ligament. The thread is now withdrawn from the eye of the needle, and the latter is removed, threaded afresh, and made to traverse the same structures in a similar manner, about a quarter of an inch internal to the first stitch. This is repeated until a sufficient number of threads have been introduced to draw the structures together and completely close the femoral ring. Sometimes one such stitch is quite enough for a permanent closure. The sutures are now drawn tight and knotted one after the other. Then the skin wound is united carefully, a drain-tube or strand of catgut being left in its lower angle. An antiseptic dressing, secured by firm bandaging, completes the operation."

3. Ball's operation has been adapted to femoral hernia by Dr. Houston, who has carried out the following operation (*Brit. Med. Journ.*, Dec. 3rd, 1887):—

The sac is exposed, and its contents reduced. It is then twisted in the manner directed by Dr. Ball, and the twisted neck is transfixed by a strong double catgut ligature, which is secured on either side. A second ligature is passed through the twisted neck above the first, and is carried through the abdominal wall above Poupart's ligament. The sac is then excised, and the neck is fixed in position by means of the second ligature. The femoral canal is closed by one or more sutures, and the superficial wound is united. It is assumed that the neck of the sac plugs the narrowed femoral canal.

4. Macewen's operation is not adapted for femoral hernia. An ingenious modification of the method has, however, been carried out by Dr. Cushing, which may prove of service (*Boston Medical and Surgical Journal*, Dec. 6th, 1888).

THE RADICAL CURE OF UMBILICAL HERNIA.

Comparatively few operations have been devised for the treatment of umbilical hernia. Certain of these—such as the ingenious procedure of Professor Wood by means of subcutaneous ligature—have been superseded.

The method already described in a previous section appears to me to possess the advantages of simplicity, completeness, and efficiency (page 532).

RESULTS OF OPERATIONS FOR RADICAL CURE.

It would be impossible to attempt to form any conclusion as to the value of one method when compared with another by criticism of the statistics of the various operations which have been from time to time published. No one method can be rigidly adhered to, or be considered to be all-sufficing. So far as published accounts extend, it could readily be maintained that no one operation is to be preferred to another. Each surgeon will select his method according to his particular surgical bias, and according to the nature of the special case in hand. In process of time it will probably be made evident that one method—either among those already described, or among such as may be evolved in the future—has claims to be considered as the best means of treatment, but at the present time it would be premature to attempt to predict in what direction this uniformity of opinion will tend.

Mr. Banks has placed on record a series of 106 cases; in thirty-eight strangulation was present, in sixty-eight there was no such complication. In the former category are three deaths, in the latter six. Out of sixty-six of these cases, in which the subsequent history could be followed, forty-four were completely successful, while seven were partially so.

Mr. Barker reports fifty operations with no death. In nearly all primary healing followed, and, indeed, *bonâ fide* suppuration occurred in only two instances. In eight cases the hernia returned, in thirty there was no recurrence, in thirteen the result is unknown.

Dr. Macewen's cases, amounting to eighty-one in all—in twenty-nine of which strangulation was present—contain no fatal result. Forty-eight of the patients subsequently wore a pad or bandage.

Dr. Ball's list of twenty-two cases also contains no death. Three of the patients subsequently wore trusses.

Part XII.

OPERATIONS UPON THE BLADDER.

CHAPTER I.

LATERAL LITHOTOMY.

History of Lithotomy.—The operation of cutting for stone is of great antiquity, and dates from a period long before the Christian era. The earliest method, and the one which was practised for some twenty centuries, was that known as the operation of Celsus, or the apparatus minor, and as cutting on the gripe. The first title is based upon the very definite description of the operation given by Celsus, and the second is derived from the fact that very few instruments were employed in the execution. In cutting on the gripe, the stone was fixed by means of two fingers introduced into the rectum. It was thus held against the neck of the bladder, and was made to bulge towards the perineum. Upon the stone thus gripped the surgeon cut through the perineum. The incision was transverse, or curvilinear, and was made without any precise anatomical knowledge.

The operation known as the Marian operation, or as the apparatus major, was described in 1524 by Marianus Sanctus. He was a pupil of Johannes de Romanis, by whom the procedure was invented. Many instruments were employed, and hence the name, the apparatus major.

The most important of these was the itinerarium, or grooved staff.

Although in the earlier operations attempts were made to avoid actual section of the neck of the bladder, yet the procedure differed but little from the modern method of lateral lithotomy. This procedure may be considered to have actually originated with Jacques Baulot, commonly known as Frère Jacques. He was born in 1651, and died in 1714.

The invention of the lithotome caché is ascribed to Frère Côsme, whose account was published in 1748.

The bilateral operation is only a modification of the lateral. As a matter of fact, the original operation of Celsus was practically bilateral, but the procedure now known by this name originated with Dupuytren in 1824. It was intended for cases of large stone. A median staff was used, and a semilunar incision, about one inch in length, was made across the rhaphe a little in front of the anus. The membranous urethra was exposed by cutting, and was opened, care being taken in the meanwhile to protect the rectum. Dupuytren's double lithotome caché was now introduced into the bladder along the groove, the blades were protruded, and the section in the prostate and neck of the bladder was made as the instrument was withdrawn.

This method is now practically abandoned.

The median operation as now practised was first performed early in the nineteenth century by Manzoni, of Verona. It was especially elaborated in England by Allarton, and the method is often known by his name.

The medio-lateral operation of Raynaud (1824) and the medio-bilateral lithotomy of Civiale (1828) have never attained any position in surgery.

The same may be said of recto-vesical lithotomy, originated by Sanson in 1817.

The high operation, or suprapubic lithotomy, appears to have been first carried out by Franco in 1556. His operation was, however, not conducted upon very precise grounds.

A more definite suprapubic method was described by Rousset in 1581, but he never appears to have performed the operation himself.

The method was brought into prominent notice by Frère Côsme, the inventor of the sonde à dard, who performed many lithotomies by this plan between the years 1758 and 1779. It was carried out in England in 1719 by John Douglas, and Cheselden's well-known memoir upon the high operation appeared in 1723. The latter surgeon performed this lithotomy many times, and ultimately abandoned it for the perfected lateral method. Although practised by such operators as Vidal de Cassis, Valette, and Morand, the procedure received little support until recent times. Its present prominent position is due to two facts—to the introduction of improved methods of treating wounds on the one hand, and to the demonstration of methods of bringing the bladder into position above the symphysis on the other. The latter investigations originated with Dr. Garson (*Edin. Med. Journ.*, Oct., 1878) and Dr. Petersen, of Kiel (*Archiv. f klin. Chirurg.*, 1880, xxv.). With the publication of the anatomical researches and experiments of these two investigators the rapid and remarkable development of the present successful operation of suprapubic lithotomy may be said to commence.

Anatomical Points.—The perineum is a lozenge-shaped space bounded by the symphysis, the rami of the pubes and ischia, the ischial tuberosities, the great sacro-sciatic ligaments, the edges of the two great gluteal muscles, and the coccyx.

This bony framework can be felt more or less distinctly all round, and in thin subjects the great sacro-sciatic ligaments can be made out beneath the gluteus maximus muscle.

The anus is in the middle line between the tubera ischii, its centre being about one inch and a half from the tip of the coccyx. The rhaphe can be followed from the anus along the middle line of the perineum, scrotum, and penis. No vessels cross this line, and therefore a median perineal incision is comparatively bloodless.

In the rhaphe, midway between the centre of the anus and the spot where the scrotum joins the perineum, is the "central point" of the perineum. The two transverse perineal muscles, the accelerator urinæ, and the sphincter ani, meet at this point, which also corresponds to the centre of the inferior edge of the triangular ligament. The bulb is just in front of it, as is also the artery to the bulb; and in lithotomy, therefore, the incision should never commence in front of this spot.

The perineal space is separated from the pelvic cavity by the levator ani muscles and the recto-vesical fascia. The depth of the perineum means the distance between the skin and the pelvic floor. This depth depends, to a great extent, upon the amount of fat under the integument. It varies considerably in different parts, measuring from two to three

inches in the hinder and outer parts of the perineum, and
less than one inch in the anterior parts of the space.

When the body is in the lithotomy position, it may be
taken that the bladder is, in the adult, from two and a half to
three inches from the surface of the perineum. The prostate
is situated about three-fourths of an inch below the symphysis
pubis.

In lateral lithotomy the parts cut in the *first incision* are
the skin and superficial fascia; the transverse perineal muscle,
artery, and nerve; the lower edge of the anterior layer of
the triangular ligament; the external hæmorrhoidal vessels
and nerves.

In the *second incision* the parts divided are the membranous and prostatic portions of the urethra, the so-called
posterior layer of the triangular ligament, the compressor
urethræ muscle, the anterior fibres of the levator ani, and the
left lateral lobe of the prostate.

The artery to the bulb is a vessel about the size of the
posterior auricular. It runs inwards between the fibres of the
constrictor urethræ muscle. It may be small, or wanting on
one side, or even double. It may arise from the accessory
pudic, in which case it lies farther forwards than usual, and is
well removed from the field of the operation. On the other
hand, it may come off from the pudic earlier than usual, and
may cross the perineum farther back, reaching the bulb from
behind. In such a case it can scarcely escape division in
lateral lithotomy.

The bulb is very small in children, is large in adults, and
usually largest in old men. The hæmorrhage that is stated
to attend the wounding of it has possibly been exaggerated,
and has most probably proceeded from a large artery to the
bulb. If the incision be kept well behind the "central
point" of the perineum, the bulb can be in little danger.

In the second incision the knife may be passed beyond
the prostate, and may so incise the visceral layer of the pelvic
fascia as to open up the pelvic cavity. It will be understood,
however, that the lateral lobe of the prostate may be cut
freely without this cavity being endangered. The gland is
enveloped by the pelvic fascia, but the incision made into the
prostate is, or should be, well below the superior reflection of

the membrane. The incision in the neck of the bladder should be strictly limited to the prostate.

The prostatic plexus of veins can hardly avoid being wounded. The left ejaculatory duct may be cut if the prostatic incision be carried too far backwards.

The actual extent by measurement of the incision in the prostate is difficult to define. The largest diameter of the gland is transverse, is at the base of the body, and measures one inch and a quarter to one and three-quarters. Vertically

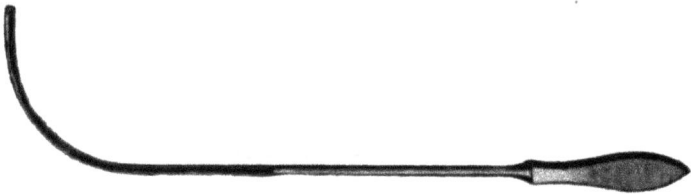

Fig. 392.—LISTON'S LITHOTOMY STAFF.

along the urethra the prostate measures from one inch to one inch and five-eighths.

Dolbeau showed that the neck of the bladder cannot be dilated to a diameter greater than 20 to 24 m.m. without producing lacerations of the prostate and vesical neck. Twenty-four millimetres is just short of one inch, and a stone with a diameter of one inch cannot therefore be drawn through the neck of the bladder without effecting some tearing of the parts.

The Instruments Employed.—The fewer the instruments employed, and the simpler they are, the better. The various special knives, staffs, scoops, forceps, and gorgets that have been introduced from time to time are legion. The lithotome caché, the lithoclast, the éclateur, and many other remarkable and ingenious productions of like character, are now only to be found in the collections of the curious.

The following list represents the full series of instruments required:—Grooved staff; lithotomy knife; probe-ended bistoury; lithotomy forceps and scoop; lithotomy tube; sound; probe; pressure forceps; syringe; anklets. To these may be added a petticoated tube or tampon, a lithotrite, and possibly a blunt gorget.

The Staff.—The curved staff with latera
known as Liston's, is the one usually en
It should be of moderate size, since a
opposes the introduction of the finger.   T
blunt. The groove should be wide, ratb
should end abruptly about one-quarter of
end of the staff. The curve of the instru
upon individual taste. Some surgeons prefe

Fig. 393.—BUCHANAN'S LITHOTOMY S

long curve (Fig. 392) ; others, and amon(
prefer a staff with not too long a curve.

Of the straight staff little is now heard.

Buchanan's rectangular staff is favour
many. The groove commences at the bene
(Fig. 393). The staff is introduced until
the membranous urethra just in front of
knife is made to hit the groove at the

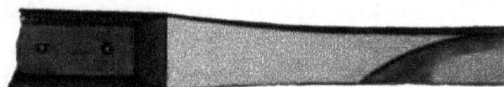

Fig. 394.—LISTON'S LITHOTOMY KNI

carried on into the bladder. The knife, i
makes the usual lateral incision. The m
the use of this staff has been termed the m

The Knife.—The best and simplest kni
Dupuytren's, or Liston's (Fig. 394). The bac
the point is central, the cutting edge exto
and a quarter from the tip. The blade is s
some three inches, while the handle is fou
This knife suffices for the whole operation
use it only for the first incision, and emplo

pointed knife for the second incision. Such a knife is represented by Blizard's well-known bistoury (Fig. 395).

The Forceps.—The straight pattern of forceps is the most useful. Curved forceps are very seldom necessary. The blades should be roughened inside or lined with linen. The blades are spoon-shaped, and the extremities of the spoons should not touch when the instrument is closed, so that any pinching of the bladder may be avoided. The ring in one handle is for the thumb, while the crook in the other handle is for the fingers. Forceps of various sizes may be required.

Fig. 395.—BLIZARD'S KNIFE.

Curved forceps are only called for in some cases in which the stone is lodged behind a large prostate.

The Scoops.—Scoops of various sizes are of service. They should be fixed in substantial handles, and should be well curved (Fig. 396). The spoon-shaped scoop usually sold is of little value; the blade is not sufficiently curved to allow of a stone, or a fragment of one, being withdrawn by traction.

The crested scoop shown in Fig. 396 has a very convenient scoop extremity. The handle-end is probe-pointed, and can

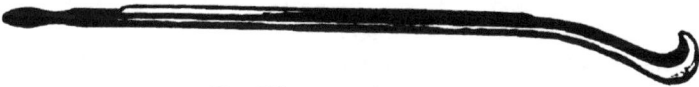

Fig. 396.—THE CRESTED SCOOP.

be passed into the bladder by following the groove on the staff, or the wall of the urethra. When the instrument has been introduced, the crest serves as a guide to the forceps, whose closed blades are yet sufficiently separate to receive the crest between them. This part of the instrument may be useful to beginners.

The Gorget.—The cutting gorget is an instrument of the past, and the same may almost be said of the blunt gorget. It can but very seldom indeed be needed. It could only be of possible service in performing lithotomy upon a large

k k

corpulent subject with a very deep perineum and a long · prostate, so that the finger could hardly reach the neck of the bladder. The most convenient form is that shown in Fig. 397. One margin is straight, the other is curved. The straight edge is entered along the staff, while the curved **border acts the part of the director.**

The Lithotomy Tube.—This tube is introduced into the bladder after the operation, to ensure rest to the bladder and

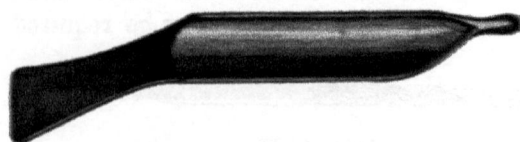

Fig. 397.—SILENT CANNULA.

perfect drainage. Cadge's tube is the best. It is a double silver can-nula, sheathed so that it can be drawn out ac-cording to the distance of the bladder from the surface. It has about the diameter of a No. 18 catheter, and has a well-bevelled end, which is perforated with numerous small holes for about an inch.

The petticoated or shirted tampon is a tube around the end of which is fastened a "petticoat" of linen, which is well oiled. In cases of persisting hæmorrhage this tampon may be employed in place of the ordinary tube. After it has been introduced, the conical space between the "petticoat" and the tube is well plugged with fine gauze. The wound can thus be plugged firmly without interfering in any way with drainage from the bladder.

The Anklets employed to fix the patient in the lithotomy position are those known as Pritchard's. Clover's crutch may be used for the same purpose. It is more quickly applied, it holds the patient more steadily, and enables the operator to do, with at least one assistant less. It has, however, the dis-advantage that the bar comes in the way of the staff and of the assistant who is responsible for holding it.

Preparatory Treatment.—Little special treatment is called for. It may be represented by absolute rest in bed for some few days before the operation, and by a simple and judicious diet. It is most desirable that the rectum should be quite empty. To effect this, an aperient should be given over-night, and an enema in the morning. It should be ascertained that the whole of the enema has been returned. A hip bath on the eve of the operation is desirable. If the urine be putrid, the bladder may be washed out twice daily during the period of resting. This is not absolutely necessary, since the removal of the stone and the drainage of the bladder will soon rectify the morbid condition of the urine.

The Placing of the Patient in Position, and the Introduction of the Staff.—The anæsthetic is administered, and as soon as the patient is insensible the anklets and wristbands may be applied. The patient is now brought down to the end of the table until the buttocks are projecting over the actual foot of the table. In this position, and while the legs are hanging towards the floor, the staff may be introduced. As soon as it is in place, the knees are very carefully brought up towards the chest, and the patient is fixed in the lithotomy position. It is very undesirable to introduce the staff while the patient is lying flat upon the table, and before any step has been taken to bring him into position. The rough movements necessary may cause the staff to damage the bladder or urethra. If the staff be introduced as above advised, all the rough movements are over, and nothing remains but to gently flex the thighs upon the pelvis.

The assistant who introduces the staff must not take his fingers off the instrument until it is finally removed from the bladder. The staff may be introduced after the patient has been placed in the lithotomy position, but the manœuvre is less easy to execute. When a Clover's crutch is used in place of the anklets, it is almost impossible.

The patient being in the well-known lithotomy position, the surgeon seats himself beyond the end of the table, his face being on a level with the patient's perineum.

Two assistants are required to support the legs, and it is their duty to see that the patient is kept immovable, that the median line of the perineum is exactly vertical, and that the knees are symmetrically separated.

A third assistant is responsible for the extremely important duty of holding the staff; and to the exact performance of this office he should devote his entire attention.

A fourth assistant may stand by the surgeon's side. to hand instruments, etc.

k k 2

The presence of the stone should be verified by the staff or by a sound previously introduced.

The position in which the staff is held is of importance.

Two positions are advised, each having vigorous advocates. By the older method the staff is held quite perpendicularly, and its concavity is drawn well up against the bony arch of the pubes. It is held rigidly and exactly in the median line. The assistant's thumb is placed upon the rough handle, while his fingers grasp the shaft. There must not be the least rotation of the instrument to one side or the other. In this position it is held throughout the operation and until it is withdrawn. The assistant at the same time holds up the penis and scrotum, and sees that the perineal rhaphe is exactly vertical.

The other position is that advised by Mr. Cadge:—" Instead of keeping the handle perpendicular, the staff-holder should incline his hand considerably towards the patient's abdomen, and gently push the convexity of the staff towards the perineum. The effect of this, as verified by dissection, is to bring the membranous urethra slightly nearer to, and almost parallel with, the surface of the perineum; the groove is more easily reached, the operator has no inducement to open the urethra too far forwards, and the bulb and its artery will probably escape being cut." The staff is steadied against the front of the pubes. This position is assumed only during the making of the first incision. While the second or deep cut is being made, the staff is held in the position first described.

That position has these two great advantages—the staff can be rigidly held, and the same position is maintained throughout the operation. It has not been shown that any special disadvantages attend the holding of the staff in this one fixed attitude.

Before the operation is commenced, it is well to ascertain that the rectum is empty, and to note the size and position of the prostate.

If the surgeon makes this examination himself, his finger must be thoroughly cleansed before he takes up the scalpel.

The Operation.—*The First* or *Superficial Incision.*— Steadying the integuments of the perineum with the fingers of the left hand, the surgeon makes the first incision. The

knife is introduced at right angles to the surface of the perineum, and at a point just to the left of the median rhaphe, and
just behind the central point of the perineum—*i.e.,* in the adult
about one inch and a quarter in front of the anus.   The
knife is thrust in the direction of the staff, and its point may
just hit the staff.   This first movement is of the nature of a
stab or a puncture.

The incision is completed as the knife is withdrawn.   It is
carried downwards and outwards into the left ischio-rectal
fossa, and ends at a point between the tuber ischii and the

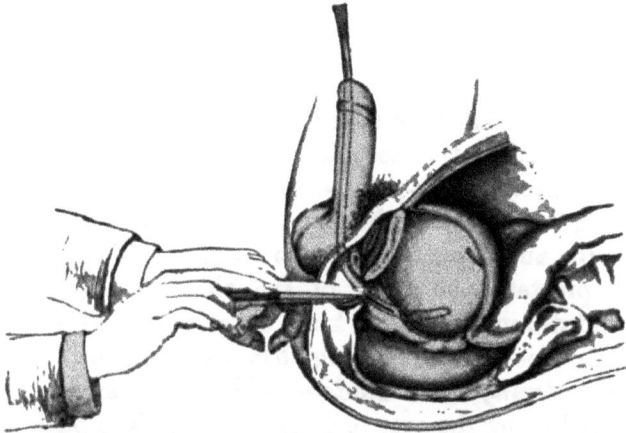

Fig. 398.—LATERAL LITHOTOMY : THE SECOND INCISION.   (*Fergusson.*)

posterior part of the anus, and one-third nearer to the
tuberosity than to the gut.

The incision will in the adult be about three inches in
length.   It becomes gradually shallower and shallower as it
proceeds outwards and backwards from the median line.

The Second or *Deep Incision.*—The left forefinger is now
introduced into the wound, and the staff felt for.   This
instrument will be perpendicular in position, and well drawn
up against the pubic arch.

The surgeon, keeping his eye upon the staff, to appreciate
its position in the depths of the perineum, slips the knife
along the back of the forefinger until it hits the groove in the
staff (Fig. 398).

There must be no doubt at this stage of the operation.

The surgeon must be assured beyond question that he has found the groove, and that the knife occupies it.

The knife is now pushed cautiously along the groove until it reaches the end of the staff and enters the bladder. The blade should be inclined laterally as it is passed along, and be kept parallel with the line of the surface wound.

The incision made in the prostate will therefore be oblique, and directed downwards and outwards.

An escape of urine and a sense of abruptly-diminished resistance will announce that the neck of the bladder has been divided.

In his anxiety not to let the knife leave the groove, the surgeon may depress the handle too much and arrest the knife by causing its sharp point to impinge against the metal. If the hand be raised a little, the knife will glide on. It is in making the second incision that some surgeons employ a special probe-pointed bistoury. (*See* Fig. 395.)

As the knife is withdrawn, its edge is pressed gently downwards and outwards, so as to enlarge the opening made in the prostate and neck of the bladder. The pressure employed diminishes as the knife is removed, and by the time the skin cut is reached the edge has ceased to cut.

The Entering of the Bladder.—The left index finger is now introduced along the groove in the staff into the bladder. As soon as the surgeon is sure that he has his finger in the viscus, but not before, the staff is removed. The finger is then employed in dilating the neck of the bladder in all directions, and in ascertaining the size and situation of the stone.

The opening made by dilatation will have to accommodate itself to the size of the stone.

The dilatation must be made in all directions, and not only in the line of the wound. In the adult considerable force may need to be employed, especially when the incision has been unduly small.

The Extraction of the Stone.—Without removing the left forefinger the surgeon introduces the lithotomy forceps along the upper or dorsal surface of the digit, and only withdraws the finger when the forceps are well in the bladder.

"The blades," writes Mr. Cadge, "should be fully intro-

duced before opening them—this is done slowly and in a
lateral direction—then, by giving a quarter turn to the
handles, one blade is made to sweep round to the lower
fundus of the bladder, and by this manœuvre the stone will
almost certainly be caught. If it is not, the process will be
repeated; and if there is still a difficulty, the surgeon will
ascertain if he has not passed over the stone, which is not
infrequently found close behind the prostate and beneath the
forceps. If this be so, he will withdraw them slightly, elevate
the handles, and repeat the rotatory movement. Sometimes,
though rarely, the stone is entangled or held by irregular contraction of the bladder at the upper fundus, in which case the
handles should be lowered and the blades directed upwards,
while an assistant makes firm pressure above the pubes. The
large size of the stone sometimes makes it difficult to grasp
it; in this case the operator will withdraw the forceps,
perhaps take a larger pair, and, having ascertained with his
finger the exact position of the stone, he will introduce them
so that the tips of the blades impinge on it; then, by slowly
opening them, they will be found to glide over each side of
the stone, and a good hold is obtained.

"All these manœuvres are to be slowly and gently conducted, and there should be no wild 'digs' at the stone, or
sudden alterations of method. The extraction should be
deliberate and steady, the direction somewhat downwards, the
blades and handles of the forceps kept in a vertical position,
and no rotation made as the stone advances, for fear of injuring the prostate and neck of the bladder. Should there be
much resistance and no sense of gradual yielding, the surgeon
will ask himself the question whether this is due to an
insufficient opening, or to the projection of the ends of an
oval stone laterally beyond the blades. The latter may be
known by observing that the bladder is brought bodily down,
so that the prostate, which is probably large, is visible near
the external wound; in this case the stone must be liberated,
the finger again introduced, and a fresh hold taken. If the
obstruction is due to a large stone and too small a wound, the
latter is to be enlarged in the direction of the first incision"
(Heath's " Dictionary of Surgery ")

Dr. Keelan (*Brit. Med. Journ.*, Oct. 15th, 1887) points out that the line of traction in removing the stone should be in the line of the outlet of the pelvis. When the body is in the lithotomy position therefore, the forceps must be drawn in a direction upwards and forwards.

The bladder is finally explored with the finger for other calculi or for fragments. If any *débris* remain, such as may be broken from a phosphatic calculus, the viscus is washed out with the syringe.

The lithotomy tube is introduced, and is secured in place by means of lateral tapes, which are fastened to the two tails of a T-bandage on a level with the perineal wound. The wound is left open and uncovered.

Lateral Lithotomy in Children.—The operation in children is much modified by the anatomical conditions of the parts. The pelvis is relatively narrower than in the adult. The bladder is more an abdominal than a pelvic organ, and the neck of the bladder is therefore high up. The viscus, moreover, is very movable, and has less substantial attachments than has the bladder in the adult. The urethra is very small, its walls are thin, and all the parts are comparatively delicate and readily torn. The prostate is wholly undeveloped, and thus much of the actual neck of the bladder has to be cut. From the small size of the gland also it happens that in some cases the knife has passed too far beyond the prostate area, and has opened up the pelvic fascia. In children also the peritoneum descends lower on the posterior surface of the bladder, and may be wounded by a careless operator.

On the other hand, the staff is in children more easily felt through the perineum, the bulb is very small and insignificant, and the bladder can be more readily steadied and manipulated by the fingers pressing deeply above the pubes, or by the forefinger introduced into the rectum.

Suitable instruments must be employed, and the surgeon must throughout exercise the utmost gentleness.

The great difficulty rests with the entering of the bladder.

If force be employed, it is possible in attempting to introduce the finger to actually tear the membranous urethra across, and to push the neck of the still undilated bladder in front of the finger into the pelvis. This accident happened to so eminently skilful a surgeon as Sir William Fergusson.

Forcible dilatation of the neck of the viscus must not be attempted. The incision of the prostatic area should be relatively freer in the child than in the adult, and the operator must within reasonable limits depend more upon the knife than upon the finger in effecting an entrance. It must be understood that the incisions, although made more freely in proportion than in the adult, must yet be strictly limited.

The *modus operandi* should be as follows:—The usual incisions are made; the staff is reached, and a relatively free incision is made into the neck of the bladder. The deep wound is examined with the finger. A pair of dressing forceps is then introduced along the staff into the bladder, and, by opening the blades, the wound in the vesical neck is cautiously enlarged. In one instance, when carrying out this step of the operation, I unexpectedly seized the stone and removed it forthwith.

The forceps are removed, and a probe-pointed director or common probe is then introduced into the bladder along the groove in the staff. The staff is withdrawn, but the probe or director is left in position, as a guide to the bladder, until the operation is completed. The finger is now introduced along the slender probe, and is slowly and cautiously wormed into the bladder. The stone may now be removed by appropriate forceps in the usual way, or its extraction may be effected by a scoop aided with the tip of the left forefinger, or the calculus may be worked out of the bladder by means of one forefinger introduced into that organ, and aided by the other forefinger inserted into the rectum.

As urinary infiltration is little to be feared in children, and as they prove restless and often unintelligent patients, the lithotomy tube may be dispensed with, and the wound left practically to look after itself.

Obstacles in the Performance of Lateral Lithotomy.

1. *A very large stone* need scarcely be considered, as it would now be dealt with by the suprapubic operation.

2. *An enlarged prostate* may cause the extraction to be very difficult. The bladder will probably be found to be almost, if not quite, beyond the reach of the finger, and the position of the stone cannot be accurately known. In most cases the suprapubic method would have been selected.

Should, however, the wound have been made, the extraction may be assisted by means of the blunt gorget, or it may be possible to tilt the stone upwards by means of the finger introduced into the rectum, so that it can be grasped by the forceps. Mr. Jacobson suggests that the rectal bag may be of service. When the median lobe is prominent, it may be accidentally or intentionally torn off and drawn away in the bite of the forceps. The post-prostatic pouch is alluded to on page 571.

3. *A deep perineum* in a very large and corpulent subject gives rise to difficulties, the neck of the bladder being scarcely within reach of the finger. Here also a blunt gorget has been advised. Some assistance may be obtained from pressure applied through the rectum, or from pressure applied to the bladder over the hypogastrium.

4. In some old subjects the *neck of the bladder* may be found to be *unduly rigid,* and to yield very indifferently to dilatation. In such cases the deep incision must be extended a little beyond the usual limits.

5. *Encysted calculus* may cause much trouble. Writing of the pouches which may engage calculi, Mr. Buckston Browne divides such pouches into three varieties (*Lancet,* April 18th, 1891).

(1) There is the ordinary sacculus, which consists of a protrusion of mucous membrane between the muscular fibres of the bladder. Such sacculi are found in the upper part, at the side, and in the floor of the bladder; and where the viscus is covered with peritoneum, they, too, are covered by the same membrane.

(2) A pouch often forms behind the trigone—*i.e.,* behind a line drawn between the vesical orifices of the ureters. It is part of the general cavity of the bladder, but is sometimes deep enough to make difficult the discovery of a stone lying within. This may be called the post-trigonal pouch.

(3) There is a post-prostatic or trigonal pouch which is often of extraordinary depth. If the patient be supposed to be lying down, it may be said to consist of the trigone of the bladder, pushed down between the enlarged and projecting prostate in front, and a thickened and firm inter-ureteral ridge behind. Where there is much intra-vesical prostatic

projection, the pouch may literally be roofed over by this prostatic outgrowth (Fig. 399).

Mr. Browne points out that the greatest difficulties in connection with the extraction of a stone may arise when it is lodged in the pouch he names the post-prostatic. If the pouch be deep, it may be absolutely impossible to find the stone by any instrument passed through the urethra. In such cases also lithotrity is more or less impracticable, and should not be attempted, and the only satisfactory means of dealing with the calculus is by suprapubic lithotomy.

When the stone is lodged in an ordinary sacculus, it may be dislodged by dilating the opening of the pouch with the finger, or by displacing it by means of the scoop or forceps. Much assistance may often be afforded by the left forefinger introduced into the rectum, and in the case of a post-trigonal pouch the stone may usually be brought into the field of the operation by that means.

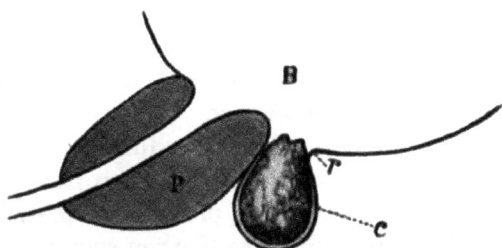

Fig. 399.—POST-PROSTATIC POUCH. (*Buckston Browne.*)
B, Bladder; P, Prostate; c, Calculus in pouch; r, Inter-ureteral ridge.

6. It is unnecessary to do more than allude to such obstacles as are presented by a testicle in the left side of the perineum, anchylosis of one or both hips, or a deformed or rickety pelvis.

Accidents and Complications of Lateral Lithotomy.

1. *Failure to find the stone* may depend upon the fact that a small calculus has escaped unobserved with the first gush of urine, or a small stone may be hidden in a blood clot, or covered with a mass of mucus. Failure to find the stone has also depended upon the circumstance that it did not exist.

2. *If the stone breaks up* during the process of extraction, especial care must be taken that every fragment is removed. The scoop may be employed in addition to the forceps, and especial use must be made of the syringe. The bladder

should be explored with the finger and the sound before the patient leaves the table.

In these cases, and in instances of multiple calculi, it may be well to examine the bladder through the perineum (under an anæsthetic) at a late period after the operation, or just before the wound is beginning to close.

3. *Hæmorrhage.*—Primary hæmorrhage, although free at first, usually ceases before the last steps of the operation are completed. Bleeding from superficial vessels may be dealt with by ligature, and from certain of the deeper vessels by means of pressure forceps, which are left in position for twenty-four or forty-eight hours. Hæmorrhage from the artery to the bulb may be checked in this manner.

There is little to be said in favour of the detachable tenacula, or of Horner's awl, or like appliances, for arresting deep-seated hæmorrhage.

In other examples of bleeding from the depths of the wound, the hæmorrhage may depend upon partial division of an artery, wound of the bulb, the prostate, or the prostatic veins.

Pressure with a fine Turkey sponge of suitable size may be tried, or the wound may be flushed with iced water, or a piece of ice may be introduced into the bottom of the incision. If all these means fail, the lithotomy tube should be introduced, and the wound plugged around it with strips of fine gauze. The "petticoated tube" should be used for the purpose, in order to ensure that no piece of gauze be left in the wound. Some surgeons prefer the special air tampon known as Buckston Browne's or Guyon's.

The plugging of the wound is not free from objection. It is painful, it prevents the escape of discharges, and may lead to extravasation in the connective tissue planes about the neck of the bladder.

When secondary bleeding occurs, the patient should be placed once more in lithotomy position, and the wound thoroughly cleansed and examined. The tube should be removed, and the clots washed out of the bladder.

When the incision has been dried, it is possible that the bleeding point may be detected, especially if the perineum be in a good light and the wound margins be well retracted. In such a case pressure forceps will meet the complication.

Failing the easy securing of the divided vessel, cold injections may be tried; but if they fail, as is most probable, the tube should be re-inserted, and the wound plugged with gauze.

Injections of powerful styptics, and especially of per-chloride of iron, are to be absolutely condemned.

4. *Wound of the Rectum.*—This accident may happen if the staff be not kept well up against the pubic arch, or if the incision be carried too little outwards, or if the rectal tissues be not sufficiently guarded with the finger during the making of the second or deep incision, or if the bowel be full or "bal-looned." The bowel is usually wounded just above the internal sphincter. In the event of such an accident it is better to leave the wound untreated. As a rule, the accidental opening closes. The same may be said of the opening into the rectum, which may result from sloughing, subsequent to the extraction of a very large stone.

5. The following *accidents* may be classed as quite excep-tional:—

The bladder has been perforated by the staff. In such cases the viscus was probably contracted, and the sound too long and too pointed.

The posterior wall of the bladder has been cut with the knife, especially when long blades have been used.

The bladder wall has been pinched up and torn with the forceps.

A false passage has been made by the staff, and upon the misplaced instrument the operator has made his incision.

The After-treatment in Lateral Lithotomy.

The patient is placed on a narrow bed with a firm horse-hair mattress, protected by a waterproof sheet. Beneath the buttocks are kept squares of old sheeting, which can be changed as often as they are wetted with urine. In addition to the sheets, large sponges may be employed to absorb the escaping urine. They can be readily changed without dis-turbing the patient, they are easily cleansed, and if plenty are employed, and each one is allowed to lie for some time in a car-bolic solution before it is used again, the same sponges can be employed over and over again. They need to be well dried by heat before being applied, and may be dusted with iodoform.

A rope and handle bar suspended above the bed will

enable the patient to raise his pelvis readily when the squares of sheeting are changed. The knees should be supported by separate pillows, with an interval between them. Nothing must obstruct the free exposure of the tube.

Clots in the tube may be removed with a moistened feather. If the escape of urine ceases, and there is pain about the bladder, the tube may be pushed a little further in, or a soft rubber catheter may be introduced through it into the bladder.

In most cases the tube may be removed in thirty-six or forty-eight hours. In some few instances—especially when there have been difficulties of micturition previous to the operation—the tube may have to be retained for three or four days, or even longer.

The parts exposed to the contact of urine should be dried as frequently as is possible. The scrotum should be kept away from the perineum by a simple suspender or "crutch pad." When the urine is alkaline and irritating, the skin of the buttocks and perineum should be smeared well with vaseline after each change of the sheets or sponges. In cases of actually putrid urine the bladder should be washed out two or three times a day with a warm solution of boracic acid. The urine begins to flow by the urethra as a rule between the eighth and twelfth day, and the perineal wound is generally healed and the patient "cured" within the month. The same care in the diet is observed as is customary after all major operations. If the bowels are not opened by the third day, a laxative should be given.

The following *complications* may occur during the after-treatment:—Retention of urine from blocking or displacement of the tube. Suppression of urine in cases in which the kidneys are diseased. Incrustation of the wound with phosphates may occur when the urine is ammoniacal, and there is much cystitis. This is especially met with in aged and feeble patients. The condition is met by frequent irrigation of the bladder with boracic acid lotion or mildly acidulated solutions, and by constant attention to the wound. Epididymitis is not infrequently met with after lateral lithotomy. Cellulitis from urinary infiltration is, of all the possible complications, one of the most serious. It is fortunately uncommon.

CHAPTER II.

MEDIAN LITHOTOMY.

In this operation the knife is entered in the middle line of the perineum, just in front of the anus. The apex of the prostate and the membranous urethra are incised in the median line.

The parts divided in the median operation are the skin and superficial fascia, the sphincter ani, the central point of the perineum, the lower border of the triangular ligament, the membranous urethra, the compressor urethræ, and the apex of the prostate.

The advantages claimed for the operation are—the smaller amount of cutting involved, the reputed lesser amount of bleeding, and the more rapid recovery. Mr. Cadge, however, states as the result of an extensive experience of both methods that troublesome bleeding is of frequent occurrence in median lithotomy, and that the rapid recovery which is claimed for the method is only to be expected when the stone is small. There are, moreover, the distinct disadvantages that both the bulb and the rectum are in greater danger of being wounded, and that the amount of space obtained for the removal of the stone is very slight. The median operation cannot be carried out in its integrity in children.

Mr. Cadge admirably sums up the present position of median lithotomy in these words:—"It is suitable only for small stones, and these, for the most part, are best dealt with by lithotrity."

The general features of the operation are identical with those of lateral lithotomy. A special staff and a special knife are employed.

The staff is of moderate size, and has a broad, deep median

groove (Fig. 400). The knife is a long, straight, narrow bistoury, with a stiff back and a double cutting point.

Little's lithotomy director (Fig. 401) is of service.

The Operation.—The method here described is that known as Allarton's.

The patient having been placed in lithotomy position, the staff is introduced, and is held in the same manner as in lateral lithotomy. The surgeon inserts the left index finger

Fig. 400.—LITHOTOMY STAFF WITH MEDIAN GROOVE.

into the rectum, and steadies the staff with the point of the finger, which is pressed against it at the apex of the prostate.

The narrow bistoury is now thrust into the median rhaphe of the perineum half an inch in front of the anus. It is introduced horizontally, and with the cutting edge directly upwards. The groove in the staff is hit at the point where it is steadied by the finger in the rectum. The groove is entered at this point, and by continuing to thrust the knife

Fig. 401.—LITTLE'S DIRECTOR.

deeper the apex of the prostate is slightly incised. The membranous urethra is cut through as the knife is being withdrawn, and the external wound is enlarged to the extent of about one inch by cutting upwards as the knife is being removed.

As the urethra is incised, the handle of the knife will be pointing almost directly downwards; as the integuments are divided, the handle will be pointing upwards. Special care must be taken to avoid wounding the bulb.

A Little's director, or similar instrument, is now introduced along the groove of the staff into the bladder. It is held in the left hand. The staff is now withdrawn.

Guided by the director, which is retained in position until the operation is completed, the operator gradually worms his right forefinger into the bladder, dilating its orifice.

The forceps are now introduced. and the stone is with drawn.

In ordinary cases no lithotomy tube need be employed.

CHAPTER III.

Suprapubic Lithotomy.

Anatomical Points.—When empty, the bladder is flattened and of triangular outline, and lies against the anterior wall of the pelvis.

Between this part of the pelvic wall and the adjacent surface of the bladder is a pyramidal-shaped space filled with a loose connective tissue. To the summit of the bladder is inserted the remains of the urachus. The peritoneal investment of the viscus, so far as its anterior surface is concerned, never extends beyond the attachment of this structure.

To the bladder at its summit the peritoneum is firmly attached, but to the anterior abdominal parietes at the site of the reflection of the membrane the attachment is remarkably lax. This loose connection of the peritoneum to the parietal tissues allows the serous membrane to accommodate itself to changes in the size and position of the bladder.

The conditions under which the fold of peritoneum at the reflection can be displaced upwards, and a portion of the bladder be projected above the symphysis pubis, free of covering from the serous membrane, vary somewhat according to the age of the patient.

In the child the bladder is still rather an abdominal than a pelvic organ, its vertical axis is elongated, and its outline is more nearly oval. When distended, the organ tends certainly to project towards the pelvic floor on the one hand, while on the other it mounts readily over the symphysis pubis, and soon presents a fair non-peritoneal surface above that bone. By means of a frozen section Symington showed (*Edin. Med. Journ.*, April, 1885) that in the case of a male child aged five, the injection of three ounces of water into the bladder caused the reflection of the peritoneum to be carried 2·7 c.m. (*i.e.*, more than one inch) above the symphysis pubis.

It will be evident therefore that in children mere distension of the bladder—without the aid of any rectal tampon—will suffice to bring the viscus into a safe position for suprapubic lithotomy.

Schmitz, who up to 1886 had operated in thirty-eight cases of children by the high operation (*Langenbeck's Archiv.*, 1886), totally discards the rectal bag, to which allusion will be subsequently made. Trendelenburg and others also make a practice of operating without the assistance of the rectal tampon.

With regard to the adult bladder, our knowledge of its relations and adjustments under distension has been greatly added to by the preparation of frozen sections, and especially by those of Pirogoff and Braune. Garson (*Edin. Med. Journ.*, Oct., 1878) was the first to describe the influence of rectal tamponade in raising the pre-vesical fold of peritoneum.

Two years later Petersen, of Kiel (*Archiv. if klin. Chir.*, 1880), published the results of his experiments in the same direction, and from this period the modern operation of suprapubic cystotomy may be considered to date.

Valuable investigations upon the effect of vesical and rectal distension upon the reflection of peritoneum have been carried out by means of frozen sections by Fehleisen (*Langenbeck's Archiv.*, vol. xxxiv.), Strong (*Annals of Surgery*, Jan., 1887), and others.

When empty, the bladder is flattened and of triangular outline, and lies against the anterior wall of the pelvis. The empty bladder may be found in one of two conditions (as demonstrated by Hart in the adult female bladder). It may be small, oval, and firm, with its upper wall convex towards the abdomen (the systolic empty bladder); or it may be larger, and soft, with its upper surface concave towards the abdomen, and fitting into the concavity of the lower wall or surface (the diastolic empty bladder).

When moderately distended, it is of rounded outline; when completely distended, it assumes a more oval outline, and rises out of the pelvis. As the bladder becomes distended its fundus extends more and more towards the perineum. Its summit is brought more and more in contact with the anterior abdominal parietes.

l l 2

When the bladder and rectum are quite empty, the apex of the bladder and the pre-vesical reflection of peritoneum are a little below the upper margin of the symphysis pubis.

When the apex of the bladder is two inches above the pubes, and the organ is pressed against the abdominal wall, the peritoneal reflection is probably not more than three-quarters of an inch above the same point of bone.

The mobility of the bladder and the laxity of the peritoneal fold vary greatly in different individuals, and are much influenced by the physical condition of the tissues. In two males, aged thirty-four and thirty-five respectively, an injection into the bladder of ten ounces raised the peritoneal fold in one case an inch and three-quarters, and in the other three-quarters of an inch. In fleshy and flabby subjects the bladder usually will rise easily out of the pelvis against the abdominal wall when alone moderately distended.

With regard to the *rectal bag* and its effect in elevating the pre-vesical fold of peritoneum, it is evident that its power is inconstant, that it varies in different individuals, and is much influenced by the physical state of the tissues.

The researches published show very varying, and often quite contradictory, results, which may be explained by the different conditions under which the experiments were performed, by the different states of the tissues, and by the time which had elapsed since death.

Distension of the rectum alone will elevate the base of the bladder, but will usually have no effect upon the reflection of peritoneum. The rectal bag provides a more or less firm base for the fundus of the bladder, and it overcomes the tendency of the dilating organ to extend towards the perineum. It also pushes forwards the posterior wall of the bladder, and tends to force the entire organ towards the anterior abdominal wall.

To avoid a number of confusing and often conflicting data, the following results of experiments may be selected as illustrative of the effect of the rectal bag. These results are examples merely. They do not represent constants, nor can they be considered as conclusive. They show the effects produced in certain individual bodies. They are the results of Fehleisen's experiments upon the adult bladder as demonstrated by frozen sections.

Experiment 1.—The rectum is quite empty; the bladder contains ten and a half ounces of fluid; the internal meatus is 1 c.m. above the lower border of the symphysis; the pre-vesical fold of peritoneum is raised only half a centimètre above the upper margin of the symphysis.

Experiment 2.—The rectum is quite empty; the bladder contains twenty-two and a half ounces of fluid. The bladder is

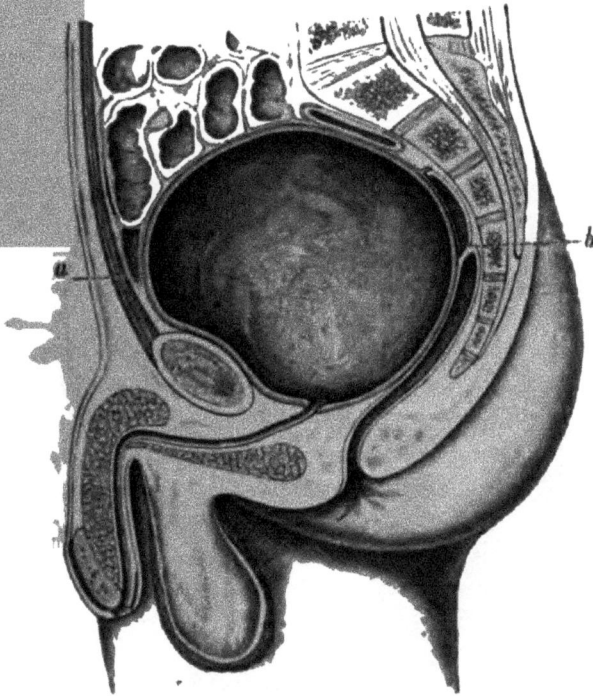

Fig. 402.—EFFECTS OF DISTENSION OF THE BLADDER UPON ITS POSITION.
a Anterior, and *b* Posterior, reflection of peritoneum. (*Fehleisen.*)

spherical, and is distended backwards rather than upwards; the prostatic urethra is nearly horizontal; the pre-vesical fold of peritoneum is raised 2 c.m. (more than three-quarters of an inch) above the symphysis pubis (Fig. 402).

Experiment 3.—The rectum contains sixteen and a half ounces of fluid injected into an oval bag; the bladder contains seven ounces. The bladder is pentagonal rather than rounded; the base of the bladder is much raised; it is close behind the anterior abdominal wall; the reflection of peritoneum has been raised four centimètres (one inch and five-eighths) (Fig. 403).

Experiment 4.—The rectum contains seventeen and a half ounces in a bag; the bladder contains fourteen and a half ounces. The bladder is of irregular outline; its base is more raised than in experiment No. 3. The internal meatus is,

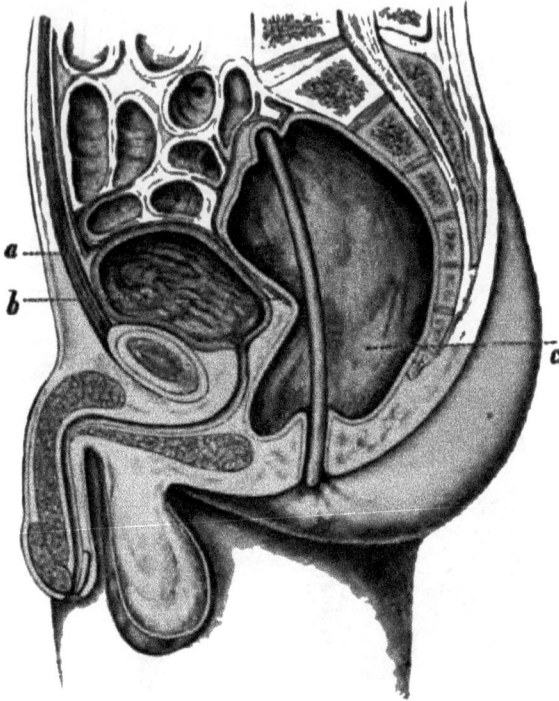

Fig. 403.—EFFECTS OF DISTENSION OF THE RECTUM AND BLADDER UPON THE POSITION OF THE LATTER.

a Anterior, and *b* Posterior, reflection of peritoneum; *c* Rectal bag. (*Pohleism.*)

indeed, elevated two and a half centimètres (one inch) above the lower border of the symphysis. The prostatic urethra is vertical. The anterior fold of peritoneum is raised eight and a half centimètres (three and a half inches) above the upper edge of the symphysis.

It would appear that the best results are obtained when the rectum is distended first and the bladder afterwards; the

the rectal bag should be inserted high up, so as to occupy the hollow of the sacrum.

In the cadaver the rectum has been ruptured opposite to the promontory of the sacrum by injecting twenty-three ounces of fluid into the rectal bag.

It must be remembered that the vesical veins which course over the apex of the bladder, and which are exposed in the operation, pass under the fundus of the organ; and that when the rectal bag is employed, these veins must of necessity be rendered unduly prominent.

The Instruments Required.—A scalpel; probe-pointed bistoury; scissors; sharp hook, blunt hooks; dissecting, artery, and pressure forceps; broad rectangular retractors; wound retractors; rectal bag; ligature for penis; syringe; sound; lithotomy forceps and scoop; drainage-tube for bladder; needles, sutures, ligatures, etc.

The rectal bag should be strong, of oval or pear shape, and of suitable size.

Preparation of the Patient.—The preparation, such as it is, has already been alluded to in the chapter on Lateral Lithotomy. If the bladder be unduly irritable, it is recommended that it should be washed out daily for some few days beforehand. The rectum must be well emptied. In the adult the pubes should be shaved. In any case, the region of the operation must be thoroughly cleansed.

The patient lies upon the back, close to the right edge of the table. The shoulders are raised. A few sponges are wedged in against the perineum, to collect any blood or fluid which may run in that direction.

The surgeon stands to the patient's right, and the chief assistant takes his place upon the opposite side of the table.

THE OPERATION.

The Distension of the Rectum and Bladder.—The rectal bag is thoroughly emptied, is smeared with vaseline, is folded in two, and when thus made conical is introduced into the rectum. It should be passed in well above the sphincters, and should lie in the hollow of the sacrum. It should be introduced by someone who is not otherwise assisting at the operation.

It is better to postpone the filling of the bag until the bladder has been injected. A soft catheter is passed, the urine is drawn off, and through the catheter the bladder is washed out with a warm boracic solution (half an ounce to the pint). This is more conveniently done with an irrigator than with a syringe. The bladder is now filled with a weak warm solution of boracic acid, or a solution of carbolic acid in the proportion of one to eighty or one to a hundred. In children from two to five years of age three ounces will probably suffice. In adults, eight to ten to fifteen ounces may be introduced. The injection should be carried out by means of an irrigator held a few feet above the level of the table. The fluid then enters the bladder with a more equable stream than when it is forced in by means of a syringe. The quantity of fluid required must be placed in the irrigator, and no more. If a piece of glass tubing be inserted in the irrigator tube close to the nozzle, the ease with which the fluid enters can be noted, as also the evidence of any backward pressure. The irrigator is detached, and, as the catheter is withdrawn, an indiarubber cord is tied round the penis to prevent the escape of the injected fluid.

The rectal bag is now distended should its use be indicated. It is filled with warm water. For an adult, some ten to twelve ounces may be injected. For a child of five, from two and a half to three ounces. In actual practice the bag is seldom needed in operating upon children, and can very well be dispensed with in such patients. In old and thin subjects also the bag can often be omitted. It not unfrequently happens that after the injection of the bladder the organ can be made out above the pubes. In such case the rectal bag is hardly needed. It may be left in place, and be distended when the bladder is exposed, if it should appear necessary.

The practice observed by some of not distending the rectal bag until the bladder has been reached has much to commend it.

As already mentioned, experiments upon the cadaver show that the best results are obtained, so far as the projection forwards of the bladder is concerned, when the rectum is distended first and the bladder afterwards. This order of proceeding is not quite so easily followed, and may possibly be not quite so safe so far as the bladder is concerned. Mr. Mayo Robson recommends it, and has found no ill from its employment (*Brit. Med. Journ.*, Oct. 11th, 1890). The bladder is emptied, and, if necessary, washed out. The catheter is not removed.

The rectal bag is introduced and distended. The bladder is then filled, the catheter withdrawn, and the cord tied round the penis.

If there be any evidence of disease of the mucous membrane or walls of the rectum, the bag should not be used at all.

A case is reported in which the bladder of a man was torn by injecting 125 grammes of water.

The Opening of the Bladder. — An incision about three inches in length is made precisely in the median line immediately above the symphysis. The incision should be extended about half an inch actually over that process of bone. There is no linea alba below the umbilicus, and after dividing the skin and subcutaneous tissues, the surgeon may find muscular fibre lying across the line of the incision. If the interval between the muscles is not readily found, the knife should be carried directly through the muscle fibres themselves, the median line being strictly observed.

The wound must be a clean one, and any tearing of the parts with the fingers or forceps, or the handle of the scalpel, to seek for an inter-muscular interval, is to be deprecated. When substantial and powerful muscles are met with, it may sometimes be advisable to divide the fibres transversely, to a slight extent, close to their attachment to the bone.

Any bleeding points are secured with pressure forceps. The transversalis fascia is reached, and is divided in the same precise manner in the median line.

The area of connective tissue overlying the summit of the bladder is now exposed. This must be cleanly and precisely divided with the scalpel, and the bladder reached by dissection.

The peritoneum may possibly be made out, and can be readily pushed upwards with the left forefinger. The dissection necessary to expose the bladder should be commenced close to the symphysis, and be continued cautiously upwards. The peritoneum has been found adherent over the symphysis, and has been wounded. If such an accident should occur, the opening should be at once closed by fine catgut sutures.

Wide rectangular metal retractors must now be used in order to extend the width of the wound to the utmost.

All bleeding into the lax connective tissue, which is exposed, must be arrested.

Several veins are met with ramifying over the apex of the bladder. They must be avoided. Should any be divided, the hæmorrhage may be very free; but it will cease when the bladder is opened, and especially when the rectal bag is emptied. The bag presses upon these veins, and tends to cause them to be prominent.

The pre-vesical fat may be considerable in quantity. It should never be torn through with the fingers or with the forceps and the handle of a scalpel. All such rough manipulations open the way for urinary infiltration. The exposure of the bladder should be, as already stated, by dissection.

All bleeding at this stage should be promptly checked, since the blood readily infiltrates the loose tissue in which the surgeon is working.

The bladder is recognised by its pinkish colour, by its rounded outline, and by the exposed layer of muscular fibres. The peritoneum, if in view, must be pushed upwards with the left forefinger, while the surgeon transfixes the bladder with a sharp hook. This hook should be introduced transversely across the median line, and should be inserted near the upper part of the exposed viscus.

The scalpel is now thrust vertically into .the bladder, exactly in the median line and just below the hook, and is made to incise the organ by cutting downwards towards the symphysis. It should be introduced with a sharp stab, lest the undivided mucous membrane be pushed inwards by its point. If any vein be in the way, it may be thrust aside, although the thinness of these vessels calls for gentle manipulation.

The actual opening of the bladder is demonstrated by the escape of the contained fluid. The bold upon the tenaculum should not be relaxed. The cut margin of the bladder on either side of the opening should now be seized neatly and symmetrically with artery or pressure forceps. These enable the operator to maintain a hold upon the organ during the remainder of the operation, and they render the position of the opening perfectly distinct.

Very little tissue need be taken up in the blades, and it has not been shown that the temporary compression of the instruments does any harm.

When the forceps are in place, but not before, the tenaculum may be removed.

Loops of silk have been employed to hold up the bladder, and to maintain the fixed position of the opening; but if drawn upon, they are apt to cut out. Certain special specula are described on page 614.

When the bladder collapses, the fold of peritoneum may present at the upper angle of the wound. The tenaculum keeps it out of the way, but it may be noted that the membrane has been inadvertently injured at this stage.

Unless means such as have been described are taken to prevent the sinking of the bladder, its anterior wall may descend into the pelvis, and much damage may be done to the soft parts in endeavouring to draw it up again. The finger should not be prematurely thrust into the opening, and should never be introduced until the margins of the orifice have been fixed. Ill-considered attempts in this direction may cause the bladder to be pushed before the finger, the opening to be closed, and the viscus to be separated from the surface of the pubes.

The hæmorrhage from the edges of the wound in the bladder may be a little free at first, but it soon ceases.

As soon as the bladder has been opened, an assistant may remove the ligature from the penis.

The surgeon holds the right-hand pair of retaining forceps, while the assistant holds the left; and with the opening thus fixed, the right forefinger is introduced into the bladder.

The opening may be enlarged with a blunt-pointed bistoury as required. There is no need to make the orifice so small that the finger has to be wormed in.

The stone is now extracted. For this purpose lithotomy

forceps may be used, or the scoop may be found to be of greater service, or the two forefingers may be employed forceps-wise. The manipulations attending the extraction may be aided possibly by emptying the rectal bag, or possibly by distending it if it has not been filled.

Should any *débris* remain, or should the urine be putrid, the bladder should be well washed out.

In a perfectly straightforward case this may be dispensed with. Before the operation is concluded, the interior of the bladder should be thoroughly explored with the finger. The retaining forceps are removed from the bladder.

Two or three sutures of silkworm gut are introduced into the upper part of the parietal wound, each suture including the whole thickness of the divided tissues.

The question of suture of the bladder and total closure of the surface wound is considered in the next section.

The ligature upon the penis will probably have been already removed.

The rectal bag is now emptied and withdrawn. All the parts concerned are dried and cleansed.

The Suturing of the Bladder.—This is an ideal method of concluding the operation whenever it can be carried out. The bladder wound may be closed by suture in children, and in healthy adults provided that the viscus itself is healthy.

It is not wise to attempt it in aged subjects, in those who have cystitis, or in cases where the operation has been protracted, and the margins of the bladder wound much bruised, as in the extraction of a large calculus.

The application of the sutures is comparatively easy in children and in thin adults. It is difficult in the corpulent. The early records show that after immediate suture of the bladder in two-thirds of the cases the wound reopens, and in one-third only primary healing takes place. Mr. Mayo Robson, in a more recent communication, records ten cases of suture, with only one failure to secure immediate healing. In this instance the bladder was so deep as to be almost out of reach of the finger.

The opening into the bladder is fixed, and is held up by

two blunt hooks, one inserted at each extremity of the wound. By means of these hooks the margins of the incision are kept steady and parallel with one another. Very fine chromicised catgut should be employed. The sutures should be interrupted, should not include the mucous membrane, should be introduced by means of a curved needle in a holder, and be very closely applied. Many forms of suture have been advised, but this appears to be the best.

A small drainage-tube is introduced into the lower part of the parietal wound, which is then closed.

A dry dressing is applied. The tube may be removed in forty-eight hours.

The bladder is left undisturbed. No catheter is tied in, nor is any drain through the perineum necessary. If the patient cannot pass water, a soft catheter must be introduced as often as required.

The After-treatment.—If the wound in the bladder has been closed by sutures, the after-treatment of the case is conducted upon the lines observed after any ordinary abdominal section.

The question of the employment of the catheter has already been alluded to. The superficial sutures may be removed at the end of a week; and if all goes well, the patient may be sitting up in ten days.

If the wound in the bladder has been left open, the after-treatment becomes very tedious, and demands infinite care. The bed must be protected by macintosh sheets, placed beneath the usual draw-sheets. A large cradle is spread across the pelvis. The care of the wound will demand the constant and undivided attention of a nurse.

The raw surface is dusted with iodoform, and left. There is no object in introducing a tube into the bladder, and the various syphon drainage-tubes are delusions and snares. There is no need to pass a catheter into the bladder, and to tie it in; nor is there in any ordinary case any reason why the bladder should be cut into from the perineum for the purposes of drainage. If the wound be simply left open, the bladder drains itself well enough. No drainage-tube will prevent the occasional escape of urine into the connective tissue around the incision.

The skin of the perineum, buttocks, and lower part of the abdomen should be kept as dry as possible, and should be smeared with vaseline to prevent the irritating effects of the contact of urine. Over the wound should be placed a large sponge, and beneath the sponge should be a large pad of absorbent wool, applied transversely, like a scarf from one side of the groin to the other.

This pad rests upon the pubes. It keeps the sponge in place, and serves to absorb any urine which may escape the sponge. It may be conveniently replaced, if expense be disregarded, by a thick scarf-like fold of Tillmann's dressing.

Not less than twenty sponges should be in use.

The arrangement of the bed-clothes over the cradle allows the part to be always in view, the patient's trunk and limbs being well covered up with blankets.

The sponges and wool pad must be changed as often as needed—possibly two, three, or four times in the hour. The pad is of course thrown away, but the sponge can be used over and over again. Each sponge is well rinsed in water, is then immersed for some hours in carbolic lotion, is once more rinsed, and is then dried ready for use. Before being applied, each sponge may be dusted with a little iodoform.

Before each sponge and scarf of wool are applied, the skin should be rapidly dried. No bandage is required. The patient must lie upon the back, and should assume, as soon as he is able, the sitting position. If he wishes to lie upon one or other side, the sponge and the wool pad must be adjusted to meet the altered position.

If this plan be carried out by intelligent and painstaking nurses, the patient's bed may be kept absolutely dry, and the skin perfectly sound and free from excoriation. The sponges can be changed during sleep without waking the patient, the wound being always in view through a " window " in the cradle.

The sooner the patient can sit up in bed the better, as the wound is much more readily dealt with when that attitude is assumed.

Any "dressing" secured with a bandage round the body is useless. By the time the dressing has been applied and the bandage secured, the whole arrangement is probably soaked with urine.

The bladder may, when necessary, be washed out with a boracic acid solution as often as required.

The bladder wound usually closes in two, three, or four weeks, and the external wound one or two weeks later. It is probable that the patient will be able to be moved into a chair by the end of the second or commencement of the third week.

No advantage appears to attend attempts to approximate the margins of the wound by strips of strapping.

The Use of the Sonde à dard.—This instrument was at one time an essential element in the suprapubic operation It is still much used by French surgeons, and has been recommended by English writers for suprapubic lithotomy in

Fig. 404.—sonde à dard.

the female or in the male when a perineal opening has already been made.

The sound has been modified from time to time since its introduction by Frère Côsme. It consists essentially of a curved hollow sound with a slightly bulbous end and a concealed sharp-pointed stylet, which can be protruded as shown in Fig. 404.

A rectum bag may be introduced if thought fit. The sound is introduced into the bladder through the urethra. The rectal bag is distended. The handle of the sound is then depressed between the patient's legs, until the point presses the apex of the bladder against the upper part of the symphysis.

The median suprapubic incision is now made, and the bladder exposed in the usual way.

It may either be opened by cutting upon the blunt point of the sound, or the stylet may be thrust through the bladder wall, and the knife be conducted into the bladder by following the groove which should mark the posterior surface of the stylet.

After the viscus has been opened, the stylet is withdrawn into the sound, and the instrument is removed.

Results of Lithotomy Operations.—Mr. Cadge gives in Heath's "Dictionary of Surgery" the results of the operations for stone performed at the Norwich Hospital.

The following is an abstract of a collection of 1,124 cases of lithotomy :—

Mortality, males	...	...	...	...	...	13½ per cent.
„ females	...	...	...	...	...	8 „
Mortality under 20 years of age	...	...	...	8 „
„ over „ „ „	...	...	...	19 „
„ „ 50 „ „	...	...	...	27·4 „

Out of 1,030 patients who were cut, only forty were subjected to a second operation and five to a third.

Sir Henry Thompson has published the results of his extensive experience of operations for stone in the *Medico-Chirurgical Transactions* for 1890. They include 115 examples of perineal lithotomy in male adults, with forty-three deaths; and twelve examples in boys, with one death. The admirable results published by Dr. Freyer (*Brit. Med. Journ.*, May 9, 1891) give but one death in fifty-four cases of perineal lithotomy.

Any attempt to estimate correctly the mortality that attends the suprapubic operation would at present be misleading. Dr. Dennis's collection of 127 cases operated on since 1879 gives a mortality of nine per cent. ; but more recent communications show that better results are being obtained from year to year, and indicate that the mortality in the future will be considerably below Dr. Dennis's estimate.

CHAPTER IV.

LITHOTRITY AND LITHOLAPAXY.

THESE operations concern the treatment of stone by crushing.

By *lithotrity* is understood the crushing of the stone by many repeated brief sittings, the fragments being left to be voided by natural means. The crushings are conducted without an anæsthetic. *Litholapaxy* concerns the entire crushing of the stone and the fragments at one sitting under an anæsthetic, the *débris* being completely removed at the time by means of a special instrument.

The latter and more modern operation has more or less completely replaced the older procedure.

The treatment of stone by crushing is of quite recent origin. Gruithuisen (a Bavarian surgeon) proposed in 1813 that the stone should be broken up by drilling, and invented some remarkable instruments, including a trephine, which do not appear, however, to have been employed on the living subject. In 1818 Civiale published an account of a litho-tripteur, but the instrument was never employed. A like fate attended the curved file introduced by Elderton (a Scottish surgeon) in 1819. During the next few years a great number of remarkable instruments were invented, including the saw, or litho-prione, of Leroy D'Etiolles, the brise-pierce of Amussat, and the brise-coque of Heurteloup. To a Danish surgeon, Jacobson, is due the credit of demonstrating in 1831 that stones might be crushed by simple pressure. Civiale's first successful operations had been performed already in 1824, but with very imperfect instruments. The development of the modern lithotrite followed very rapidly, and is associated with the names of Weiss, Heurteloup, L'Estrange, Brodie, Charrière, Thompson, and others. To Brodie, Coulson, and Sir Henry |

Thompson are mainly due the final elaboration of the operation, and its ready establishment in Great Britain.

No description of the perfected instrument is called for. It is the outcome of innumerable experiments and of infinite ingenuity, and as an example of applied mechanics is without an equal in the surgeon's armamentarium.

In 1878 Professor Bigelow proposed the method of lithotrity with which his name is associated, and to which he gave the title of litholapaxy. The ground had been prepared by the researches of Otis, who had demonstrated that the urethra could take with safety instruments of infinitely larger calibre than had ever been supposed. The way was thus made clear for the employment of large evacuating catheters, by means of which the bladder could be cleared of all *débris*. The use of anæsthetics, and the demonstration of the tolerance of the bladder and urethra to the long-continued contact of instruments, completed the bases for the operation.

Heurteloup and others had many years previously advocated the removal of the calculus at one sitting, but this advice had no practical issue.

In Ashhurst's "Encyclopædia of Surgery," vol. vi., page 234, will be found a full account of the development of the evacuator—from the crude aspirating bottle of Crampton, used in 1846, to the elaborate and efficient instrument devised by Bigelow after many experiments and many modifications. In the article in question figures are given of no less than sixteen different evacuators, many of which, however, are merely the earlier forms of more perfect instruments.

LITHOLAPAXY.

In the following account the more modern method of dealing with the stone—viz., by litholapaxy—will be dealt with. A brief notice of the older operation will be found at the end of the present chapter (page 604).

Preparation of the Patient.—In an ordinary case no special preparation is needed. It is well, however, that for some days before the operation the patient should rest quietly in bed, and should sleep well. His diet should be simple and non-stimulating, and the action of the bowels should be attended to. It is assumed that the urethra is in a condition to admit a sufficiently large lithotrite and evacuating catheter. There is no need that the bladder should be injected with fluid before the operation. The patient should not empty the viscus; and if three or four ounces of urine be retained at the time of the operation, so much the better.

The patient should lie flat upon the back upon the operating-table, and close to the right-hand edge. The pelvis should be raised above the level of the shoulders by means of a firm pillow. This has the effect of causing the stone to gravitate towards the fundus of the bladder.

The surgeon stands to the patient's right. The assistant takes up his position upon the opposite side of the table, and attends to the filling and adjusting of the evacuating apparatus. The thighs should be so separated that there is an interval of a foot or more between the knees. The patient is anæsthetised. In suitable cases Dr. Freyer performs the operation without an anæsthetic. If any doubt exists as to the capacity of the urethra, a sound of suitable size may be passed. In some instances it may be necessary to incise the meatus.

Before using the lithotrite the surgeon should have made himself thoroughly familiar with the instrument, and should have practised crushing operations with it outside the body.

The **Operation.**—No better account of the manipulations involved in lithotrity can be given than is provided in the description by Sir Henry Thompson, whose skill with the lithotrite is probably unequalled. The account appended is derived from Holmes's " System of Surgery," third edition, vol. iii., page 294 :—

" The operator places himself on the right side of the patient, and stands with his back turned partly towards the head of the couch, his left side being to the patient's right. Having well oiled the lithotrite, he holds it lightly with his right hand, in a horizontal position, the blades pointing downwards, and raises the penis with his left; and as he introduces the blades into the urethra, the left draws the penis gently over the angular end of the instrument, which descends in this manner down to the bulbous portion of the urethra, the shaft rising gradually towards the perpendicular. Having arrived there, it is not now to be depressed as in catheterism, since this movement raises the point of the blades against the roof of the urethra in front of the deep fascia above the narrow orifice of the membranous portion, while the large capacity of the bulbous urethra favours the malposition described, and, if force is used to overcome the difficulty, laceration will probably take place. . . . In order to pass the blades easily and safely through the narrow membranous portion, it is necessary to maintain the lithotrite a few seconds at or near the perpendicular, permitting it to progress slowly in that position. This proceeding is accomplished by permitting a part of the weight of the instrument to act as the propelling power, while the penis is drawn upwards a little, in the same—that is, the vertical—direction. In this position the blades slide through the bulbous portion, enter and traverse the membranous portion, and arrive at the prostate. Then, and not before, the operator gradually depresses the instrument towards the patient's thighs; the blades rise up through the prostatic portion into the bladder—a movement which is rendered more easy if a very slight lateral rotary motion is given to the instrument at this part of its progress. In ordinary—that is, normal—conditions the shaft of the lithotrite at the entry into the bladder forms an oblique line, and an angle of about twenty to thirty degrees with the horizon; and this it continues, as it slides easily and freely down upon the trigone to the posterior wall of the viscus. It will be obvious that the urethra now entirely loses its curve, being occupied throughout by the straight shaft of the lithotrite. The jaws being now closed, and lying at the bottom of the cavity, or nearly so, the finding and seizing of the stone have to be achieved. . .

" First, nothing is more important at the onset to remember than this—namely, that quiet and slow movements of the jaws of the lithotrite in searching the bladder are desirable, because rapid movements produce currents in the urine, which keep the stone more or less in motion, so that it is less easily seized than when the surrounding fluid is in a state of rest. . .

" Let it be understood that the blades of the lithotrite have entered the cavity of the bladder, and that the instrument slides easily and smoothly down the trigone, which in the living and healthy organ is an inclined plane, although quite otherwise in the atonied and in the dead bladder. In many cases the instrument in thus passing grazes the stone, and the slightest lateral movement of the blades, right or left, will determine on which side it lies. Whether the stone is felt or not, when the blades have passed gently down in the middle line until a very slight check to their movement is perceived, the lithotrite should rest there for three or four seconds, and then the male blade should be slowly withdrawn, without moving any other part of the instrument, towards the neck of the bladder, until a very slight check is perceived in that direction, followed by another three or four seconds' rest, for currents to subside. Now the operator should quietly press back the male blade, without changing the position of the lithotrite, and almost certainly the stone will be seized. In other words : open ; pause ; close—that is all. It is necessary always to remember, when withdrawing the male blade, that it is never to be drawn out roughly, since in this action the sensitive neck of the bladder may easily be irritated.

"But if no stone is thus found, the operator again withdraws the male blade as before, but inclining to the right side about 45°, and closes without disturbing the central position of the instrument ; if nothing is felt, he turns to the left in like manner, and closes. It is often right to open the blades before turning, for this reason : if the turn is first made and the blades are subsequently opened, the male blade as it is withdrawn will often move the stone away ; whereas if the blades are inclined while open, the stone, if there, is almost certainly seized. It is not very common for the stone to elude the search thus far ; but if it does, depress the handle of the lithotrite an inch or so, an act which raises the blades slightly from the floor of the bladder, and turn them another 45° to the left—bringing, in fact, the blades horizontal to the left ; close ; if unsuccessful, turn them gently to the horizontal on the right, and close. In all these movements, if properly executed, there has been barely contact of the lithotrite with the vesical walls : at all events no pressure, nothing to occasion injury to the bladder. But if there is an enlarged prostate, causing an eminence at the neck of the bladder, or the stone is very small, or we are exploring for some fragment suspected to be present, the blades are to be reversed so as to point downwards to the floor, and the object sought may then often be

secured with ease. It
ments, we may empl
can therefore be rev
long blades.

"In order to do th
depressed another inc
so that the shaft of th
little upwards, is level
blades, being still clos
reversed position, an
manner of a sound in
carefully opened and
varied directions, bu
bladder; after which
ought to have been
when the prostate is
fragments have to be
be reversed without d

"As a rule, all the
beyond the centre of
operating, without hu
partakes of the natu
common cause of fail
close proximity to
position is given to
being drawn up agai
In these circumstance
stone, without suspe
withdraws the blade,
to seize it when he cl
it is essential to drav
the neck of the bladd
neck and the stone w

"The rules alread
more or less to lithol
rule may be borne in
trite—that is, the la
readily are we to add
and the more fluid is
large and fenestrated

of breaking up a large stone into fragments, it is obvious also
that there is less occasion for the horizontal and reversed
movements, since a large stone may almost certainly be seized
by the right or left incline.

" Now, supposing that a hard stone of an inch and a half in
diameter has fallen into the grasp of a powerful lithotrite, the
screw is to be gradually turned at first, to make the blades
bite, since a sharp turn at this moment may drive the stone
out either right or left. As the power is increased, the resistance
is felt to relax, sometimes by degrees, sometimes suddenly with
a crack, and the stone is broken—usually into four or five large
pieces, besides some small *débris*. This done, the male blade
is again drawn out, taking care not to shift the situation or
alter the axis of the lithotrite, and, almost certainly, one of
the large fragments will be picked up.   It is then only necessary to screw home, release the screw, and open as before.
This process may be repeated several times at the same spot,
for the area within which the larger fragments fall is very
limited, and is unchanged if all remains quiet. . . .

" Having now broken up the stone, and crushed well
the largest fragments, and thus occupied perhaps from ten
to fifteen minutes, it should be time to employ the
aspirator and remove a good quantity of *débris*.   Accordingly, the screw of the lithotrite is driven well home,
to close the blades, between which some calculous matter
probably is engaged, and the lithotrite is withdrawn.
An evacuating catheter of the size known to be necessary—
No. 15 or 16 amply suffices for small stones ; No. 17 or 18
may be employed for larger ones, if the urethra fairly admits
it—is then introduced, and all the urine withdrawn. An
aspirator previously filled (with a warm boracic solution) is
then attached, the connection-tap opened, and a small portion
of its contents pressed by the right hand into the bladder, the
left hand supporting and directing the evacuating catheter.
On relaxing the pressure, an immediate current outward
follows, carrying with it very probably a fair quantity of
débris. Wait some three or four seconds after expansion has
finished, and the current apparently ceased, as at that precise

perhaps by too rapidly resuming the pressure. This process is repeated several times, according to the amount of *débris* observed to enter the trap.

"If the patient is breathing heavily under the influence of ether, it is desirable to inject during the act of his expiration, and let the fluid flow outwards into the aspirator during his inspiration, which act assists the evacuation of the bladder.

"After a large crushing, the end of the evacuating catheter should not rest on the floor of the bladder, as it is then likely to be choked with *debris*. But after most of the fragments have been removed, it is advantageous to lower the end of the catheter, in order to catch the last fragments.

"If the outflow of the current is felt to be suddenly checked, and the aspirator ceases to distend, the operator may be almost certain that a fragment of a rounded or cubical form, or a small calculus, nearly fitting the interior of the catheter, blocks the passage and prevents further egress. The piece must be expelled by making smart pressure on the india-rubber bottle, after which the action of the aspirator will probably be resumed.

"If after crushing all the stone, so far as the operator is able to judge, and removing the *débris* largely, nothing is heard or felt in contact with the end of the evacuating catheters, notwithstanding that three or four successive pressures have been made, there is ground for believing that all the fragments may now have been removed. Perhaps there can be no better proof that the bladder has been emptied than is afforded by the fact that a succession of outward and inward currents through the aspirator shows no sign, either to the eye or to the ear, of the presence of another fragment.

"It may be added here that evacuating catheters of different patterns should be within reach. The curve, the situation of the opening, may vary advantageously in different cases; the latter may be either terminal or lateral.

"If all has not been removed, the sound of a large piece perhaps making itself heard and felt at each outward current against the end of the catheter indicates that this must be withdrawn, and a lithotrite introduced. If the fragments are not of considerable size, a lighter and handier lithotrite may succeed with advantage to the heavy fenestrated one originally used, and the crushing continued. Of course if more stone remains, the process is repeated once or more."

The following practical observations by Dr. Keyes may find a place here:—As the tube is moved from side to side, and particularly when the curved tube is inverted, the bladder wall often flaps with a sharp click against the eye of the tube, and then flutters spasmodically with dull thuds against the open end of the instrument. When the bladder is empty, the sharp click may be so hard in quality as to resemble the sound given by a fragment of some size.

Should air enter the bladder, it churns up the water, distends the bladder, interferes with the efficient washing-out of the viscus and with the recognition of small fragments. To dislodge the air, the bladder should be fully distended, and then the handle of the tube be fully depressed between the thighs, so that the open end may be raised to the top of the bladder. The evacuator is now worked slowly, the air escapes into the bottle, and, remaining at the top, can be allowed to escape.

Dr. Keyes advises that the last fragment be sought for by auscultation. Water is gently passed to and fro in the bladder, while the operator places his ear directly over the lower part of the abdomen. "The tube is turned in various directions, and the operator listens. The swish of the water as it rushes in and out is heard with startling distinctness, and if the management of the tube be skilful, any fragment of stone lying loose in the bladder is sure, in a short time, to be driven against the metallic tube, and to announce its presence by a characteristic click."

The time occupied by the operation varies. From twenty to forty to seventy minutes will suffice for all ordinary cases. In one instance Bigelow operated continuously for upwards of three hours. The stone weighed 744 grains. The patient did well.

Complications.—As a rule, the bleeding is very trifling. It may, however, be severe, and depend upon damage to the urethra, bladder, or prostate, or be due to the presence of a vesical growth.

Complete clogging of the instrument with *débris* has

occurred. This is only possible with the non-fenestrated lithotrite.

If the blades cannot be cleared, nor the instrument removed, it must be cut down upon from the perineum, and when cleared must be withdrawn. The operation is then completed as a perineal lithotomy.

After-treatment.—The patient must lie in bed. An india-rubber hot-water bottle or a warm fomentation may be applied to the hypogastrium. Some opium may be required.

There may be some urethral fever, or retention of urine from atony of the bladder. Sir Henry Thompson points out that a little subacute cystitis not infrequently appears on the fourth or fifth day. These complications are treated in the usual way. A warm hip bath daily adds greatly to the patient's comfort. The urine ceases to be bloody, as a rule, between the second and the fourth day; and in the majority of cases the patient may be allowed to get up on the seventh day.

According to Dr. Freyer (*Brit. Med. Journ.*, May 9, 1891), the average number of days spent in hospital or under treatment is, in adult males, six; in boys, five and a half; and in females, four.

Results of Litholapaxy.—Sir Henry Thompson's cases of lithotrity since 1878 number 378, including 325 treated at one sitting. The mortality is a little over $3\frac{1}{2}$ per cent. (*Med.-Chir. Trans.*, 1890).

Dr. Keyes has reported a splendid series of 108 cases of litholapaxy in males above puberty, with a mortality of only 3·7 per cent. (*Lancet*, February 28th, 1885).

He has since reported (*Brit. Med. Journ.*, December 24th, 1887) 77 cases of litholapaxy without a death.

Dr. Keegan, in 160 operations upon male children, had a mortality of only 4·37 per cent. (*Lancet*, October 4th, 1890).

Dr. Freyer reports (*loc. cit.*) 342 litholapaxies—221 in male adults, 5 in female adults, 115 in male children, 1 in a female child. Out of this large number there are only four deaths.

Mr. Cadge has expressed his belief that the relapses after simple lithotrity reach to nearly 20 per cent., if the cases of phosphatic deposits and concretions common after this operation are included among the examples of recurrence of the stone. Litholapaxy is attended with no such proportion of unsatisfactory results; and, indeed, if the evacuator be carefully and thoroughly employed, the relapses after litholapaxy will probably include few cases of recurrence due to the actual retention and subsequent increase of a fragment.

LITHOLAPAXY IN MALE CHILDREN.

Lithotrity and litholapaxy have been condemned as unsuited for the treatment of stone in male children upon the following grounds :—(1) The smallness of the bladder ; (2) the delicate character of the mucous membrane of the bladder and urethra, rendering it liable to laceration ; (3) the small calibre of the urethra ; and (4) the great success of lithotomy operations in children.

Dr. Keegan (*Indian Medical Gazette*, June and September, 1885) was the first to systematically demonstrate the fallacy of these objections, and in his hands it very soon became evident that litholapaxy offered an excellent means of treating stone in children.

(1) The bladder of a child, even if only two or three years of age, is large enough to allow of the manipulation of suitable lithotrites and evacuators. In Dr. Keegan's lists of cases will be found several successful instances of litholapaxy in children of three, two and a half, and two years of age. One child's age is given as one year and three-quarters. The stone weighed eighteen grains, and the child left the hospital in four days.

(2) The mucous membrane is certainly delicate, but it is exposed to no especial risk of laceration if due care be employed. Dr. Keegan very properly insists that no one should attempt to perform litholapaxy in boys until he has first gained some experience of the operation in male adults.

(3) The urethra in male children is of much greater calibre than was supposed. The meatus is often very small, and has to be incised. Dr. Keegan states that the urethra of a boy from three to six will admit a No. 7 or No. 8 lithotrite (English), and that of a boy from eight to ten will admit a No. 10, No. 11, or possibly even a No. 14

Dr. Freyer has passed a No. 6 instrument with ease in a male child aged nine months.

(4) Dr. Keegan (*Lancet*, October 4, 1890) has performed since December, 1881, 160 litholapaxies in male children, with a mortality of 4·3 per cent. This represents seven deaths, in four of which there was extensive organic disease of the kidneys.

In the actual performance of the operation the following points need special note:—

(a) The lithotrite must be completely fenestrated. For litholapaxy in boys Dr. Keegan advises a set of fenestrated lithotrites, running from No. 6 to No. 10. He states that with a No. 8 lithotrite and a No. 8 evacuating catheter it is quite possible to dispose of a mulberry calculus, weighing between 200 and 300 grains, in an hour's time.

(b) The evacuating catheter should be provided with a stylet, so that any fragment lodged in the eye may be displaced.

(c) The stone must be very thoroughly crushed, since the small size of the catheter will only allow comparatively fine fragments to pass. It is well that the first crushing should be as complete as possible, in order to avoid the unduly frequent passage of instruments.

The results of the operation in children are alluded to in the previous section (page 602).

THE OLD OPERATION OF LITHOTRITY.

No anæsthetic is required, and no assistant. The lithotrite is used precisely in the manner already described. At the first sitting the stone may be taken up and crushed some four or five times.

The sitting is repeated in a few days. The number of sittings required will vary; from three to six is the average. Cadge mentions cases requiring seventeen and twenty sittings.

The length of the sitting must depend upon the patient's endurance. Three minutes has been considered a reasonable limit.

After each sitting the patient should lie in bed until the irritation of the bladder or the mild cystitis induced has passed off. The general treatment after the operation would be that

f irritable bladder. He should pass his water lying upon the
back, or while rolled over upon the side, for at least twenty-
our hours.

The diet must be simple and non-stimulating. At the
and of forty-eight hours the patient would probably be able to
get up. Possibly a week's rest may be required between the
irst and the second crushing; but after that, sitting would
follow sitting at intervals of about three or four days.

Allusion has been already made to the frequency of rocur-
rence after lithotrity by the old method (page 602).

CHAPTER V.

THE TREATMENT OF STONE IN WOMEN.

1. In the case of quite small stones the urethra may be dilated, and the stone removed by suitable forceps.

The dilatation of the urethra is best accomplished by Hegar's uterine dilators while the patient is in lithotomy position and under an anaesthetic. The canal can soon be sufficiently dilated to admit the forefinger, the amount of laceration is reduced to a minimum, and the subsequent incontinence is of short duration. The process of dilatation should be slowly carried out, and each dilator be introduced gently.

2. In the case of larger stones, which could not be removed by the above method, the urethra should be dilated by Hegar's dilators until the canal will admit the forefinger: a lithotrite is then introduced, and the stone crushed at one sitting, the fragments being removed by a large evacuating catheter.

The comparative large size to which the urethra may be dilated renders the operation of litholapaxy simple and efficacious. The pelvis should be well raised while the lithotrite is being used.

By this method stones up to the weight of one and a half or two ounces may be dealt with.

3. The largest vesical calculi—those weighing three or more ounces—should be dealt with by suprapubic lithotomy.

In no operation upon the adult female for the removal of stone is it necessary to incise the neck of the bladder.

Vaginal lithotomy is probably now an operation of the past. It is a simple measure, and one attended by a low immediate mortality, but in a large proportion of the cases—especially when large stones have been dealt with—a vesicovaginal fistula has followed.

The operation has been replaced by litholapaxy and supra-pubic lithotomy.

The actual procedure involved in vaginal lithotomy is very simple. The patient is placed in lithotomy position, and the thighs are separated by a Clover's crutch. The posterior wall of the vagina is retracted, and the anterior wall well exposed by means of a duck-bill speculum. A short, straight, grooved staff or director is passed into the bladder, and is pressed downwards, so that the grooved surface can be felt through the anterior vaginal wall.

The surgeon cuts down upon the staff with a sharp-pointed bistoury. The incision will be from half an inch to two inches, will be precisely in the median line, and will be commenced behind the neck of the bladder. This part of the viscus should never be included in the cut. The stone is removed by means of the finger, a suitable scoop or hook, or by lithotomy forceps.

If the bladder be healthy, and the wound have not been contused, the vesical incision may be closed, as in a case of vesico-vaginal fistula.

If the bladder be unhealthy, or if much difficulty have attended the extraction of the stone, then the wound should be left open.

In any case, before the operation is completed the bladder should be thoroughly washed out with a warm boracic solution, which, entering through the urethra, will escape by the vaginal wound.

If the wound remain open, the case must be treated as one of vesico-vaginal fistula.

A valuable paper by Mr. Walsham upon the treatment of vesical calculus in female children will be found in the eleventh volume of the *St. Bartholomew's Hospital Reports.*

CHAPTER VI.

CYSTOTOMY.

THIS term does not involve a special operation. It is conveniently employed in connection with cases in which the bladder is opened for other reasons than the removal of a calculus, the excision of a growth, or the elimination of a projecting lobe of the prostate.

Cystotomy, in the residual sense in which it is here employed, is carried out in certain cases of cystitis and of irritable bladder, and for the purpose of dealing with certain ulcers of the bladder—notably the tubercular—by means of scraping.

The organ may be opened by (1) the suprapubic incision (page 585); (2) the lateral perineal incision (page 564); (3) the median perineal incision (page 576); and (4) by external urethrotomy (page 625). The last two are the methods usually employed; and when drainage of the organ only is called for, the simple urethrotomy will usually suffice.

When it is desirable to thoroughly explore the bladder, or when it is intended to treat an ulcerated surface by scraping, the suprapubic method is made use of. A speculum may be used to keep open the incision in the bladder (page 614), and a small electric lamp in a convenient handle will be found of great service.

The scraping of the ulcer is conducted in the same manner as is observed in dealing with like ulcers elsewhere. A Volkmann's spoon with a long shaft is employed. The ulcer may be brought conveniently into view by means of two fingers introduced into the rectum. In some cases the rectal bag may be of service.

After the bleeding has ceased, the scraped surface may be rubbed with a little iodoform.

The lateral perineal operation is seldom called for, and when drainage of the organ only is required—and these represent the majority of the cases—the simple median incision answers admirably. The staff is passed, the prostatic urethra is divided, and probably, without further manipulation, a tube

t once introduced into the bladder, and the operation
>mpleted. To this simple operation the term external
hrotomy is commonly applied. The term includes also
more serious operations which are carried out when
atractable or complicated stricture exists. (*See* page 625.)

CHAPTER VII.

REMOVAL OF TUMOURS OF THE BLADDER.

WITHIN recent years certain cases of vesical tumour have been very successfully dealt with by operation, and many have been followed by complete cure. In instances in which the operation has been of necessity incomplete, or in which a rapid recurrence of the growth has supervened, considerable relief has usually been given to the patient, and the more distressing symptoms have been got rid of.

The method of treating vesical growths by deliberate operation was prominently brought before the notice of surgeons by Sir Henry Thompson, who in 1883 published an account of twelve cases so treated (*Med.-Chir. Trans.*, vol. lxvi., page 349).

Various methods of reaching the tumour may be employed:—(1) By median perineal cystotomy ; (2) by lateral perineal cystotomy ; (3) by suprapubic cystotomy ; (4) by suprapubic cystotomy associated with a median or lateral perineal incision.

When the growth is single, of small size, and situated near to the neck of the bladder, the viscus may be opened by the median perineal incision.

When the tumour is large or the growths numerous, when it is suspected that the trouble is malignant in character, when the perineum is deep, or the prostate unduly large, the suprapubic method should be followed. This procedure should also be carried out in all cases of recurrent growth.

The perineal operation is of limited application, the access to the bladder is through a narrow strait, the manipulations necessary for the removal of the growth must needs be restricted, and no actual inspection of the part is permitted.

The suprapubic operation, on the other hand, allows of a free exposure and a ready inspection of the growth, and permits the necessary manipulations to be carried out with ease. It is the more complete and satisfactory method, and the one applicable to the larger series of cases.

Lateral perineal cystotomy is advised by those who consider that the bladder should be reached through the perineum, and that the median incision does not supply sufficient room.

Combined suprapubic and perineal incisions have been effected in many cases. In some of these an attempt to remove the growth through the perineum had failed; in others it was

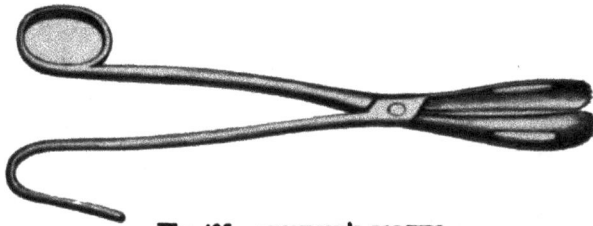

Fig. 405.—THOMPSON'S FORCEPS.

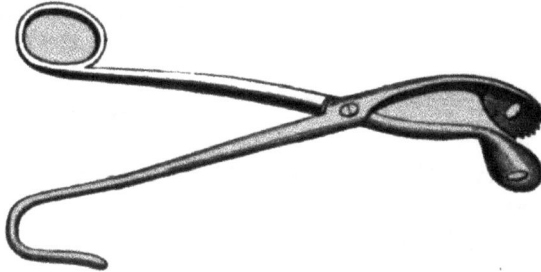

Fig. 406.—THOMPSON'S FORCEPS.

considered desirable to drain the bladder through the perineum; and in a third series of cases the surgeon's manipulations through the suprapubic wound were aided by a finger or forceps introduced into the bladder from the perineum.

Increased experience has not encouraged the development of the combined incisions.

Two operations will be described; viz., the median perineal and the suprapubic.

1. **By the Median Perineal Method.**—This is the operation advised and carried out by Sir Henry Thompson.

Certain special forceps are required. The more useful patterns are shown in Figs. 405 and 406.

n n 2

A blunt gorget may be of service.

The patient is placed in lithotomy position, and the bladder is then opened precisely in the manner described in the chapter on Median Lithotomy (page 576). The finger is introduced into the bladder, and the exact size, situation, consistence, and outline of the tumour are ascertained.

A director is employed, as in the operation for stone. In the place of lithotomy forceps the surgeon introduces the special instruments for dealing with the growth.

The following is Sir Henry Thompson's account :—

"If the surgeon finds a polypoid growth, he should introduce a pair of forceps into the cavity of the bladder, and use them without aid from the finger. The forceps should have wide and serrated margins where the blades meet, so as to crush, but without power to cut, the tissues seized, and should be provided in different forms. The simplest should be like an ordinary lithotomy forceps (Fig. 405). Others

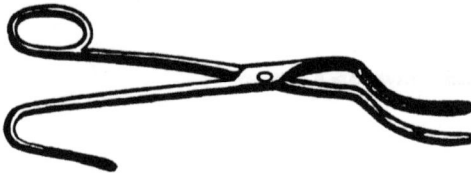

Fig. 407.—THOMPSON'S FORCEPS.

should be curved (Figs. 406 and 407), for seizing tumours which are situated laterally, and near to the neck of the bladder, in which last-named position the forceps is powerless to grasp the tumour. When the blades are free, if they are opened easily and widely, the polypus is almost sure to be within their grasp. No suprapubic pressure, as a rule, should be made during this act, so as to disturb the contour of the bladder. He should never drag or pull forcibly, but rather 'bite' off the growth with the blades, twisting it somewhat, perhaps. After this the finger alone may often remove it safely. Every time the forceps has removed a portion, the finger should examine the interior before the forceps is introduced again. · And in no case where the tumour is a flattened growth with broad base should an attempt be made to separate it very near to the walls of the bladder, which might thus be fatally injured."
The writer warns the surgeon against strong suprapubic pressure during the operation. He points out that such

pressure forces the upper wall of the bladder into the cavity of the viscus, and causes the growth to appear more prominent and larger in contour than is in reality the case. If a growth thus distorted be seized, a double fold of the bladder wall may be picked up at the same time and crushed between the blades of the forceps.

" To avoid such a catastrophe it is only necessary, first, to decline the attempt to destroy any growth which is clearly not sufficiently salient to admit of complete, or nearly complete, removal; and secondly, never to employ the forceps while forcible suprapubic pressure is made—at least, no more pressure than is desirable just to steady and support the bladder and the parts adjacent."

In some cases the surgeon's manipulations may be assisted by employing a blunt probe-pointed gorget (Fig. 409).

In certain instances the growth may be scraped away by means of a suitable spoon or curette, or the special instrument devised by Sir Henry Thompson for de-taching vesical growths may be employed (Fig. 408).

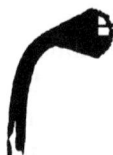

Fig. 408.

In other cases the detachment of the growth may be accomplished by one of the various forms of loop devised by Mr. Berkeley Hill and others. These loops are also of use in removing portions of the growth that have been already detached.

It has been possible by dragging upon a firm polypoid tumour to bring its pedicle within easy reach of the fingers, and in women such a manipulation of the growth can fre-quently be effected through the dilated urethra.

After the tumour has been dealt with, the bladder is washed out, and the case is treated upon the same lines as a case of perineal lithotomy. It is seldom necessary to introduce a tube. Bleeding may be checked by pressure of the finger upon the spot from which the growth was removed, or by the injection of cold water.

2. **By the Suprapubic Method.**—The precise method of opening the bladder has been described in the chapter on Suprapubic Lithotomy.

As soon as the bladder has been opened, means such as those already mentioned (page 587) must be employed to secure the margins of the vesical wound.

Various specula have been invented for the purpose of keeping the opening in the bladder sufficiently patent to allow of a view of the interior being obtained. The speculum devised by Dr. Watson, of Boston, and described in the *Lancet* for October 18. 1890, is an ingenious instrument. In its general features it somewhat resembles an eye speculum. The blades are of strong wire, and are readily introduced. They can be accurately adjusted. and are self-retaining. They serve to separate and fix the margins of both the vesical and the abdominal wounds.

The speculum, being two-bladed, fails, however. to keep back the posterior wall of the bladder, and the same may be said of the two-bladed speculum of Keen's.

The most serviceable instrument of this class is the three-bladed speculum invented by Mr. Bruce Clarke, and described in the *British Medical Journal* for July 4. 1891.

The growth, when exposed and carefully examined by the finger, and also by inspection, may be dealt with in the same manner as like growths in more accessible parts would be treated. A small electric lamp is of considerable service. Growths with slender pedicles may be pinched or twisted off. If the pedicle be stouter, it may be grasped and fixed close to the bladder wall by means of a pair of pressure forceps bent at a suitable angle. The neck is then grasped by a straight pair of pressure forceps at a little distance from the first pair, and is twisted off by rotating the instrument last introduced.

In other instances an écraseur, carrying a fine cord or a fine cold wire, may be employed.

If the growth have a broader base. it may, if it be well defined, be transfixed close to the bladder wall by means of a rectangular needle in a handle, and be then ligatured with silk in two segments.

Some of the softer and more diffused growths can be scraped away with the finger-nail, or with a curette or sharp spoon.

Others, of greater substance. can be removed piecemeal with Thompson's forceps. and the resulting stump then well scraped with Volkmann's spoon. This is the method which would be applied to epitheliomatous growths.

After the removal of extensive growths the bladder may be well rubbed out with a Turkey sponge, which will remove all detached or partly-detached fragments.

Bleeding may be checked by the pressure of a firm piece of sponge, or by cold injections. The cases must be few in which an appeal to the actual cautery is necessary. The pressure of the rectal bag causes venous engorgement, and the sooner that appliance can be dispensed with the better. Two fingers introduced into the rectum by an assistant will often bring the growth more readily into view than will the rectal bag.

The after-treatment of the case is the same as is observed after suprapubic lithotomy.

Growths of the Female Bladder can, in the great majority of instances, be dealt with through the urethra. The urethra is most conveniently dilated by means of Hegar's uterine dilators. The process is a little slow, but it is satisfactory, and leads to the minimum amount of laceration of the part. The finger can be introduced, and the growth examined.

Pedunculated tumours have been dragged sufficiently far forwards to enable a ligature or the loop of an écraseur to be applied to their pedicles.

Other tumours may be torn or bitten off with forceps, while the softer and more diffused growths may be scraped.

Larger and multiple vesical tumours are better dealt with through a suprapubic incision.

The results of operations for the removal of vesical growths may be said to be on the whole distinctly satisfactory. The period has not yet been reached when any substantial value can attach to the publication of statistics.

Dr. Stein's table, published in 1885, gave the general mortality of all operations for vesical growths as 39·8. Since 1885 the aspect of the operation has been much altered, and the mortality has been greatly reduced.

It may be said that while a certain number of cases are entirely cured, a large number show a recurrence of the growth, but that even in the worst cases the operation affords the patient very substantial relief and prolongs life.

Resection of Portions of the Bladder.—This operation has been performed in some four cases of malignant disease, but the results have at present not been sufficiently good to give the procedure a definite place in surgery. Mr. Gilbert Barling has given an excellent *résumé* of the operations performed up to the present time, in an article published in the *Birmingham Medical Review* for March, 1890.

The operation of resection of the bladder is still in the experimental stage.

CHAPTER VIII.

OPERATIONS ON ENLARGED PROSTATE.

THESE operations, which are sometimes known by the questionable title of "prostatectomy," are carried out in cases of hypertrophy of the prostate, to effect the following objects:—1. To drain the bladder for a time, and to give the organ complete rest. 2. To remove the obstructing portion of the prostate, and to restore to the patient, when the wound has healed, the power of normal micturition.

Perineal drainage—i.e., the drainage of the bladder through a wound made in the perineum—has long been employed as a means of affording relief in prostatic cases. By such drainage the more urgent and distressing symptoms are assuaged, but the relief continues only so long as the urinary fistula is maintained. The obstruction is untouched; and if the wound be allowed to close, the patient's symptoms will, after a varying period, return.

The operations about to be described aim at more than temporary relief, and have for their object a permanent cure of the condition.

McGill points out that the severity of the symptoms in a case of hypertrophy of the prostate bears little or no relation to the apparent size of the gland as felt through the rectum. He points out also that probably only about fifty per cent. of the subjects of hypertrophied prostate suffer from urinary symptoms. The symptoms when present depend upon the extent of the intra-vesical growth. McGill describes the following varieties of the intra-vesical growth:—(1) A projecting middle lobe, pedunculated or sessile. (2) A middle lobe, with lateral lobes forming three distinct projections. (3) The lateral lobes alone. (4) A pedunculated growth springing from a lateral lobe. (5) A uniform circular projection surrounding the internal orifice of the urethra like a collar.

PROSTATECTOMY.

The intra-vesical part of the enlarged prostate may be reached and removed in one of three ways:—

    A. By perineal incision.

    B. By suprapubic incision (McGill's operation).

    C. By combined perineal and suprapubic incisions.

Attempts to deal with the obstructing mass through the urethra have proved to be entirely unsatisfactory.

A. **By Perineal Incision.**—The bladder is reached and opened by the method described in the chapter on Median Lithotomy (page 576). According to Belfield (*Internat. Journ. of the Med. Sciences*, Nov., 1890), this method has been employed in some thirty cases, and small median tumours ("middle lobes") and lateral lobes have been removed, and the obstruction relieved. The projecting growth has been torn away with the finger or with special forceps. It has been excised by cutting, and has been removed with a curette or sharp spoon.

The operation is not quite satisfactory, since when the prostatic urethra is greatly lengthened, the finger often fails to reach the vesical orifice, and, moreover, the rigidity of the prostate seriously restricts the use of instruments. Dr. Watson, of Boston ("Operative Treatment of Hypertrophied Prostate," 1888), states that in two-thirds of the cases of enlarged prostate needing treatment the intra-vesical growth could be successfully reached and incised, or partially or wholly removed through a perineal incision, "by any one possessing an index-finger which has a working length of three inches or more." In his comment upon this, McGill observes that it is unwise to commence an operation with the probability of failing in one-third of the cases, and that it is undesirable to limit the performance of the operation to gentlemen with preternaturally long fingers.

McGill states further that in only three cases out of twelve upon which he operated (by the suprapubic method) would it have been possible to have removed the obstructing growth through the perineum. As it is impossible to tell beforehand the condition of the intra-vesical projection, it is obvious that the perineal operation must carry with it a great element of uncertainty.

In performing lateral lithotomy, prostatic outgrowths have been met with, and have been removed with the finger. Reginald Harrison describes such a case (*Med.-Chir. Trans.*, 1882, page 39), and alludes to like experiences at the hands of Fergusson, Bickersteth, and others. Prostatectomy by this route does not seem to have ever been deliberately performed. It has been so far an accidental incident in lithotomy.

The general treatment of a case of prostatectomy by a median perineal incision is conducted upon the same lines as a case of perineal lithotomy. (*See* page 573.)

B. **By Suprapubic Incision.**—This very successful operation we owe to McGill, of Leeds.

It has these advantages over the perineal operation:—It allows of a minute and exact exploration of the vesical surface of the prostate, and of the easy and complete removal of the obstructing mass. It is simple and precise. It allows at the same time of complete and most efficient drainage.

The operation of exposing and opening the bladder is carried out in the manner already described in the account of suprapubic lithotomy (page 583).

McGill details the following special points in the *technique* of the operation, and in the method to be adopted in actually removing the obstructing mass (*Lancet*, Feb. 4th, 1888; and " Address at Leeds," August, 1889):—

" 1. The quantity of water injected into the rectal bag, especially in cases where the prostate is abnormally hard, should be smaller than is usually recommended. In one case there was profuse rectal hæmorrhage, only stopped with considerable difficulty. Each case must be decided on its merits, but six or ten ounces are usually sufficient.

" 2. The bladder should be irrigated till the antiseptic solution used is perfectly clear. The quantity left in the bladder varies from ten to twenty or more ounces. The hand placed on the hypogastrium will show when the distension is sufficient.

" 3. In cases where the bladder is contracted, with thick non-distensible walls, it will usually be inadvisable to perform this operation.

" 4. It is better to leave a catheter in the bladder till its cavity is opened, as it is a guide that expedites the operation.

Care must be taken not to hook the peritoneal fold (superior false ligament) into the wound with the point of the instrument.

"5. The linea alba is best divided by incising it immediately above the symphysis, and then dividing upwards on a director.

"6. Care must be taken to secure the bladder before proceeding to remove the prostate. This is best done by inserting two sutures through each lip of the wound, and fastening it securely to the deeper part of the abdominal wall. When the operation is completed, a third suture passed through the lower angle of the wound is an additional security against urinary extravasation into the retro-pubic space.

"7. A pedunculated middle lobe can be removed with ease, its pedicle being divided with curved scissors. A sessile middle lobe can be removed in the same way, helping the scissors by tearing with forceps. The collar enlargement is removed with greater difficulty. It is advisable to **divide it** longitudinally, by inserting one blade of the scissors into the urethral opening and dividing the portion above, and then passing the other blade into the same opening and dividing the portion below. That part of the gland which projects into the bladder is now divided into two lateral halves; these can be removed separately by scissors curved on the flat, or enucleated with the tip of the forefinger. Care must be taken not to leave any portion of the projecting valve untouched.

"The prostate should be removed as far as possible by enucleation with the finger, and not by cutting. The mucous membrane over the projecting portion having been snipped through, the rest of the operation is completed with finger and forceps. In this way excessive hæmorrhage is prevented. Hæmorrhage is best arrested by irrigation with water so hot as to make it unpleasant for the hand.

"When the operation is complete, whichever form of growth has been removed, it is advisable to see that the urethra is patent, and to pass the forefinger as far as the first joint into its canal.

"8. A large tube should be inserted into the bladder, and the wound united above the tube by a deep and superficial row of sutures. The tube is to be removed in forty-eight hours.

" 9. The after-treatment consists in keeping the parts clean, and washing the bladder and the wound—in exceptional cases—with a boracic solution."

The masses of prostatic tissue removed by this operation are described in McGill's tables as the size of " a bean," " a filbert," " a large walnut," " a cricket-ball." One tumour was removed in seven pieces. Dr. William White, of Philadelphia, removed in one case a mass weighing three ounces. In several instances the substance removed has weighed over two ounces.

c. **By Combined Perineal and Suprapubic Incisions.**— This method is advocated by Dr. Belfield, who points out that the urethra may be distorted by growths both imperceptible and inaccessible from the bladder. Especially frequent is a great thickening of the sub-urethral prostate, whereby the vesical orifice is displaced upwards.

In many reported cases the suprapubic operation has not been entirely successful, owing to the fact that the prostatic urethra was left still obstructed.

In any case, therefore, in which it is not made evident that the urethral canal is entirely patent, the suprapubic operation may be supplemented by a median perineal urethrotomy. Through this wound the urethra can be explored, the prostatic part of the canal well stretched, and any growths in that part of the tube more conveniently dealt with.

Results.—Dr. Belfield gives the mortality of prostatectomy as thirteen per cent., that of the perineal operation as nine per cent., and of the suprapubic as sixteen per cent. He gives the following table :—

	Cases.	Restoration of Voluntary Urination.		Deaths.
		Successes.	Failures.	
By perineal incision ...	41	17	7	4
By suprapubic incision ...	88	29	12	12
By combined incisions ...	4	3	0	1
Totals ...	133	49	19	17

The discrepancy in the totals in the second and third columns depends upon the fact that in estimating the result of the operation the author has omitted all cases in which the history after the operation is imperfect.

CHAPTER IX.

RUPTURE OF THE BLADDER.

THE treatment of rupture of the bladder by operation is of quite recent date. The most valuable contribution to this branch of surgery is afforded by Sir William MacCormac's paper, published in the *Lancet* for December 11th, 1886, and containing an account of two successful cures.

Benjamin Bell suggested suture of the bladder for rupture in 1789; and in later times Grandchamps, Gross, Cusack, and Holmes advocated the same measure. The first operations in England were performed by Heath (*Med.-Chir. Trans.*, vol. lxii.) and Willett (*St. Bartholomew's Hospital Reports*, vol. xii.), but in both instances without success.

MacCormac's first operation was performed on September 22nd, 1885.

Norton has collected twenty-seven examples of the operation. Of this number, ten recovered and seventeen died—a mortality of 62·9 per cent.

Operation.—An incision is made in the median line, immediately above the pubes, and the abdomen is opened in the usual way. The incision must be free, and in MacCormac's cases was six inches in length. Blood-stained urine and serum will probably escape as soon as the peritoneal cavity is opened. The depths of the wound should be exposed as well as is possible by means of strong rectangular retractors, and assistance may be obtained from a small electric lamp.

The posterior surface of the bladder is well exposed. The intestines are pushed upwards, and are kept out of the way by means of suitable sponges.

Search is made for the rent, which will most usually be found upon the posterior surface, midway between the summit and the base of the viscus. If a catheter has been already

introduced, it will be felt through the rupture. If the rent be
low down in the bladder, some assistance may be derived from
the use of the rectal bag, which will probably bring the parts
better into view. In one case MacCormac divided the parietal
peritoneum transversely on either side of the bladder, and
then found that the organ could be brought further towards
the surface wound.

The parts having been well cleaned with a sponge, the
sutures are at once introduced. The sutures should be inserted by Lembert's method. The best suture material is fine
carbolised silk, and each stitch is introduced by means of a
curved needle, held in a needle-holder. The sutures must be
applied closely. About four to the inch will suffice. In one
of MacCormac's cases the rent measured four inches, and required sixteen sutures; in the other case the wound was two
inches long, and twelve sutures were applied. The threads
should include only the serous and muscular coats, and must
on no account involve the mucous membrane. In tying the
sutures, care must be taken that the edges of the wound are
so inverted as to bring the two serous surfaces in even contact.
It is well to begin the closure of the rent at its lowest point.
The margins of the rent may perhaps be steadied by means
of a blunt hook introduced into one end of the fissure.
MacCormac advises that the sutures should be continued for
some little way beyond the angles of the wound, in order to
add to the length of infolded tissue, and to strengthen the
suture line.

When all the sutures have been tied, a warm boracic
solution should be injected into the bladder, in order to test
the soundness of the seam. Any weak or suspicious spot in
the suture line should be strengthened by the insertion of
additional sutures.

The peritoneal cavity, and especially the pelvis, must now
be thoroughly flushed out. (*See* page 231.) Care must be
taken that no sponges are left behind.

The parietal wound is then closed with sutures in the
usual way.

If the rent in the bladder has been securely closed,
and if the peritoneal cavity has been well flushed out, there is
no need to employ a drainage-tube in the parietal wound.

There is also no need to drain the bladder, either by a perineal incision or by a retained catheter. MacCormac advises that the bladder should be left alone. If the patient cannot readily pass water, a soft catheter may be used as often as is required.

CHAPTER X.

Urethrotomy.

EXTERNAL URETHROTOMY.

The operations known by this name include several methods of opening the urethra by an incision in the perineum.

They are carried out in certain cases of stricture of the urethra which have resisted other methods of treatment, and which are, for one reason or another, unsuited for less severe surgical measures.

The following are the operations described :—

1. *Syme's Operation.*—In this operation a staff can be passed through the obstruction, and upon it the stricture is divided.

2. *Gouley's Operation.*—In this method a small conductor is passed through the stricture, and, guided by this, the stricture is divided, and a catheter conducted into the bladder. This operation is applicable to cases in which a Syme's staff could not be passed.

3. *Wheelhouse's Operation.*—Here the urethra is opened upon the distal side of the stricture. The orifice of the narrowed canal is exposed, a director is passed into it, and guided by this instrument the stricture is divided.

4. *Cock's Operation,* or *Perineal Section.*—In this procedure the urethra is opened behind the stricture, and just in front of the prostate. No staff or artificial guide of any kind is used. The operation is applied to cases in which the urethra is practically impermeable.

The term external urethrotomy is also employed in connection with the opening of the normal urethra through the perineum, for the purpose of draining the bladder.

This measure is alluded to on page 608. It consists merely in opening the urethra immediately in front of the prostate

s s

by cutting upon a staff. After the incision is completed, the staff is withdrawn, and a perineal tube is passed into the bladder.

The general details of this simple operation are considered in the chapter on Median Lithotomy (page 576).

1. **Syme's Operation.**

Instruments required.—Syme's staff. (This instrument has a narrow terminal part, which is passed through the stricture. Where this part joins the rest of the staff, there is a "shoulder," which rests against the distal surface of the stricture. The narrow segment is grooved, and the groove is continued on to the shoulder.) Manacles or Clover's crutch; scalpel; probe; director; Teale's probe gorget (Fig. 409); perineal tube; catheter.

The Operation.—The patient is placed in lithotomy position, and the staff is introduced with the care already advised in that operation (page 563). An incision is made precisely in the median line of the perineum, and the knife is so directed that its point shall hit the shoulder of the instrument. The

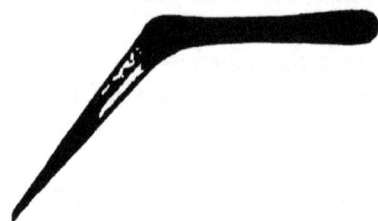

Fig. 409.—TEALE'S PROBE GORGET.

surgeon must convince himself that this portion of the staff is laid bare. He then engages the point of the knife in the groove of the staff, and, keeping most carefully to the groove, thrusts the knife towards the neck of the bladder until he has divided the whole of the stricture. A director or probe, or Teale's probe gorget, is now introduced along the convexity of the staff into the bladder, and the staff is removed. A gum-elastic catheter may then be passed into the bladder through the penis, and be guided into position by the director or probe gorget, aided by the finger inserted into the wound.

Should the irritability of the bladder prevent the retention of a catheter, a tube should be passed into the bladder from the perineum, and should be retained in position by tapes. (*See* pages 562 and 568.)

Syme's curved perineal catheter may be employed for this purpose, or a portion of a gum-elastic catheter be made use of.

Whitehead's perineal tube, with sliding adjustable shield, is a useful instrument.

As soon as possible, however, a catheter should be passed by the meatus, and the perineal wound allowed to close.

2. Gouley's Operation.

This operation was described in the *New York Medical Journal* for August, 1869.

Instruments required.—Manacles or Clover's crutch; Gouley's catheter staff (Fig. 410, A); flexible bougie; capillary whalebone bougies; Gouley's beaked bistoury (Fig. 410, B); scalpel; curved needles and needle-holders.

The Operation.—The exact seat of the stricture having been ascertained, the urethra is filled with olive oil, and a capillary probe-pointed whalebone bougie is introduced into the canal,

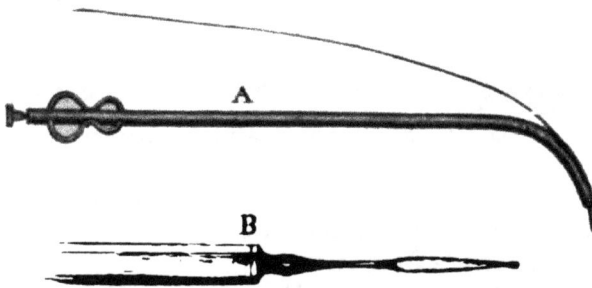

Fig. 410.—A, GOULEY'S CATHETER STAFF; B, GOULEY'S BEAKED BISTOURY.

an attempt being made to pass it through the stricture. If it enters a false passage, it is retained *in situ* by the left hand, while another is passed by its side. If this second guide finds its way into a false passage, it is treated precisely as was the first, and the operation is repeated until one bougie has been passed through the obstruction into the bladder. The other guides—often five or six in number—are then withdrawn.

The next step is to introduce a No. 8 grooved metallic catheter staff (Fig. 410, A), with a quarter of an inch of its extremity bridged over, so as to convert the groove into a canal, the bridged portion itself being also grooved. Its introduction is accomplished by passing the tunnelled point over the free end of the retained guide, then holding the latter steadily between the thumb and index-finger of the left hand, and pushing the catheter staff gently into the urethra until its point comes in contact with the face of the stricture.

The staff and guide are then kept in position by an assistant, who supports the scrotum, and the patient is brought into the lithotomy position.

The surgeon makes a free incision in the median line of the perineum, and brings into view the urethra, which is opened upon the bridged portion of the staff, the knife following the groove on the instrument. A loop of silk is then passed through each edge of the incised urethra, close to the face of the stricture, and serves to enable the canal to be held open by an assistant. The catheter staff is now withdrawn a little, so as to bring into view the black guide; then the stricture, with about half an inch of the uncontracted canal behind it, is divided by means of the beaked bistoury. The last step consists in passing the staff, guided by the whalebone bougie,

Fig. 411.—STAFF FOR WHEELHOUSE'S OPERATION.

into the bladder. The subsequent treatment of the case is conducted upon ordinary principles.

3. Wheelhouse's Operation.

Instruments required. — Manacles or Clover's crutch; Wheelhouse's hooked staff (Fig. 411); two pairs of fine-nibbed forceps; scalpels; catheters; probe; probe-pointed director; Teale's probe gorget (Fig. 409); curved needles; needle-holder; artery and pressure forceps; sponges in holders.

The Operation.—The patient is placed in lithotomy position. " The staff is to be introduced with the groove looking towards the surface, and brought gently into contact with the stricture. It should not be pressed much against the stricture, for fear of tearing the tissues of the urethra and causing it to leave the canal, which would mar the whole after-proceedings, which depend upon the urethra being opened a quarter of an inch in front of the stricture. Whilst an assistant holds the staff in this position, an incision is made into the perineum, extending from opposite the point of reflection of the superficial perineal fascia to the outer edge of the sphincter ani.

The tissues of the perineum are to be steadily divided until the urethra is reached. This is now to be opened in the groove of the staff, not upon its point, so as certainly to secure a quarter of an inch of healthy tube immediately in front of the stricture. As soon as the urethra is opened, and the groove in the staff fully exposed, the edges of the healthy urethra are to be seized on each side with straight-bladed nibbed forceps, and held apart. The staff is then to be gently withdrawn until the button-point appears in the wound. It is then to be turned round, so that the groove may look to the pubes, and the button may be hooked on to the upper angle of the opened urethra, which is then held stretched open at three points, and the operator looks into it immediately in front of the stricture. While thus held open, a probe-pointed director is inserted into the urethra, and the operator, if he cannot see the opening of the stricture—which is often possible —generally succeeds in very quickly finding it, and passes the point onwards through the stricture towards the bladder. The stricture is sometimes hidden amongst a crop of granulations or warty growths, in the midst of which the probe-point easily finds the true passage. The director having been passed into the bladder (its entrance into which is clearly demonstrated by the freedom of its movements), its groove is turned downwards, the whole length of the stricture is carefully and deliberately divided on its under-surface, and the passage is thus cleared. The director is still held in the same position, and a straight probe-pointed bistoury is run along the groove, to ensure complete division of all bands or other obstructions. These being thoroughly cleared, the old difficulty of directing the point of a catheter through the divided stricture and onwards into the bladder is to be overcome. To effect this, the point of a Teale's probe gorget (Fig. 409) is introduced into the groove in the director, and, guided by it, is passed onwards into the bladder, dilating the divided stricture and forming a metallic floor, along which the point of the catheter cannot fail to pass securely into the bladder. The entry of the gorget into the latter viscus is signalised by an immediate gush of urine along it. A silver catheter (No. 10 or 11) is now passed from the meatus down into the wound, is made to pass once or twice through the

divided urethra, where it can be seen in the wound, to render
certain the fact that no obstructing bands have been left
undivided, and is then, guided by the probe-dilator, passed
easily and certainly along the posterior part of the urethra
into the bladder. The gorget is now withdrawn, the catheter
fastened in the urethra, and allowed to remain for three or
four days, an elastic tube conveying the urine away. After
three or four days the catheter is removed, and is then passed
daily, or every second or third day, according to circumstances, until the wound in the perineum is healed; and after
the parts have become consolidated, it requires, of course, to
be passed still from time to time, to prevent re-contraction "
(Wheelhouse, *Brit. Med. Journ.*, June 24th, 1876).

The operation requires a good light and infinite patience.
There is often some difficulty in detecting the orifice of the
stricture, and matters may be complicated by a false passage.

The hooking of the button of the staff on to the upper
angle of the opened urethra is not always of service. The
instrument has to be held by an assistant, and is apt to be in
the way. The margins of the urethral wound may be conveniently held aside by long threads which have been passed
by means of curved needles in holders.

4. Cock's Operation.

This operation consists in opening the urethra behind the
obstruction, and at the apex of the prostate, unassisted by
a guide. It is a modification of the old *boutonnière* operation, is sometimes spoken of as " perineal section," but is more
correctly represented by the title " external urethrotomy without a guide."

Instruments required.—Manacles or Clover's crutch; a
broad double-edged knife with a very sharp point; a probe-
pointed director in a handle (the handle and the shaft of
the instrument should form such an angle as is observed
in Teale's probe gorget); a perineal cannula; a gum-elastic
catheter, to be retained in the bladder through the perineum.

The Operation.—The operation is thus described in the
Guy's Hospital Reports for 1866 :—

"The patient is to be placed in the usual position for
lithotomy; and it is of the utmost importance that the body
and pelvis should be straight, so that the median line may be

accurately preserved. The left forefinger of the operator is then introduced into the rectum; the bearings of the prostate are next examined and ascertained, and the tip of the finger is lodged at the apex of the gland. The knife is then plunged steadily and boldly into the median line of the perineum, and carried on in a direction towards the tip of the left forefinger, which lies in the rectum.

"At the same time, by an upward and downward movement, the vertical incision may be carried in the median line to any extent that is considered desirable. The lower extremity of the wound should come to within half an inch of the anus.

"The knife should never be withdrawn in its progress towards the apex of the prostate, but its onward course must be steadily maintained until its point can be felt in close proximity to the tip of the left forefinger. When the operator has fully assured himself as to the relative position of his finger, the apex of the prostate, and the point of his knife, the latter is to be advanced with a motion somewhat obliquely, either to the right or the left, and it can hardly fail to pierce the urethra. If, in this step of the operation, the anterior extremity of the prostate should be somewhat incised, it is a matter of no consequence.

"In this operation it is of the utmost importance that the knife be not removed from the wound, and that no deviation be made from its original direction until the object is accomplished. If the knife be prematurely removed, it will probably, when re-inserted, make a fresh incision and complicate the desired result. It will be seen that the wound, when completed, represents a triangle; the base being the external vertical incision through the perineum, while the apex, and consequently the point of the knife, impinges on the prostate.

"The knife is now withdrawn, but the left forefinger is still retained in the rectum. The probe-pointed director is carried through the wound, and, guided by the left forefinger, enters the urethra and is passed into the bladder."

Along the groove of the director the cannula or perineal tube is passed into the bladder.

It only remains to secure this drainage-tube in place

by means of two tapes, which are attached to the sides of the tube on the one hand, and to the perineal strips of a T-bandage on the other.

Through the tube the bladder may be washed out. The stricture may now possibly be dealt with by such means as appear advisable. The operation is, however, usually carried out in cases in which the urethra is permanently obstructed or destroyed, in which urinary extravasation has taken place, and in which the perineum is infiltrated with inflammatory exudations, and probably riddled with sinuses.

The perineal opening is, therefore, as a rule, a permanent one; but should the urethra be once more restored to its normal calibre, the artificial opening in the perineum soon heals up.

There is no doubt that this operation may prove to be exceedingly difficult. It needs to be carried out with the utmost patience, care, and precision.

Repeated stabs in the dark may lead to severe bleeding; and if the urethra be not reached at the first or second attempt, the operation had better be abandoned.

INTERNAL URETHROTOMY.

In this method of treatment the stricture is divided by means of an instrument introduced through the urethra. The measure, as an operative one, consists of little more than a knowledge of the mode of manipulating the particular instrument employed.

The instruments used or recommended in internal urethrotomy are legion.

In the American "Armamentarium Chirurgicum" figures are furnished of thirty-six forms of urethrotome, and a great many more instruments are alluded to in the descriptions.

One of the most convenient urethrotomes, and the one which is probably most extensively used in England, is Maisonneuve's. This instrument has been the subject of many modifications; and of these, the modification introduced by Teevan appears to have resulted in the most successful instrument.

The precautions to be taken in performing internal urethrotomy have been well considered by Mr. Southam

(*Lancet,* June 14th, 1890), and the surgeon cannot do better than observe the following directions, which are given in the paper alluded to :—

Operation.—The urethrotome is carefully carbolised. The patient having been anæsthetised, about a drachm of carbolic oil (1 in 16) is injected into the urethra. The urethrotome is inserted, and the constriction is divided in the usual way. The instrument is then withdrawn, and the stricture is afterwards dilated by passing Lister's sounds, 9—12 to 12—15. A full-sized silver catheter is then introduced into the bladder, and the urine having been drawn off, the viscus is thoroughly washed out several times by injecting a saturated solution of warm boracic acid. About two ounces of the solution are left in the bladder, and as the catheter is withdrawn the urethra is also flushed out with the lotion. An iodoform bougie is then passed down the canal as far as the neck of the bladder, so that it may lie in contact with the urethral wall at the seat of division of the stricture. During the operation especial care is taken to protect the patient from exposure to cold ; and in addition to the ordinary precautions, the lower extremities are wrapped up to the hips in thick woollen bandages.

After-treatment.—As soon as the patient recovers from the anæsthetic, ten minims of liquor opii sedativus are given, and the dose is repeated in a few hours if he is at all restless and complains of pain. He is directed to hold his urine for six or eight hours, if possible; at the end of this period, when he is allowed to pass it himself, the urine will generally come in a good stream. For a time micturition is attended by more or less pain and smarting, and in most cases the urine will be slightly stained with blood for the first day or two after the operation. On the fourth morning, either a cocaine bougie or a drachm of a ten per cent. solution of cocaine is introduced into the urethra, and after an interval of ten or fifteen minutes Lister's sounds, 9—12 to 12—15, well carbolised, are passed through the stricture. By means of the cocaine the pain which usually attends the passage of an instrument for the first time after operation is more or less completely prevented. During the remainder of the treatment Lister's sounds are passed daily, and the patient is himself instructed how to pass a No. 9—12, which he is allowed to take away with him, so that in the future he may keep the stricture dilated by the occasional passage of an instrument, and therefore be independent of further surgical assistance. The average length of time spent in hospital after the operation is twelve days.

Part XIII.

OPERATIONS UPON THE SCROTUM AND PENIS.

CHAPTER I.

OPERATIVE TREATMENT OF VARICOCELE.

Anatomy of the Cord.—The vas deferens lies at the posterior aspect of the cord, and is to be easily recognised by its whipcord-like density when rolled between the thumb and finger. A considerable amount of connective tissue surrounds the vas and the blood-vessels of the cord. Three arteries occupy the cord: the spermatic, from the aorta, lies in front of the vas; the deferential artery, from the superior or inferior vesical, lies by the side of the vas; the cremasteric artery, from the deep epigastric, lies among the superficial layers of the cord and in its outer segment (Fig. 412).

The first-named vessel is the size of the posterior auricular, and the two latter the size of the supra-orbital.

The veins of the cord have been elaborately investigated by Mr. Walter G. Spencer, to whom I am indebted for the section from which Fig. 412 is drawn.

The veins are divided roughly into two sets. The anterior, and by far the larger set, runs with the spermatic artery, is bound together by a good deal of connective tissue, and forms the pampiniform plexus. The posterior set is small, and surrounds the vas deferens, running with the deferential artery. A few isolated veins, independent of these sets, are found among the tissues of the cord.

It would appear from Mr. Spencer's inquiries that the veins in the left cord are always larger than those of the right; and in connection with this point it may be observed that the congenital origin of varicocele is very generally allowed.

In severe cases of varicocele all the veins of the cord would appear to be involved. In ordinary cases the veins only of the pampiniform plexus are sufficiently dilated to require treatment.

In the operation of excision I have been in the habit of removing only the veins forming the pampiniform plexus, and have left those accompanying the deferential artery.

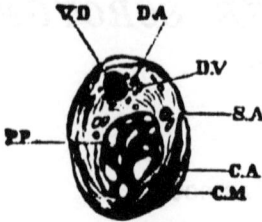

It must be remembered that the testicle is a vascular gland, and that it is possible to so far occlude the veins returning from the organ as to lead to gangrene (page 641).

Many operations have been proposed and performed for the relief of varicocele. Three only are here given.

Fig. 412.—SECTION OF THE LEFT SPERMATIC CORD OF AN ADULT, AT THE LEVEL OF THE EXTERNAL ABDOMINAL RING, VIEWED FROM ABOVE. (*From a specimen prepared by Mr. W. G. Spencer.*)

V.D, Vas deferens; D.A, Deferential artery; D.V, Deferential veins; S.A, Spermatic artery; C.A, Cremasteric artery; C.M, Cremaster muscle; P.P, Pampiniform plexus.

OPERATIONS.

Ligature with Wire. — Erichsen's Modification of Vidal de Cassis' Operation.—"The vas deferens, readily distinguished by its round cord-like feel, is first separated from the veins, and entrusted to an assistant to hold; an incision, about half an inch long, is then made in the front and back of the scrotum; a needle, so threaded with silver wire that the wire will follow without any dragging, is then passed between the vas and the veins, and brought out behind. The needle is then re-entered, and carried out in front, but this time is passed between the veins and the skin, thus including the veins in a loop of wire without implicating the scrotum. The loop is then tightly twisted, so as to constrict the enclosed vessels. From day to day the wire is tightened up afresh, until it has completely cut its way through the veins by ulceration—a process that takes about a week or ten days. Meanwhile there is much plastic matter thrown out around the veins, which finally contracts and obliterates their channels" (Holmes's "System of Surgery," vol. iii., page 570—Mr. Jacobson's article).

Galvanic Écraseur.—Pearce Gould's Operation.—"The

vas deferens is to be carefully separated from the veins at the upper part of the scrotum, and the skin, pinched up between the two, is to be transfixed with a tenotome, and divided parallel with the vas for one-third of an inch.

"Through this incision a needle, armed with a platinum wire, is to be passed and returned through the same skin apertures, but between the skin and the veins. The veins are thus secured in a loop of the wire. The ends of the loop are to be affixed to an écraseur, and the current of one cell of a Grove's battery or of a small bichromate battery passed through it. The heated wire quickly severs the veins, and securely sears the cut ends. A moderate traction should be kept up on the wire, so as to draw the veins out of the scrotum as much as possible, and in this way the action of the hot wire is limited to the veins. The wire must be heated to a dull red colour only. The patient must subsequently rest quiet and still in bed, with the scrotum supported, and with a small pledget of iodoform wool over each skin wound. The veins will be felt to become filled with clotted blood, which gradually becomes absorbed. As a rule, the patients are kept in bed for a week, and are able to resume active duties in ten to fourteen days. They should wear a suspender for another month " (Heath's "Dictionary of Surgery," vol. ii., page 778).

Excision.—Howse's Operation.—Mr. Howse has given an account of this operation in the *Guy's Hospital Reports* for 1887.

The procedure has been a little modified, and I have been in the habit of carrying it out in the following manner:—

The bowels should be well cleared out before the patient is placed on the table. A large sponge fixed against the perineum will absorb any blood lost during the excision. The surgeon stands on the side upon which the operation is to be performed. The hair having been shaved from the parts, the scrotum and surrounding skin are well washed with some antiseptic solution.

Two assistants are required. Both stand upon the opposite side of the table to the surgeon. One assistant attends to the wound; the other takes firm hold of the testicle, and draws it horizontally downwards, so as to make the cord tense. He should not relax his hold until the operation is completed.

An incision, about one inch and a half in length, is made over the most prominent part of the varicocele. The edges of the wound are held asunder by suture retractors, the ends of which are made fast around the thighs (Fig. 413). The coverings of the cord are now carefully dissected from the varicocele, the vertical line of the original incision being followed. No fibres

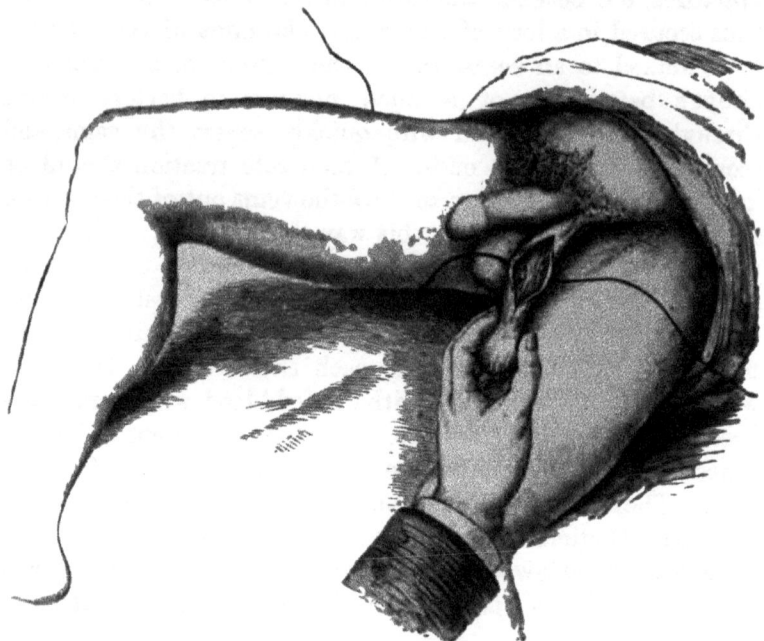

Fig. 413.—EXCISION OF VARICOCELE.

of the cremaster muscle need be cut. The veins composing the varicocele should be well and cleanly exposed over an extent equal to about one inch and a half. The vas deferens is identified, and, together with the small column of veins attending it, very carefully avoided. No attempt should be made to expose it by dissection. If the testis be well held, and moderate traction be kept up upon the cord, there is no disposition for the vas to protrude at the field of the operation.

The veins forming the pampiniform plexus are isolated, and are hooked up by two aneurysm needles. If they have been well exposed, there is no difficulty in clearly separating them from the other tissues of the cord. I have never been able to identify and isolate the spermatic artery.

The two aneurysm needles are now threaded with stout chromic catgut or with carbolised tendon, and withdrawn. The veins are then ligatured in two places, about one inch and a half apart. The lower ligature should be tied first. The vessels so isolated are divided with scissors close to the ligatures, and removed.

The amount excised will be represented by about one inch —the scissors being applied about a quarter of an inch from the ligature.

There is no need to clamp the veins above the site of the proposed excision in order to render them distinct.

If two pairs of dissecting forceps are gently used in clearing the varicocele from the surrounding tissues, there is little risk of damaging the vessels. The action of the forceps must be supplemented by the scalpel.

There will probably be no bleeding points to secure.

The cavity of the wound having been well washed out with an antiseptic solution, and a blunt hook having been inserted at each extremity of the wound, in order to bring the edges of the incision parallel, the sutures are introduced.

As a rule not more than two sutures will be needed, so that there may be a gap in the wound for drainage.

No drainage-tube is required. The wound is dressed in the same manner as after castration (page 653).

The first dressing need not be changed until the fourth day, and the sutures may be removed on the seventh.

Healing by first intention is the rule after this operation.

The patient should be kept in bed for about fourteen days. At the end of three weeks he will probably be able to resume his work.

He should wear a suspender for at least a month after he is moving about.

Bennett's Modification.—Mr. W. H. Bennett (*Lancet*, February 9th, 1889) points out the importance of not only excising the dilated veins, but of effecting at the same time an immediate and permanent shortening of the elongated cord.

"The precise extent of the varicocele," he writes, "which it is desirable to resect in any given case is best determined by placing the patient in the standing position, and roughly estimating with the eye—or, better still, by measuring with a tape—the degree of elongation of the cord: for instance, should the testis be three inches lower than normal, then certainly not less than three inches of the veins should be included between the two ligatures, as it will be desirable to excise at least two inches and a half."

The operation is conducted after the manner already described, but with these modifications :—

The veins are not actually denuded. "By leaving the sheath of fascia which immediately surrounds the varicocele intact, and including it with the veins in the ligature, two objects are attained—(a) the certainty of passing the ligature around all the affected vessels, as none of these ever lie outside the fascia ; and (b) the prevention of any material chance of recurrence of the abnormally dependent position of the testicle, which is probable if the veins are actually denuded before the ligatures are applied, and the stumps brought together in the manner described below, since it is manifest that the weight of the testis would tend to drag the veins considerably out from the sheath above, whereas this fascia, if included in the ligatures, not only obviates this tendency, but, in fact, also carries the weight of the dependent organ without stretching it to any appreciable extent.

"The portion of the varicocele included between the ligatures is divided above and below, about a quarter of an inch (not less) from the corresponding ligature, and removed. . . . The cut ends of the stumps left by the division of the varicocele are brought together, and retained in permanent apposition by knotting the ends of the upper ligature to those of the lower, thus at once raising the testis to about its natural level. The ligature-ends are cut off quite short."

Comment.—Of these various procedures, that by excision is undoubtedly the best.

In the wire operation, as well as in any of the operations by ligatures or pins, the surgeon must be acting a little in the dark, and cannot be sure of the precise amount and character of the tissue included within his loop.

It is possible for a vein to be transfixed in the passing of the wire or the ligature, and moreover, if a wire be retained, as in the method first described, the risk of phlebitis is not inconsiderable.

The subcutaneous method has been followed by erysipelas, by repeated hæmorrhages, by sloughing of the skin, and by abscess. These complications are mentioned by Mr. Lee (*Clin. Soc. Trans.*, vol. i., page 73), who practised this mode of treatment.

It does not appear, moreover, that the duration of the treatment is shortened by the subcutaneous method. It can not be claimed—so far, at least, as the first two described methods are concerned—that the procedure is painless. The results obtained by the subcutaneous methods are by no means remarkably successful.

The treatment by excision has much to commend it. The affected vessels are actually exposed, and the ligatures can be passed with the greatest precision. No complex appliances are required. The operation involves little more than a clean cut, and the simplest instruments are called into use.

So far as my experience goes, the result of the operation is certain; and the procedure may claim to effect a radical cure. The wound heals well, and I have never met with a single case of secondary hæmorrhage, abscess, or phlebitis. The after-treatment is not painful. There may be some œdema of the scrotum, and a little engorgement of the testis; but among a now considerable number of cases I have never met with an example of true orchitis.

I think it is important that the pampiniform plexus only should be dealt with. Mr. Jacobson (Holmes's "System of Surgery," vol. iii., page 571) mentions a case where some gangrene of the testis followed the excision, due, he believes, to the inclusion of too many veins in the ligatures. The veins which accompany the vas deferens should be left untouched.

There is not the least doubt but that the main trunk of the spermatic artery is often included with the veins, and is divided.

I can entirely endorse Mr. Bennett's statement (*Lancet*, March 7th, 1891) that no harm follows this division. The testicle does not slough, as some have surmised, nor does it

P P

become violently inflamed, nor does it undergo atrophy. The artery to the vas deferens certainly escapes injury, and appears to bring enough blood to the testicle by means of its anastomosing branches with the spermatic to maintain the healthy life of the testicle.

The value of Mr. Bennett's modification of the operation is undoubted. So far as I have observed, the testicle has in due course become braced up after the operation of simple excision; but it is obvious that the process may be helped by the knotting together of the two ligatures. It is not claimed however, that any direct union of necessity takes place between two masses of tissue included in the ligatures.

It is probable that the cremaster muscle, the vas deferens and the dartos have more to do with the holding up of the testicle than has the pampiniform plexus.

CHAPTER II.

The Operative Treatment of Hydrocele.

The chief palliative measure consists of repeated simple tappings. The curative measures have for their object the obliteration of the hydrocele sac.

Under this head will be considered the treatment by injection, by incision, and by excision of the parietal part of the sac.

In the subsequent sections it is considered that the hydrocele of adults is referred to. In the treatment of the hydrocele of infants and young subjects certain especial points are involved which need not be dealt with here.

Simple Tapping.—The position of the testicle must be made out by means of the patient's sensation, the use of transmitted light, and by following the vas deferens into the scrotum. In inversion of the testis—a condition where the epididymis lies to the front—the gland may be applied to the anterior wall of the sac, and be immediately pierced in tapping at the usual site. The patient should stand with his back against a wall; or, if he be old or nervous, may lie on his side at the edge of a bed. I have seen this little operation attended by alarming faintness.

The scrotal tissues are grasped from behind with the left hand, and the skin over the front of the swelling thus made as tense as possible. The trocar should be bright and well oiled, and should have been lying in a carbolic solution for some minutes before being employed. It is important that the cannula fits close. The nail of the right forefinger is placed on the trocar one inch from the point, to prevent too deep a plunge. The instrument is stabbed sharply into the sac at about the junction of its middle and lower thirds. The site of any visible vein is avoided. The instrument is first directed backwards, and then, when it is well into the sac, is sharply turned upwards to avoid the testicle. All tho

p p 2

fluid should be removed, and then a little tuft of iodoform wool should be applied over the puncture.

The patient should wear a suspender. He should, if possible, rest in the recumbent posture for the remainder of the day of the operation.

Some of the fluid may escape into the scrotal tissues and lead to a little œdema, which soon subsides. If a vessel be pricked, a considerable ecchymosis of the entire scrotum may result. If the trocar be blunt, or the cannula ill-fitting, or if the sac be thick, and the puncture be made in a hesitating manner, the tunica vaginalis may be pushed in front of the point of the instrument. Hæmatocele has in comparatively rare cases followed simple tapping. In such instances probably the testis has actually been pricked, or has been the subject of disease, or the patient has engaged in active work directly after the operation. If a foul trocar be used, suppuration of the sac may follow, especially in old and weakly subjects. A fresh tapping will probably be required at an interval of from three to six months.

Treatment by Injection.—The sac having been entirely emptied by tapping, the nozzle of a special syringe is applied to the cannula, and some irritant injected. The operation is most conveniently done while the patient stands. Iodine and carbolic acid are the substances most frequently used for the injection.

Iodine.—The following solution may be employed :—Iodine, forty grains ; iodide of potassium, thirty grains ; water, one ounce. Neither the ordinary tinctura iodi nor the liquor iodi are strong enough for efficient use in the majority of cases.

From three to four drachms should be injected and retained, and be brought into contact with all parts of the sac by rubbing the walls together after the cannula has been removed. The puncture may be covered by a piece of strapping or a tuft of iodoform wool. Some surgeons inject a larger quantity of fluid, and allow half of it to escape after it has been brought well in contact with the interior of the sac. Mr. Jacobson injects two to three drachms of the tincture of iodine of the Edinburgh Pharmacopœia, and allows the whole to remain.

Little pain, or only a feeling of heat, may follow the operation. On the other hand, the pain may be severe and nauseating, and may spread to the perineum, the loins, or the neck of the bladder. The patient may faint.

Within twelve hours the scrotum will probably be swollen to its previous size, the parts are red and tender, and the reaction is attended with some fever. The patient should lie in bed with the scrotum well supported. He will probably have to keep his bed for four or five days, and then will have to wear a suspender for a considerable time. Some three or four weeks will elapse before the parts will be restored to their normal condition. The inflammation excited may be of so insignificant a degree as to produce no curative result. On the other hand, it may assume serious proportions, and call for the use of ice-bags and the free administration of opium.

I have noticed that the inflammatory swelling that follows the successful use of iodine injection is sometimes tympanitic on percussion—an occurrence possibly due to the conversion of some of the iodine into vapour.

Carbolic Acid.—Five to ten drops of pure solid carbolic acid liquefied with the least amount of water are injected ; or a drachm of crystallised carbolic acid liquefied by the addition of 5 per cent. of glycerine is employed. The injected fluid is retained. It is claimed that carbolic acid excites less pain than iodine, and is more uniform and certain in its results.

Other injection materials are rectified spirit, port-wine,

The patient must lie in bed for from ten to fourteen days. The scrotum is kept well slung up in a scarf of carbolic gauze, and the actual wound is dressed with a sponge or a pad of Tillmann's dressing dusted with iodoform. A depression is cut in the sponge or pad to receive the end of the drainage-tube. The hollows around the sponge are packed with loose gauze or cotton-wool, and the whole dressing is secured by a T-bandage.

· The parts should be washed and irrigated with boracic lotion night and morning. Care must be taken that no bagging occurs. The drain should be shortened every day (commencing with the morning of the second day), and removed by the sixth or seventh day. The catgut sutures should be removed on the fourth or fifth day. The patient will probably be able to return to his usual mode of life by about the twenty-first day, but he should wear a suspender for some months after the operation. Some orchitis may follow the incision, but I have never seen it assume a severe grade.

Another method consists in incising the hydrocele, in securing the cut margins of the tunica vaginalis to the skin, and in then lightly plugging the exposed cavity with iodoform gauze.

I have been in the habit, in suitable cases, of exposing the hydrocele sac by free incision, and of then swabbing out the whole of the cavity of the tunica vaginalis with a plug of cotton-wool dipped in pure (liquefied) carbolic acid. The endothelium is destroyed, and suppuration follows. The after-treatment consists in very free drainage and in frequent irrigation.

Treatment by Excision of the Parietal Part of the Sac. —This operation was first introduced by Von Bergmann (*Berlin. klin. Woch.*, 1885, page 209). It has been fully described also by Henry Morris (*Internat. Journ. of the Med. Sciences*, Aug., 1888). An incision three inches long is made over the front and outer part of the tumour and through the tunica vaginalis. The sac is peeled and dissected away from the structures of the cord and scrotum, and cut off as close as possible around the testicle. In this excision the fingers are freely used, assisted by scalpel, scissors, and forceps. There is, as a rule, but little bleeding.

A drainage-tube is inserted in the cellular tissue space from which the hydrocele sac has been removed, and the edges of the external wound are brought together by sutures. An iodoform dressing is applied, and the scrotum is kept well raised. The operation may not involve a confinement in bed for more than ten days. Some patients have been laid up for periods of three to four weeks.

Comment.—The only known method of effecting a certain, absolute, and permanent cure of a hydrocele is to bring about the complete obliteration of the cavity of the tunica vaginalis. This is effected by the inflammatory process, and is shown either by the firm universal adhesion of the two surfaces of the sac together, or by the filling-up of the cavity of the sac by cicatricial tissue. Relapse may follow a partial obliteration of the sac, and, indeed, a hydrocele may reappear after treatment in any little cavity of the sac which may persist and have escaped the obliterating process.

On the other hand, cure may occur without this effacement of the sac cavity. This is seen in cases where a hydrocele has disappeared after a simple tapping, and in the very large series of hydroceles that have been subjected to some form of operation, and have disappeared, in spite of evidence that the cavity of the tunica vaginalis still existed.

At the present time it cannot be claimed that we possess an infallible method of treating hydrocele. To no operative process can the term "radical cure" be applied.

Of the operations described, the two most extensively practised are those by injection or by incision.

While each method has met with a certain degree of success, each has been attended by a certain proportion of failures.

The obstinacy of some cases of hydrocele is very marked. Mr. Pollock has alluded to a case (*Lancet*, March 3, 1888) that had been tapped and injected twice, with a recurrence of the collection. A seton was then passed through the tunica, and retained for three weeks. The hydrocele again recurred. The sac was then incised and dressed from the bottom. Profuse suppuration followed, but in due course the wound healed. The hydrocele returned again for the fourth time, and further attempts to effect a cure were abandoned.

Mr. Henry Morris refers to an instance where a hydrocele returned twenty-four years after it had been "cured" by tapping and injection.

Both the methods named appear to be attended by about the same percentage of failures. Mr. Jacobson (*Lancet*, September 1, 1877) has shown that the iodine injection, as usually practised, fails in nearly twenty per cent. of the cases. He believes that this average may be very considerably lessened, and thinks that failure is too often courted by want of attention to the following points :—(*a*) The use of a too dilute solution; (*b*) not bringing the solution in contact with the whole of the sac ; (c) not withdrawing all the hydrocele fluid ; (*d*) injecting large hydroceles immediately after they are emptied; (*e*) making use of iodine in unsuitable cases, viz., hydroceles with thick walls.

The incision operation, as usually practised, appears to be attended with about the same proportion of failures.

In one case of incision mentioned by Mr. Southam (*Lancet*, September 10, 1887) a sinus was discharging at the end of four months.

In comparing the two operations, the following advantages may be urged on behalf of the injection method :—There is no cutting and no open wound; no anæsthetic is required; the period of convalescence is comparatively short.

The especial advantage to be noted in favour of the incision method is that it enables the testis to be examined in cases of a suspicious nature.

In choosing between these two procedures, the advice given by Mr. Jacobson ("The Operations of Surgery," page 912) may be followed :—

The *Iodine Injection* should be the first mode of treatment. It is applicable to the great majority of cases.

The *Antiseptic Incision* would appear to be especially applicable to cases "(*a*) of previous failure with iodine; (*b*) with a sac very large or with very thick walls ; (c) where, on account of ill-health or premature age, the risk of inflammation after iodine injection is especially to be dreaded ; (*d*) in cases of congenital hydrocele a careful incision with antiseptic precautions will be safer than any other method, if the pressure of a truss for the obliteration of the peritoneal communication cannot be persevered with; (e) where the surgeon is desirous of exploring the sac of the tunica vaginalis, as in cases where enlargement of the testis, of a doubtful nature, co-exists with hydrocele, and does not yield to ordinary treatment; (f) where two hydroceles co-exist—e.g., vaginal and encysted hydroceles; (g) in some cases of hydrocele complicated with hernia—e.g., when the bowel is irreducible, and where, especially in unhealthy patients, there is a risk of the inflammation set up by the iodine extending to the hernial sac."

The value of *the treatment by excision* of the parietal part of the tunica vaginalis has been much disputed. In two cases reported by Mr. Henry Morris the hydrocele returned, and from that surgeon's account it would appear that the after-treatment may extend to four or seven weeks. Mr. Southam, on the other hand (*Lancet*, September 10, 1887; October 26, 1889; and July 25, 1891), regards this operation as the one with the greatest claim to be considered as a means of radical cure. He supports his statement with an account of ten cases attended with excellent results.

CHAPTER III.

CASTRATION.

The Instruments Required.—A median-sized scalpel; scissors; razor; dissecting forceps; artery forceps (several pairs); a clamp; two large blunt hooks; aneurysm needle; catgut ligatures; straight needle (two and a half inches); suture material; drainage-tube.

Position.—The patient lies upon the back, with the thighs extended and a little apart. The surgeon stands on the right-hand side of the patient. This position he may occupy both when operating upon the right and upon the left testicle. The one assistant required stands on the other side of the table, opposite the surgeon. His most important duty is to keep hold of the cord after it has been divided. Some surgeons advise that the patient should be brought to the foot of the table, and that the operator should stand between the patient's legs. This position, however, is not so convenient.

The Operation.—The pubes must be shaved, and the hair removed from the scrotum as far as possible. The parts should have been washed several times before the operation, first with soap and water, and then with carbolic lotion (1 in 20), or corrosive sublimate solution (1 in 100). This washing should include the perineum, and should be repeated when the patient is anæsthetised.

The bowels must have been well evacuated by purge and enema. The upper part of the scrotum and the inguinal canal are examined for hernia, and any history of previous hernia inquired into.

The testicle may rest upon a large sponge placed between the thighs. The skin of the scrotum is steadied by the left hand in this manner: the thumb and fingers are separated; the thumb lies on the right side of the swelling, the fingers on the left, the wrist is towards the abdomen, and the finger-tips towards the bottom of the scrotum. The incision is made between the thumb and the fingers, and by the separation of these the skin is well steadied and stretched.

A vertical incision is carried from a point about one inch below the external abdominal ring to the bottom of the scrotum.

When the skin is involved by the growth, or when it has become adherent to the testis or is the seat of sinuses, two elliptical incisions that clear the affected skin and meet above and below should be made. The position of these elliptical cuts must obviously depend upon the position of the implicated skin, and they may have to be made upon the lateral or even the posterior aspects of the scrotum. In dividing the tissues between the skin and the tunica vaginalis, the soft parts should be gently moved to and fro by the left hand, which still keeps its position on the scrotum. The mobility of the superficial layers is striking, but the tunica as it is approached is recognised by its perfect immobility.

When the skin is involved, this means of noting the progressive depths of the incision is lost.

The testis may be removed without opening the tunica vaginalis. In such case the tunica, as a simple bag, may be separated from the scrotal tissues with the fingers. While this is being done, the assistant should hold the scrotum and the testicle of the opposite side. In a large number of cases, however, it is desirable that the tunica should be opened : first, for diagnostic reasons ; second, to lessen the bulk of the swelling when the sac is distended with much fluid ; third, when the tunica is adherent, owing to the progress of the growth or the disease.

The testis is now shelled out of the scrotal tissues with the fingers. It is practically torn out, and at this step all cutting should be avoided, except when a point resists the fingers.

Even after the serous sac has been opened, the tunica vaginalis can very usually be shelled out together with the testis, to which it clings.

If the testis alone be disturbed, the connections between the visceral and parietal layers of the tunica must be cut with scissors.

In exposing the tumour, care should be taken not to cut

into it. The operation is complicated by opening an abscess cavity or a cyst, or by cutting into a mass of soft growth.

The cord is now well isolated with the fingers, and drawn down. It is then secured by a clamp. The best clamp for the purpose is a Spencer Wells's large pressure forceps. The assistant holds the clamp, and the surgeon, grasping the testicle, divides the cord with the knife about three-quarters of an inch below the clamp. The vessels of the cord can now be secured. Their position has been indicated (page 635). Three arteries must be included in the ligatures—the artery to the vas deferens, the cremasteric, and the spermatic. The deferential artery is found close to the vas. With it are a few veins (the posterior set, page 635). The cremasteric artery lies towards the outer part of the cord and nearer its surface. The spermatic artery is in front of the vas, and is surrounded by the veins of the pampiniform plexus. It is impossible to identify the arteries from the veins. The mouths of the latter vessels gape when grasped by the clamp; they are thereby rendered obvious, and are readily secured. Both veins and arteries are picked up with artery forceps, and secured with catgut. The two sets of veins may be tied each in a mass. Three or four ligatures may be required, but very seldom more.

Before removing the clamp a couple of bull-dog artery forceps should be temporarily fixed into the cord, in order that it may be readily drawn down again, should bleeding follow the removal of the clamp.

Any bleeding points in the scrotal incision must be secured. The following vessels are divided—superior and inferior external pubic, superficial perineal, and the artery to the scrotal septum. As a rule, none of these need a ligature.

In applying sutures, it is best to use a straight needle and silkworm gut. In order to obtain an even line of union, the edges of the incision should be stretched between two blunt hooks, inserted at the extremities of the wound and held by the assistant. This will prevent the in-turning of the edges of the incision, due to the contraction of the dartos, and will allow of accurate adjustment of the parts. It is well to introduce all the sutures before tying the first one. A drainage-tube one inch and a half long may be secured by means of the last suture.

The After-treatment.—The scrotum is well slung up by a light roll of loose gauze applied as a suspender. This gauze clings to the skin better than any other dressing. The wound may be then dressed with a sponge dusted with iodoform, or with a pad of Tillmann's dressing packed all round with gauze, and secured by means of a T-bandage or a spica. If this be properly applied, the sponge or pad exercises firm but gentle pressure upon the wound. The drainage-tube should be removed in twenty-four hours, and the dry dressing continued.

In the first twenty-four hours after the operation retention of urine may exist.

The scrotum is easily inflamed by the use of irritant lotions; *e.g.*, strong carbolic lotions.

Should suppuration occur, constant care must be taken to prevent bagging.

The sutures are removed on the fifth to the seventh day. The patient will probably complain of the hard tender swelling which usually appears at the external ring, and which is due to inflammatory changes in the stump of the cord.

As the wound heals, the cicatrix becomes depressed, from the obliteration of the scrotal pouch.

If primary union be not obtained, the edges of the wound may need to be retained in contact by strapping.

Comment:—In some cases the descent of a hernia after castration has forced open the wound, the rupture having been previously kept up by the enlarged testicle. During the operation, moreover, hernial sacs have been inadvertently opened up. If a scrotal hernia exists, the rupture should be reduced, the sac excised, and its neck ligatured. The procedure is described in the chapter on the Radical Cure of Hernia (page 539).

The skin incision should be carried to the bottom of the scrotum, in order to secure good drainage.

When the skin is implicated, the incisions should extend beyond the diseased area, and involve sound skin only.

It is not necessary to remove redundant skin, unless it be excessive in amount and much atrophied.

Lafage employed in all cases an elliptical incision. Amussat made his wound on the posterior aspect of the scrotum. Jobert employed a curved incision, with the convexity turned downwards and inwards. Rima advised the cutting of a U-shaped flap by transfixion from the posterior wall of the scrotum.

If any sinuses be left behind, as after the removal of a tubercular testis, they should be most carefully scraped with a Volkmann's spoon. The cord should be secured about one inch from the testis. If it be involved, it should be divided higher up. It can seldom be necessary to open up the whole inguinal canal to secure the cord, as advised by some. If the disease has extended to the external ring, the expediency of any operation may be questioned. Before the cord is secured and divided, the anæsthetic may be discontinued for a while, as the section is sometimes attended by a very marked and possibly alarming sinking of the pulse.

It is to be remembered that the cord is very much dragged down by a large growth; and if secured very high up, the stump, after section, may be withdrawn beyond easy reach when the heavy tumour is removed.

The chief bleeding to be feared after castration cases is venous rather than arterial.

It is unwise to include the cord in one ligature; the vessels are not well secured by this means. The loop of thread may slip off when the clamp is removed. A substantial ligature must be employed, and it is to apt to excite suppuration until it is discharged. Secondary hæmorrhage may follow the loosening of the single ligature. Neuralgia of the cord may also attend the procedure.

The same objections apply, but in a less degree, to the practice of transfixing the cord with a needle, and ligaturing it in two segments. The simple searing of the stump with the cautery, or the division of the cord with the écraseur, are measures which are, I believe, out of date, and which certainly have little to recommend them.

CHAPTER IV.

AMPUTATION OF THE PENIS.

THIS operation is required principally for cases of epithelioma. As the penis is well supplied with vessels, and as the cavernous tissue that forms the main part of its substance lends itself readily to the spread of a malignant growth, an early operation and a very free excision are necessary to ensure a complete removal of the disease.

The procedure is attended by these complications—hæmorrhage, the retraction of the orifice of the divided urethra within the stump, the narrowing of that orifice by the contraction of cicatricial tissue, the wetting of the wound with urine, and the infiltration of urine into the tissues of the scrotum, when the part is removed far back.

The Instruments Required—For the operations to be described, the following instruments are required :—An elastic band tourniquet ; a gum-elastic catheter ; a scalpel ; a narrow straight bistoury ; straight and curved scissors ; a tenaculum ; dissecting, toothed, and artery forceps ; small curved needles and needle-holder for the urethra ; straight needles ; a periosteal elevator ; sutures ; ligatures.

Amputation of the Free Portion of the Penis.—1. *By Simple Section.*—The hair about the root of the penis having been shaved off, the parts all well washed with a solution of carbolic acid (1 in 20), or of corrosive sublimate (1 in 100), the patient is placed in the lithotomy position, and the surgeon stands between his legs. Previous to the operation the rectum and bladder should have been emptied. An elastic tourniquet—a No. 9 soft rubber catheter answers admirably—is tied around the root of the penis. The glans is held in the left hand and drawn gently forwards. (If drawn too vigorously from the body, too much integument may be removed.) A circular cut—involving the skin only—is now

made round the penis with the scalpel. As the knife traverses
the urethral region, the traction on the organ may be relaxed,
so that the skin over the corpus spongiosum may be cut a
little longer than the rest.

A straight piece of gum-elastic catheter is now introduced
into the urethra down to the tourniquet, and the corpora
cavernosa are divided vertically. The limits of the corpus
spongiosum are defined, and the catheter having been removed,
that body, with the urethra, is cut one inch longer than the
rest of the stump.

The urethra thus projects like a shoot. It is slit up with
scissors along the dorsum, and the lower wall is attached by
a suture to the skin of the under-surface of the penis, while
the cut edges of the upper wall are sutured to the corpora
cavernosa. This is effected with a small curved needle,
carrying catgut. The vessels are now secured. They are at
least four in number—the two dorsal arteries and the arteries
of the corpora cavernosa (lying in the centre of those bodies).
These vessels are the size of the posterior auricular, and the
last-named are more readily secured when picked up by a
tenaculum. The tourniquet is now removed, and any other
vessels are secured. In the corpus spongiosum a fair-sized
branch of the artery to the bulb may be found, and other
vessels may follow the septum in the body of the penis. · The
general oozing from the cut surface usually stops in a while
spontaneously.

The wound is dressed with iodoform, and is packed round
with cotton-wool, supported by a T-bandage. A soft rubber
catheter attached to a tube, which enters a receptacle beneath
the bed, should be kept in the bladder for three days. If after
or before its removal any urine escapes, the parts should be at
once washed with boracic lotion.

The scrotum should be kept supported, and smeared with
vaseline to prevent excoriation. The wound should be well
irrigated twice a day with boracic lotion. The sutures on the
urethra may be left to cut their way out. The cut surface
granulates, the skin turns in and becomes puckered over the
face of the wound.

The patient may expect to be confined to bed for some
weeks. When cicatrisation is taking place, care should be

observed that a stricture does not form at the urethral orifice. If no catheter is retained, a long silk ligature may be stitched to the urethral floor, to form a guide to that opening; for when a few days have elapsed, the urethral orifice is often very difficult to find, and the patient may be troubled with retention. The catheter, if retained, can be secured to the groin by strapping.

2. *By Section, with Flap.*—Hæmorrhage having been pro vided against, a rectangular flap of skin is cut from the dorsum and sides of the penis, and the dorsal arteries are secured. The flap may be compared, in miniature, to the anterior flap in an amputation of the thigh. A narrow-bladed knife is then made to transfix the penis at a point on a level with the base of the above flap, between the corpora cavernosa and the corpus spongiosum, and then is made to cut forwards, out-wards and downwards, for about three-quarters of an inch. From this smaller inferior flap the urethra is dissected out. The corpora cavernosa are then cut vertically upwards, on a level with the point of transfixion. The tourniquet is re-moved, all bleeding points are tied, and the upper or skin flap is punctured at a point opposite to the divided urethra. That tube is drawn through the punctured hole in the flap, is slit up, and stitched *in situ.* The two flaps, upper and lower, are then joined by sutures.

It is claimed for this operation that a natural skin covering is secured for the severed corpora cavernosa, and thus the irritation and delay which the healing of these bodies by granulation entails are avoided.

3. *By the Galvanic Écraseur.*—A gum-elastic cathetor having been introduced into the urethra, a straight needle—carrying the platinum wire—is introduced between the catheter and the corpora cavernosa. The two ends of the wire are then drawn upwards round the penis. Before they are tightened the skin is incised along the line that the wire will occupy. The wire having been connected with the battery, the corpora cavernosa are divided. The catheter is now removed, and the corpus spongiosum and urethra are divided in like manner, but at the distance of half an inch nearer the glans. The wire should be only at a dull heat, and be very slowly tightened.

The method cannot be recommended. It is mentioned

merely because it is still frequently employed. It is not always bloodless, as claimed. I have seen it attended by free primary bleeding, and also by secondary hæmorrhage when the sloughs separated.

It would seem as if the actual cautery was not well adapted to close the peculiar blood channels of erectile tissue. Moreover, the wound left is a sloughy one, and healing is slow and tedious. In old and debilitated patients this sloughing, ill-conditioned wound becomes a serious element.

Amputation of the Entire Penis.—The best procedure for the removal of the entire penis is that devised by Pearce Gould (*Lancet*, vol. i., 1882, page 821). It ensures a very complete removal of the diseased organ. The new opening of the urethra is well established. There is no risk of an infiltration of urine into the tissues of the scrotum, and the skin of the part is not irritated by the trickling of urine over it.

The Operation is performed as follows:—

The patient having been placed in the lithotomy position, the skin of the scrotum is incised along the whole length of the rhaphe. With the finger and the handle of the scalpel the two halves of the scrotum are then separated, quite down to the corpus spongiosum. A full-sized metal catheter is now passed as far as the triangular ligament, and the knife is inserted transversely between the corpora cavernosa and the corpus spongiosum.

The catheter having been withdrawn, the urethra is cut across. The deep end of the urethra is then detached from the penis quite back to the triangular ligament. An incision is next made round the root of the penis, continuous with that in the median line; the suspensory ligament is divided, and the penis separated, except at the attachment of the crura. The knife is now laid aside, and with a stout periosteal elevator, or rugine, each crus is detached from the pubic arch. This step of the operation involves some time, on account of the very firm union of the parts to be severed. Four arteries—the two arteries of the corpora cavernosa and the two dorsal arteries—require ligature.

The corpus spongiosum is slit up for about half an inch, and the edges of the cut stitched to the back part of the incision in the scrotum.

The scrotal incision is closed by sutures, and a drainage-tube is so placed in the deep part of the wound that its ends can be brought out in front and behind. No catheter is retained in the urethra.

In Mr. Gould's case—the operation was performed for epithelioma in a man aged seventy-three—there was no complaint of pain after the operation. The temperature reached the normal line on the fourth day, and on the sixth day the patient had regained complete control over the bladder. The skin wound healed by first intention, the deeper wound by granulation. The parts were completely healed in forty-six days.

CHAPTER V.

THE OPERATIVE TREATMENT OF SCROTAL ELEPHANTIASIS.

THE question of operation in cases of elephantiasis of the penis and scrotum is admirably discussed by Dr. McLeod, of Calcutta, in Heath's "Dictionary of Surgery" (vol. ii., page 399).

Mere bulk is no bar to operation, as tumours weighing 100 to 120 lbs. have been removed with success.

The following are the chief contra-indications to operation —old age; organic disease of the heart, kidneys, or intestines; anæmia; diabetes; recent and acute enlargements of the liver or spleen; incurable urethral fistulæ; the existence of large herniæ.

Before the operation any stricture of the urethra should be relieved, and abscesses and sinuses cured.

The main points in the operation are—rapid execution, the removal of every trace of the disease, the prevention of bleeding, the preservation of the essential parts of the organs of generation, and the encouragement of rapid healing.

The Operation is thus described by Dr. McLeod :—

The patient is placed in the recumbent posture and anæsthetised. To anæmiate the tumour, the mass is elevated and compressed by an elastic bandage for ten to twenty minutes, according to the size of the mass.

To prevent bleeding during the operation, an elastic cord about three feet long is taken, and the centre of it is passed round the loins, the ends are brought over the brim of the pelvis, are crossed twice over opposite sides of the neck of the tumour, and finally are brought together below the navel. The neck of the tumour will thus be tightly embraced by two turns of the cord on each side, crossing each other on the pubes, and just in front of the anus.

No portion of diseased tissue must be left behind. Even although the prepuce appears to be healthy, it should be removed close to the corona; and as thickening is peculiarly apt to commence in the rhaphe of the perineum, that part should, in most cases, be freely removed by a V-shaped incision up to the verge of the anus. If any attempt is made to cover the penis and testes with flaps, these should be taken from the skin of the abdomen or thighs, and not from the neck of the tumour; but a satisfactory result can be secured in all cases without resort to flaps, which are prone to slough and suppurate.

The first step consists in decorticating the penis. The prepuce is slit up, and a skin incision continued from this slit along the whole dorsum of the penis to the root. The penis is then freed by finger and knife, the mucous membrane of the prepuce being carefully detached at the line of its reflexion. The isolation of the penis is completed as far as its suspensory ligament, which should not be injured. A vertical incision is now made from the pubes to the fundus of the tumour, over one cord and testis. By successive bold strokes these are exposed, and then dissected out by fingers and knife, and subsequently held out of the way by an assistant. The other testis is similarly dealt with. The three vertical incisions are then connected at their pubic terminations by two transverse cuts, which must be beyond the limit of the diseased tissue.

A circular or oval incision is now made round the rest of the circumference of the neck of the tumour, and by rapid strokes the whole mass is removed. Vessels are now looked for. The largest will be found in the centre of the perineum and on each side of the pubes. By gradually loosening the cord, others will be observed to spring. As many as thirty or forty ligatures may be required. The parts may now be trimmed, if any diseased tissue has been left behind. The testes may now be stitched together by means of catgut, and fastened in proper position by sutures of the same material. Depressions or pockets can be very easily made for their reception, by separating the deep layer of the superficial perineal fascia from the subjacent fat and areolar tissue. The skin can then be drawn over them from each side to a considerable extent by means of a continuous catgut suture.

The prevention of putrefaction in such an extensive wound is difficult. Free and frequent irrigations and careful drainage must be persisted in. Dr. McLeod is in favour of the use of boracic dressings.

The wound fills up by granulation, and the process of repair occupies from six weeks to two months. Care must be taken to keep the penis free, as it is apt to become embedded in the mass of granulation tissue. The ultimate result of the operation is in the great majority of cases satisfactory. Skin is dragged by the process of cicatrisation from the thigh to form a seemly substitute for the scrotum, and the penis acquires a fresh covering of epidermis. The sexual functions are restored, and both health and comfort re-established.

If the skin of the penis is quite healthy, the scrotum may be removed alone by a circular incision round its neck, the testes being dissected out as the incision is deepened.

CHAPTER VI

CIRCUMCISION.

IN performing the operation for a redundant prepuce, the following method will be found convenient:—

The end of the penis is lightly seized with a pair of circumcision forceps or dressing forceps. The forceps are so applied that their lower margins fall exactly across the line of the corona. As the blades are closed the glans slips out of the way, and at last nothing is held but the prepuce. The size of forceps employed must vary with the age of the patient. They should hold the skin firmly and squarely.

As the glans slips out of the grip of the forceps, the skin at the orifice of the prepuce may become turned in, and too much of the integument of the penis be drawn between the blades of the instrument. To avoid this, the foreskin should be firmly held with a pair of sharp-toothed forceps, which are applied at the preputial orifice, exactly where the skin and mucous membrane join. They serve to keep the prepuce in position while the clamp forceps are acquiring a hold. As already stated, the latter are applied exactly along the line of the corona; they will thus, when fixed, be obliquely placed with reference to the long axis of the penis.

More skin is removed from the dorsal than the frænal aspect of the part. To ensure a most correct adjustment of the forceps, an ink mark may be made on the skin of the penis, precisely around the line of the corona, as the parts lie before being disturbed. When the blades are closed, this ink line should not be visible beyond them.

The skin being now put upon the stretch by drawing on the forceps, the prepuce is divided with a fine straight bistoury just beyond the forceps blades—i.e., on the penis side of the instrument.

The mucous layer left behind is now slit up along the

dorsal median line. This is best done with straight scissors, while the membrane is held with toothed forceps. The slit must go well back to the corona. The two flaps of mucous membrane are now stripped off the glans until the corona is reached. The membrane is often very adherent, and has to be forcibly peeled off by forceps and a director. Any collection of smegma preputii is removed. The edges of the mucous flaps may be trimmed, and then allowed to fall over on to the cut skin surface. In infants no sutures are required; and as no bleeding points will require attention, the operation is complete. In lads and adults the cut edges of the mucous membrane and skin must be united by sutures. The finest catgut should be employed, and should be inserted as close as possible to the free margins of both the skin and the mucous membrane. If this is done, the sutures will cut their way out, and need not be removed unless they are still retained on the seventh day. Not more than three suture points on each side will be required.

In adults there may be free bleeding, and a vessel or so may have to be secured. Before the operation (in adult subjects) an india-rubber catheter may be tied around the root of the penis as a tourniquet.

The wound is best dressed by a narrow strip of quite dry lint dusted with iodoform, and secured around the penis.

By the use of the dry dressing oozing is checked; and as the lint sticks to the part, the wound edges are kept in contact. Oiled dressings of any kind are objectionable. The dressing slips about, and is very apt to come off.

The first dressing is left untouched for twenty-four or thirty hours; it is then allowed to soak off as the patient sits in a warm hip-bath.

Dry lint and iodoform make, I think, the best dressing throughout the case. The patient—if an adult—should remain in the recumbent position for two or three days, and should not move about much until the part is nearly healed. He should have a warm hip-bath once a day, or, if possible, night and morning. On each occasion the wound is re-dressed.

It is important that no tight band should surround the penis, since the extremity may become congested and œdematous. As the patient lies in bed, the penis must be kept supported, and not allowed to hang down. A cradle will be required. In infants, the following method of dressing the wound—as proposed by Paul Swain—will be found very convenient (Heath's " Dictionary of Surgery," vol. i., page 308) :—

" A long strip of dry lint, six or eight inches long and half an inch wide, is applied as follows :—The glans being well pulled forward by an assistant, the middle of the strip of lint is applied to the under-surface of the penis, immediately behind the glans. The two ends are then passed over and around the organ in successive turns until the root is reached, when they will lie crossed on the lower part of the abdomen, and must be secured in that position by a couple of strips of adhesive plaster. The orifice of the urethra is thus left free, the cut edges of the mucous membrane and skin are retained in apposition, and the child is unable to pull off the dressings."

Often a good deal of thickening remains about the frænum, and there may result therefrom a permanent lump. This is entirely due to the leaving of too much tissue about the frænum. It is to a great extent avoided if the wound line faithfully follow the corona. It is a common mistake to divide the prepuce in a line at right angles to the long axis of the penis.

In adults, where the preputial orifice is very narrow, but the foreskin itself is not unduly redundant, nothing requires to be cut away. A director is thrust under the prepuce, and carried well back to the corona. A narrow curved bistoury with a sharp point is made to follow the director, and the point to pierce the skin at the level of the corona. The foreskin is thus slit up along the median dorsal line. The mucous membrane is peeled back, the two flaps are rounded off, and the cut edges are united by a few suture points, as in the more complete operation.

Part XIV.

OPERATIONS UPON THE RECTUM.

CHAPTER I.

OPERATIVE TREATMENT OF HÆMORRHOIDS.

The Anatomy of the Rectum.—The length of the rectum is estimated at about eight inches. Its upper part for about three inches is entirely invested by peritoneum. The serous membrane gradually leaves its posterior surface, then its sides, and lastly its anterior surface. Anteriorly, the peritoneum, in the form of the recto-vesical pouch, extends in the male to within about three inches of the anus. This distance is lessened when the bladder and rectum are both empty, and is increased when they are distended. On the posterior surface of the gut there is no peritoneum below a spot five inches from the anus.

Below the point where the serous membrane ceases, the rectum is connected to surrounding parts by areolar tissue. It is in close relation behind with the sacrum and coccyx, at the sides with the levatores ani, and in front (in the male) with the trigone of the bladder, the seminal vesicles, and the prostate. Below the prostate the rectum becomes invested by the internal sphincter, and is embraced by the levatores ani muscles. In the female the lower part of the rectum is firmly attached to the posterior wall of the vagina.

The internal sphincter surrounds the lower part of the rectum an inch above the anus, and extends over about half an inch of the intestine.

Mr. Harrison Cripps has shown that the posterior edge of the levator ani muscle forms a distinct free border, which crosses the rectum, at very nearly a right angle, at a point from

one and a half to two inches from the anus, and therefore
above the upper limit of the sphincter ani.

Of the arteries of the rectum, the most important is the
superior hæmorrhoidal. It runs down behind the rectum,
lying slightly to the left of the median line, and breaks up
into its terminal branches about four or four and a half inches
from the anus.

Over the lower part of the rectum—the last four inches—
the arteries are arranged as follows:—" The vessels, having
penetrated the muscular coat at different heights, assume a
longitudinal direction, passing in parallel lines towards the end
of the bowel. In their progress downwards they communicate
with one another at intervals, and they are very freely connected near the orifice, where all the arteries join by branches
of considerable size " (R. Quain). This longitudinal arrangement of the arteries explains the fact that when the rectum is
incised in the line of its long axis, the bleeding is comparatively
slight; while it is copious if the bowel be divided transversely.

The fact that the lower part of the rectum is mainly
supplied by these vertical branches which descend in the coats
of the bowel, explains the comparatively slight bleeding that
attends the separation of the gut from its lateral connections
in the operation of excision.

The veins have an arrangement closely resembling that of
the arteries. For the first three inches or so beyond the anus
they run between the mucous and muscular coats, and then,
perforating the muscular tunic, pass up external to the bowel.

OPERATIVE TREATMENT OF HÆMORRHOIDS.—INTERNAL PILES.

The indications for operating in cases of internal piles are
admirably given by Mr. Harrison Cripps in his work on
" Diseases of the Rectum and Anus," page 96.

The operative measures which have been from time to
time proposed or carried out in the treatment of hæmorrhoids
are legion. In few departments of surgery has there been a
more remarkable or a more restless activity.

Among the numerous operations which are at the present
time employed, a certain number do not call for description in
a work like the present. Such are the treatment by caustics
and acids, the injection of carbolic acid or other fluids, the

puncture of the pile with a fine cautery point, the treatment by dilatation of the sphincter, as advocated by Verneuil, and the employment of electrolysis.

The following operative measures will be here described:—

1. Treatment by ligature.
2. Treatment by excision.
3. Treatment by crushing.
4. Treatment by the cautery.

Preparation of the Patient.—A few days' rest before an operation for piles is carried out is very desirable, although it is not often afforded. During these few days the patient should limit himself to a very simple and moderate diet, should avoid stimulants, and should attend to the action of the bowels. The man who is working hard and living "well" up to the very eve of the operation, and who concludes the preliminary treatment with a "good" dinner, on the plea that it will be some time before he will have another such repast, is not a good subject for operation.

The bowels must be well opened by an aperient—preferably, castor oil—administered thirty-six hours before the operation is performed. Just before the surgeon's arrival the rectum should be thoroughly cleared out by a warm water enema, and the nurse should be careful to see that all the fluid injected is returned. A hot bath should be taken on the evening before the operation.

The Instruments Required. — *Ligature Operation.*— Clover's crutch; pile-holding forceps (there are many forms of these forceps—some resemble the volsella, others are constructed on the principle of the pressure forceps, and another series follow the mechanism of artery torsion forceps, and are provided with a sliding catch—it is desirable that the instrument should be self-holding); scissors — sharp and blunt-pointed, straight, and curved on the flat—(special forms of hæmorrhoid scissors, such as the well-known scissors or shears introduced by Salmon, are not specially convenient); pressure and artery forceps; silk.

Excision Operation.—The same instruments, with the addition of dissecting forceps, volsella, needles and needle-holders, catgut ligatures, sponges in holders. A rectal speculum may be of use.

The Operation by Crushing.—In addition to the chief instruments already mentioned, a special crushing clamp is required; and in the *Treatment by the Cautery*, Smith's clamp and Paquelin's cautery are needed.

1. **The Operation by the Ligature.** — The patient is anæsthetised, Clover's crutch is applied, and the patient is placed in the lithotomy position, the buttocks being brought close to the lower end of the table. The surgeon sits facing the perineum.

The first step consists in dilating the sphincters. Both index fingers are introduced, and the anus is slowly and gradually stretched. The process will require at least two minutes to accomplish, and when complete the anus will be patulous, and the sphincter will have lost its tendency to contract. If a hasty dilatation be effected, the sphincter may relax suddenly, and a laceration of the parts be brought about. The surgeon should maintain a watchful control over the dilating fingers.

The parts are now in a convenient condition for operation. The piles, which may previously have been entirely withdrawn from view, are now readily exposed, and the whole of the lower part of the rectum can be inspected and explored. The surgeon, after a careful examination of the district, should decide on the number of piles which may require removal.

It is desirable to commence with the hæmorrhoids on the lower or posterior wall of the rectum, since, when the piles on the opposite wall are being dealt with, these are obscured by the blood. Small piles, which are evident enough before the actual operation is commenced, may be lost sight of after some of the main ligatures have been applied. As a preliminary step, it is well to seize each of these smaller excrescences with pressure forceps, which are left in position, as a guide to the site of the pile, until the surgeon finds it convenient to deal with them. These forceps hang loose, and are not in the way.

Each pile is seized with the pile-holding forceps, held in the left hand, and is gently drawn away from the anus and towards the middle line. Its base is thus rendered tense, and the line of junction of the skin with the mucous membrane is brought well into view.

By a series of snips with the scissors the surgeon severs

all the *lower* attachments of the pile, cutting along the line of junction of the skin and mucous membrane.

By a few light snips, aided with a little pressure from the blunt points of the scissors, the pile is dissected up from the submucous tissue until it is attached only by the healthy mucous membrane above it, and by the vessels that are descending to enter it. As the vessels come from above and run just beneath the mucous membrane, and enter the upper part of the hæmorrhoid, this detachment is readily and safely accomplished, and the bleeding is very trivial.

The detachment should be sufficiently extensive to form a deep groove.

The forceps are now handed to an attendant, who maintains the traction upon the pile, while the surgeon places a silk ligature round its pedicle, which he at once proceeds to tie as tightly as possible.

The ligature should not be too thick, and it should not be applied with such violence as to cut the pedicle of the pile entirely through. Before tightening the knot, the ligature should be so manipulated as to include the highest part of the mucous membrane left attached to the pile.

The number of ligatures to be applied will of course vary More than five will seldom be required.

The operation is completed by cutting the ligatures off, and by snipping away the strangulated hæmorrhoidal tissues which project beyond the knot. The parts are lightly dried with wool, are dusted with iodoform, and returned.

When the hæmorrhoids form a complete circle within the anus, the most prominent portions must be isolated by means of incisions made through the mucous membrane; and when the pile mass has thus been divided into segments, each part is ligatured separately.

This method of employing the ligature is that introduced by Salmon at St. Mark's Hospital.

Some surgeons prefer that the patient should lie during the operation upon one side, and with the knees well drawn up.

The plan of drawing forward a pile and of transfixing its pedicle with a needle in a handle carrying a ligature, and of then securing the pile in two parts, is to be condemned. A great deal more tissue is taken up than is necessary, the vein in the excrescence may be transfixed by the needle, bleeding may follow, and a certain risk of septic infection is incurred.

2. The Operation by Excision.—Of the various methods of treating piles by excision which have been from time to time employed, the most precise, and probably the most successful, is that introduced by Mr. Walter Whitehead (*Brit. Med. Journ.*, February, 1882; and February, 1887). The operation is carried out on sound surgical principles, and has been attended with considerable success.

The patient is secured in the lithotomy position by Clover's crutch, and the sphincters are fully dilated. "By the use of scissors and dissecting forceps the mucous membrane is divided at its junction with the skin round the entire circumference of the bowel, every irregularity of the skin being carefully followed. The external, and the commencement of the internal sphincters are then exposed by a rapid dissection, and the mucous membrane and attached hæmorrhoids, thus separated from the submucous bed on which they rested, are pulled bodily down, any undivided points of resistance being nipped across, and the hæmorrhoids brought below the margin of the skin.

"The mucous membrane above the hæmorrhoids is now divided transversely in successive stages, and the free margin of the severed membrane above is attached as soon as divided to the free margin of the skin below by a suitable number of sutures" (*Brit. Med. Journ.*, February 26, 1887, page 449).

In this way the complete ring of pile-bearing mucous membrane is removed. All bleeding vessels encountered throughout the operation are treated by torsion. As a rule, only one or two need torsion.

It is best to commence with the separation of the mucous membrane at the lowest point, and then at the two sides, completing the circle above.

The separation of the mucous membrane is accomplished with the fingers and the end of a pair of blunt-pointed scissors.

The sutures employed are of carbolised silk, and are allowed to come away of themselves. The parts are dressed with iodoform powder.

In the paper from which the above quotation is made Mr.

Whitehead reports 300 consecutive cases of hæmorrhoids which he has treated by excision alone, without a death, without a single case of secondary hæmorrhage, and without any instance of complication or relapse.

Mr. Coates, of Salisbury, excises internal .piles with the assistance of a special clamp (Fig. 414).

The operation having been commenced in the usual way, a pile is seized with forceps, is drawn down, and to its pedicle the little clamp is applied. A few sutures of the finest catgut are then passed underneath the clamp, and the pile is excised. The clamp is now opened a little. The needles which have transfixed the growth prevent retraction. All bleeding having been checked, the clamp is entirely removed, and the catgut sutures

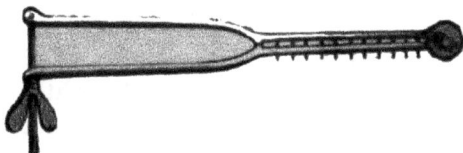

Fig. 414.—COATES'S CLAMP.

are tied. The remaining piles are then treated in like manner one by one. This substitutes for the contused wound produced by the ligature a cleanly-incised cut neatly adjusted by sutures.

3. The Operation by Crushing.—The treatment of piles by crushing was introduced by Mr. George Pollock (*Lancet*, July 3, 1880). The operation has been advocated by Mr. Benham, Mr. Allingham, and many others.

Of the many pile-crushers devised, the most convenient is that known as Allingham's (Fig. 415).

The patient having been placed in position, and the sphincter dilated (*see* page 670), a pair of pile-holding forceps is passed through the open square of the crusher, a pile is seized with the forceps, and is then drawn into the crusher, the blade of which is at once screwed down. The instrument should be screwed up as tightly as possible, and should be left in place for a minute or two. The portion of the pile projecting beyond the clamp is then either cut away or destroyed by the cautery. The clamp is now slowly unscrewed and removed, and it will usually be found that no bleeding follows. Any bleeding vessel may be secured by a ligature or be twisted. Care must be taken not to include any skin in the crusher.

4. The Operation by the Cautery.—The method of treating piles by means of the actual cautery is of very ancient date. The elaboration of the present means of employing the cautery is due to Mr. Lee and Mr. Henry Smith, both of whom devised special clamps for holding the pile and limiting the action of the heated iron.

The best clamp is that invented by the latter surgeon.

The patient having been placed in position, and the sphincter having been dilated as above described (page 670), each pile is seized in turn, and is drawn between the blades of the clamp, which are then screwed tightly together. The part of the pile projecting beyond the clamp is then cut off, and the stump, which should be at least one-eighth of an inch in depth, is well charred with the Paquelin's cautery. The cautery point should be heated only to a dull-red heat; the clamp is slowly relaxed, and the surgeon follows with the cautery point the charred tissues as they slip out between the blades. Bleeding very seldom occurs. The parts must not be roughly manipulated after the clamp has been removed, as the eschars are readily detached.

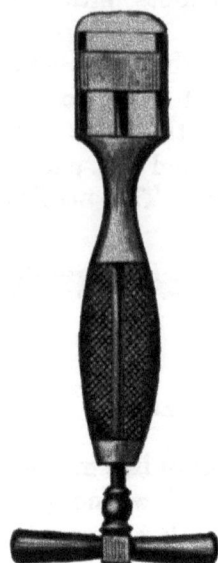

Fig. 415.—ALLINGHAM'S PILE-CRUSHER.

Comment.—Out of the operations above described it would be impossible to select one as the best if it were attempted to found the selection upon the writings of those surgeons who have more especially concerned themselves with this branch of surgery. Each operation has its own vigorous advocate, and in the hands of these special pleaders such excellent results are obtained as to make a safe criticism difficult.

Personally, I would share the opinion expressed by many, that the ligature offers on the whole the best means of dealing with internal piles. It is simple and of wide application. It involves the employment of no complex instruments. It is but very rarely attended by secondary hæmorrhage, and its results are certain.

When the hæmorrhoids, however, are very extensive and involve the whole of the circumference of the anus, then there is no better method of dealing with them than is provided by Whitehead's operation. Crushing is well suited to small piles which involve no part of the actual skin, and the cautery is adapted for simple venous piles of moderate size.

From my experience of these various operations, I should say that for no one method can a particular exemption from pain be claimed, nor can it be shown that the after-treatment is always less protracted after one operation than after another.

The pain after operations for piles depends rather upon whether the anal margin is encroached upon, or is the subject of acute inflammation during the after-treatment, than upon the particular operation carried out. Of the methods described, the after-treatment is perhaps a little more prolonged after the use of the ligature than after the use of any one of the other measures detailed.

The risk involved by operations for piles is quite trifling. The statistics of St. Mark's Hospital show that the mortality during the past forty years was only at the rate of 1 in 670 cases.

Mr. Allingham reports 1,600 cases operated upon by himself, without a single death.

The After-treatment.—After the stumps left by the operation have been returned, the parts should be well dried, and then dusted with iodoform.

A pad of cotton-wool may be placed over the anus, and be fixed in position by a T-bandage. Or in the place of the pad and bandage, a " sanitary towel " may be worn.

The pad or the towel supports the part during coughing or vomiting, absorbs any blood which may escape from the anus, keeps the buttocks apart, and prevents the involuntary straining which is common after these operations.

It may be discarded in a few days.

A morphia suppository inserted at the time of the operation is of very doubtful service. After extensive operations it is probable that but little is absorbed. Pain is much more effectually relieved by opium administered as required by the mouth or by a hypodermic injection of morphia. If no skin

r r 2

has been included in the operation area, if the sphincters have been well dilated, and if no inflammation of the anal region follows, the amount of pain may be slight. A little opium at night-time is, however, always desirable. The patient is often troubled by violent spasms—apparently of the levatores ani— which may be relieved by opium, aided, if there be no objection to the contrary, by a hot fomentation to the anus.

The patient should retain strictly the recumbent position. The anus should be washed night and morning, dried, and dusted with a little iodoform; or the part may be dressed with iodoform ointment. In some cases the patient has derived most comfort from a wet pad soaked with boracic or spirit lotion, and pressed firmly against the anus.

It is well that the bowels should not act until the morning of the fifth day. A dose of castor oil, or of any other suitable aperient, may be given, and just before the bowels act it is well to inject into the rectum some two ounces of warm olive oil. The patient may possibly take a warm hip-bath on the sixth day. The ligatures usually come away about the sixth or seventh day, and at the same time the sloughs left by the crushing or cautery operations may be expected to be expelled.

After the sixth day the bowels should be made to act every day, an aperient being administered as often as required.

Until the bowels act, the patient should be limited to a slop diet. Stimulants should be entirely avoided, except in the case of the aged or cachetic.

After the bowels have acted, the patient may commence with fish, and later with meat. A liberal allowance of fruit and of suitable vegetables will be found to be of service. In the matter of diet, the patient's own inclination and appetite are usually surer guides than certain arbitrary rules which are founded upon the tastes and powers of an abstract stomach.

It is impossible to indicate precisely the duration of the after-treatment. It will depend largely upon the extent of the operation and upon the disposition of the patient. In a case of average severity the patient will probably be moved on to a sofa on the tenth day, and will be up between the fourteenth and the twenty-first day. It is most undesirable to allow the patient to get up too soon. No one single factor in the management of the case is more likely to protract the recovery than is a too early "getting-up." Time is always a most important element in the management of operations for piles.

It is well to remember that on the second or third day after the operation some œdema of the anus is usually met with, and that this is apt to give the patient unnecessary alarm, and to induce a belief that the piles have "returned" in full force.

Undue irritation about the anus—which may in some cases be caused by iodoform—may usually be relieved by calomel ointment.

The chief complications which may occur during the after-treatment are retention of urine, hæmorrhage, tedious ulceration, and contraction of the anus.

CHAPTER II.

Operative Treatment of Fistula.

The Varieties of Fistula in Ano are conveniently divided as follows :—(1) Complete, in which there are distinct external and internal openings. (2) Blind external, in which an external opening alone exists. (In not a few of these cases there is an internal opening, but from its being very small or situated in an unexpected place, it is overlooked.) (3) Blind internal, in which the internal opening alone exists, the skin being sound.

Both the openings are usually situated within an inch of the anus, and most commonly within half an inch of that part. The external opening may be very small, may be obscured by a fold of the skin, and may only be detected by squeezing pus out of it. The tract of the sinus can often be made out as a hard cord running in the wall of the bowel.

The site of the internal opening may sometimes be detected as a slight depression or papilla, or it may be demonstrated by the probe. In any case of doubt the finger may be dried and introduced into the bowel, and retained there while a little iodine is injected into the sinus. A brown stain upon the finger would prove that an internal opening existed, although it may not have been actually demonstrated.

The examination of a fistula should be very carefully conducted ; small pliable probes should be used, and in any case of difficulty a speculum should be employed. It must never be forgotten that the connection between the mucous and muscular coats of the bowel is comparatively lax, and that a large steel director, roughly used, will pass with great readiness through the submucous tissue, and will give rise to conceptions of burrowing sinuses, which exist only as results of the surgeon's bungling.

To Percival Pott is due the credit of introducing the present method of operating. It was a common practice in his time to excise the entire sinus. It is still common to hear the uneducated classes speak of having a fistula " cut out." Pott demonstrated the possibility of curing fistula by simple incision.

Operation.—The patient is prepared in the same manner as is described in the previous chapter (page 669).

He is placed in lithotomy position, and is secured there by a Clover's crutch. It is assumed that an external opening exists. A Brodie's probe-pointed fistula director is introduced into the fistula, and is passed into the bowel through the internal opening. Not the very least force must be employed. The internal opening might have been already examined, and the passing of the probe may be carried out while a speculum keeps the inner opening in view. If the director does not easily pass, a flexible or especially bent probe may be introduced. If the probe is found to present under the thinned mucous membrane in a case in which no internal opening exists, the point of the director should be thrust through the mucous membrane at the thinnest spot. In every case, when possible, the probe should be passed while the left forefinger occupies the rectum and acts as a guide.

In a simple case in which the inner orifice is low down the point of the director may be engaged upon the top of the left forefinger (lying in the rectum), and may be cautiously brought outside the anus. Nothing then remains but to slit up the fistula with a sharp-pointed curved bistoury.

When the inner opening is high up, persistent attempts to bring the point of the director out of the anus may lead to undue laceration of the part.

In such case a plug of soft wood (a rounded piece of firewood, for example) about the size of the forefinger may be introduced into the rectum, and the probe brought into contact with it. A sharp-pointed bistoury is passed along the fistula until it enters the bowel. Its point is then driven into the wooden plug, and as the two are brought out together, the tissues which separate the length of the sinus from the bowel cavity are divided.

After the division of the fistula comes the most delicate part of the operation—the search for secondary fistulæ, for burrowing tracts, and for diverticula from the primary sinus. For this examination a speculum may be needed. Rapid sponging, a good light, and suitable probes are, however, of more value; and if the sphincter have been dilated before the cutting operation was commenced, a speculum can usually be dispensed with.

The finger should search for any tracts of indurated tissue, and the surgeon should note if the escape of a bead of pus follows pressure in any direction.

Any secondary sinuses must be treated as their condition indicates. Those which burrow beneath the mucous membrane should be slit up for their entire length. No object is gained by sparing the mucous membrane, and hesitating and incomplete incisions will nearly always be regretted. Secondary sinuses, which pass away from the rectum, may sometimes be slit up. When this involves too great a division of the soft parts, they may be freely opened into the original wound, may be dilated with dressing forceps and the finger, and well scraped with a sharp spoon or seared with the actual cautery.

All the pulpy granulation tissue which is met with about fistulæ should in every case be scraped away. The surgeon should endeavour to leave as clean and fresh a wound as possible.

In the division of the fistula the anal margin is of necessity in every case divided, and in order that the section of the muscle fibres should be as slight as possible, the knife should always cut its way into the bowel at right angles to the anal margin.

If any piles exist, they should be removed at the time of the operation, and all ill-nourished flaps and tags of inflamed and undermined skin should be cut away.

In old-standing cases, when the edges of the fistula are very indurated and callous, Salmon's "back cut" may be carried out. After the usual division of the fistula, a linear cut is made through the dense tissue of the fistula, and through that portion of the sphincter muscle which is outside the tract of the fistula.

In certain *Blind External Fistulæ* the sinus extends as far as the levator ani, and then turns abruptly away from the rectum, instead of burrowing down between the sphincters. In such cases division of the sphincter would effect no good, but the sinus, on the other hand, should be very freely laid open from the external orifice, should be scraped out, and then dressed from the bottom.

In *Blind Internal Fistulæ* the site of the threatened external opening may be indicated by a little redness of the skin, or by induration or fluctuation, or the tract of the sinus may be marked by an indurated cord.

In any such case a knife thrust through the skin at the point indicated would open the sinus, and allow of a director being introduced, and of the operation being concluded in the usual way.

Failing such indication, a speculum should be introduced, and the inner aperture sought for. When it is found, the end of a probe bent very much upon itself is introduced, and the point is made to project towards the skin. Upon this projecting point the first incision is made.

In cases of *Horseshoe Fistula*, in which an external opening on either side of the anus communicates with a single internal opening, usually at the back of the bowel, it is undesirable to cut through the sphincter on both sides. If this be done, much loss of power will result. It is better to divide the sphincter on one side, and to dilate the other side of the fistula to its utmost from the wound thus made. The cavity thus produced can then be dressed from the bottom. If, later, it should become necessary to cut through the anal margin upon the opposite side, much less loss of power results than is the case when the sphincter is divided in two places at one sitting.

When the *sinus extends far up along the bowel*, it may be possible still to slit up the undermined tissues. When, however, the thickness of the structures to be divided renders it probable that much bleeding may ensue, the knife can be carried up as far as appears desirable, and the highest part of the sinus may then be treated by means of the elastic ligature, which is introduced along the fistula by the aid of Allingham's special director.

The ligature is made of a solid cylindrical rubber cord one-tenth of an inch in diameter. It should be of good length. One end of the loop occupies the sinus, while the other hangs in the rectum. A pewter ring is then threaded

over the two ends, and as the ligature is drawn upon, the ring
is forced against the soft parts, and is made to clamp the cord
by compressing the ring with necrosis forceps. The ligature
is allowed to cut its own way out. This it will effect, on an
average, in six days.

When *multiple fistulæ* exist, burrowing in various
directions, it is well to adhere to the rule of dividing the
sphincter in one place only. The sinuses are slit up in all
directions, granulation tissue is scraped away, undermined
skin is excised, fistulæ which cannot be cut open are dilated,
scraped, and dressed from the bottom. In these cases one or
even more subsequent operations may be called for.

In *women*, Mr. Cripps points out that, owing to the
manner in which the sphincter ani and the sphincter vaginæ
decussate beneath the perineal rhaphe, a complete division of
the former muscle at the site of decussation causes loss of
the point of resistance from which it acts, and consequently a
considerable loss of power. Mr. Cripps is of opinion that the
sphincter ani should never be completely divided in this
situation.

The After-treatment.—It may almost be said that the
after-treatment of the case is of more importance than the
operation. When all bleeding has been checked, the parts
should be well dried, and a folded piece of lint, or, better
still, a strip of iodoform gauze, should then be lightly packed
into the incision. A large pad of wool is applied over the
part to maintain pressure, and to overcome any inclination to
strain, and is fixed in place by a T-bandage. This outer
dressing can be replaced later by a sanitary towel only. A
morphia suppository will be found to be of little use, and need
not be employed. In forty-eight hours the first dressing
should be removed, the part well washed, and re-dressed. The
dressing consists of a folded piece of lint or of gauze lightly
packed in the wound. It may be covered with boracic,
iodoform, or eucalyptus ointment, or be merely dusted with
iodoform.

The part should be dressed night and morning, and after
each action of the bowels. Scrupulous cleanliness must be
insisted upon. A hip-bath may be taken daily after the action
of the bowels.

The bowels should at first be kept confined, but should be opened by means of a dose of castor oil on the fourth day. It must be seen that they act regularly after this.

The discharge will be free for about the first ten days.

The dressing may need to be changed from time to time, and the lint may be soaked with sulphate of zinc lotion, with a nitrate of silver solution, with the compound tincture of benzoin, with weak iodine, or with such other drug as the surgeon employs in like cases.

The parts may be over-dressed, and the skin around be kept in a condition of irritable inflammation. Every care must be taken that the skin does not heal over prematurely, and a constant watch must be kept for burrowing sinuses and for undermining of the skin. "Pockets" for pus soon form, and good drainage should be maintained throughout.

The diet should be simple, but not meagre. Every means should be taken to improve the general health.

The operation will probably involve, in an ordinary case, confinement in bed for some fourteen days, followed by another week or so in the house. In a complex case, with many deep sinuses, the after-treatment may extend over many months. Rest is all-important, and the healing process is very distinctly retarded by too early movement. Change of air will often do more for an indolent sinus than will the most elaborate dressing. Some loss of power over the sphincter will be noticed for a little while. It is generally regained within three weeks. A permanent weakening of the anus may result, and Mr. Harrison Cripps has pointed out that in some cases this may depend upon the implication of some fibres of the sphincter in the cicatricial tissue left by the wound.

Other Methods of Operating.—Some surgeons employ specially-constructed scissors for dividing the fistula, but no particular advantage can be claimed for them.

The division of the tissues about a fistula by the thermo-cautery, the galvanic écraseur, or the wire écraseur, has little to recommend it.

The treatment of fistula by the elastic ligature has been extensively employed. It is attended by no hæmorrhage, and is best adapted for cases of deeply-extending fistulæ.

In individuals suffering from hæmophilia, I imagine that the risks of bleeding would be as great after the use of the ligature as of the knife.

The ligature is applied very tightly, and cuts its way out. Mr. Allingham states that the average time occupied in the cutting-out of the ligature is about six days. It has not been shown that the after-treatment is shortened by this method, nor that it is less painful. The method of using the elastic ligature has been already alluded to (page 681).

CHAPTER III.

OPERATIVE TREATMENT OF PROLAPSE.

IT is usual to divide prolapse of the rectum into two classes :—

The. partial form, in which the mucous membrane is alone extruded, and in which the muscular coat remains unchanged in position.

The complete form, in which all the coats of the rectum, including the peritoneal covering, are extruded, and are involved in the prolapse. The partial prolapse is usually of slight extent, and may measure but an inch or two in length. In the complete variety the protrusion is more extensive; and may measure as much as six inches, or even more.

The methods of treating prolapse by operation are numerous. Many of these have fallen entirely into disuse, while some appear to have commended themselves to few other than the actual inventors.

It is needless to describe the treatment by the injection of various fluids into the ischio-rectal fossa, nor to do more than allude to the treatment by excising elliptical folds of skin and mucous membrane from the margin of the anus. Removal of the mass by the galvanic or cold wire écraseur has not proved to be an encouraging procedure; and the same may be said of the " radical cure " by means of elastic ligatures, aided by the liberal application of chloride of zinc.

Dr. K. McLeod has carried out the operation of stitching the upper part of the rectum to the anterior abdominal parietes, a wound being made through the abdominal wall for the purpose. In the single case recorded, a good result followed this very extreme measure (*Lancet*, July 19th, 1890).

Two operations will be described—the operation by caustics or the cautery, and that by excision.

1. **The Treatment by Caustics or the Cautery.**—The bowels having been evacuated according to the method

advised in preparing a patient for operation for hæmorrhoids (page 669), the subject is placed in the lithotomy position, and the thighs are secured by a Clover's crutch.

With a little manipulation the prolapse can usually be made to protrude, or it may be drawn down with forceps. It is then well dried with cotton-wool, and is ready for the application of the caustic or cautery.

The usual caustic employed is strong nitric acid. This is painted over the whole of the exposed surface, care being taken that none of the acid touches the verge of the anus or the skin. The part is then well oiled and returned, and the rectum is lightly stuffed with wool. Outside the anus a supporting pad of wool is fixed firmly in position by a T-bandage.

If the actual cautery be employed, the iron, heated to a dull-red heat, is applied to the whole length of the prolapse, in the form of a series of lines in the long axis of the bowel. Four of such linear burns at equal distances from one another will suffice. The width of each line will be about one-fourth of an inch. The burn should be sufficiently deep to sear, but not actually destroy, the mucous membrane.

Most surgeons use Paquelin's cautery for this purpose. Mr. Cripps, however, advocates the use of the old actual cautery iron. The operation should be performed quickly, and the prolapse at once returned, before any swelling takes place.

When the prolapse cannot be readily extruded, a duck-bill speculum may be introduced into the rectum, and the mucous membrane may be then seared *in situ* along four vertical lines, each extending upwards for a distance of from two to four inches from the anus.

The After-treatment advised by Mr. Harrison Cripps should be adopted. It is described by him in the following words :—

" A thick india-rubber tube, with a third of an inch calibre, seven inches in length, is passed up the bowel for about five inches. Strips of oiled lint are then arranged round the interior of the bowel, extending as high as possible. Cotton-wool thoroughly well dusted with iodoform is then evenly and carefully packed into the bowel between the tube in the centre and the oiled lint on the sides. This gives a firm, even support to the lower few inches of the bowel, while the escape of flatus, etc., is provided for by the tube. The success of the operation depends on the care that is taken to prevent the descent of the bowel during the early stages of healing, before the adhesions have become firm. After forty-eight hours the whole dressing is gently removed, the part thoroughly washed, and a clean dressing replaced. The desire to strain has generally passed off by this time, and it does not seem necessary to pass the dressing far up the bowel. After the first few days internal dressings can be dispensed with, but the tube, cleaned daily, is kept in for ten days or more. It allows the easy passage of flatus without straining effort. By a small nightly dose of opium the bowels can be kept confined for ten days. Small doses of castor oil can then be given, together with an enema if necessary. The patient must on no account sit up or strain, and the motion is to be passed lying on the side, and the anus drawn up a little from the middle line; and this should be enforced for at least six weeks, whilst consolidation is taking place, otherwise the whole advantages of the operation may be lost."

2. **The Treatment by Excision.**—This operation may be illustrated by two actual cases—one of partial and the other of complete prolapse, both treated by excision.

I have given an account of this operation, with three illustrative cases, in a paper published in the *Lancet* for March 1st, 1890. Cases of excision of the prolapsed bowel have been reported by Mr. S. Partridge, Mr. Raye, and others. (See *Indian Annals of Medical Science*, No. xxvii., page 237; and *Lancet*, July 10th, 1886.)

Case of Partial Prolapse.—Man aged thirty-seven; length of prolapse five inches. The patient was prepared as for the operation for piles, was placed in lithotomy position, and secured by Clover's crutch. The buttocks were well raised, partly for the purpose of bringing the region in more convenient position for operation, and partly that the coils of small intestine might be to some extent withdrawn from the pelvic floor in the event of there being any protrusion of the peritoneum. The first step of the operation consisted in demonstrating the full extent of the prolapse. The mucous

membrane within the lumen of the prolapse was seized, at
some height above the aperture in the bowel, with tongue
forceps, and pulled down. Three pairs of such forceps were
employed, and were applied at different points on the rectal
wall; and when it was evident that the whole of the relaxed
mucous membrane was entirely drawn down, the forceps were
allowed to remain attached. They served to indicate the real
apex of the protrusion, and to allow a hold to be taken of the
part, while their weight prevented any great recession of the
everted mucous membrane.

I now made a circular cut around the base of the prolapse,
at the exact spot where the skin joined the mucous membrane. The incision involved the mucous membrane only.
This mucous membrane I next proceeded to dissect off, turning the whole of it down like a cuff.

It was dissected up with scissors and forceps only. When
the separation was complete, the prolapse had an hour-glass
shape, the waist of the hour-glass corresponding to the site of
the apex of the protrusion. Nothing but a raw surface was
visible, and the prolapse was, of course, doubled in length.
The bleeding was quite insignificant. The object of this dissection was to clearly demonstrate the nature of the tissues
forming the prolapse, which were about to be excised.
Both sphincters could be defined. I now introduced my left
forefinger into the lumen of the prolapse, and ascertained that
the protrusion was composed of mucous membrane only. The
layer of mucous membrane—the inner layer—I next divided
at the level of the anus with scissors. As each inch or so
was divided, the cut margin was seized with pressure forceps.
This allowed of the immediate arrest of all bleeding, and also
prevented the mucous membrane from being withdrawn into
the rectum. The prolapse was in this way completely excised,
and some six or eight pressure forceps were left attached to
the cut mucous membrane of the rectum. The forceps were
removed, bleeding points were ligatured, and the mucous
membrane was then attached to the skin at the margin of the
anus with sutures of silkworm gut. Eight vessels were ligatured, and fifteen sutures were applied.

The part was dressed with wool dusted with iodoform.
The bowels were opened on the fifth day; the sutures were

removed on the tenth. At the end of four weeks the parts were sound, and the function of the anus entirely restored.

Case of Complete Prolapse.—Man aged thirty-six; prolapse measured five inches in length. Its circumference at the base was no less than ten and a half inches. The operation was commenced in the manner already described. The mucous membrane forming the outer wall of the prolapse was separated all round, as in the above case, the knife traversing the skin close to its line of junction with the mucous membrane. The protrusion, quite bared of mucous membrane, was now exposed.

It felt hard and firm, except at its anterior part, close to the anus. Here there was evidence of a protrusion of peritoneum. The wall of the cone was at this point flaccid, and compared very markedly with the firm wall presented by the rest of the prolapse. The buttocks had been well raised, to hinder the protrusion of any coils of small intestine, and no evidence of such a hernia existed. I then cut across the prolapse at the level of the anus—*i.e.*, at the very base of the cone. I divided the anterior wall first, and opened the peritoneal cavity ; the opening was at once plugged with a sponge. The rest of the prolapse was then severed rapidly with scissors in the manner already described. The peritoneal wound was closed by seven points of the finest catgut. The divided end of the bowel was then attached to the margin of the anus, all hæmorrhage having been arrested. The sutures involved the skin, the whole thickness of the wall of the rectum, and as much as possible of the subcutaneous structures about the anus. Silkworm gut was employed. The bowels were opened on the seventh day ; no sutures were removed until the thirteenth day. The patient got up on the nineteenth day. The wound healed soundly, without a drop of pus. Control over the anus was slowly regained, and the patient was discharged " cured " at the end of six weeks.

Comment.—Of the value of the measures above described considerable differences of opinion have been expressed. A valuable article upon this subject, by Mr. Harrison Cripps, will be found in the *Lancet* for October 11th, 1890.

Speaking from my own experience of these operations, I would venture the opinion that the treatment by strong nitric acid is barbarous and uncouth, and a survival of the surgery of past ages. It is very painful. It has been followed by sloughing and acute inflammation of the rectum, and has led to severe, and even fatal, hæmorrhage, and also to stricture.

The after-treatment, moreover, is apt to be protracted, and, indeed, Mr. Cripps alludes to a case in which it extended over four months.

The treatment by means of the actual cautery is highly commended by so sound an authority as Mr. Cripps. This measure appears to be well enough suited to mild forms of the trouble which have resisted all modes of treatment short of those by operation. The measure is painful, a severe degree of inflammation is excited, some sloughing is inevitable, and the special dangers of a burn are introduced. A long confinement in bed is also necessary.

For severe cases, I would venture to think that the treatment by excision is distinctly the best.

A clean incision is made, the operation area is reduced to a minimum, no damaged bowel is left in the pelvis, hæmorrhage may be rendered practically impossible, and the after-treatment is of comparatively short duration.

Inasmuch as the parts are cleanly excised, and as the whole of the operation is conducted without the anus, the risk of subsequent stricture must be exceedingly small.

691

CHAPTER IV.

EXCISION OF THE RECTUM.

EXCISION of the rectum, or proctectomy, is carried out in certain cases of malignant disease involving the anus or lower part of the rectum. The term is a little misleading, inasmuch as the rectum is never excised, but only a comparatively small part of it. The cases suited for this mode of treatment must be most carefully selected. They will be found to be comparatively few in number, and the indiscriminate practice of the operation has done much to bring proctectomy into disrepute.

The growth should be of recent origin and of limited extent, be capable of being entirely isolated, and of being removed together with a not inconsiderable portion of the adjacent bowel. It must of necessity be free from attachments, and still limited, so far as palpation can testify, to the wall of the rectum. The patient should be in good health.

The best results follow—other things being equal—when the growth is upon the posterior wall of the gut.

The amount that may be safely excised cannot be estimated by anatomical data. Very rarely does the excised portion measure more than three inches in length.

If much more of the bowel has to be excised, the case must be one of so extensive a growth as to raise the question as to whether the operation is justifiable. In no case should the peritoneum be deliberately opened, or a portion of the vagina, or bladder, or prostate excised. Experience has condemned these extensive operations. If the malignant growth has reached the peritoneum, or has even approached very near to it, and if it has invaded any of the adjacent viscera, it may be safe to say that it is of such extent as to render an operation conducted upon sound surgical bases an actual impossibility.

The operation was originally performed by Faget in 1763. It was, however, little noticed by surgeons until the procedure was revived by Lisfranc in 1830.

Among the earlier operators were Velpeau, Recamier, and Chassaignac. The operation underwent a rapid development in the hands of German and French surgeons, but it was regarded with some suspicion in England until the matter was elaborately reviewed by Mr. Harrison Cripps in an admirable essay written in 1876.

Since this time excision of the rectum has become an established operation in a certain series of selected cases.

The operation described below is founded upon that originally performed by Lisfranc. It has undergone many modifications, and has been the subject of many improvements; and among those who have been especially concerned in the elaboration of the operation, as it is now usually carried out, must be mentioned the names of Denonvillier and Harrison Cripps.

Instruments Required.—Clover's crutch; curved sharp-pointed bistoury; straight probe-pointed bistoury; scalpels; straight blunt-pointed scissors; scissors curved on the flat; two pairs of volsella forceps; dissecting forceps; a liberal supply of pressure forceps; artery forceps; sponges in holders; rectum speculum; syringe; Paquelin's cautery; ligatures.

Curved needles in holders may be required.

The Operation.—The patient is prepared in the manner described on page 669, is anæsthetised, and is placed in the lithotomy position, the lower limbs being secured by means of Clover's crutch.

A good light is required, and at least one thoroughly efficient assistant. The left forefinger is passed into the rectum, and the position of the coccyx is defined; a curved sharp-pointed bistoury is now introduced into the rectum by the side of the left finger, and is made to cut directly backwards and precisely in the median line. In this way all the soft parts between the rectum and the coccyx are cleanly and completely divided. The lateral incisions are now made. The position of each will depend upon the distance between the growth and the margin of the anus. Whenever possible, these lateral incisions should be made through the mucous membrane. When the growth actually reaches the anus, they must of necessity be made through the skin.

Each incision is commenced behind, at the posterior wound already made, and is carried boldly into the ischiorectal fossa. The corresponding buttock is steadied and held aside as the cut is being made. All bleeding points are at once seized with pressure forceps.

The finger, thrust into the incision on each side, will readily separate the rectum, except at the insertion of the levator ani. The fibres of that muscle must be divided with scissors. The two lateral incisions are crescentic, and are so carried round the bowel as to meet in front. As each one is finished, and as the separation on each side and behind is completed, the deep wound outside the rectum thus left by the scalpel and the finger is plugged with a sponge.

The lateral and posterior parts of the rectum are thus freed.

The next step is the difficult one of separating the bowel from its anterior connections. In the case of a male subject, this is much facilitated by having a full-sized catheter passed into the urethra, and held in the position of the staff in lithotomy. In the female, the finger introduced from time to time into the vagina will afford valuable guidance. The portion of the bowel already detached is held by an assistant, who draws it downwards. The surgeon proceeds to separate the gut from its anterior connections by means of blunt-pointed scissors, aided by the left forefinger. A digital examination per rectum and per vaginam from time to time will assist in estimating the position of the line of separation.

When the rectum has been freed all round well above the upper limits of the disease, the gut is cut across transversely by scissors. The division should be made cautiously and in sections, and all bleeding vessels are secured at once with pressure forceps. These forceps serve also to maintain a hold upon the divided intestinal wall. The wound cavity is now syringed out and dried. The sponges in the ischiorectal fossa are removed, and the vessels held by the pressure forceps are secured as required; some will have been already closed by pressure, others can be dealt with by torsion, and the remainder by ligature.

The hæmorrhage varies a great deal; but as the chief bleeding vessels are situated in the wall of the bowel, they are readily secured. Such venous oozing as exists will usually yield to pressure, and in any case will cease, more or less completely, when the body is put out of the lithotomy position.

The use of the cautery should be avoided whenever possible. It obscures the anatomical details of the parts, involves sloughing, and necessitates much after-contraction of the wound.

Much difference of opinion exists as to the manner in which the operation should be completed. Volkmann and others advise that the mucous membrane should be drawn down, and attached to the skin at the anal margin by means of a close row of sutures. Harrison Cripps strongly condemns this proceeding. He states that the stitches are sure to give way; that so long as they hold they prevent a free discharge from the wound, and permit spaces to form outside the bowel.

Those who advise the suturing of the divided parts claim that the wound surface is thus greatly diminished, that the duration of the after-treatment is shortened, and that the tendency to stricture is obviated. That the slow closure of a long tract in the rectum by the process of granulation may lead to stricture cannot be denied.

Ball points out that a great deal depends upon the manner in which the sutures are introduced. If the skin and the margin of the gut be merely sutured together, then pouches will certainly form outside the bowel, and the hold of the sutures will be slight. If, on the other hand, the threads be passed deeply through the surrounding pelvic structures as well as through the skin and mucous membrane, then the stitches will be scarcely able to cut their way out, and no pockets for pus can be left outside the bowel.

In connection with this subject, it is impossible to avoid drawing attention to the excellent results obtained by Mr. Cripps, which compare very favourably with the results obtained by many German surgeons who carry out the plan of suturing.

The operation as above described applies to the removal

of the whole circumference of the bowel. It differs in no essential particular when a part only of the circumference is removed.

It is needless to say that no more should be removed than is consistent with a free, complete, and proper excision of the growth, and that the preservation of any part of the anal margin is always desirable.

For these partial operations, which are often more difficult than the complete procedure, a large duck-bill speculum will as a rule be found useful.

The median posterior incision should always be made whenever the growth approaches· the hinder wall of the bowel. It must be confessed that the results of the partial operations have not been very satisfactory, and the surgeon must feel perfectly confident in the wisdom of the course he has marked out before he proceeds to remove the growth, and to leave a considerable part of the circumference of the bowel behind.

If, however, only a little of the anal margin can be preserved, the amount of the after-contraction is considerably lessened.

The After-treatment.—The parts should be well dried, and then freely dusted with iodoform. A pad of wool is placed over the anus, and retained in position by a T-bandage. This pad is only of service to support the perineum, and to absorb such blood and fæcal matter as escape.

No rectal plug is necessary, nor is there any advantage in inserting a tube. The anus will be found to be patulous enough. Pain may be relieved by hypodermic injections of morphia.

There will probably be retention of urine.

The patient should lie upon the back, with the shoulders well raised, and every facility should be afforded for free drainage.

After the first twenty-four hours the T-bandage may be discarded, and the discharge collected by a large pad of cotton-wool placed beneath the buttocks. Any bandage only tends to retain discharge, and to prevent ready access to the parts. On, or soon after, the third day the discharge from the wound will probably be copious.

The after-treatment consists in the most scrupulous cleanliness. The case will require the exclusive services of one or possibly two nurses. The wound should be irrigated with a warm weak antiseptic solution every three or four hours. This should be directed upon the part by an irrigator throwing a large and gentle stream. The fluid is collected in a kidney-shaped receiver, or is allowed to escape through such a hole in the bed as is provided in certain special beds for fractured thigh.

After each washing, the part is dried and dusted with iodoform, creolin powder, or like application. It should be a matter of duty with the nurse that no smell arises from the wound.

If the bowels do not act spontaneously, an aperient may be given on the fifth or sixth day.

The parts must be irrigated after each action of the bowels.

As soon as the patient is able, the use of a daily hip-bath will be found of service, so long as care is taken that no muscular effort is made by the patient in moving into or from the bath.

The patient should keep in bed until the deep part of the wound is sound, and the surface portion is granulating.

At the end of two or three weeks the rectum should be examined for stricture. If any evidence of narrowing be forthcoming, a bougie should be introduced, and should be subsequently passed every other day, so that any further contraction may be prevented. The use of the bougie may have to be continued occasionally for many months after the operation.

The incontinence of fæces and flatus is at first absolute, but after a period of from eight to ten weeks some control over the anus returns. In thirty-six recorded cases collected by Mr. Cripps, defæcation became normal in twenty-three instances; fæces could be retained, when not too fluid, in six cases; and in only seven instances did the inconvenience persist.

Results.—Mr. Ball, in his admirable work on "The Rectum and Anus," has collected 175 cases of excision of the rectum, which show a mortality of 16·5 per cent. Mr. Cripps has performed the operation in thirty cases, with only two deaths—a death-rate of less than 7 per cent.

In general terms it may be claimed for the operation that in those who recover from the immediate effects it prolongs life and increases the patient's comfort. With regard to the question of cure, the operation of excision of the rectum occupies the same position as is held by like operations for malignant disease. Cases of cure—or, rather, of non-recurrence of the growth after periods of years—are reported, and also many instances in which the progress of the disease has been distinctly arrested. As in other parts of the body, these successes depend upon early operation, complete removal, ready healing of the wound, and good health in the patient.

Part XV.

OPERATIONS ON THE HEAD AND SPINE.

CHAPTER I.

OPERATIONS ON THE SKULL AND BRAIN.

THE operations here dealt with include those carried out for the relief of depressed or splintered fracture of the skull, for the evacuation of pus or blood between the dura mater and the bone, for the removal of cerebral tumours, for the evacuation of abcesses of the encephalon, and for the removal of foreign bodies (such as bullets) from within the skull.

No especial description is needed of the operation carried out in certain cases of epilepsy.

In the present category is included the operation of opening the frontal sinuses, and of trephining the antrum of the mastoid.

The term trephining is not used always in a very precise sense. In the operation which is usually termed "trephining for depressed fracture of the skull" the trephine is, in many cases, not used, but the necessary opening in the skull is made by removing loose fragments, or by cutting away projecting parts of the bone with Hey's saw, the chisel, or the rongeur.

The various operations which are now performed upon the brain constitute one of the most remarkable elements in the surgery of the century.

Anatomical Points. — *Position of the Sutures.* — The bregma, or point of junction of the coronal and sagittal sutures, is in a line drawn vertically upwards from a point just in front of the external auditory meatus, the head being in normal position. The lambda, or point of junction of the

lambdoid and sagittal sutures, lies in the middle line, about
two inches and three-quarters above the occipital protuberance. The lambdoid suture is fairly represented by the
upper two-thirds of a line drawn from the lambda to the
apex of the mastoid process.

The coronal suture lies along a line drawn from the bregma
to the middle of the zygomatic arch. On this line, at a spot
about on a level with the external angular process of the
frontal bone, and about one inch and a half behind that
process, is the pterion. The summit of the squamous suture
is one inch and three-quarters above the zygoma.

The Thickness of the Skull varies greatly, not only in
different parts of the same skull, but also in corresponding
parts in different individuals. The average thickness is one-fifth of an inch. The thickest parts are at the occipital protuberance (where the section may measure half an inch), the
mastoid process, and the lower part of the frontal bone. The
bone over the inferior occipital fossæ is very thin, while it is
thinnest over the squamous bone. Here the bone may be no
thicker in parts than a visiting-card. The skull is also
thinned over the sinuses and the grooves for the meningeal
vessels. It is important to remember in trephining that the
inner table is not always parallel with the outer.

The Middle Meningeal Artery is a frequent source of
bleeding after fracture of the skull. The vessel having passed
through the foramen spinosum, divides into two branches : the
anterior—the larger—runs upwards across the anterior inferior angle of the parietal bone : the posterior runs backwards,
with a horizontal sweep, across the squamous bone.

The branches of the artery are more frequently ruptured
than the trunk, and a laceration of the vessel as it crosses the
anterior angle of the parietal bone is very common.

The Relations of the Brain to the Skull.—Into this
subject it is unnecessary to enter in a book like the present.
It is needless to say that in dealing with troubles involving
the brain very precise localisation is all-essential.

The diagram shown in Fig. 416 depicts the relations of the
chief sutures and convolutions, as defined by Dr. Reid. As
in the following pages allusion will often be made to " Reid's
base line," it may be said that this is a line drawn across the

skull from the inferior margin of the orbit backwards through the centre of the external auditory meatus (Fig. 416).

The positions of the two great fissures may be indicated. *The Fissure of Sylvius.*—A line is drawn from a point one

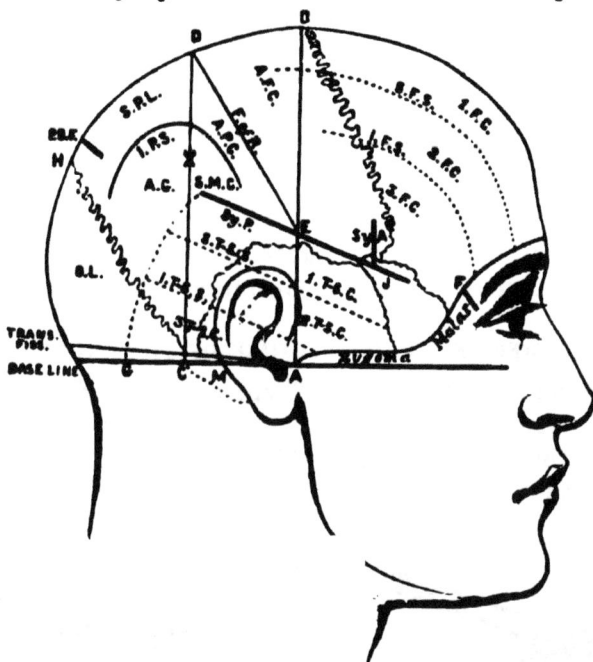

Fig. 416.—DIAGRAM TO SHOW THE RELATIONS OF THE BRAIN TO THE SKULL. (*Modified from Reid.*)

F.R, coronal suture; B, bregma; F, external angular process; H. lambda; H.C, lambdoid suture; J, pterion; M, mastoid process; X, parietal eminence; SY.A, SY.P, anterior and posterior limbs of Sylvian fissure; F. of R, fissure of Rolando; A.F.C, A.P.C, ascending frontal and ascending parietal convolutions; S.F.S, I.F.S, superior and inferior frontal sulci; 1 F.C, 2 F.C, 3 F.C, frontal convolutions; S.T-S.S, superior and inferior temporo-sphenoidal sulci; 1 T-S.C, 2 T-S.C, 3 T-S.C, temporo-sphenoidal convolutions; I.P.S, intraparietal suture; S.P.L, superior parietal lobule; S.M.C, supramarginal convolution; A.G, angular gyrus; P.O.F, parieto-occipital fissure; O.L, occipital lobe.

inch and a quarter behind the external angular process (Fig. 416, F) to a point three-quarters of an inch below the most prominent part of the parietal eminence (x). The first three-quarters of an inch of the line will represent the main fissure, and the rest of the line will indicate the horizontal limb. The ascending limb will start from the anterior end of the line indicating the main fissure, and run vertically upwards for about one inch (Fig. 416, SY.A).

The Fissure of Rolando.—From the base line draw two vertical lines upwards—one (Fig. 416, A B) from the depression in front of the meatus, and another (C D) from the posterior border of the mastoid process at its root. There is thus formed a four-sided figure, bounded above and below by the median line and the horizontal limb of the Sylvian fissure respectively, and in front and behind by the two vertical lines. A diagonal line (D E) drawn from the posterior superior angle to the anterior inferior angle of the space will be over the fissure of Rolando.

The situation of the chief convolutions is indicated in Fig. 416. In this matter the surgeon should consult Professor A. Frazer's admirable " Guide to Operations on the Brain."

TREPHINING IN FRACTURE OF THE SKULL.

Instruments Required.—Trephines of various sizes; a quill; a trephine brush; a pair of Hey's saws; a small pair of bone-cutting forceps; slender chisel and mallet; a pair of gouge forceps, such as Hopkins's rongeur (Fig. 417); an elevator; periosteal rugine; necrosis forceps; scalpels; dissecting, pressure, and artery forceps; scissors; dressing forceps; fine-toothed forceps, and fine scissors for the dura mater;

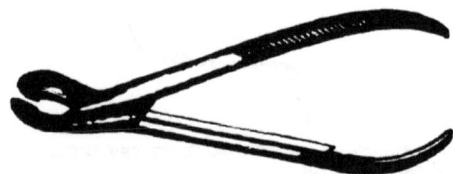

Fig. 417.—HOPKINS'S RONGEUR.

small tenaculum or slender curved needle in a handle for bleeding vessels; probe; needles and sutures.

Trephines are made in various sizes; one with a crown three-quarters of an inch in diameter is the most convenient. The so-called " old-pattern " trephine is shown in Fig. 418. It is the form of instrument still usually employed in Great Britain. American surgeons largely employ the conical trephine or Galt's trephine (Fig. 419). It is claimed that the instrument is steadier and safer, since it is almost impossible for it to be driven on to the brain when the last portions of the inner table give way unexpectedly. This accident has happened with the old-pattern trephine. Horsley employs a trephine for operations upon the brain which is provided with a very convenient handle. It has also such a thin cutting edge that the buttons of bone when replaced fit much better than when cut by the more substantial instrument.

The rongeur is of great service in cutting away projecting rims of bone, and in smoothing sharp edges.

A fine chisel may be employed for the same purposes by those who are familiar with the use of this instrument.

All the instruments must be scrupulously clean, and are

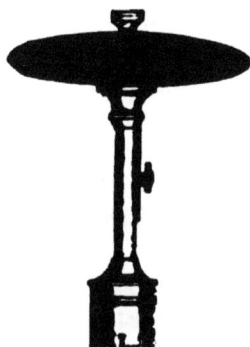

Fig. 418.—OLD-PATTERN TREPHINE. Fig. 419.—CONICAL TREPHINE.

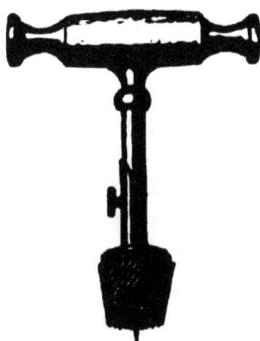

placed in a tray containing a 1 in 20 solution of carbolic acid some little time before the operation is commenced.

Preparation of the Patient.—The head is shaved, then washed with soap and water, and scrubbed with a nail-brush. It is next washed with ether, and finally with a 1 in 20 solution of carbolic acid. Lint soaked in this solution is placed over the scalp, and is kept moistened and in place until the surgeon is ready. In operations that are not of an urgent character this cap of carbolised lint should be worn for some twelve hours before the operation. Such preparation is possible in most cases of operation upon the brain.

The head is conveniently supported upon a sand-bag covered with thin macintosh sheeting.

Chloroform will be the anæsthetic probably selected. In some cases of depressed fracture no anæsthetic is required.

The Operation.—When any wound already exists, the fracture is exposed by enlarging it as required. When the scalp is sound, a semilunar flap may be raised, the free end of which points vertically downwards. It should form a shallow curve, and be so planned as to avoid the main scalp arteries.

Or a V-shaped incision may be employed, with the apex of the V pointing downwards. In any case, the flap should be of ample size. The old-fashioned crucial incision is most inconvenient. Four small flaps result, which have to be held out of the way, and the after-adjustment of the wound is tedious and complex.

A weak part will be left where the four flaps meet, and this spot will probably be just over the centre of the fracture.

The incision should be carried at once down to the bone, and the pericranium having been detached with a curved rugine, the flap as it is turned up will be composed of all the soft parts covering the skull.

A long silk suture should be inserted into the free end or apex of the flap, and by means of this thread the flap is drawn up, and held out of the way.

The bleeding from the scalp tissues is usually free. The more conspicuous bleeding points are neatly secured by pressure forceps ; sponge pressure will check mere oozing.

The fracture is now exposed and examined. It may be found to be at once possible to introduce an elevator beneath the depressed bone, and to elevate it. Fragments at the same time may often be readily removed by means of dressing forceps or necrosis forceps.

In other cases a rim of projecting bone—belonging to the sound part of the skull—may be removed with a narrow chisel and mallet, or with Hey's saw, or with the gouge forceps, and a little space is at once provided between the bones which will allow of an elevator being introduced. In raising the depressed bone, it is needless to say that the elevator must be supported upon the sound part of the skull.

Sometimes when the bone is much comminuted one fragment will be found to be so tilted outwards that it can be seized and removed, and through the gap thus left the elevator or the blade of the dressing forceps or necrosis forceps can be introduced.

In a comparatively few cases the trephine will be needed. The centre-pin of the instrument is protruded about one-sixteenth or one-tenth of an inch, and is firmly fixed by the screw; the crown is then applied to the sound bone near to the fracture. As a rule, it is so applied that two-thirds or three-fourths of the circle will be upon the sound skull, and the remaining third or fourth over the fractured area. The trephine should not be placed so far over the injured area as to produce trouble by jarring any fragment which may be lying in contact with the dura mater.

The point is bored into the bone, and then the trephine is made to cut into the skull by light sharp movements from left to right, and from right to left.

At first the instrument may be steadied by the left fore-finger, which rests upon the skull. As soon as a groove has been cut all round, the pin may be withdrawn, and the instrument will be found to maintain a steady hold of the part. The pressure must be evenly maintained throughout, and will be found to be chiefly exercised when the hand is turned from left to right (the supination movement). At first the bone-dust is dry, but as soon as the dense outer table is cut through it becomes soft and bloody. As the trephine enters the diploë the softer character of the resisting medium is at once recognised.

The wound in the bone must be kept constantly clear of dust by frequent irrigation, and the use of the trephine-brush or the quill. The trephine itself is rinsed in a warm carbolic solution from time to time, to free it from *débris*. Those who have only experimented with the dry skull of the cadaver will be surprised at the ready manner in which the trephine cuts its way into the living bone. The depth of the groove in the skull must be estimated from time to time with the quill. Inasmuch as the skull is spheroidal, it is exceedingly difficult to make the groove of equal depth all round. The shallower parts must be especially cut down to the level of the deeper parts, by bearing pressure upon the bone at the points where the division has been less complete. As the inner table is penetrated, increased caution must be exercised, and still more care is needed when once the groove has been ex-tended right through the skull. It must be remembered that the bone will probably be of unequal thickness even over the small area covered by the trephine.

When the groove is of sufficient depth, the disc of bone

t t

may be removed by gently rocking the trephine to and fro
while it is still in position, or by cautiously introducing an
elevator at a spot where the bone is entirely divided. Not
infrequently the disc of bone can be grasped with forceps,
and lifted out. In any case, some little portion of the inner
table will have to be broken through.

Should any portions of the inner table be left behind,
they can be removed by the elevator or the cutting gouge.

In removing large discs of bone it is important that the
dura mater be carefully stripped from the inner table as the
button is being cautiously lifted up with the elevator.

The trephine disc, as well as any fragments of bone subsequently removed, should be at once put in a china receptacle
containing a warm solution of corrosive sublimate (1 in 2,000),
and maintained at a temperature of 100° F.

In the case of a punctured fracture it is well to employ an
inch trephine, and to let the pin of the instrument fall near to
the puncture, in order that the whole of the damaged area
may be removed, and the possibly wide-spreading com-
minution of the inner table be fully exposed.

If in any case the hole made is not sufficient for the
purpose, it may be enlarged by means of Hey's saw, the
rongeur, the chisel, or a fresh application of a smaller trephine
to an adjacent segment of bone.

In all cases every splinter and loose fragment of bone must
be cautiously removed. Depressed fragments which still
retain a hold upon the sound bone are left in position after
they have been elevated.

The edges of the opening in the bone are finally smoothed
off with the rongeur or the file edge of the elevator.

The treatment of any hæmorrhage that may arise is dealt
with on page 707.

The trephine disc, and any other fragments of bone which
have been preserved, are replaced as near as possible *in situ.*

Should they be too small to fill up the gap, they may be
perforated with the centre-pin of the trephine, placed with one
portion of their edge in contact with the sound bone, and
sutured to the scalp by passing a catgut thread through the
perforation, as advised by Dr. W. Keen. If a large gap be
still left after the adjustment of the available fragments, some

surgeons recommend the pulverising of the smaller bone fragments, and the dusting of them over the exposed dura mater.

The flap or flaps of scalp are now brought into place by silkworm-gut sutures, and drainage is secured by introducing a bunch of fine catgut threads here and there between the stitches. The skin is well cleansed, a moist sponge, dusted with iodoform, is placed over the part, to keep the catgut drains moist, and to absorb any discharge; and over this may be placed a pad of gauze which has been wrung out in a suitable antiseptic solution. The whole dressing is secured by means of a tight flannel bandage. If small drainage-tubes or half drainage-tubes be employed in the place of catgut drains, a dry dressing, composed of Tillmann's linen or of cotton-wool, may be employed. When many fragments of bone have been replaced in the skull wound, drainage with catgut is safer.

Complications.—When the dura mater has been wounded, it should be carefully sutured with the finest catgut whenever possible.

Hæmorrhage throughout the course of the operation may be free, but it seldom gives much trouble. Oozing from the diploë, as a rule, soon ceases spontaneously. Should one of the diploic veins have been cut across, and bleed persistently, in spite of sponge pressure, a little of the bone tissue around the divided vessel may be crushed into the mouth of the opening by means of the point of an elevator. Bleeding from the dura mater, if obstinate, may need to be checked by a fine catgut ligature. The vessel will have to be picked up, most probably, by means of a delicate tenaculum.

Hæmorrhage from the middle meningeal artery is dealt with on page 709.

If bleeding take place from a sinus, pressure should at once be applied by means of a piece of fine Turkey sponge or lint. Mr. Jacobson points out that bleeding from even a large venous sinus is readily arrested by quite moderate pressure. The piece of sponge or lint may need to be kept in position for some time, and in extreme cases has been left *in situ* for two or three days. In several instances hæmorrhage from a sinus has been arrested by lateral ligatures, and cases are recorded in which lacerations of both the superior longitudinal

t t 2

sinus and of the lateral sinus have been successfully treated
by these means.

"Certain precautions must be observed," writes Dr. Nancrede, "when the fracture is near a sinus which we suspect
has been wounded by depressed fragments. Thus the
trephine-cut must be planned so as to give access to any
bleeding point rather than merely to admit easy elevation of
the fragments. One is often tempted to draw out a long fragment driven some distance beneath sound bone, whose concealed extremity lies in close proximity to a large sinus,
possibly wounding it. . . . In such case it is far safer to
trephine over the site of the concealed extremity of bone,
when, if its withdrawal is followed by hæmorrhage from a
wound of the sinus, instant compression may be effected."

When in certain cases—probably cases of operation for
disease—it appears imperative to trephine over a sinus, two
smaller trephine discs should be removed from either side
of the sinus, and the intervening bridge of bone be then
cautiously cut away.

The After-treatment is considered on page 718.

TREPHINING FOR MIDDLE MENINGEAL HÆMORRHAGE.

The whole subject of hæmorrhage from the middle meningeal artery has been thoroughly dealt with by **Mr. Jacobson in**
a most able article published in the *Guy's Hospital Reports*
for 1886. So far as operative interference is concerned in
cases of intra-cranial hæmorrhage, it is practically limited to
blood collections arising from rupture of this artery.

The artery crosses the anterior inferior angle of the parietal
bone at a point one inch and a half behind the external
angular process of the frontal bone, and one inch and three-
quarters above the zygoma. These measurements apply to
the adult skull. Mr. Jacobson advises that the centre of the
wound made for the trephine should be on a spot one inch
and a half behind the external angular process, and one inch
above the zygoma.

Kronlein recommends the following guides for the application of the trephine (*Deutsche Zeitschrift für Chirurgie*,
1886, *Hefte* 3 *und* 4). Unless specially contra-indicated by
some very decided localising symptoms, which point to a

collection of blood pressing upon a definite centre, the trephine-holes should be determined as follows:—A line is drawn around the skull at the level of the upper margin of the orbit, and is throughout parallel with Reid's base line (Fig. 420). (*See* also page 701.) The trephine is first placed at a spot upon this line, which is from one inch and a quarter to one inch and a half, according to age and the size of the head, behind the external angular process of the frontal bone (Fig. 420, A).

Should the opening reveal no blood clot and no bleeding vessel, a second trephine-hole is made upon the same line, just below the parietal eminence, and at a point where a vertical line, carried up from the posterior border of the mastoid process, bisects the horizontal line already indicated (Fig. 420, B).

When any external injury or fracture of the skull exists, this should be first explored. The hæmorrhage will very probably be found beneath the damaged bone, and one operation may suffice to elevate depressed fragments, and to allow extravasated blood to escape.

In many cases no anæsthetic is required.

The operation of opening the skull is carried out precisely in the manner already indicated.

The clot, when exposed, is removed by forceps, or a small scoop, aided by free irrigation.

If bleeding continue, any accessible vessels in the dura mater should be secured by catgut ligatures, passed by means of a fine curved needle. Single bleeding points have been checked by a touch from a red-hot probe. Bleeding from the trunk of the middle meningeal artery, as it lies in its bony canal, may be arrested by plugging the canal with wax or a little strip of gauze, or a thread of catgut well softened.

More general oozing, or such hæmorrhage as arises from inaccessible sources, may be dealt with by the application of ice to the skull, or by pressure maintained by plugging the wound with antiseptic gauze. In a few instances a ligature of the external or common carotid artery has been deemed necessary, and has been carried out with success.

The operation is concluded as already described. The question of drainage is alluded to on page 707. It is possible,

according to Fluhrer, rebounds at an angle equalling that of incidence, and becomes embedded in the brain about one inch above, below, in front of, or behind the point of bone struck, according to the direction pursued by the ball. If the probe show that the cerebral mass has been completely traversed, and that the ball has struck the bone, a large counter-opening is to be made, the membranes carefully incised, and the ball first sought for in the positions which the above-mentioned rule of Fluhrer would indicate. If neither ecchymosis nor a deeper-seated hardness indicate the presence of the missile

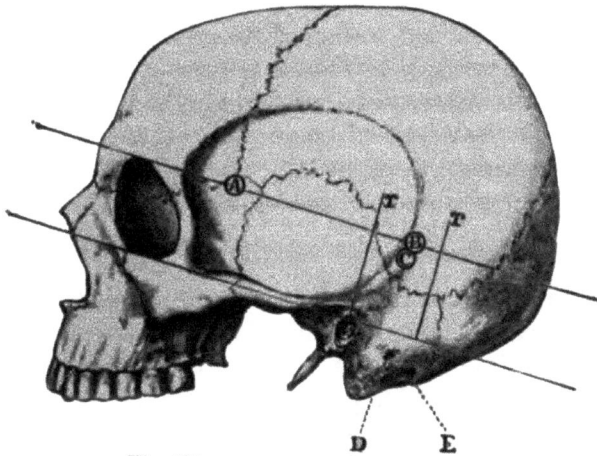

Fig. 420.—POINTS FOR TREPHINING.
A, B, spots for trephining in middle meningeal hæmorrhage ; c, spot for trephining in abscess of the temporo-sphenoidal lobe ; E, spot for trephining n abscess of the cerebellum ; D, mastoid foramen. (*After Nancrede.*)

at this point, careful methodical search must be made in various directions, remembering the possibility of the ball having lost so much of its initial velocity that, instead of penetrating the brain by its rebound, it may be merely lying between the dura mater and the cerebrum, from which point it may gravitate out of reach, if the brain be carelessly depressed or manipulated. In other words, the periphery of the space exposed by the elevation of the membrane should be carefully scrutinised, unless local ecchymosis or manifest penetration of the brain exists.

" When the ball has been found and extracted, and its track carefully disinfected, there remains only the drainage of passage made by the missile.

" A fine antiseptic thread is to be attached to one end of the gravity probe, when the opposite extremity must be introduced at the wound entrance, and the instrument withdrawn through the trephine opening, leaving the thread in the ball track. By attaching a fine rubber drainage-tube to this thread, the tube can be readily drawn through the track."

The flaps of scalp tissue are now brought into place, and the operation completed as already described (page 707).

Should the ball not be discovered, the exploration will have at least provided for efficient drainage, and for the disinfection of the track made in the brain. In straightforward cases, where the ball is found but a short distance beneath the skull, its exposure and removal by forceps become a very simple matter. Arrangements for suitable drainage should be made.

The after-treatment of these cases will be conducted upon the lines indicated in page 718, especially in so far as they concern cases of abscess of the brain treated by operation.

TREPHINING FOR ABSCESS OF THE BRAIN.

When the abscess of the brain is the result of injury, or depends upon the lodgment of a foreign body, the situation of the external lesion and the nature of the symptoms may serve to indicate the probable position of the purulent collection.

In any case, when the trephine has been placed over the most probable spot, and no abscess has been exposed, the necessity for multiple trephining may be obviated by the use of a slender aspirating needle attached to a large hypodermic syringe. If the needle be thoroughly disinfected, it may be pushed into the brain at many points, and may reach many different levels. It has been shown that such an examination can do but little harm. The needle must be pushed in in a direct line at each examination. There must be no lateral movement of it, and no attempt to pass it from one point of the brain to another without removing it and re-introducing it. The piston of the syringe must be repeatedly withdrawn during the exploration. An abscess of the brain is usually at least as large as a walnut, and may, of course, be of much greater size.

In many instances the abscess of the encephalon is dependent upon suppurative disease of the middle ear. The

pus in these cases is very commonly
sphenoidal lobe, and next in freque
It is estimated that three abscesses
cerebrum to one situated in the cerebe

Mr. Barker states that nine-tenths
temporo-sphenoidal lobe occupy a sp
inch in diameter, whose centre is one
and the same distance behind the cen
tory meatus (*Brit. Med. Journ.*, 1887,

The abscess of the temporo-sph
found (according to Mr. Barker's resea
drawn at right angles to Reid's bas
about one inch and a quarter apart ;
meatus, the other about one inch and
opening (Fig. 420, *x x*).

The trephine should be introduc
space marked out by these two lines, a
one inch and a quarter above the base

A needle introduced through suc
thrust inwards, forwards, and a little c

Dr. Birmingham has suggested th
lateral sinus in all circumstances, th
should be made a little higher up
(*Brit. Med. Journ.*, September 20th, 1

In dealing with an abscess of the c
to select is, in the adult, one inch and
of the meatus, and one inch below the

The Operation for Cerebral Abs
carried out in the manner already des
an abscess in the temporo-sphenoidal
with its base above and behind, will b
This is held up by means of a ligature

The dura mater is exposed, and v
be without pulsation, and to bulge
This change in the membrane is a cer
of pus, but of increased intra-cranial t

The dura mater is incised with
opened by the aid of fine scissors and
The division should be so made as to
closure of the rents with sutures possi

will probably be the most convenient. The aspirating needle having been introduced and pus discovered, the next step is to insert a pair of slender sinus forceps by the side of the needle, and to thus enlarge the track along which the pus may escape.

Along the passage thus made a drainage-tube of india-rubber or of silver is introduced. Mr. Barker advises a silver tube, provided with a proper flange or shield, and of the diameter of a No. 8 catheter. The length of tube within the skull should measure about one inch. The tube must be secured in place by sutures. The flap is now adjusted, but the sutures must be omitted at the apex of the flap, so that the trephine-hole may not be entirely covered up, but that there may be every opportunity offered for the escape of matter.

The wound is now cleaned, dusted with iodoform, and covered with a dressing of loose gauze. The part should be frequently irrigated.

The tube will require to be removed and cleaned once or twice a day, as it soon becomes blocked with soft cerebral granulation tissue. The tube will be gradually shortened, and the surgeon should not be in great haste to remove it finally, since a re-accumulation of pus may occur. It will probably have to be retained for two or three weeks.

If a branch of the middle meningeal artery be exposed in the trephine-hole, it should be secured between two ligatures before the membrane is divided.

The Operation for Cerebellar Abscess.—The trephining is conducted upon the same lines. The point for the insertion of the trephine has been already indicated (Fig. 420, E). Mr. Barker recommends that the point be reached by means of an incision parallel with Reid's base line, and half an inch below it. The cut starts from the posterior border of the mastoid process, and extends backwards for two inches. Through this incision the superior curved line of the occipital bone is exposed.

All the soft parts, together with the pericranium, are peeled downwards with a rugine until the inferior curved line is reached. Care must be taken not to wound the trunk of the occipital artery. The spot already indicated as most suited for the introduction of the trephine will lie just below the latter line. The bone here is very thin. The lateral sinus lies opposite to the superior curved line above and the mastoid process in front. The spot for the trephine is a little behind and below the mastoid foramen. The bone may be removed with the trephine, or, if more convenient, with the gouge.

The dura mater is incised, the needle is employed, and the abscess is opened and drained in the manner already described (page 714). If the skin and soft parts on being released are found to overlap the trephine-hole, they must be divided in such a way as to leave the latter quite clear.

Mr. Barker recommends that as soon as the bone is exposed it is well to examine the mastoid foramen. If pus have found its way along the groove of the lateral sinus, it may induce symptoms akin to those of cerebellar abscess, and an examination of the foramen may reveal pus escaping, since that opening leads direct into the groove for the sinus.

A sufficient enlargement of this foramen to allow of free drainage may render further operation unnecessary.

TREPHINING FOR CEREBRAL TUMOUR.

On May 12th, 1885, a paper in every way remarkable was read before the Royal Medical and Chirurgical Society by Dr. Hughes Bennett and Mr. Godlee. In this communication an account was given of the accurate diagnosis and the successful removal of a tumour of the brain. The operation was performed on November 25th, 1884. The patient lived four weeks. The account of the case forms an admirable exposition of scientific precision and surgical acumen.

From this case cerebral surgery as a practical measure may be said to date.

In the autumn of 1888 Dr. Macewen, of Glasgow, in an address delivered before the British Medical Association, gave an account of a series of successful operations which he had performed upon the brain or its meninges. Among these cases was one of removal of a "syphilitic tumour" from the precentral lobe. The operation had been performed in June, 1883, and the patient made a good recovery (*Lancet,* August 11th, 1883).

These pioneer operations were rapidly followed by many

others. The further development and elaboration of the details of cerebral surgery depend mainly upon the genius of Mr. Victor Horsley, whose work in this department of practice has been brilliant and of infinite value. In a paper published in the *British Medical Journal* for December 6th, 1890, Mr. Horsley gives a table of no less than forty-four cases of operation upon the brain performed by himself. Out of this number, ten died.

A very remarkable and successful case of the evacuation of a sub-tentorial hydatid tumour is recorded by Dr. Maunsell (*New Zealand Med. Journ.*, April, 1889).

The trephine-hole was made in the occipital bone below the superior curved line.

The following account is based mainly upon Mr. Horsley's instructions and descriptions of various operations, and especially upon his articles in the *British Medical Journal* for October 9th, 1886, and April 23rd, 1887.

Instruments Required.—In addition to the instruments already mentioned as used in trephining (page 702), the following are employed :—Very large trephines with a diameter of 1½ or 2 inches; a circular saw worked on a Bonwill's surgical engine; strong bone-cutting forceps; fine curved needles and a needle-holder for suturing the dura mater ; wire serres-fines; scoop or enucleator ; sharp spoon ; Horsley's flexible knife.

Preparation of the Patient.—The head is shaved and cleaned as already described. A cap of lint soaked in a 1 in 20 carbolic solution is worn over the scalp for at least twelve hours before the operation. The situation of the growth is marked out upon the scalp, and after the anæsthetic has been administered, this surface-marking is transferred to the skull by boring small holes here and there with the finest trephine pin. Very strict antiseptic precautions must be observed throughout.

The Anæsthetic.—A hypodermic injection of morphine is administered, in suitable dose, one hour before the operation. The anæsthetic advised is chloroform, on the ground that it induces less cerebral excitement. The morphine has the effect of contracting the arterioles of the central nervous system, and hence of lessening hæmorrhage. At the same time, it allows less chloroform to be given.

The Scalp Incisions.—A single flap is raised, the outline of which is a shallow curve. It is free below, and is so planned as to avoid the main scalp arteries, and to permit of free drainage when the patient is recumbent. The pericranium is separated by the rugine over the area exposed, and is turned back together with the other structures of the scalp. All bleeding must be arrested before the trephine is applied.

The Exposure of the Brain.—This is effected by the large trephines. An opening may be made at the two extremes of the area to be removed, and the intervening bridge of bone may then be divided by means of Hey's saw or the chisel and mallet. The dura mater during the process will be protected by a thin metal spatula. All the bone fragments removed are preserved in the manner already described (page 706).

The dura mater is now divided around about four-fifths of the margin of the aperture in the bone. The incision is made about one-eighth of an inch from the bone, so as to leave room for suturing. The incision may be conveniently commenced with the scalpel, and with slender blunt-pointed scissors.

All arteries lying in the line of the proposed incision must be tied, and this is most readily done by passing the ligature with a fine curved needle in a handle. The brain is now exposed, the flap of dura mater being held aside by a suture passed through its margin.

The Removal of the Tumour.—Incisions into the brain must be clean cut, be vertical to the surface, and be directed into the corona radiata when necessary, so as to avoid damage to fibres coming from other portions of the cortex. The growth may be enucleated by means of Horsley's flexible knife, or by a scoop or sharp spoon. In all cases, adherent or altered dura mater must be excised.

When a portion of brain has been cut away, the underlying cerebral tissue soon bulges up, and obliterates the hollow left by the loss of substance.

Hæmorrhage from the brain tissue is seldom troublesome. The arterioles for the most part run perpendicular to the cerebral surface. Most of the bleeding is soon checked by sponge pressure. Failing this, the application of very fine pressure forceps should be tried. For this purpose Nunneley's artery forceps have been employed, but more convenient and lighter are serres-fines of wire. The actual cautery should never be employed to arrest bleeding from the brain. Extensive divisions of surface blood-vessels may be avoided by lifting them out of the sulci between the convolutions, and replacing the pia mater after the tumour has been removed.

The treatment of bleeding from large meningeal arteries and also from the venous sinuses has been already alluded to (page 707).

The Closure of the Wound.—The flap of dura mater is brought into place, and is secured to the unwounded part of the membrane by a few fine catgut sutures ; space, however, must be left for drainage. The bone discs and portions of skull removed by the saw are now arranged and secured in the manner already described (page 706).

This step can only be taken when the dura mater is intact. If any of the brain area be left uncovered, it is unwise to attempt to replace the lost pieces of bone. The scalp flap is now brought into place and secured by silkworm-gut sutures, room being allowed for drainage. The drainage-tube reaches to the surface of the wound in the brain, and is placed at the most dependent part of the wound when the patient lies supine. This tube is retained only for twenty-four hours. A voluminous antiseptic dressing is then applied.

THE AFTER-TREATMENT OF CASES OF TREPHINING.

The patient is kept absolutely at rest, and the room occupied should be perfectly quiet. The head is kept a little raised. The wound is dressed upon ordinary surgical principles. In cases of fracture, or in cases of trephining for epilepsy, etc., where no lesion of the dura mater exists, draining by catgut will suffice. In cases of trephining for the removal of a brain tumour, or the evacuation of a cerebral abscess, drainage with a tube is necessary. In the former case the tube is retained for twenty-four hours only ; in the latter it is retained until the abscess cavity has practically closed, and is shortened as often as required. In a few instances of intra-cranial suppuration a second opening in the skull may be necessary to ensure perfect drainage.

If, after the removal of the drainage-tube in any case, pain and throbbing in the wound be complained of, and if the scalp flap appear to be raised up, it may be necessary to reopen the track of the drainage - tube to allow pent-up discharges to escape.

Sutures may be removed at any time after the fifth or sixth day, or be retained as long as appears needful. If a hernia cerebri form, it can best be treated, so far as my own experience goes, by means of a pad of gauze and wool, kept constantly wet with absolute alcohol. The surface of the protrusion hardens, and forms a species of scab or cuticle, which in time becomes quite tough, and affords an efficient covering to the exposed brain.

The patient will need to remain in bed until the wound is soundly healed. From two to three weeks will represent an average time.

The diet is such as is advised after any grave operation.

CRANIECTOMY.

The operation so named has been advised and has been carried out with success by Professor Lannelongue, of Paris (*L'Union Médicale*, July 8th, 1890). It is employed in cases of microcephaly and some other conditions, such as hyperostosis due to congenital syphilis, and hydrocephalus with thickening and premature closure of the skull; and consists in the excision of a strip of the skull, with the idea that by this means an obstacle to the natural growth of the enfeebled brain is removed. As an American surgeon expresses it, the operation is intended to allow the growing brain more "elbow room." Craniectomy is obviously applicable to only quite young children. Up to the present time most of the subjects operated upon have been under the age of five years. In M. Anger's case the child was an idiot of eight years old. One of Mr. Horsley's patients was seven. Dr. Keen objects to the term "craniectomy," and proposes that of "linear craniotomy."

The vertex of the skull is exposed by means of a single incision in its long axis. A narrow strip of bone is then removed from the parietal bone, close to the sagittal suture. In both of Professor Lannelongue's first cases the excision concerned the left bone, the left side of the skull being smaller than the right. The strip of bone is parallel with the sagittal suture, and its inner margin is a finger's-breadth from the median line, so as to avoid damage to the superior longitudinal sinus. The length of the piece removed corresponds to the antero-posterior measurement of the parietal bone. The width of the strip is a quarter to half an inch. The bone is removed by a small trephine, assisted by bone-cutting forceps.

The incision in the scalp is made in such a way as not to correspond to the incision in the bone. The dura mater is not opened. The excision of bone may be extended into the frontal or the occipital bones, bridges of bone being left to carry the coronal and lambdoid sutures. The scalp wound is closely united by sutures. No drains other than catgut drains are required. The operation is apt to be attended by considerable shock.

Dr. W. W. Keen exposes the skull through a slight flap, and divides the bone by means of special bone-cutting forceps which are a modification of Hoffmann's forceps. His first operation occupied one hour and a quarter, but with the forceps the procedure can be completed in thirty minutes.

Mr. Horsley also employs a flap, but removes the bone with a trephine and bone-cutting forceps (*Brit. Med. Journ.,* September 12th, 1891).

M. Lannelongue in a more recent paper (*Rev. Mens. d. Mal. de l'Enfance,* May, 1891) brings forward twenty-eight cases of craniectomy—twenty-five by himself and three by other French surgeons. Out of this number there was one death. In a large number of the patients a great improvement followed the operation.

In addition to the linear craniectomy M. Lannelongue now carries out a *craniectomie à lambeaux,* in which the bones of the skull are s , cut as to produce osseous flaps of various shapes, such as the U-shape, V-shape, or T-shape.

Dr. Keen has carried out the operation in three cases. He has collected eight examples of the operation. Six of these are not included in M. Lannelongue's list. In two cases death followed speedily. Of the six that survived, there has been in four a very decided improvement, while in two the after-history of the cases is incomplete. In all the cases rapid healing followed (*Med. News*, November 29th, 1890 ; and *Amer. Journ. of the Med. Sciences*, June, 1891). Mr. Horsley has operated in two cases ; one patient was improved, and one died (*Brit. Med. Journ.*, September 12th, 1891).

There are thus thirty-six cases recorded up to the present time, with four deaths.

TREPHINING THE FRONTAL SINUSES.

The frontal sinuses are opened up with the trephine in certain cases of disease of the lining membrane of those cavities, and especially in such affections as are associated with occlusion of the infundibulum.

In cases of necrosis, also attended by the retention of fœtid pus, this operation has been carried out with success.

These cavities are absent in the infant, are very small in children, and hardly have an existence, from a surgical standpoint, until after puberty.

A single vertical incision is made down to the bone in the median line of the forehead. It will commence at the root of the nose, and measure about an inch or an inch and a half. The pericranium having been divided and turned back, a trephine of suitable size is applied to the anterior wall of the sinus. The opening can be subsequently enlarged by means of the rongeur or the chisel and mallet.

The subsequent treatment of the case will depend upon the condition found. Diseased mucous membrane may be scraped, retained secretions are allowed to escape, necrosed fragments are removed, the opening into the nose, if occluded or insufficient, is reopened or enlarged.

The cavity may very often be drained from the nose, or partly from the nose and partly from the surface wound

CHAPTER II.

TREPHINING THE MASTOID ANTRUM.

THIS little operation is called for in those cases of suppurative disease of the middle ear in which the pus has spread to the mastoid process, and being retained, is producing more or less serious symptoms.

The operation does not consist of merely opening the nearest cells of the mastoid process, or of driving a boring instrument vaguely into that bone, but is represented by a definite and precise opening of the space known as the antrum of the mastoid. Into this central cavity the mastoid cells open, and it is, moreover, in direct communication with the cavity of the tympanum.

The bone can only be efficiently drained when this particular cell-space is opened up.

The operation is therefore not so much a "trephining of the mastoid cells" as an opening into the mastoid antrum.

Anatomical Points.—In the infant the mastoid as a distinct process has no existence; but in the mastoid segment of the petrous bone is a single air-cell, the mastoid antrum, which communicates by a large opening with the posterior part of the tympanum. Its outer wall is very thin, and thus it happens that in infants pus in the antrum can very readily reach the surface, or be still more readily evacuated by operation. A small incision, extending some two lines into the bone, is all that is necessary. Across the roof of the antrum at this period runs the petro-squamous suture. About the second year the mastoid process becomes visible. As the bone increases, its growth mainly involves its external parts, so that as years pass on the antrum becomes more and more deeply placed. In a child aged nine this cell is about 1 c.m. from the surface. At this period no other air-cells exist, but at puberty an extensive series of such cells develop.

In the adult the mastoid cells extend upwards to within half an inch of the temporo-parietal suture. Anteriorly they extend forwards over the external meatus. Posteriorly they cease abruptly at the masto-occipital suture, although in rare cases they are continued beyond that suture into the occipital bone.

About the centre of the mastoid spaces is the antrum. It is about the size of a pea. Its roof is only separated from the cranial cavity by a layer of bone about 1 m.m. in thickness. The distance of the posterior end of the antrum from the lateral sinus is from 3 to 6 m.m., while its outer wall is from half to three-fourths of an inch from the external surface of the mastoid process.

According to Dr. Birmingham (*Brit. Med. Journ.*, September 20th, 1890), the antrum is directly beneath a point as near as possible to the posterior margin of the meatus, and on a line with the roof of that aperture. According to the same writer, the lateral sinus starting from the protuberance ascends above Reid's base line, until it reaches a point one inch and a half behind and three-fourths of an inch above the centre of the bony meatus. It here makes the bend, and runs down in front of the posterior margin of the mastoid process about half an inch behind the meatus.

Wilde's Incision.—This incision is convenient for opening abscesses behind the ear and for exposing the mastoid process. The incision is quite vertical, and extends from the apex of the mastoid to its base. The apex of the bone is the guide to the position of the incision. If the knife be carried too far up, branches of the posterior auricular artery are divided. The incision is carried well down to the bone.

The Opening of the Mastoid Antrum.—Of the many special instruments employed or advised for this operation, few have much claim to serious consideration.

Drills of any kind are to be avoided as dangerous. The surgeon has little control over their movements ; they are apt to cut deeper than was intended, and are most readily carried beyond their mark.

Trephines are clumsy and needlessly destructive. In

u u 2

children the orthodox "mastoid trephine" would cut away the greater part of the mastoid bone.   They are not under very complete control, and there is no indication conveyed to the hand of the moment when the antrum is reached.

The instrument I have always employed is a carpenter's gimlet of suitable size.   This instrument is simple, and is very easily employed.   Its movements can be regulated with the greatest precision, a sense of diminished resistance at once indicates when the antrum is reached, and the groove on the instrument affords an immediate exit to the pus.

Many surgeons use a sharp gouge.   The instrument is much more serviceable than any form of drill or trephine, but I venture to think that it is inferior to the gimlet.

The parts having been well cleansed and well washed with a carbolic solution (1 in 20), Wilde's incision is made.   The knife is carried to the bone.   The periosteum is turned aside by means of a rugine.

An imaginary line is drawn through the roof of the auditory meatus at right angles to the line of Wilde's incision, and where these two lines meet the gimlet is applied.

The instrument is bored forwards and inwards parallel with the long axis of the meatus.   It is convenient to introduce a short piece of pencil or of gum-elastic catheter into the meatus as a guide, and to keep the gimlet exactly parallel with it.

If the instrument be directed inwards at right angles to the surface of the skull at the point indicated, the antrum will certainly be missed, and the lateral sinus almost as certainly opened.   The direction followed by the gimlet is therefore of the utmost importance.

In the adult the antrum will be reached at a depth not exceeding three-fifths of an inch.   The loss of resistance and the escape of pus indicate when the cavity is opened.

The gimlet is withdrawn, and the opening enlarged to the extent desired by means of a sharp gouge.   If any necrosis be present, the gouge will need to be liberally employed.

The tunnel in the bone having been well syringed out, a suitable drainage-tube is inserted, and the parts are well dusted with iodoform.

A boracic fomentation forms the most suitable dressing.

CHAPTER III.

EXCISION OF THE EYE-BALL.

The Instruments Required. — Eye speculum; strabismus hook; strabismus scissors; toothed forceps; blunt-ended scissors curved on the flat; small sponges.

The Operation.—The patient's head is a little raised, and the surgeon stands in front, facing the patient.

The speculum is introduced between the lids and opened.

With the blunt-pointed scissors the surgeon snips through the conjunctiva just behind the corneal margin. The toothed forceps are used to pick up the membrane and to steady the globe. The division of the conjunctiva is complete all round.

By the further use of the scissors Tenon's capsule is freely opened, and each of the rectus tendons are then picked up in turn with the strabismus hook, and are divided close to the sclerotic with the strabismus scissors. It is convenient to begin with the external rectus, then to divide the superior and inferior recti, and to finish with the inner rectus. If the speculum be now pressed back into the cavity of the orbit, the eyeball starts forwards. The blunt-ended scissors curved on the flat are then introduced into the orbit to the outer side of the globe, and are carried back until the optic nerve is reached. It is divided by one cut of the blades.

The eye-ball being drawn forwards with the fingers, the oblique muscles are divided, together with any soft parts which may still hold the globe in place.

A piece of Turkey sponge is then pressed into the cavity of the orbit, and is allowed to remain there for a few minutes.

The first dressing consists merely of an aseptic sponge pressed into the cavity of the orbit, and retained in position by a pad and bandage. This is taken out at the end of twelve hours or earlier, and the subsequent treatment consists of daily irrigations, and the dressing of the part with a pad of wool soaked in boracic lotion.

If the globe be collapsed, as is frequently the case when excision is carried out, the operation becomes a very meagre affair, scarcely removed from the humble procedure of detaching a slough with scissors and forceps.

It is well in these cases, however, to take care to remove the globe alone, and to leave the muscles with as little of their substance displaced as possible.

CHAPTER IV.

Operations upon the Spine and Spinal Cord.

On June 12th, 1888, a paper was read before the Royal Medical and Chirurgical Society by Dr. Gowers and Mr. Horsley, which dealt with the case of a man from whose spinal cord a tumour had been removed with success. This paper may be said to form the foundation or starting-point of the more modern phase of spinal surgery.

Operations upon the spine in certain cases of injury are of some antiquity. In instances of fracture in which broken or displaced portions of bone were pressing upon the cord, the injured region has been exposed, and the fragments removed. This procedure, known usually as " trephining the spine," was attended, before the days of antiseptic surgery, with such lamentable results as to cause the measure to be regarded by many as totally unjustifiable.

One of the earliest of the more formal operations was carried out in 1814 by the younger Cline. The patient died; but the method of treatment excited considerable notice, and drew forth much adverse criticism. A successful case operated upon by Dr. Macewen in 1885 (*Brit. Med. Journ.*, August 11th, 1888) marks a new era, and since then a large number of successful cases has been recorded.

Dr. William White, of Philadelphia, has given an admirable *résumé* of these earlier cases in a paper published in the *Annals of Surgery* for July, 1889. He has collected thirteen recent examples of operation for fracture, with only one death.

Operations upon the spine in cases of paralysis due to pressure by inflammatory exudations, or displaced or deformed bone in Pott's disease, are of much more recent date.

On May 9th, 1883, Dr. Macewen removed the laminæ of

the fifth, sixth, and seventh dorsal vertebræ in a case of complete paraplegia of two years' duration, depending upon angular deformity of the spine. The patient made a complete recovery. The number of cases of like character operated upon since this date has been numerous. Mr. Horsley reports seven as performed by himself, with one death from exhaustion at the end of six weeks (*Brit. Med. Journ.*, December 5th, 1890).

Among other cases to which reference may be made are those of Mr. Lane (*Lancet*, July 5th, 1890), Mr. Herbert Page (*Lancet*, December 6th, 1890), Dr. William White (*Annals of Surgery*, vol. ix., page 425), and Kraske (*Centralblatt für Chirurgie*, November 25th, 1890). Out of twenty-three cases collected by Mr. Herbert Page (*loc. cit.*), an improvement more or less considerable followed in about half the cases. M. Chipault (*Arch. Gén. de Méd.*, December, 1890) has brought together thirty-five cases of operation in Pott's disease, the examples of improvement showing a somewhat higher percentage.

The examples of operation for tumour have, up to the present time, been very few.

The surgeon interested in this branch of operative surgery should consult Thornburn's valuable work on " The Surgery of the Spinal Cord."

The Instruments Required. — Stout and fine scalpels: trephine: bone-cutting forceps: rugine: elevator: necrosis forceps: chisel and mallet: retractors: blunt hooks: probe: Volkmann's spoons: fine tenaculum-pointed forceps: fine scissors: small curved needles and needle-holder; straight needles: ligatures: sutures. etc.

The Operation.—One of the most lucid accounts of the operation is that given by Dr. William White, and it has been, to a great extent, followed in the appended description:—

The patient lies in a prone or semi-prone position, and a gentle curve is given to the spine by means of a small hand pillow placed under the lower ribs.

A long incision is made in the median line, exactly over the spines of the vertebræ, in the region it is desired to expose.

The incision is carried deep down, and the muscles are

freely separated from the sides of the spinous processes and the posterior surfaces of the laminæ by the knife, aided by the rugine. One side is cleared, and all the bleeding arrested, before the other side is exposed in like manner.

A considerable portion of the spine being now exposed, the periosteum is divided along the angle between the spinous processes and the laminæ, and is then reflected from the surfaces of the vertebral arches by means of a curved rugine. Firm rectangular metal retractors are needed at this stage of the operation. Mr. Horsley divided the deep fascia at right angles to the line of the incision in one or more places. Gordon severed the muscular bundles attached to the articular processes, in order to obtain a fuller view of the neural arches.

The spinous processes are now divided close to their bases by means of large, strong, bone-cutting forceps, with blades set at an obtuse angle. It is now necessary to divide the laminæ on each side, in order to expose the vertebral canal. Some surgeons have used a trephine for the purpose—a not very convenient instrument ; others have employed Hey's saw, or the chisel and mallet, or bone-cutting forceps. The method employed must depend upon the surgical habit of the individual surgeon.

. In any case, some trouble may be anticipated from the very tough ligamentum subflavum. The laminæ should be divided as near to the transverse processes as possible. When the neural arch has been removed to a sufficient extent, the dura mater is well exposed. The operation may end here. The excision of the laminæ may have removed the injurious pressure from the cord, or displaced fragments of bone may be taken away, or pus or an extra-dural collection of blood may be evacuated, or an extra-dural tumour may be excised.

The hæmorrhage in this part of the operation has never been so extensive as arguments, based upon theoretical grounds, had predicted. It has been in nearly every instance easily and permanently arrested by moderate pressure.

If it be determined to open the dura mater, it is seized in the middle line with fine tenaculum-pointed forceps, and is opened vertically—either by a small scalpel, or, better, by means of fine scissors. When the divided parts are retracted upon either side, the whole of the posterior surface of the cord is well exposed.

Any tumour detected is dealt with by simple excision. (*See* the section on tumours of the brain, page 717.)

The opening in the dura mater is closed by many points of fine catgut, introduced by means of a curved needle in a needle-holder.

A drainage-tube is now placed along the whole length of the wound, in its deepest part. The muscles are brought together above it by means of catgut sutures; after which the superficial parts are united by sutures of silkworm gut.

An escape of cerebro-spinal fluid has continued for some days or weeks after the operation. A careful suturing of the dura mater should prevent this.

The length of time during which the patient must remain in the recumbent position will depend upon the nature of the case, and the extent and character of the operation. It will usually be advisable that a spinal jacket or spinal support should be worn for some little time after the patient gets up.

CHAPTER V.

THE TREATMENT OF PSOAS ABSCESS.

IN a paper read before the Royal Medical and Chirurgical Society in June, 1884 (*Med.-Chir. Trans.*, vol. lxvii.), I urged the evacuation of psoas abscesses through an incision in the loin, and gave the details of the operation, which is described below. The incision is so placed as to open the abscess directly, and at its most dependent spot (when the patient is recumbent). At the same time it allows of the bodies of the vertebræ being examined with the finger, and enables the surgeon to remove carious and necrosed bone by such means as are employed in like affections elsewhere. In the first case operated upon (June 1st, 1883), I removed from the body of the first lumbar vertebra a sequestrum measuring one inch by half an inch, which represented all that remained of the centrum. Since that time I have removed smaller fragments of dead bone, and have been able, by means of long and conveniently-shaped gouges and sharp spoons, to scrape away carious bone from the anterior surface of the column.

The incision allows of a direct exposure of the diseased area, and of the evacuation of the pus by the shortest possible route. The wound, moreover, is made through a comparatively unimportant district.

I have carried out the method of treating psoas abscess in a large number of cases with most excellent results.

At first I merely evacuated the abscess and drained it. In later years I have treated the cavity in the manner herewith described.

The Opening of the Abscess.—The patient's loin having been exposed, a vertical incision some two and a half inches in length is made through the integuments. The centre of this cut should lie about midway between the crest of the ilium and the last rib, and the cut should be

so placed as to correspond to a vertical line parallel
with the vertebral side of the outer border of the erector
spinæ. I find that the average width of the erector spinæ
in this situation is, in the adult, from two inches and three-
quarters to three inches. The incision, therefore, should be
situated about two and a half inches from the lumbar spinous
processes.

After cutting through the superficial fascia the dense
aponeurosis is exposed that covers the posterior surface
of the erector spinæ, and which is variously known as the
superficial layer of the lumbar fascia, as the aponeurosis of the
latissimus dorsi and serratus posticus inferior muscles, and as
the inferior part of the vertebral aponeurosis. The part of
this layer exposed in the lower half of the incision is wholly
tendinous, but from that seen in the upper half of the cut
arise some of the fibres of the latissimus dorsi. These fibres
are thin, and pass from below obliquely upwards and outwards.
The dense aponeurosis with its attached muscular fibres
having been divided in the full length of the incision, the
erector spinæ is exposed. This muscle is at once recognised
by the vertical direction of its fibres. The outer border of the
muscle should now be sought for, and the whole mass drawn
by means of retractors as far as possible towards the middle
line of the back. In this way the anterior part of the
sheath of the muscle, known as the middle layer of the
fascia lumborum, is readily exposed. Neither in front nor
behind has the erector spinæ any direct adhesion to its sheath
at this part.

The anterior layer of the sheath, as now exposed, is seen
to be made up of dense white glistening fibres, which are all
more or less transverse in direction. Through this sheath the
transverse processes of the lumbar vertebræ should be sought
for. The longest and most conspicuous process is that belonging to the third vertebra. It is readily felt. The erector
muscle having been drawn as far as possible towards the
middle line, the anterior layer of its sheath must be divided
vertically as near to the transverse processes as convenient.
By this incision the quadratus lumborum muscle is exposed.
The muscle as here seen is very thin. It is composed of
fibres, which run from above obliquely downwards and

outwards. Between the fibres are tendinous bundles which spring from the tips of the transverse processes. The muscle should be divided close to the extremity of a transverse process, and the incision cautiously enlarged until the muscle is divided to the full extent of the skin wound. It is at this stage that there is danger of wounding the abdominal branches of the lumbar arteries. The inner edge of the quadratus is overlapped by the psoas muscle, so that when the former is divided the latter is exposed. The psoas fibres, as now seen, take about the same direction as the posterior fibres of the quadratus: *i.e.*, run downwards and outwards. The interval between the two muscles is marked by a thin but distinct layer of fascia, known as the anterior lamella of the fascia lumborum. Some of the tendinous fibres of the psoas having been divided close to a transverse process, the finger is introduced beneath the muscle, and gently insinuated along the process until the anterior aspect of the bodies of the vertebræ is reached. The incision in the psoas can be enlarged to any extent.

If the patient were stout or very muscular, the length of the skin wound would have to be increased, or a transverse cut might be made into the erector spinæ to allow of its more effectual retraction.

With common care there should be no danger of opening up the subperitoneal connective tissue, much less of wounding the peritoneum. All risk on this score will be avoided by making the incision in the quadratus as near to the transverse processes as possible.

Great care must be taken not to wound the lumbar arteries. The abdominal branches of these vessels run for the most part behind the quadratus lumborum. That, however, from the first vessel runs in front, and not infrequently those from one or two of the lower arteries follow its example. These vessels may be of large size—often as large as the lingual. They may be avoided, as well as the trunks from which they arise, by keeping close to a transverse process. The main vessel curves around the spine between the transverse processes, and between these processes also the division of the artery occurs. If, therefore, the rule be observed of always reaching the spine along a transverse process, the

lumbar arteries and their abdominal
to no risk.

In actual practice the operation i
may appear from this description.
young and thin—often very thin. If
any length of time, the muscles abou
atrophied; and if any moderate de
render the morbid region more easy
moreover, that the quadratus is inci
and here will in all probability be
which will immediately conduct th
seat of the disease. As to which loi
right or the left—it matters little
somewhat more conveniently perfo
while upon the left the risk of dam
an accidental slip is reduced to a mi:

It must be borne in mind th
deformity exists the space between
crest becomes much encroached up
touch and even overlap the pelvic
where the space available for this o
rowed are not common, are most
extensive disease in the dorsal spi
reasons, unsuitable for active treatm

The Treatment of the Absce
the abscess cavity is well open
duced, and the anterior surface (
examined as far as is possible. Such
only called for in cases of disease of
bar section of the column. It is eas
and slender adults. In individuals (
impossible.

The surgeon will have all ready a
solution of corrosive sublimate (1 in
perature of 100° F., a Leiter's gla
receptacles to take the water as it e
of waterproof sheets is needed.

A tube of a Leiter's irrigator is i
of the abscess, and the cistern being
to six feet above the level of the ta

mercurial solution is allowed to run through the abscess. During this process of irrigation the abscess is frequently emptied by pressure applied to it from the front, and is allowed to fill again and to be emptied again. The patient's position, also, is altered many times. He is turned over towards the sound side, and is then turned almost upon the back, in order that every part of the abscess sac may be well and vigorously flushed.

The surgeon now proceeds to remove as much of the lining membrane of the abscess as is possible. The finger is the safest and most useful instrument.

It is introduced as far as possible. Diverticula from the main abscess are opened up, collections of caseous matter are scraped away with the nail, and here and there the action of the finger may be helped by a sharp spoon. This instrument, however, must be used with caution. It causes bleeding, and produces often a needlessly extensive raw surface. Moreover, the anterior wall of the abscess cavity is usually thin, and the steel instrument may inflict a serious injury upon that part of the parietes.

Next to the finger, the most valuable means of clearing out the abscess cavity is a piece of fine Turkey sponge held in a slender long-bladed holder.

This should be passed in all directions over every part of the abscess wall. The wall should be literally scrubbed with it. It should be gently bored by a rotatory movement into every pocket and diverticulum. The sponge must be changed very frequently.

After a vigorous use of the finger and sponge, the irrigator is again brought into action, and the abscess cavity is once more flushed out, and such *débris* as the sponge has left is swept away. Once again the finger and thumb search out all the recesses of the abscess, and once again the stream from the irrigator follows.

This is done until the abscess cavity appears to be clean, and until the sponge is returned practically unsoiled. The process is slow and tedious, but it is very effectual. It leaves the abscess cavity bare, and freed entirely of the curdy pus, of the caseous masses, and of the ill-conditioned *débris* which filled it.

A very considerable quantity of the solution of corrosive sublimate is required.

Finally, the interior of the abscess is wiped dry with the last set of sponges used, and the wound is closed by a series of silkworm-gut sutures, passed sufficiently deep to include the greater part of the muscular and tendinous structures with the skin.

A pad of Tillmann's dressing or of wool dusted with iodoform is placed over the little wound, and is secured in position by a broad flannel bandage.

The After-treatment.—The subsequent treatment consists of absolute rest in the recumbent position for a period of months—a period which may easily be too short, but hardly too long. The actual number of months during which the recumbent posture should be observed must depend upon the nature, extent, and stage of the disease. In adults it will probably extend beyond twelve months in the hands of those who wish to exercise a wise caution. It is not the abscess which is in need of treatment—it is rather the diseased condition which has produced it.

If the period of rest can be carried out at the seaside, and the patient spend the greater part of the time out in the open air (winter and summer) in a spinal carriage, so much the better.

The abscess may re-fill, and may need to be evacuated, washed, and scrubbed out and closed a second time. In no case have I had occasion to carry out a third operation.

If the wound should break down and pus escape at the site of the incision, free drainage and a most liberal irrigation must be the plan of treatment. This has occurred in a few of my cases, and in every instance the patients who have been the subject of this complication have done well. The wound, even in these cases, will heal by first intention, and signs of pus beneath the surface will usually not be observed until a fortnight or more has passed by.

Mr. Barker has recently employed in these cases an ingenious instrument, which he terms the hollow or flushing gouge. It consists of a gouge with a tubular handle and shaft, through which water can be conducted into the hollow of the gouge. (*See* page 704, vol. i.) The water, running continuously through the instrument, washes away all *débris* as soon as it is loosened by the gouge.

The *modus operandi* is thus described (*Brit. Med. Journ.* Feb. 7th, 1891):—

A two-inch incision is made through sound structures over the lower end of the swelling. Through this opening a hollow gouge is inserted, which is connected with a reservoir of hot water at 105° to 110° Fahr. by a rubber tube some six feet long. This reservoir (a three-gallon can) is raised about five feet above the operating-table. When the water is now turned on, it rushes through the long gouge to the fundus of the abscess with considerable force, and the reflux carries the contents of the cavity out by the incision. By gently scraping with the flushing-scoop, the more solid caseous matter is dislodged, the hot water carrying it clear of the cavity at once. Then the walls of the cavity are gently scraped in a methodical manner until the soft lining is loosened and carried away from every part of the abscess. In order to effect this thoroughly, the scoops are made of varying length, so that the deeper parts can be reached. With hot water the bleeding is but slight, if the peeling be done cautiously.

When the water runs out clear after having been carried to all the recesses of the cavity, the instrument is withdrawn. Then any excess of water is squeezed out; and if the deeper parts are accessible, sponges are used to dry out the last traces of moisture. Then two or three ounces of fresh iodoform emulsion are poured into the deepest part of the abscess, and stitches are inserted in the edges of the incision. Before these are knotted, all excess of emulsion should be squeezed out of the cavity. The knotting of the silk sutures then completes the procedure. As no drain-tube is used, a simple dry dressing of salicylic wool is alone required; but it should be laid on in considerable quantity, so as to exert elastic pressure over the whole area of the abscess when bandaged. Such a dressing may be left on for about ten days, when it is time to remove the stitches, and the wound should then be firmly healed. A piece of salicylic wool secured by collodion at the edges should, however, be laid over it, to keep it from chafing, for a few days longer, and the elastic pressure should also be kept up.

It appears to me that in less skilled hands than Mr Barker's some risk may be run in using this sharp-edged instrument in such an abscess as that found in the psoas muscle. The anterior wall of the abscess is often thin, and little force would be needed to perforate it. The instrument is passed deeply, and is a little removed from direct control. It is in every way admirably suited for intramuscular abscesses nearer to the surface, and especially in suppurative adhesions in or about large joints.

Part XVI.

OPERATIONS ON THE THORAX AND BREAST.

CHAPTER I.

OPERATIONS ON THE THORAX.

Anatomical Points.—The ribs are placed so obliquely that the anterior end of one rib is on a level with the posterior end of a rib some way below it in numerical order. Thus the first rib in front corresponds to the fourth rib behind, the second to the sixth, the third to the seventh, the fourth to the eighth, the seventh to the eleventh. If a horizontal line be drawn round the body at the level of the inferior angle of the scapula while the arms are at the side, the line would cut the sternum in front at the attachment of the sixth cartilage, the fifth rib at the nipple line, and the eighth rib at the vertebral column. The second rib is indicated by the transverse ridge on the sternum. The lower border of the pectoralis major leads to the fifth rib, and the first visible serration of the serratus magnus corresponds to the sixth.

The intercostal spaces are wider in front than behind, and between the upper than the lower ribs. The widest of the spaces is the third, then the second, then the first. The narrowest spaces are the last four. In normal conditions the first six spaces are wide enough to admit the whole breadth of the index finger.

Beyond the angle of the rib the intercostal vessels lie in a groove on the inferior border of the rib forming the upper boundary of a space. The vein lies nearer to the rib than does the artery.

The lower border of the lung corresponds to a slightly

convex line drawn round the chest
sternal articulation in front to t
behind. In the mammary line this
sixth rib, in the mid-axillary line
line continued vertically downward:
the scapula with the tenth rib. 1
down than the lung, reaching in
seventh chondro-sternal union, beh
spine, and at the sides to a poi
inches above the lower margin of t
in relation with the eleventh rib p
with the twelfth.

The following operations will be

1. Incision of the thorax,
    of a portion of rib.—
2. Esthlander's operation.—
3. Incision and drainage of
4. Treatment of hydatid cy
5. Incision and drainage of

1. INCISION OF THE THORA

This operation is carried out
consists of opening the suppurating

As a surgical measure, it diffe
ordinary method of treating puru
i.e., by free incision and drainage.

Among the many excellent
recently published upon this subj
be directed to an admirable mo
the *Lancet* for 1886 (vol. i.).

Site of the Incision.—This mu
by the physical signs afforded by t]

If pus be actually pointing at an
the incision may be made there
to make a second wound to afford :

The sites commonly selected
space, just in front of the posterior
space immediately external to the
ninth space just external to the
scapula. The latter situation is th

In children it is perhaps always the best, while in adults it is usually the most favourable.

As Mr. Godlee points out, an opening in the lowest part of the space where the cavity is soonest obliterated is less efficient than one made higher up, opposite to the part of the cavity which is the last to close.

The opening in the sixth or seventh space at the point indicated has the advantage afforded by a very thin covering of soft parts.

The Operation.—The skin around the site of the operation must be well cleansed and thoroughly disinfected.

Chloroform is the best anæsthetic.

The patient is brought to the extreme edge of the table, and is allowed to lie as nearly as possible upon the back.

It is more convenient to the surgeon if the patient be rolled over upon the sound side; but such a position is apt to seriously interfere with the breathing, especially when the patient is under the influence of the anæsthetic.

The arm must be raised, but not beyond a right angle. The lifting of the arm involves a displacing upwards of the skin. Before making his incision the surgeon must note to what extent the integument is displaced by raising the limb, and must make his incision so far above the spot at which it is intended to divide the intercostal muscles as will correspond to that spot when the limb is brought to the side. It is essential that the incision be not valvular, and that the opening into the thorax be quite direct, the skin wound and the deeper wound exactly corresponding.

An incision, from one and a half to three inches in length, is made transversely, so as to correspond to the upper border of the lower rib bounding the space.

The intercostal muscles are divided close to the rib; a director is then gently thrust through into the pleural cavity; the opening made is subsequently enlarged with dressing forceps and the finger.

The pus, if considerable in quantity, should be allowed to escape slowly. The abscess cavity may be examined with the forefinger as the fluid is escaping, or after it has been entirely evacuated. All thick curdy material within reach of the finger should be removed.

Experience has shown that it is unwise to wash the cavity of the empyema out at the time of the operation. All that can be done at first is to provide a free opening for the escaping pus.

If for any reason the incision has not been quite conveniently placed for, drainage, a counter-opening lower down in the thorax should be made.

A steel bladder-sound, or other suitable instrument, is introduced into the incision, and its point is made to project in one of the lower spaces upon the instrument thus held. A cut with the knife is made. Two drainage-tubes should, in such cases, be inserted. There is nothing to recommend the plan of passing a single tube from one opening to the other.

The drainage-tubes employed should be large and not too rigid. They should not be inserted at great depth. It is only necessary that their open ends should project into the pleural cavity, and that they should not impinge directly upon the lung. No object can be served by a long drainage-tube.

A great and remarkable variety of drainage-tubes has been employed for these cases. They have been made of very varied materials, and in very varied shapes.

During the earlier days of the after-treatment, a short length of common drainage-tube answers admirably, and later, when the cavity is contracting, a bent rubber tube, like a soft tracheotomy cannula, answers the purpose.

Above all things, it is most necessary that the tube be well secured, and that every precaution be taken to prevent it from slipping out of sight into the pleural cavity. This accident has occurred over and over again. Flanged tubes, tubes with shields, or tubes held in place by sutures and "buoyed" by long ligatures, are consequently to be recommended.

In removing every dressing during the after-treatment, the first care should be to note the position of the drainage-tube. In more than one case an extensive operation has been carried out in order to search for a chimerical drainage-tube, reported to be in the pleural cavity, but, in reality, thrown away with the dressings.

If during the operation an intercostal artery be cut, the surgeon's first care should be to see that the vessel is entirely severed, and not partly divided. This object is attained by passing a small scalpel down to the bone at the bleeding point. I venture to think that the most serious hæmorrhage in these cases comes from partly-divided arteries. If cleanly cut, the little vessel soon retracts. Failing this, pressure may be kept up for a while with the finger or a plug of fine sponge. Should the bleeding still continue, a portion of the adjacent rib should be excised, when there will be no difficulty in directly securing the bleeding point.

After the tube is in place the skin is cleansed, the wound dusted with iodoform, and the dressing applied. The latter must be of considerable proportions, and may consist of a loose pad of Tillmann's linen covered with fine gauze. This may be powdered with iodoform. Over the whole is placed a covering of protective or oiled silk, or fine waterproof sheeting, secured in place by a bandage.

The dressing will need to be changed frequently.

When the discharge has subsided a little, and especially when the escaping matter is offensive, the empyema cavity may be washed out once or twice daily. This is best done by means of a funnel and long tube. A very weak antiseptic solution, at a temperature of about 100° F., should be used. The most usual injections are solutions of corrosive sublimate, 1 in 8,000 or 10,000 ; of tinctura iodi, 1 in 1,000 ; and of boracic acid—a cold saturated solution made warm.

Later in the progress of the case a counter-opening may be called for, should none have been made at the time of the operation.

Incision, with Removal of a Portion of a Rib.—In some cases the simple incision described does not permit of a free enough opening being made into the pleural cavity, or does not permit of as extensive an examination being carried out as is necessary. In such instances a small portion of one, or even two, ribs may be excised. The rib is exposed through the incision already made, and is completely bared of periosteum by a curved rugine. By thus baring the rib the intercostal artery is avoided. The rib is then steadied with lion forceps or flat-bladed necrosis forceps, and is divided in two places with a fine saw. The section may be completed with cutting forceps, but any attempt—especially in adults—to divide the entire rib by forceps is to be deprecated. By such division the bone is unduly crushed and splintered. About one inch and a half of the rib should be removed.

After its excision the sac of periosteum left behind is cut away. It is at this step of the operation that the intercostal artery is probably divided. It can, however, be most readily secured. By first stripping off the periosteum a division of the intercostal artery at an inconvenient time is avoided. The vessel is turned back with the periosteum. It is well to excise the periosteum thus left isolated, since it may produce, at a later period, an inconvenient mass of ill-formed bone.

2. ESTHLANDER'S OPERATION.—THORACOPLASTY.

This operation is carried out in certain cases of empyema of long standing—cases in which no healing follows, in spite of long-continued and free drainage of the purulent cavity.

In such instances the chest walls have contracted to their utmost, the lung lies unexpanded, the pleura is greatly thickened, and although the diaphragm has risen to an exceptional position, there still remains a cavity with rigid walls which can contract no further, and which could never close by the slow and exhausting process of granulation. The operation is a plastic measure, which has for its object the speedy obliteration of this cavity. This is effected by cutting away the rigid part of the wall of the space—i.e., the whole of its costal boundary.

Resection of ribs is an operation of some antiquity, but the procedure has only of recent years become a precise and widely-employed measure.

Esthlander, who paid especial attention to the removal of ribs as a plastic measure, published his account of the operation in 1879 (*Revue Mens. de Méd. et de Chirurg.*). A very practical contribution to the subject is afforded by an article of Mr. Pearce Gould's, published in the *Lancet* for February 11th, 1888.

The Operation.—The patient having been placed in position and anæsthetised (*see* page 741), the cavity to be treated is thoroughly examined, its full extent is ascertained, and the condition of its interior is determined.

The cavity will be found in the upper or central parts of the pleural space, rather than in the lower.

A special operation must be planned for each case, and it is impossible beforehand to determine how many ribs will have to be resected, or how much of each one will have to be removed.

Success depends upon the removal of the whole of the unyielding bony wall of the cavity, and the limits of the excision are identical with those of the suppurating hollow which has to be closed.

As soon, therefore, as the extent of the cavity is known the extent of the excision is defined.

The ribs usually removed are the second, third, fourth, fifth, sixth, and seventh. The amount excised will vary from an inch or so to nearly the whole length of the bony part of the rib.

In the case of a female aged twenty-five, Mr. Pearce Gould (*loc. cit.*) removed considerable lengths of the ribs from the second to the ninth inclusive. The total length of bone resected was fifty-four inches, giving an average of six inches to each rib. The pleura in this case was nearly an inch thick.

. Various plans are adopted for exposing the costal walls. Mr. Godlee recommends a flap composed of all the soft parts covering the ribs. This flap is marked out by a **V**-shaped or **U**-shaped incision, and is free below, so as to allow for drainage. This procedure is somewhat serious, involves a great wound, and possibly much hæmorrhage.

Esthlander makes a transverse cut over the centre of an intercostal space, and through this wound excises portions of the two ribs which bound the space. If, therefore, six ribs have to be removed, three of such incisions will be called for.

Jacobson advises the formation of two, three, or more small flaps.

Gould recommends a vertical incision over the central part of the cavity, and this, probably, will be found as convenient a way of exposing the ribs as any.

Each rib is exposed in turn, and is bared of periosteum with the curved rugine. It is then excised in the manner already described (page 743). The periosteum is removed after each excision.

"If the cavity extends far back towards the spine," writes

Mr. Gould, "it will be found convenient, after removing the front portion of the rib in the usual way, to remove the posterior part from the inside, peeling the thickened pleura off the bone, and applying the cutting forceps from within the chest. The dense cicatricial tissue which will usually be found lining the ribs, and the greatly-thickened pleura, must be cut away with scissors and forceps."

The hæmorrhage attending the operation is often considerable, but is readily controlled.

The operation should be completed with as little delay as possible.

The cavity should be then washed out with a weak solution of corrosive sublimate. Very small cavities may be stuffed with fine gauze, and allowed to close up from the bottom.

In dealing with the ordinary cavity, the skin is brought into place by silkworm-gut sutures, and the wound thus closed. A large drainage-tube is introduced into the most dependent part of the cavity; or, if necessary, a special drainage incision may be made.

The operation produces much shock.

There is nothing especial to note in the after-treatment. It is that of an extensive and deep wound made in tissues that have been long the seat of inflammatory action.

3. INCISION AND DRAINAGE OF LUNG CAVITIES.

The whole subject of the surgical treatment of pulmonary cavities has been very fully dealt with by Mr. Godlee in an admirable series of lectures, illustrated by numerous cases, published in the *Lancet* for March, 1887.

For precision and completeness these lectures leave little to be desired. Mr. Godlee discusses the history of the operation from the early part of last century, when the surgical treatment of lung cavities was discussed in a somewhat wild and nebulous manner by Sir Edward Barry.

As exact methods of treatment, these operations are of quite recent date.

The cases in which surgical measures may be or have been attempted are thus classified by Mr. Godlee :—(1) Tubercular cavities. (2) Cavities resulting from gangrene of the lung. (3) Cavities resulting from the bursting into the lung of abscesses or other collections of irritating matter from without. (4) Bronchiectases, from whatever cause arising.

The Operation.—The anæsthethic selected is chloroform, which is slowly and cautiously administered, to avoid coughing. The patient should lie as nearly as possible upon the back.

The exact position of the cavity must be made out, and in cases of doubt the aspirating needle should be freely used. Mr. Godlee insists upon "the unwisdom of incising the lung until the presence of pus is ascertained."

A free incision, some one and a half or two inches long, is made over the site of the cavity or by the side of the exploring needle, and is carried down to the intercostal space. The lung tissue, with the overlying pleura, is most conveniently opened with a medium-sized trocar and cannula, the puncture being subsequently dilated with sinus forceps or dressing forceps.

The cavity should be well opened up, and should, when possible, be explored by the finger. If gangrenous lung tissue be met with, it may be removed. It may be necessary to make a second opening in the cavity at a lower level, in order to secure more efficient drainage. A long soft drainage-tube of full size is employed, and is passed well into the cavity.

It is seldom necessary to excise a portion of the exposed ribs, and when the pus is offensive this course is not advised.

If the cavity should be missed, a tube should be placed in the incision made in the lung, in the hope—which was realised in one case—that the pus might find its way later into the opening.

In the majority of cases adhesions will be found to have fixed the lung, and to have practically obliterated the pleural cavity at the site of the operation.

When no such adhesions exist, the following course is advised by Mr. Godlee:—

"The right method of procedure—though I confess it is not a very easy one—is carefully to stitch the lung up to the opening which has been made in the chest walls. It is a difficult proceeding, because the parts are in a constant state of movement from the act of respiration, and because the lung itself is but ill-suited to retain the stitches that are placed in it, and also because the hole in which the manœuvres have to be carried on is a rather deep one, and mostly obscured by the

presence of blood. I have only once had to put this plan
into practice, and though here it was only partially successful,
it was sufficiently so to show that, with a little more care, the
closure of the pleura might have been effected. We found, in
this case, at the end of a few days, that a part of the stitching
had given way; but as no cavity was reached, no evil consequences as regards the pleura resulted, the wound remaining
aseptic. Of course, after the stitches have been placed, the
attempt to open the cavity must be postponed for at least a
week, and at the end of that time the instruments used must
be sharp, and their employment gentle, lest the accident which
it is intended to avoid may, after all, happen."

Should foul pus escape into the pleural cavity, the case
must be treated as one of empyema.

Hæmorrhage is seldom troublesome after incision of the
lung under the conditions met with in these operations. Any
serious bleeding would be met by plugging the cavity with
aseptic gauze.

The After-treatment.—The cavity is syringed out with a
suitable antiseptic solution—preferably, carbolic acid—until
all fœtor has disappeared. The drainage-tube must be
retained until the discharge has almost, and the expectoration
quite, ceased. This rule should be closely adhered to, as the
most serious relapses have attended a too early removal of
the tube.

It is unnecessary to dwell upon the questions of rest,
liberal diet, and the necessity of plenty of fresh air. The
sooner the patient can be moved out of doors the better.

4. THE TREATMENT OF HYDATID CYSTS OF THE LUNG.

The following account has been kindly written for me by
Dr. W. Gardner, Lecturer on Surgery at the University of
Adelaide. Dr. Gardner's exceptional experience of hydatid
disease gives authority to his remarks. The subject is very
fully dealt with by Dr. Gardner and others in the *Transactions
of the Second Inter-Colonial Medical Congress* (Melbourne,
1889) :—

"The site of the cyst having been mapped out by auscultation and percussion as carefully as possible, an incision
about four inches long is then made in the line of the ribs

through the skin, which is retracted by means of two loops of silk passed through the divided edges. The periosteum over two ribs is then divided and peeled off with a raspatory, and at least three inches of the ribs are removed. Any bleeding points must now be ligatured or twisted, and all oozing stopped by sponge pressure.

"The next step in the operation is to pass a long and fine trocar and cannula in the direction in which the cyst has been localised. If this fail, the needle must be driven in again, altering the direction; but this is rarely required. It must then be noted at what depth the cyst is reached, as evidenced by the escape of clear fluid, or of pus if suppuration has occurred. To facilitate this step, the trocar should be marked off in inches and quarter-inches. If not so marked, the finger must be used to measure, as the cannula is withdrawn, the distance to which it penetrated.

"A long narrow-bladed knife must then be thrust in the same direction into the cyst, and an incision large enough to admit two fingers rapidly made. Two fingers of the left hand are then introduced and the cyst hooked up, the knife laid down, and a Hagedorn's needle, which is held by an assistant, and threaded with wallaby tendon or silk, is passed through the cut edge of the cyst, visceral and parietal layers of the pleura and intercostal muscles, and handed to an assistant, but not tied. The same manœuvre is then repeated on the side which is held up by the fingers of the left hand; and this loop is also held, but not tied.

"If the cyst be situated at the base of the lung, a drainage-tube must now be passed into the pleura by the side of the cyst; but if it is situated higher up, it is better to take out a piece of rib in a convenient situation, and pass a drainage-tube into the bottom of the pleura. The two stitches are then tied, and several others inserted in the same way and tied at once. With the finger as a guide, a pair of rat-trap forceps are introduced, and made to take hold of the mother-cyst. The finger is then withdrawn, and, with the forceps in the left hand, the surgeon gently draws on the cyst—and as it frequently tends to break, he must be prepared with another pair of strong catch-forceps to take a fresh hold—and a little delicate manipulation will deliver the mother-cyst entire. In the process of removal, the rent in the mother-cyst may allow daughter-cysts to escape into the cavity; but it is better to allow them to be washed out later by douching than to run the risk of injury to the wall of the external capsule. A large drainage-tube is then introduced into the cavity, and the extremities of the skin incision are approximated by sutures of gut or horsehair."

5. INCISION OF THE PERICARDIUM IN PURULENT PERICARDITIS.

This subject has been fully dealt with by Dr. Samuel West (*Med.-Chir. Trans.*, vol. lxvi., page 260; *Brit. Med. Journ.*, February 21st, 1891), by Professor Rosentein (*Berliner klinische Wochenschrift*, 1881), and by Dr. Hermann Bronner (*Brit. Med. Journ.*, February 14th, 1891), and the operation has been now illustrated by a number of most successful cases.

The amount of pus evacuated has in some cases been remarkable. In one of Dr. West's cases "fully two quarts" were evacuated in a few seconds.

The pericardial sac is more safely opened by means of an incision than by means of aspiration in cases of suppurative pericarditis.

The incision is made in the fourth or fifth intercostal space of the left side, and about one inch to the outer side of the edge of the sternum, in order to avoid the internal mammary artery.

The incision is at first small, and is cautiously deepened. The opening in the pericardium may be at first a mere puncture, and may then be enlarged by cutting, or dilated with sinus forceps.

When all the pus has escaped, a soft drainage-tube is inserted. The cavity exposed must be kept well drained, and should be well washed out as often as required. The after-treatment differs in no essential from the after-treatment of purulent collections elsewhere.

No advantage has attended the approaching of the pericardium through a trephine-hole made in the sternum, nor does any advantage attend the resection of a rib or costal cartilage.

CHAPTER II.

REMOVAL OF THE BREAST.

Anatomical Points. — The female breast normally extends from the third to the fifth rib. It is supplied by the following arteries, which are divided in excision of the organ:—The second, third, fourth, and fifth intercostal branches of the internal mammary. Of these, the branch from the third interspace is often of comparatively large size. All these vessels enter upon the inner margin of the gland. Entering the outer margin of the gland, there are, from above downwards, a branch of the acromio-thoracic, the long thoracic artery, which closely follows the anterior fold of the axilla, and the external mammary, which is near the middle of the hollow of the axilla. Several branches issuing from the great pectoral muscle pierce the fascia and enter the breast. The branches of the third intercostal and the long thoracic, or possibly the external mammary, are the vessels which are usually the most conspicuous as bleeding points. The chief blood supply of the breast comes from the axillary side.

Some of the lymphatics of the mamma accompany the intercostal arterial branches, and enter the anterior mediastinal glands. The majority, however, enter a set of axillary glands, which are placed behind the edge of the pectoral muscle and upon the serratus magnus. They accompany the long thoracic artery.

The Instruments Required.—A large scalpel; a small scalpel; dissecting forceps; six to ten pressure forceps; artery forceps; a tenaculum; scissors; long straight needles; ligatures and sutures; a kidney-shaped receiver; drainage-tube.

Position.—The patient is brought to the edge of the table, and lies with the head and shoulders raised. The arm of the affected side is raised, and is so placed that the hand lies behind the nape of the neck.　It is retained in this position by the anæsthetist.

The lower part of the trunk is covered with a macintosh sheet.　Three or four coarse sponges are wedged in between the scapula and the operating-table to absorb the blood, which tends to run down over the patient's back.

In dealing with the right breast, the surgeon faces the patient.　In dealing with the left gland, he faces towards the hip of the opposite side.　The chief assistant in either case places himself opposite to the surgeon, and upon the other side of the table.　He leans over the patient's trunk. He helps to retract the parts, to hold up the breast when required, and to grasp any bleeding point with pressure forceps.　A second assistant may stand by the surgeon's side.　Both assistants should have pressure forceps close at hand.

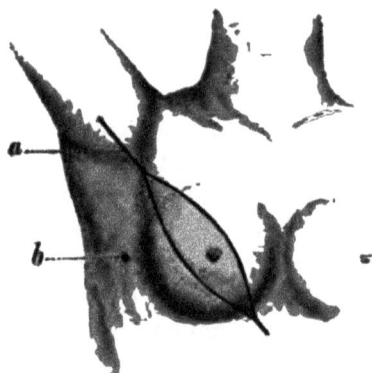

Fig. 421.—EXCISION OF THE BREAST.
a, Axillary incision ; b, Drainage opening.

When the patient is in position, the mammary and axillary regions should be well washed with an antiseptic solution, and the axillary hair should be shaved off.

The Operation.—An elliptical incision is made, the dimensions, and especially the width, of which will depend upon the size of the mass to be removed.　The centre of the ellipse will be about the nipple.　The long axis of the ellipse will be parallel with the anterior fold of the axilla in the position in which the limb is fixed.　The upper end of the incision will be opposite to the centre of the axilla on the pectoral side ; the lower end of the incision will be just beyond the mamma (Fig. 421).

In dealing with the right side, the surgeon commences the incision over the axilla and cuts toward the chest.

In dealing with the left breast, it is convenient to commence the incision at its lower part, and cut towards the axilla.

As the cut is made, the surgeon steadies the part with his left hand, which is made to press in the opposite direction to that followed by the knife, so as to keep the skin tense.

The whole of the incision should be completed at once.

The knife should at first involve the skin and superficial tissues only, and should just pass down into the subcutaneous fat. As soon as the ellipse has been completed the surgeon should turn to the V-shaped point at each extremity of the wound, and should see that the skin is entirely free at these points. It is very common for the mass to be held here, owing to a faulty division of the skin.

The chief assistant, who stands upon the opposite side of the table, now draws the skin up on the sternal side of the mamma towards the median line, while the surgeon lightly presses the breast downwards with his left hand. While the parts are in this position the upper limb of the incision is carried down to the pectoral muscle. If the skin be fully retracted by the assistant, a division of the deeper parts well beyond the limits of the breast is ensured.

The surgeon now grasps the mamma and drags it away from the thorax, while he severs its deep attachments in such a way as to lay bare the great pectoral muscle. In this stage of the operation the breast is as much torn away as cut away.

The chief assistant secures any bleeding points with pressure forceps. Nothing now remains but the attachments of the breast on the axillary side. The assistant should grasp the breast and draw it upwards and towards the middle line, while the surgeon retracts the skin in the opposite direction. The inferior part of the incision is now carried down to the thorax.

The breast is now only attached by the part just beyond the anterior fold of the axilla—*i.e.*, on its axillary side. The surgeon, grasping the tumour in his left hand, drags it away from the thorax, while he rapidly severs the few remaining connections of the part. In this way the chief vessels going to the mamma are divided last.

If an attempt be made to remove the whole breast by one continuous dissection from above downwards, the skin beyond the lower incision becomes turned in, and is very easily button-

w w

holed. The vessels which come from the axillary artery are also divided at an inconvenient time.

The removal of the mamma should be complete, and the great pectoral muscle should be laid quite bare. If the carcinoma has spread into the fibres of the muscle, the whole of the affected part must be liberally cut away.

The next step consists in *the treatment of the axillary glands.*

If no glands can be detected through the skin, the finger may be passed into the axilla, through the upper part of the incision, and the region of the mammary chain of glands examined. If no enlargement can be detected, there is no need to open the axilla further, provided that the tissues right up to the fatty base of the axilla have been very liberally removed. It must be borne in mind that accessory lobules of the mammary gland may be found between the breast and the axilla, and should be removed. If any glands exist in the axilla, the incision should be continued upwards into the armpit, as shown in Fig. 421, *a*. But little cutting is required. The glands may be most conveniently removed with the fingers. Great care must be taken not to damage the axillary vein, and the nerves which cross the outlet of the axilla should also be preserved. The heroic evacuation of the axilla which involves the laying bare of the whole of the axillary vein, the removal of the fatty tissue of the entire space, and the exposure of the upper ribs, has nothing to recommend it. (*See* page 757.)

It is now convenient to mention the following *general points* with regard to excision of the breast:—(1) All bleeding points should be picked up neatly, and not grabbed up together with a mass of the surrounding tissue. (2) The wound should not be scrubbed with a sponge. It barely needs to be sponged at all. (3) Weak antiseptic solutions should be used to wash the wound. It should be cleansed by washing, and not by sponging. A kidney-shaped receiver is placed beneath the wound, and a stream of weak carbolic lotion (1 in 40) is allowed to run over the raw surface until all clots have been washed away.

The bleeding points are now dealt with. In the majority of cases the long-continued pressure of the forceps will suffice to close the larger number of the vessels, others are occluded by twisting the pressure forceps before they are removed. It is rare that any artery requires to be ligatured. Trouble is often given by little vessels which emerge from the substance of the pectoral muscle. A tenaculum may be required before these can be ligatured.

The wound is gently dried by patting, the arm is brought down until it forms a right angle with the trunk, and the sutures are then introduced. The wound margins are put upon the stretch by means of blunt hooks (page 59, vol. i.). The needles employed are straight and long, and the sutures are of silkworm gut. The upper and lower sutures are applied first, the middle ones being left to the last. The sutures are not tied until the upper and lower series are completed. They are then knotted, and the assistant follows the closing wound with sponges, so applied as to maintain considerable pressure over the recently-united incision, and to obliterate the wound cavity. This pressure must not be relaxed. An opening for a drainage-tube is now made in the hollow of the skin below the wound (Fig. 421, *b*). A tube is inserted and secured by a suture.

The middle sutures—*i.e.*, those in the central part of the wound—are now inserted and, when they are all in place, tied. The assistant with the sponges still follows the sutured incision, and obliterates by pressure the wound cavity. The dressing is prepared. It consists either of sponges, cotton-wool, or, better still, Tillmann's dressing. The material employed should be dusted with iodoform, and be large enough to fully occupy the whole axilla and cover the entire wound. A momentary removal of the sponges already in place allows the wound to be dusted with iodoform ; and then, in the place of the first sponges used, the fresh sponges or the pad are applied. The arm is now brought across the chest, and it should be the duty of one assistant to maintain it in place during the application of the bandage. He must rigorously carry out the order, " Keep the elbow to the side, and the hand upon the opposite shoulder."

Between the hand so placed and the chest a layer of cotton-wool is inserted. A four- or five-inch flannel bandage is now firmly applied. It must hold the arm in place. If it be

w w 2

properly applied, the arm acts as a splint, which keeps the parts at rest, and which, through the extensive axillary dressing, maintains such complete pressure over the whole of the operation area that the wound cavity is entirely obliterated. In such circumstances no effusion can take place, and such oozing as occurs finds an exit through the drainage-tube.

The space between the upper arm and the chest must be well packed with wool.

The bandage must be applied while the patient is raised in the sitting position, and it is needless to say that the skin of the chest, arm, and back must be cleaned before it is put on.

The bandage is first carried several times around the arm

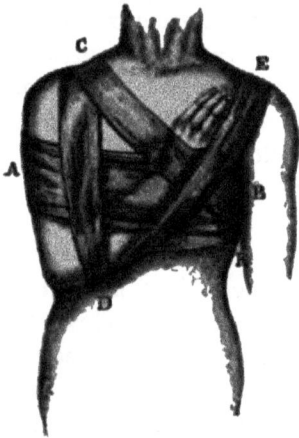

and chest, so as to bring the limb very firmly to the side (Fig. 422, A to B). Then from B it passes under the opposite axilla and across the back to the summit of the affected shoulder at C. It is then made to pass down under the forearm at D, so as to support the upper arm. From D it is carried up behind the axilla to C; thence across the front of the chest to B, whence it returns behind the back to C, and down again on the front of the body to D, to strengthen the supporting

Fig. 422.—ADJUSTMENT OF DRESSING AFTER EXCISION OF THE BREAST.

sling. It passes in the next place across the back from D to E (the summit of the opposite shoulder). Thence it is taken across the front of the chest and under the axillary dressing, and, finally, round the body behind the back to end at F. At least two bandages will be required, and some of the turns may be repeated several times, especially in the case of heavy and corpulent patients. A liberal supply of safety-pins is needed to fix the bandage at different points. This bandage serves practically to seal the wound, and to support the part perfectly.

After-treatment.—If there be any pain, a hypodermic of morphia may be given. As a rule, the patient complains only of the tightness and irksomeness of the bandage, and for this inconvenience she should be prepared. The wound should be dressed and the drainage-tube removed in forty-eight hours. The parts are washed and dried, and dressed in the same manner as on the first occasion. It is rarely necessary to disturb the dressing again until the fifth or sixth day, when it is washed, dried, and powdered, and the arm put up as before. The sutures may be removed on the eighth or ninth day, and the forearm may then be liberated. The patient may usually be ordered up on the eleventh day, and may leave the hospital on the fourteenth. Primary healing may be depended on, and of late years I have had exceedingly few exceptions to this rule.

There is never any need to syringe out the wound if firm pressure be maintained. The maintenance of this pressure, irksome as it is, is all-essential. In persons who perspire much, the iodoform powder may cause some irritation, especially around the axillary part of the wound. In such case some other dusting powder may be used.

Silkworm-gut sutures may be left in for fourteen days if necessary, and in no ordinary cases is it ever needful to support the wound by strapping.

Comments upon the Operation and Modifications of the Procedure.—In dealing with large tumours, such as some sarcomata, the skin incision must be planned with much care, or the operator will fail to adjust the margins of the wound. If any tension fall upon the sutures in consequence of an unusual amount of skin having been removed, a hare-lip pin had better be introduced at the point where the greatest strain comes.

It appears to be totally unnecessary in ordinary cases of malignant disease to remove the *whole* of the skin covering the breast, whether sound or unsound, as some advise. Such skin as is implicated by the disease or adherent thereto must, of course, be freely removed ; but if the case be so advanced that all the integument covering the mamma is involved, then it is probable that the case is not suited for treatment by operation.

Influenced by the advice of more than one eminent surgeon, I at one time cleared out the contents of the axilla in all cases of excision of the breast, including those in which no glandular swellings could be discovered in that space. This practice I have discontinued. The results obtained have appeared to me to be in no way more satisfactory than those which follow the lesser operation.

The operation has been rendered more tedious and more dangerous. Some patients, after recovery from the operation, have complained of stiff and painful shoulders, of neuralgia involving the nerves of the limb, and of considerable œdema of the hand and forearm.

There is little evidence to support the value of some of the more extensive operations carried out in cancer of the breast —operations which involve the complete evacuation of the axilla, the removal of so large a tract of skin that the wound must close by granulation, and the excision of considerable portions of the pectoral muscle. In many instances I am convinced that, although the patient has recovered well from the actual operation, the duration of life has not been prolonged. This is noticeable in cases of slow-spreading atrophic cancer, which may cause little trouble, and may last for years. It is removed at a late period. The wound heals, and in a very short time the malignant disease returns. It comes back, however, in an altered character. In the place of the feeble unobtrusive growth, there appears a ruddy cancerous mass, rampant and aggressive, which soon brings life to an end.

Small innocent tumours of the breast are removed through a simple incision, which should follow a line radiating from the nipple. If much thickness of mammary tissue is cut through, a drainage-tube should always be retained for twenty-four or thirty-six hours.

It is sometimes possible to remove an innocent growth by an incision which follows the crease between the lower segment of the mamma and the thorax. Excellent drainage is provided by such an incision, and the scar is entirely hidden from view.

The Results of Excision of the Breast.—The actual mortality following the operation of excision of the breast is very low, and is at the present day probably less than five per cent. When the amputation is performed for malignant disease, recurrence is unfortunately the rule. The average date of recurrence after the operation is about twenty months.

In most cases the excision gives to the patient great temporary relief of both mind and body; and in instances in which the operation is performed early, life is undoubtedly prolonged. Mr. Butlin believes that in excising the breast for mammary cancer, a cure—*i.e.*, a freedom from recurrence for full three years—may be expected in twelve to fifteen per cent. of the patients operated upon; and that in cases of sarcoma, somewhat more satisfactory results may be anticipated. Mr. Williams, in an analysis of the cancer cases at the Middlesex Hospital, gives the following averages (*Lancet*, January 12th, 1889):—The average duration of life, dating from the time when the disease was first noticed, is 60·8 months for those who undergo operation, and 44·8 months for those in whom the disease runs its natural course. The average duration of life subsequent to amputation of the breast is 40·3 months. The average interval between the first operation and the first recurrence is 26 months; the maximum, 130 months; the minimum, 2·5 months.

THE END.

INDEX OF SUBJECTS.

x x

9 781330 278192